Living Nutrition

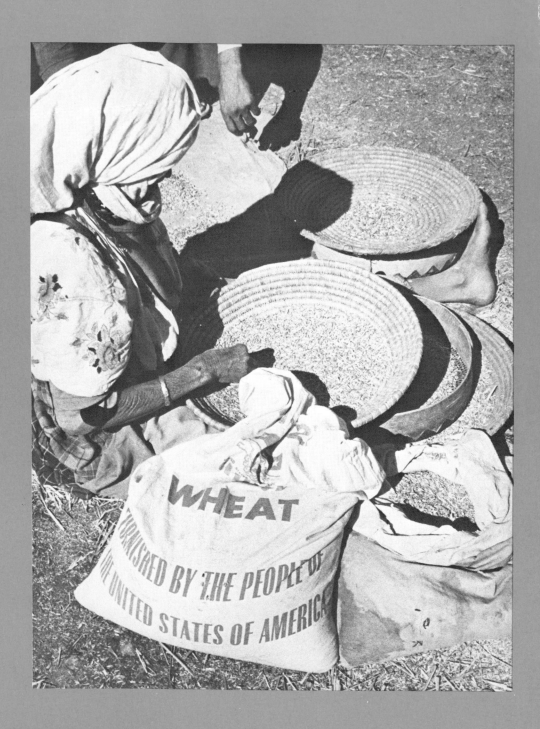

LIVING NUTRITION

SECOND EDITION

FREDRICK J. STARE,
Harvard University

MARGARET McWILLIAMS,
California State University, Los Angeles

John Wiley & Sons. New York, Santa Barbara, London, Sydney, Toronto

COVER AND BOOK DESIGNED BY ANGIE LEE

Copyright © 1973, 1977, by John Wiley & Sons, Inc.

All rights reserved. Published simultaneously in Canada.

No part of this book may be reproduced by any means, nor transmitted, nor translated into a machine language without the written permission of the publisher.

Library of Congress Cataloging in Publication Data:

Stare, Fredrick John.
   Living nutrition.

   Includes bibliographies and index.
   1. Nutrition. I. McWilliams, Margaret, joint author. II. Title.
TX354.S82   1977   641.1   76-17821
ISBN 0-471-82081-4

Printed in the United States of America

10 9 8 7 6 5 4 3 2 1

Preface to the Second Edition

1963028

This edition was written with a keen awareness of the immensity of the problems of producing and distributing an adequate supply of food for the world's still-expanding population as well as the need for motivating modifications in food patterns if the goal of optimal nutrition is to be achieved. As with the first edition, we have given considerable attention to the sociopsychological aspects of nutrition so that the interdisciplinary context of nutrition can be brought into focus.

The sequence of presentation has been modified to enable the student to gain insight into the physiological aspects of nutrition, in addition to the sociopsychological aspects, prior to studying the special nutritional needs at various stages in the life cycle. This provides the setting for an entirely new section, "Applying Nutrition." The two new chapters in this section help make basic nutrition knowledge become a working reality in daily life.

We acknowledge the assistance of Dr. James H. Shaw, Professor of Nutrition at the Harvard School of Dental Medicine, in the sections on dental development and health and Jelia Witschi, Assistant Professor of Nutrition at Harvard's Department of Nutrition, in developing the new tables.

Fredrick J. Stare, M.D.

Margaret McWilliams, Ph.D.

Preface to the First Edition

With the increasing awareness of the importance of the individual and the greater appreciation of sociopsychological influences on groups and individuals, there is a critical need for studying nutrition in the interdisciplinary context of the world today. Our book has been written from this viewpoint.

A brief introduction of the nutrients provides the foundation for a global look at the numerous aspects of the social sciences that shape the dietary patterns of people throughout the world. When interest and awareness of nutrition have been developed in this context, we then progress to the technical discussions of the nutrients—carbohydrates, fats, proteins, water, minerals, and vitamins. The presentation of the general subject of vitamins as the final chapter of a nutrition book is unique; we feel that the technical portions achieve a greater depth of understanding when they are based on the sociological and applied aspects of nutrition. This approach is new. In our experience this framework generates enthusiasm for nutrition among students who will become tomorrow's nutrition educators, citizens, and parents.

The problems of feeding the present and future populations of the earth are crucial and burdened with political importance. The knowledge and skills of nutritionists, biochemists, agriculturists, economists, social scientists, physicians, other professionals, and politicians are the keys to solving the developing food crisis. The interrelated contributions of these people are explored here. The environmental factors that influence food preferences are examined. Practical matters, such as inadequate diet resulting from cultural or religious practices and poor nutrition caused by economic restrictions that inhibit food purchasing or limit farm productivity, are discussed from the vantage point of the social sciences. The contribution that technology can make by developing more nutritious forms of existing foods, enhancing storage life, or creating acceptable foods from exotic sources is also considered.

People as individuals need to understand the numerous factors that determine food preferences and biases. Students gain a broader understanding when they examine these aspects of nutrition as well as the biochemical and metabolic roles of the numerous nutrients in the body. Now is the time to incorporate the pertinent information of the social and biologic sciences into an integrated and meaningful whole —the science of applied nutrition. We hope this textbook is a step forward in accomplishing just that.

We take pleasure in acknowledging the many professionals who have reviewed and criticized portions of the manuscript, particularly Dr. Nancy Bowden, Dr. Gene Calvert, Dr. Susan Calvert, Dr. Howard Jacobson, Mrs. Ruth Johnson, Dr. Constance Jordan, Mrs. Mary Kramer, Dr. Pearl Swanson, and Mrs. Jelia Witschi. We especially appreciate the food composition tables that have been compiled and prepared by Mrs. Jelia Witschi of Harvard's Department of Nutrition. Our special thanks are given to the students in nutrition classes at Framingham State College in Massachusetts and at California State University, Los Angeles, for testing the manuscript. We also wish to thank Mr. Earl Shepherd for serving as editor for us in this project.

Fredrick J. Stare, M.D.

Margaret McWilliams, Ph.D.

Contents

Living Nutrition

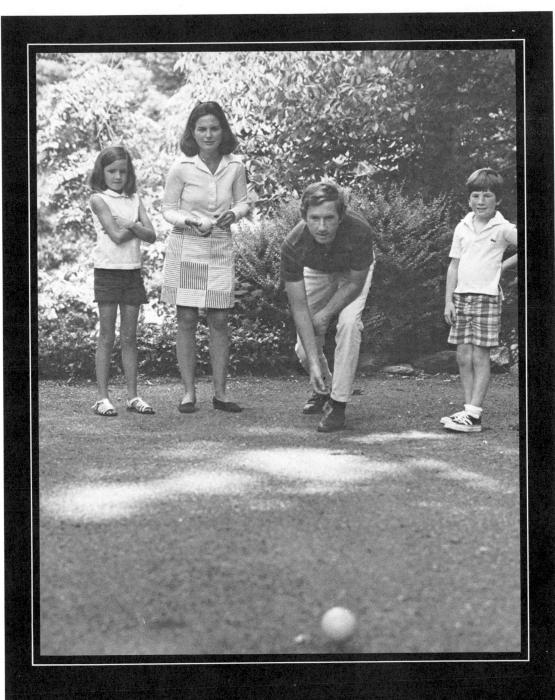

Chapter 1

Introduction to Nutrition

Nutrition is the study of the food man eats and the use of this food in the body. The broad nature of this study requires exploration into the social, biological, and physical sciences. Psychology, sociology, anthropology, geography, and education are all influential in determining the diet of man as a group and as an individual. Agriculture, economics, and commerce further define the availability of food. The functions of nutrients and the utilization of food in the body are the realm of the nutritionist, dietitian, biochemist, microbiologist, and physical scientist. This book is a concerted effort to bring the full scope of nutrition into perspective through discussions that draw upon these related disciplines.

Nutrition for each individual represents an accumulation of the habits formed throughout his lifetime. These food preference patterns tend to become increasingly rigid as an individual ages. Dietary patterns vary markedly from individual to individual and from one cultural and geographic environment to another. Food preferences, cultural heritage, and the availability of foods are fundamental in establishing and molding food patterns of individuals. These patterns can be altered, but usually only with considerable effort and patience.

The improvement of the general nutritional status of a population is a long-range goal that can best be achieved through the joint efforts of concerned physical and social scientists and educators. A key to improving the nutrition level in a population is the development of an understanding and appreciation of the psychological and sociological factors determining food consumption patterns. Further progress can be achieved through nutrition education programs intensively directed to students throughout their school years, particularly in the early years. By teaching applied nutrition to children of school age (and even younger), good dietary patterns are encouraged at a time when food habits are being established. Over an extended period of time, such education will begin to influence nutrition habits in all segments of the population.

A study of food preferences and dietary patterns gains depth and perspective when considered in the context of the interrelated social sciences. However, full understanding of the discussions in the following sections requires some knowledge of the nutrients and their food sources. The remainder of this chapter provides a brief look at these topics. Each nutrient is considered in much greater depth in Chapters 6 through 11. Application of this information for daily living is presented in Chapters 17 and 18.

The Nutrients

Carbohydrates, fats, and proteins are the three classes of organic compounds that occur abundantly in various foods. In addition to these nutrients, foods contain lesser amounts of inorganic elements known as minerals. Vitamins are yet another class of organic compounds required for growth, good health, and life itself. However, vitamins are needed in much smaller quantities than carbohydrates, fats, and proteins. No single food contains all of the nutrients in amounts sufficient to maintain life and promote optimum growth. Man must eat a varied diet if he is to consume all the nutrients his body needs.

Carbohydrates

Starches, sugars, and cellulose (dietary fiber) are all common forms of carbohydrate. Carbohydrates are essential in the diet. Starches and sugars supply the body with a relatively inexpensive and important source of energy. Cellulose plays the unique role of providing bulk in the intestinal tract, thus encouraging motility of food through the digestive tract. Since cellulose is not digested, it is not a source of energy for humans.

In typical American diets, carbohydrates provide between 45 and 55 percent of the day's calories.[1] Thus, approximately half of the energy in the typical American diet is supplied by carbohydrates, of which sugar provides about one-third and starch about two-thirds. In other parts of the world as, for example, in the rice-eating population of Asia, the percentage of carbohydrate is much higher, and more of the carbohydrate is in the form of starch. Foods such as pastas, breads, cereals, legumes, potatoes, and corn are particularly good sources of starch, although they also contain protein, minerals, and vitamins. The obvious sources of sugar are sugar and candy of all types. Sugars also are found in a wide range of fruits and in honey. Soft drinks, cakes, and other sweet foods and desserts are other sources of sugar in the diet.

Cellulose is present in varying amounts in fruits and vegetables, particularly in the non-digestible portions of the skins; also in grains, primarily in the bran, which is largely removed in milling. Cellulose is only a portion of what is referred to as dietary fiber. Other constituents include hemicelluloses, mucilages, pectins, and a noncarbohydrate known as lignin. While the importance of dietary fiber has long been known in relation to providing bulk to help in eliminating body wastes and influencing the bacterial flora of the lower intestine, it was believed to contribute little nutritionally. Epidemiologic studies of the early 1970s suggest it may have important roles in the health of man.

---

[1] A calorie is the amount of heat required to raise the temperature of 1 gram of water 1 centigrade degree at 1 atmosphere of pressure. A kilocalorie is 1000 times as large, that is, the heat required to raise 1 kilogram of water 1 centigrade degree. Caloric values of specific foods or diets always refer to kilocalories (also correctly written as Calories).

Fats

Fats in foods contribute significantly to the palatability of the diet. Few people appreciate a piece of bread without butter or margarine. Pastries and other baked products are more tender and flavorful as a result of their fat content. From the nutritionist's viewpoint, fat performs several vital physical functions in the body. It is a concentrated source of energy, providing 9 kilocalories per gram in contrast to the 4 kilocalories per gram from carbohydrates and proteins. Fats also are important as carriers of the fat-soluble vitamins, vitamins A, D, E, and K. Some fats contain linoleic acid, the essential polyunsaturated fatty acid needed by the body for growth and for healthy skin. In addition, linoleic acid, when it replaces a portion of the saturated fats of the diet, helps to lower the cholesterol content of the blood. Yet another function of fat is to provide satiety value. Because fat moves slowly through the stomach, a meal containing some fat gives the diner a satisfied feeling for a relatively long period of time and staves off hunger pangs.

Rich sources of fat include meats, butter, margarine, cream, cheese, and salad dressings. Whole milk and its products are good sources of fat, but nonfat and low-fat milks are not. The fat content of fried foods and baked products may be less evident, but it is still there in ample quantity. The typical American diet provides usually between 40 and 50 percent of the total calories from fats, but most nutritionists recommend that this be reduced to between 30 and 35 percent.

Proteins

Proteins are unique organic compounds containing nitrogen. Protein-containing foods are required in the diet to provide the essential amino acids and nitrogen required for growth and maintenance of body tissues. In addition, antibodies, enzymes, and hormones (such as thyroxine, insulin, and adrenaline) are protein-aceous compounds manufactured in the body from proteins available in the diet. Protein in blood plasma is essential for regulating the amount of water present in the space between the body's cells. Too little protein is one of the reasons why tissues become puffy (edematous) because of the accumulation of fluid. Proteins, because of their ability to act either as acids or bases, are essential in maintaining the neutral reaction of the body. Like carbohydrate and fat, protein also is a source of energy (4 kilocalories per gram). The 22 amino acids that make up the various protein molecules are classified as either essential or nonessential amino acids. If an amino acid must be included in the diet to maintain life and promote growth, it is classified as essential. Eight amino acids are dietary essentials for adult man, and one more is required by human infants. The other amino acids found in proteins are classed as nonessential, a designation that unfortunately tends to reduce their apparent importance in the diet. Nonessential amino acids are necessary to meet the body's total need for dietary protein. Proteins containing all of the essential amino acids are termed "complete" proteins, and those containing an inadequate amount of one or more of the essential amino acids are "incomplete" proteins.

Proteins are found in both animal and plant foods. The protein from animals, with the exception of gelatin, is complete protein. Animal protein sources include beef, veal, pork, lamb, poultry, fish, eggs, milk, and cheese. Plant proteins are found in legumes, wheat, corn, rice, and other cereals. Legumes (soybeans, navy beans, black-eyed peas, lentils, lima beans, pinto beans, peas, and red beans) are particularly good sources of protein and contribute significantly to the dietary intake of protein. Although plant proteins are low in at least one or more of the essential amino acids, they can be used as a relatively inexpensive source of protein, requiring only a little supplementation with animal protein. In fact, adequate protein can be consumed entirely from plant foods if a proper variety of plant proteins is eaten daily.

Approximately 12 to 15 percent of the day's calories should be available from protein in the diet.

Minerals

Minerals are the substances remaining in food after water and the carbon-containing compounds (protein, carbohydrate, fat, and vitamins) have been removed. These inorganic elements are needed daily by the body in small amounts to perform vital roles in the body. The minerals that are present in the body and required in the diet in the largest quantities include calcium, iron, phosphorus, potassium, sulfur, sodium, chloride, and magnesium. The micronutrient or trace elements essential for humans include zinc, selenium, manganese, copper, iodide, molybdenum, cobalt, chromium, and fluoride. Vanadium, barium, strontium, bromide, gallium, aluminum, silver, gold, tin, mercury, and bismuth are also present in the body in trace amounts, but their significance is uncertain at the present time.

Two very important reactions in the body are attributed to certain minerals: (1) maintenance of acid-base balance and (2) support of proper osmotic pressure to preserve the optimum fluid levels in the blood, between the cells, and within the cells. Specific minerals are essential for the transmission of nerve impulses, regulation of muscular contraction and relaxation, growth of body tissues, catalysis of numerous biological reactions, and formation of certain hormones, enzymes, and other essential compounds, including such different compounds as hydrochloric acid and hemoglobin. Calcium and phosphorus, for example, are known for their contribution to the growth and maintenance of bones and teeth. Iron and copper are two minerals needed for the formation of hemoglobin in the blood.

As a total group, minerals are available in fruits, vegetables, meats, milk, eggs, cereals, water, and nearly all other foods except such refined foods as granulated sugar and various oils. Specific minerals are found in large quantities in some foods; examples are calcium in milk and iron in liver. Other important food sources of minerals are outlined in detail in Chapter 10.

Vitamins

Vitamins have assumed almost a supernatural or magical aura in the minds of many people. There is a distinct tendency to equate vitamins with good nutrition and to use these two terms virtually as synonyms. Certainly vitamins are essential to human life, but life also depends on the many other nutrients discussed earlier in this chapter. Minerals, proteins, fats, and carbohydrates are also components of good nutrition.

Vitamins, like minerals, do not provide calories for energy. They are, however, necessary for the reactions that release energy from car-

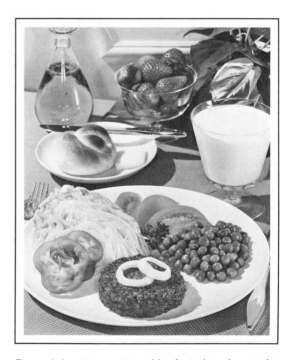

By regularly eating a variety of foods, such as those in this well-balanced meal, all of the vitamins, minerals, protein, carbohydrate, and fat needed for good health will be available to the body.

bohydrates, fats, and proteins in the body. As a group, vitamins function in very small amounts to maintain life and promote growth. Individual vitamins are needed for specific metabolic reactions in the cell. Various deficiency diseases occur when the intake of a vitamin is inadequate; examples include night blindness (when vitamin A intake is low over a prolonged period), beriberi (thiamin deficiency), pellagra (niacin deficiency), rickets (vitamin D deficiency), and scurvy (vitamin C deficiency).

The water-soluble vitamins include ascorbic acid (vitamin C) and the B-complex vitamins. The B vitamins are thiamin, riboflavin, niacin, vitamin B_6 (pyridoxine), pantothenic acid, biotin, folacin (folic acid), and vitamin B_{12} (cobalamin). Vitamin C is found in particularly large quantities in citrus fruits. The B vitamins are found in varying amounts in meats, cereals, vegetables, fruits, and milk. The specific foods that are especially rich sources of the various vitamins are discussed in Chapter 11.

Vitamins A, D, E, and K are classified as fat-soluble vitamins. Butter, other animal fats, and margarine are useful sources of the various fat-soluble vitamins. Vitamins A and D, unlike the water-soluble vitamins, are stored in the body, and excessively large supplements of these two vitamins may be harmful. However, persons in good health who select a varied diet based on consumption of meats, milk, fruits and vegetables, and breads and cereals will obtain all the vitamins they need for optimal growth and maintenance.

Water

No discussion of nutrients is complete without including water. Approximately two thirds of the body's weight is water. Water serves as a solvent and mode of transport for nutrients and waste products that result from the utilization of food.

Water is needed for the numerous reactions that must take place within living cells. The various essential body fluids, including blood, saliva, perspiration, and digestive juices all contain large quantities of water. In the case of saliva and other digestive fluids, water is important as a lubricant to ease the movement of food. In blood, water is the medium for transporting numerous compounds through the body. In perspiration, water serves as a temperature-regulating substance; the evaporation of water from the lungs and skin removes heat from the body.

Water is supplied by fluids in the diet. Many foods, particularly fruits and vegetables, contain a high percentage of water. For example, cantaloupe is about 90 percent water, and lettuce is more than 95 percent water. The body itself also makes some water as carbohydrates, fats, and proteins are utilized in the cells. Since the amount of water needed by the body varies with such factors as climate and amount of physical activity, the recommendation to drink six to eight glasses of liquid daily is merely a guideline.

Guides to Good Nutrition

Daily food guides

The food one eats is a very personal matter. Normally, most people resist eating a diet outlined completely and specifically by someone else. The comments and complaints about food that are so common in college dormitories and other institutionalized settings illustrate the emotional and personal value people place upon selecting their own foods. Menus planned for groups of people may be nutritionally adequate in every way, and yet these menus may fail to allow for the fact that one or more of the foods included may not be eaten for cultural or personal reasons. Planned, but uneaten food serves no nutritional purpose in a diet! Clearly then, it is necessary to provide a complete easy-to-use guide for the individual to use in planning his daily food intake. The merits of good nutrition are gaining ever-increasing recognition, but it is the application of this knowledge to daily living that must be achieved.

Nearly three decades ago the U.S. Department of Agriculture devised the "Basic Seven" to explain the variety needed in the diet to achieve good nutrition. The seven food groups enumerated included milk, meats, citrus fruits, green and yellow vegetables, other fruits and vegetables, breads and cereals, and butter or margarine. This plan was a simplification of the "Basic Eleven" that was presented several decades earlier! Despite this improvement, it soon became apparent that a system with seven categories still presented more of a challenge than most people wished to accept. Therefore, Harvard's Department of Nutrition suggested a daily food guide comprised of four basic food groups (Hayes et al., 1955). At about the same time the U.S. Department of Agriculture also settled on the same "Basic Four"; this plan was subsequently adopted by most groups interested in nutrition education in the United States.

The "Basic Four" is a simple device for planning adequate nutrition on a daily basis to outline the variety of foods that will provide a "balanced diet" that includes the essential nutrients. Although not structured to enumerate all foods needed daily, it does provide a very practical framework for meal planning. Sugar or refined fats and oils are not included because these substances, although they are important in nutrition, mainly provide energy and are usually not lacking in American diets.

The food groups mentioned in the Basic Four are (1) milk and its products; (2) meats, poultry, fish, eggs, and other excellent protein sources; (3) vegetables and fruits; and (4) cereals and their products. The recommended servings for each category are outlined on a daily basis in Table 1.1. The consumption of food according to this plan will provide adequate amounts of the nutrients, with the exception of iron and energy. The problem of an adequate intake of iron is discussed in Chapter 10. Many people require more calories than will be provided by the minimum servings suggested in the Basic Four. These calories are available from many foods including additional carbohydrate (sugar) and some fat (butter or margarine), that are customarily included in the diets of active people.

There has been criticism of the Basic Four by a few nutritionists who feel that the present system of nutrition education does not specify all important dietary requirements. They suggest that the public should be using a meal-planning system (as yet undefined) that specifies all aspects of the diet needed for good nutrition. The Basic Four is not all-inclusive in its outline of dietary needs, but the four groups are easier for people to remember than plans listing six or more groups. Furthermore, consuming a variety of foods from within each of the Basic Four food groups will essentially assure a good or balanced diet for most individuals. Since even this streamlined listing of four categories has been difficult for some people to remember and utilize, there is valid reason to question the wisdom of shifting back to a more complex plan.

Milk group

Milk is valued particularly for its content of calcium, riboflavin, and protein of high quality. In addition, milk is an excellent source of phosphorus and thiamin. Vitamin A, a fat-soluble vitamin, is found in whole milk. Some low-fat and nonfat milks now have vitamin A added, a practice of significant nutritional value. Much of the milk on the market today also is fortified with vitamin D, making fortified milks the major source of this vitamin in the diet. Two nutrients that are notably low in milk are iron and ascorbic acid. The significance of milk as a source of calcium and the great need for calcium during growth are reflected by the servings of milk and

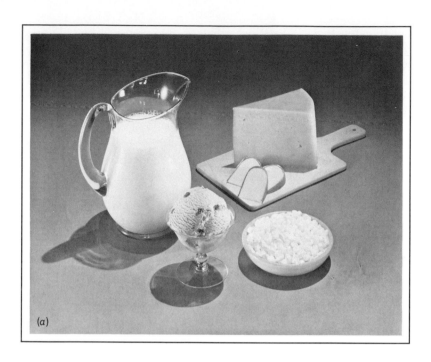

(a)

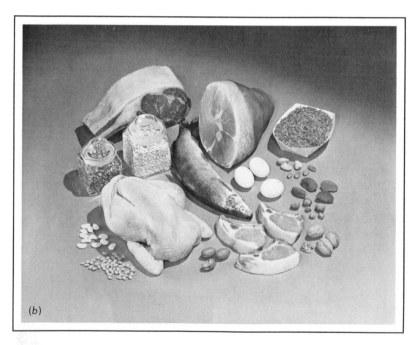

(b)

The Basic Four is a simple daily plan dividing the foods needed for good health into (a) milk and dairy products, (b) meats, poultry, fish, eggs, legumes, and nuts, (c) fruits and vegetables, including citrus and dark green, leafy or yellow vegetables (d) breads and cereals.

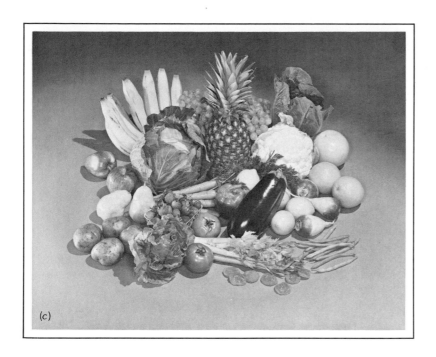

(c)

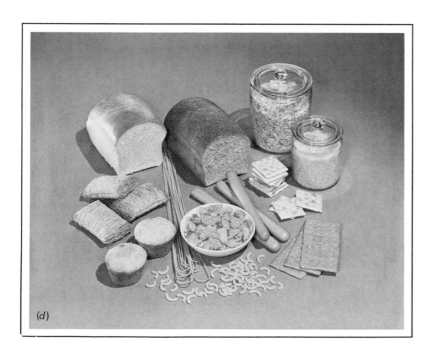

(d)

Table 1.1   The Basic Four[a]

Milk group (8-oz. cup)[b]	2 to 3 cups for children under 9 years 3 to 4 cups for children 9 to 12 years 3 to 4 cups or more for teen-agers 1 to 2 cups or more for adults 3 to 4 cups or more for pregnant women 4 cups or more for nursing mothers
Meat group 2 or more servings. Count as 1 serving	2 to 3 oz. lean, cooked beef, veal, pork, lamb, poultry, fish (without bone) 2 eggs 1 cup cooked dry beans, dry peas, lentils 4 tbsp. peanut butter
Vegetable-fruit group (½-cup serving or 1 piece fruit, etc.)	1 serving of citrus fruit, or other fruit or vegetable as a good source of vitamin C, or 2 servings of a fair source 1 serving, at least every other day, of a dark green or deep yellow vegetable for vitamin A value 2 or more servings of other vegetables and fruits, including potatoes
Cereal group 4 or more servings daily (whole grain, enriched, or re-stored) Count as 1 serving	1 slice bread 1 oz. ready-to-eat cereal ½ to ¾ cup cooked cereal, corn meal, grits, macaroni, noodles, rice, or spaghetti

[a] Modified by the authors from **Consumers All, Yearbook of Agriculture, 1965.** U.S. Department of Agriculture. Washington, D.C., 1965, p. 394. Sizes of servings obviously must be adjusted to the weight one wishes to reach and then maintain.

[b] Alternatives providing equivalent calcium values:

> 1 cup milk = cheddar cheese slice 1 in. x 1 in. x 2 in.
> 1 cup milk = 1¼ cup cottage cheese
> 1 cup milk = 1⅔ cup cream cheese
> 1 cup milk = 1½ cup ice cream

milk products recommended for people of different ages (Table 1.1).

Although it is not difficult to meet the recommended numbers of servings daily by drinking milk, variety can be added by substituting various dairy products for part of the milk servings. If weight control is a problem or if a person simply prefers a different type of milk, whole milk can be replaced entirely by any of the low-fat milks, skim (nonfat) milk, reconstituted evaporated milk, or buttermilk (Table 1.2). Dry milk solids, either whole or nonfat, are comparable to their fresh counterparts when properly reconstituted and are usually less expensive.

Low-fat milks, usually containing 1 or 2 percent fat, are becoming very popular. These milks are intermediate in fat content between whole and skim milk, and hence are suitable choices for people who like the flavor of fat in milk without the greater number of calories in whole milk. These low-fat milks may have extra

Table 1.2 *Nutrient Value of Milk in 1 Cup (8 oz) Portions*[a]

	kcal	Protein (g)	Fat (g)	Carbohydrate (g)	Calcium (mg)	Vitamin A (I.U.)	Thiamin (mg)	Riboflavin (mg)	Niacin (mg)
Fresh milk									
Whole (3.5% fat)	160	9	9	12	288	342	0.07	0.41	0.2
Skim (0.5% fat or less)	90	9	Trace	12	295	Trace	0.10	0.44	0.2
Fortified low-fat[b]	145	10	5	15	349	195	0.10	0.51	0.2
Chocolate	205	8	8	27	269	315	0.07	0.39	0.2
Chocolate drink[c]	185	8	6	27	264	195	0.10	0.39	0.2
Cultured milk									
Buttermilk[d]	90	9	Trace	12	295	Trace	0.10	0.44	0.2
Yogurt, plain[e]	195	11	3	30	122	108	0.08	0.43	0.2
Yogurt, sweetened, flavored	260	10	2	47	98	106	0.06	0.36	0.2
Partially dehydrated milk									
Evaporated (undiluted)	345	18	20	24	635	806	0.10	0.86	0.5
Condensed (sweetened)	980	25	27	166	802	1102	0.24	1.16	0.6
Dry milk solids									
Nonfat[f]	90	9	Trace	13	323	8	0.09	0.44	0.2

[a] Data adapted and calculated from *Composition of Foods—Raw, Processed, Prepared,* Agriculture Handbook No. 8, U.S.D.A., 1963; *Nutritive Value of Foods,* Home and Garden Bulletin No. 72, U.S.D.A., 1971; manufacturers' information; and *Nutritive Value of American Foods,* Agriculture Handbook No. 456, U.S.D.A., 1975.

[b] Partially skim milk with 2% milk solids added.
[c] Skim milk with chocolate and sugar added.
[d] Bacteria cultured skim milk.
[e] Low-fat Swiss style.
[f] "Instantized" crystals—⅓ cup reconstituted to 1 cup skim milk.

protein added in the form of skim milk solids, which are rich in protein and minerals.

Regardless of the type of fluid milk selected, all fresh milks should be pasteurized. The heating of milk (either to 145°F for 30 minutes or to 161°F for 15 seconds) is sufficient to kill microorganisms that might be harmful to man. In addition to pasteurization, whole milk commonly is homogenized, a process that breaks up fat globules and makes protein more digestible. Milk enriched with vitamin D (400 International Units[2] per quart) is recommended, particularly for children, pregnant and lactating women, and adults beyond middle age.

Two types of canned milk are commonly available in the market. Evaporated milk is a canned milk that has had approximately half of its water removed prior to canning. When this product is mixed with an equal amount of water, its nutrient content is comparable to fresh milk. Sweetened condensed milk is a canned milk that is prepared by evaporating about half of its water and then adding sugar. Sweetened condensed milk is not recommended as a beverage because the high caloric content resulting from the added sugar may lead to a weight problem when consumed on a daily basis.

Cheeses of various types and milk-containing beverages are well-accepted items in the diets of many people. These may be used to meet part of the recommendation for milk in the diet. For example, about 1¼ ounces of cheddar cheese may be substituted for a glass of milk (Table 1.3). One-half cup of cottage cheese provides about the equivalent amount of calcium provided by one-third glass of milk. Approximately 1½ cups of ice cream will provide the amount of calcium contained in a glass of milk. Unfortunately, this amount of ice cream will add three times as many calories to the diet as will a glass of milk. The use of ice cream and milk-containing beverages in place of milk causes a definite increase in the calories

consumed. Such substitutions must be done sparingly if a person does not wish to gain weight.

Meat group

Although the nutritional contributions of the meats, poultry, fish, eggs, legumes, and nuts that comprise this group are somewhat varied, most of these foods provide useful amounts of protein, iron, and the B vitamins (Table 1.4). Servings of the various cuts of beef, veal, pork, and lamb compare favorably with the amount of protein available in a serving of poultry or fish. Legumes and nuts contain about 30 percent of the amount of protein available in a serving of these animal protein foods. Differences in nutritive content of the various foods that are included in this group are of interest, particularly in light of the proportionately high cost and frequently variable price of meat cuts. The food budget can be relieved somewhat by including legumes and eggs in menus to replace some of the higher-priced cuts of meat. Further savings can be made without sacrificing nutrition by buying local fish and poultry. In fact, greater use of these foods helps to reduce the intake of saturated fat that is abundant in meats.

Vegetable-fruit group

As indicated in Table 1.1, there are specific nutrients that are supplied by appropriate selections within the vegetable-fruit category. The serving of citrus fruit or an appropriate substitute provides adequate ascorbic acid. A good source of ascorbic acid (see Table 1.5) is recommended, because this vitamin is not stored in appreciable quantities in the body.

Vitamin A (in the form of carotene) is also specified in the vegetable-fruit group (Table 1.6). This vitamin, being fat soluble, is stored in the body for long periods of time and need not be supplied on a daily basis. The recommendation that a good source of vitamin A be included at least on alternate days assures that

---

[2] One International Unit of vitamin D equals 0.025 micrograms.

Table 1.3 Nutrient Value of Foods Made from Milk[a]

	Amount	kcal	Protein (g)	Fat (g)	Carbohydrate (g)	Calcium (mg)	Vitamin A (I.U.)	Thiamin (mg)	Riboflavin (mg)	Niacin (mg)
Cheese										
Cheddar	1 oz	110	7	9	1	213	371	0.01	0.13	Trace
Swiss	1 oz	105	8	8	1	262	323	Trace	0.11	Trace
Blue	1 oz	105	6	9	1	89	352	0.01	0.17	0.3
Brick	1 oz	105	6	9	1	207	352	0.01	0.13	Trace
Camembert	1 oz	85	5	7	1	30	286	0.01	0.21	0.2
Cottage, creamed	1/2 cup	120	15	5	3	106	191	0.03	0.28	0.1
Cottage, uncreamed	1/2 cup	95	19	Trace	3	101	11	0.03	0.32	0.1
Cream	2 tbsp	105	2	11	1	18	437	0.01	0.07	Trace
Processed cheese										
American	1 oz	105	7	9	1	198	346	0.01	0.12	Trace
Cheese food	1 oz	90	6	7	2	162	278	0.01	0.16	0.1
Cheese spread	1 oz	80	5	6	2	160	247	Trace	0.15	Trace
Frozen desserts										
Ice cream	1/2 cup	145	3	9	15	88	369	0.03	0.13	0.1
Ice milk	1/2 cup	100	3	3	15	104	141	0.03	0.15	0.1
Sherbet	1/2 cup	130	1	1	29	15	58	0.01	0.03	Trace
Beverages										
Egg nog (nonalcoholic)	1 cup	230	13	13	18	242	843	0.12	0.45	0.2
Hot chocolate	1 cup	230	9	12	26	269	363	0.07	0.41	0.2
"Instant" breakfast	1 cup	290	18	9	34	413	1400	0.30	0.58	2.7
Liquid diet beverage	1 cup	225	18	5	28	500	1250	0.50	0.75	3.8
Milkshake, vanilla	8 oz	220	9	12	19	285	509	0.07	0.41	0.2
Milkshake, malted	8 oz	330	9	13	47	276	586	0.12	0.43	0.3

[a] Data selected and calculated from *Composition of Foods—Raw, Processed, Prepared,* Agriculture Handbook No. 8, U.S.D.A., 1963; *Nutritive Value of Foods,* Home and Garden Bulletin No. 72, U.S.D.A., 1971; manufacturers' information; and *Nutritive Value of American Foods,* Agriculture Handbook No. 456, U.S.D.A., 1975.

Table 1.4 Nutrient Value of Representative Foods of the Meat Group[a]

	Amount	kcal	Protein (g)	Fat (g)	Iron (mg)	Vitamin A (I.U.)	Thiamin (mg)	Riboflavin (mg)	Niacin (mg)
Beef									
Rump roast, roasted, fat and lean	3 1/2 oz	345	24	27	3.1	50	0.06	0.18	4.3
Rump roast, roasted, lean	3 1/2 oz	210	29	9	3.7	20	0.07	0.22	5.2
Sirloin steak, broiled, fat and lean	3 1/2 oz	385	23	32	2.9	50	0.06	0.18	4.7
Sirloin steak, broiled, lean	3 1/2 oz	205	32	8	3.9	10	0.09	0.25	6.4
Ground beef, regular	3 1/2 oz	285	24	20	3.2	40	0.09	0.21	5.4
Ground beef, lean	3 1/2 oz	220	27	11	3.5	20	0.09	0.23	6.0
Veal, medium fat class									
Leg roast, roasted	3 1/2 oz	215	27	11	3.2		0.07	0.25	5.4
Loin chop, broiled	3 1/2 oz	235	26	13	3.2		0.07	0.25	5.4
Pork									
Loin chop, broiled, fat and lean	3 1/2 oz	420	24	35	3.2	0	0.92	0.27	5.6
Loin chop, broiled, lean	3 1/2 oz	270	31	15	3.9	0	1.13	0.33	6.8
Center ham slice, roasted, fat and lean	3 1/2 oz	290	21	22	2.6	0	0.47	0.18	3.6
Center ham slice, roasted, lean	3 1/2 oz	185	25	9	3.2	0	0.58	0.23	4.5
Lamb									
Leg roast, roasted, fat and lean	3 1/2 oz	280	25	19	1.7		0.15	0.27	5.5
Leg roast, roasted, lean	3 1/2 oz	185	29	7	2.2		0.16	0.30	6.2
Loin chop, broiled, fat and lean	3 1/2 oz	360	22	29	1.3		0.12	0.23	5.0
Loin chop, broiled, lean	3 1/2 oz	190	28	8	2.0		0.15	0.28	6.1
Poultry									
Chicken breast, fried	3 1/2 oz	205	33	6	1.7	90	0.05	0.22	14.7
Turkey, light meat, roasted	3 1/2 oz	175	33	4	1.2		0.05	0.14	11.1

Table 1.4 (continued)

	Amount	kcal	Protein (g)	Fat (g)	Iron (mg)	Vitamin A (I.U.)	Thiamin (mg)	Riboflavin (mg)	Niacin (mg)
Variety Meat									
Calf liver, fried	3 1/2 oz	260	30	13	14.2	32,700	0.24	4.20	16.5
Beef tongue, braised	3 1/2 oz	245	22	17	2.2		0.05	0.29	3.5
Luncheon meats									
Bologna	1 slice	90	4	8	0.5		0.05	0.07	0.8
Salami	1 slice	95	5	8	0.8		0.08	0.07	1.2
Frankfurter	1 medium	125	7	10	0.6	0	0.08	0.09	1.2
Fish and shellfish									
Halibut, broiled	3 1/2 oz	170	25	7	0.8	680	0.05	0.07	8.3
Tuna, oil pack	3 1/2 oz	190	29	8	1.9	80	0.05	0.12	11.9
Swordfish, broiled with fat	3 1/2 oz	175	28	6	1.3	2,050	0.04	0.05	10.9
Clams, raw	3 1/2 oz	75	13	2	6.1	100	0.10	0.18	1.3
Shrimp, cooked	3 1/2 oz	115	24	1	3.1	60	0.01	0.03	1.8
Egg, whole	1 medium	80	6	6	1.1	562	0.04	0.12	
Legumes and nuts									
Baked beans	1/2 cup	155	7	4	2.4	74	0.08	0.05	0.7
Mixed nuts, oil roasted	1 oz	175	5	17	1.0	6	0.17	0.04	1.1
Peanuts, oil roasted	1 oz	160	8	13	1.0		0.07	0.07	4.8
Peanut butter	2 tbsp	175	8	15	0.6		0.04	0.04	4.7

[a] Data selected from *Composition of Foods—Raw, Processed, Prepared*, Agriculture Handbook No. 8, U.S.D.A., 1963 and *Nutritive Value of American Foods*, Agriculture Handbook No. 456, U.S.D.A., 1975.

Table 1.5 *Ascorbic Acid Content of Fruits and Vegetables in Portions Commonly Served*[a]

Fruits, fresh	Amount	Ascorbic Acid (mg)	Vegetables	Amount	Ascorbic Acid (mg)
Guava	1/2 medium	120	Broccoli, cooked	Medium stalk	90
Orange	1 medium	75	Brussels sprouts, cooked	1/2 cup	80
Cantaloupe	1/2 small	60	Turnip greens, cooked	1/2 cup	55
Honeydew	1/4 medium	60	Mustard greens, cooked	1/2 cup	50
Orange juice	1/2 cup	55	Collard greens, cooked	1/2 cup	40
Papaya	1/3 medium	55	Cauliflower, cooked	1/2 cup	35
Grapefruit	1/2 medium	50	Kale, cooked	1/2 cup	35
Strawberries	1/2 cup	45	Kohlrabi, cooked	1/2 cup	30
Grapefruit juice	1/2 cup	40	Sweet red pepper, raw	1/4 shell	30
Mango	1/2 medium	25	Spinach, cooked	1/2 cup	30
Tangerine	1 medium	30	Tomato, raw	1 medium	25
Watermelon	1 slice	30	Sweet potato, baked in skin	1 medium	25
Tangerine juice	1/2 cup	25	Asparagus spears, cooked	1/2 cup	25
Lemon wedge	1/8 lemon	10	Tomato juice, canned	1/2 cup	20
Banana	1 medium	12	Potato, baked in skin	1 medium	20
			Cabbage, shredded	1/2 cup	15

[a] Data compiled and adapted from ***Composition of Foods—Raw, Processed, Prepared,*** Agriculture Handbook No. 8, U.S.D.A., 1963 and ***Nutritive Value of American Foods,*** Agriculture Handbook No. 456, U.S.D.A., 1975.

sufficient vitamin A is available under this plan.

The total servings of fruits and vegetables will provide nutritionally important quantities of the B vitamins, ascorbic acid, and vitamin A (as carotene), as well as many of the minerals needed for good health. Furthermore, fruits and vegetables contribute roughage to the diet, an important factor in promoting motility in the digestive tract. This roughage comes largely from cellulose, which is not digested and used as a nutrient, but is eliminated as bulk in the feces.

Cereal group

The cereal group contributes not only carbohydrates, B vitamins, and iron, but also adds generous amounts of protein to the diet when

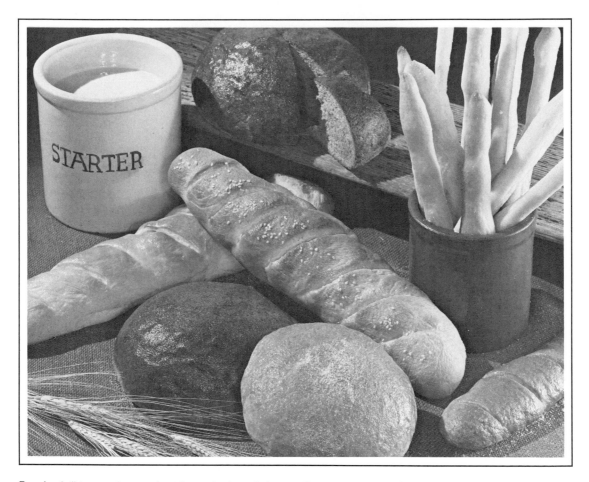

Breads of all types, when made with enriched or whole-grain flours, are important for their flavor and textural contributions to the diet as well as for their nutritional contributions.

consumed in large quantities. Foods selected in this group should be either whole-grain or enriched products. Whole-grain cereals contain valuable amounts of thiamin, riboflavin, niacin, iron, and other minerals. However, a large proportion of these nutrients is lost during processing when the bran layers are removed. Since breads and cereals are relied upon as traditional sources of the B vitamins and iron, federal standards have been established for the enrichment or replacement of these nutrients in refined products. When thiamin, riboflavin,

niacin, and iron are added to wheat, rice, corn, and pasta products, the package states that the food has been enriched or fortified. Several states are establishing laws requiring fortification of cereal products. Since this practice is not yet universal, it is important for the consumer to read labels to insure that the breads and cereals he eats are either enriched or whole-grain products. Table 1.7 gives key nutrient values of representative foods from the cereal group. The bran of cereals, when not removed, is an important source of dietary fiber.

Table 1.6 *Carotene Content of Deep Yellow and Dark Green Vegetables and Fruits*[a]

Food	Amount	Carotene, (I.U.)
Sweet potato, baked in skin	1 medium	9720
Carrots, cooked, diced	1/2 cup	8400
Spinach, cooked	1/2 cup	8100
Kale, cooked	1/2 cup	7544
Pumpkin, cooked	1/2 cup	7400
Cantaloupe, ripe, 5 in. diameter	1/2 small	6290
Mustard greens, cooked	1/2 cup	5800
Carrot, raw	1 small	5500
Swiss chard, cooked	1/2 cup	5157
Turnip greens, cooked	1/2 cup	5135
Mango, ripe	1/2 medium	4800
Collard greens, cooked	1/2 cup	4590
Winter squash, cooked	1/2 cup	4270
Broccoli, cooked	Medium stalk	2500
Papaya, ripe	1/3 medium	1750
Peach, raw (yellow)	1 medium	1330
Apricot, raw	1 medium	1134

[a] Data selected and calculated from **Composition of Foods—Raw, Processed, Prepared,** Agriculture Handbook No. 8, U.S.D.A., 1963 and **Nutritive Value of American Foods,** Agriculture Handbook No. 456, U.S.D.A., 1975.

Dietary standards and recommendations

Various standards for evaluating the nutritional adequacy of individuals have been developed around the world. In the United States, standards have been developed: (1) minimum daily requirements (MDR) were established by the Food and Drug Administration to provide a legally accepted standard for labeling the amounts of nutrients in foods; and (2) the recommended dietary allowances (RDA) were established and published by the Food and Nutrition Board of the National Research Council in 1943. The philosophy underlying the recommendations of the Food and Nutrition Board (Table 1.8) is to identify the amounts of nutrients needed by healthy,

Table 1.7 Nutrient Value of Representative Foods of the Cereal Group[a]

	Amount	kcal	Protein (g)	Carbohydrate (g)	Iron (mg)	Thiamin (mg)	Riboflavin (mg)	Niacin (mg)
Bread								
White, enriched	1 slice	60	2	12	0.6	0.06	0.05	0.6
Whole wheat	1 slice	55	2	11	0.5	0.06	0.03	0.6
Dinner roll	1 medium	115	3	20	0.7	0.11	0.07	0.8
Biscuit	1 medium	130	3	16	0.6	0.07	0.07	0.6
Cereal, cooked								
Cream of wheat	1 cup	105	3	21	1.4	0.12	0.07	1.0
Oatmeal	1 cup	130	5	23	1.4	0.19	0.05	0.2
Cereal, ready-to-eat								
Cornflakes	1 cup	110	2	25	0.4	0.12	0.02	0.6
Puffed rice	1 cup	50	1	12	0.2	0.06	0.01	0.6
Shredded wheat	1 biscuit	100	3	22	1.0	0.06	0.03	1.2
Special K	1 cup	60	3	13	2.5	0.22	0.28	2.9
Cereal grains, cooked								
Rice, enriched	1 cup	225	4	50	1.8	0.23	0.02	2.1
Bulgur wheat	1 cup	245	8	44	1.9	0.08	0.05	4.1
Corn grits	1 cup	125	3	27	0.7	0.10	0.07	1.0
Crackers								
Saltines	1 square	15	Trace	2	Trace	Trace	Trace	Trace
Graham	1 square	25	1	5	0.1	Trace	0.01	0.1
Pasta, cooked								
Macaroni, enriched	1 cup	155	5	32	1.3	0.20	0.11	1.5
Noodles, enriched	1 cup	200	7	37	1.4	0.22	0.13	1.9
Spaghetti, enriched	1 cup	180	5	37	1.4	0.22	0.13	1.8
Sweet breads								
Pecan roll	1 medium	240	5	32	0.7	0.07	0.08	0.4
Cream donut	1 medium	235	3	14	0.5	0.06	0.09	0.4

[a] Data compiled and adapted from *Composition of Foods—Raw, Processed, Prepared,* Agriculture Handbook No. 8, U.S.D.A., 1963; *Nutritive Value of Foods,* Home and Garden Bulletin No. 72, U.S.D.A., 1971; manufacturers' information; and *Nutritive Value of American Foods,* Agriculture Handbook No. 456, U.S.D.A., 1975.

Table 1.8 Recommended Daily Dietary Allowances, Revised 1974[a]
(Designed for the maintenance of good nutrition of practically all healthy people in the U.S.A.)

	Age (years)	Weight (kg)	Weight (lbs)	Height (cm)	Height (in)	Energy (kcal)[b]	Protein (g)	Fat-Soluble Vitamins			Water-Soluble Vitamins							Minerals					
								Vitamin A Activity (RE)[c] (IU)	Vitamin D (IU)	Vitamin E Activity[e] (IU)	Ascorbic Acid (mg)	Folacin[f] (µg)	Niacin[g] (mg)	Riboflavin (B2) (mg)	Thiamin (B1) (mg)	Vitamin B6 (mg)	Vitamin B12 (µg)	Calcium (mg)	Phosphorus (mg)	Iodine (µg)	Iron (mg)	Magnesium (mg)	Zinc (mg)
Infants	0.0-0.5	6	14	60	24	kg × 117	kg × 2.2	420[d] 1,400	400	4	35	50	5	0.4	0.3	0.3	0.3	360	240	35	10	60	3
	0.5-1.0	9	20	71	28	kg × 108	kg × 2.0	400 2,000	400	5	35	50	8	0.6	0.5	0.4	0.3	540	400	45	15	70	5
Children	1-3	13	28	86	34	1300	23	400 2,000	400	7	40	100	9	0.8	0.7	0.6	1.0	800	800	60	15	150	10
	4-6	20	44	110	44	1800	30	500 2,500	400	9	40	200	12	1.1	0.9	0.9	1.5	800	800	80	10	200	10
	7-10	30	66	135	54	2400	36	700 3,300	400	10	40	300	16	1.2	1.2	1.2	2.0	800	800	110	10	250	10
Males	11-14	44	97	158	63	2800	44	1,000 5,000	400	12	45	400	18	1.5	1.4	1.6	3.0	1200	1200	130	18	350	15
	15-18	51	134	172	69	3000	54	1,000 5,000	400	15	45	400	20	1.8	1.5	2.0	3.0	1200	1200	150	18	400	15
	19-22	67	147	172	69	3000	54	1,000 5,000	400	15	45	400	20	1.8	1.5	2.0	3.0	800	800	140	10	350	15
	23-50	70	154	172	69	2700	56	1,000 5,000		15	45	400	18	1.6	1.4	2.0	3.0	800	800	130	10	350	15
	51+	70	154	172	69	2400	56	1,000 5,000		15	45	400	16	1.5	1.2	2.0	3.0	800	800	110	10	350	15
Females	11-14	44	97	155	62	2400	44	800 4,000	400	12	45	400	16	1.3	1.2	1.6	3.0	1200	1200	115	18	300	15
	15-18	54	119	162	65	2100	48	800 4,000	400	12	45	400	14	1.4	1.1	2.0	3.0	1200	1200	115	18	300	15
	19-22	58	128	162	65	2100	46	800 4,000	400	12	45	400	14	1.4	1.1	2.0	3.0	800	800	100	18	300	15
	23-50	58	128	162	65	2000	46	800 4,000		12	45	400	13	1.2	1.0	2.0	3.0	800	800	100	18	300	15
	51+	58	128	162	65	1800	46	800 4,000		12	45	400	12	1.1	1.0	2.0	3.0	800	800	80	10	300	15
Pregnant						+300	+30	1,000 5,000	400	15	60	800	+2	+0.3	+0.3	2.5	4.0	1200	1200	125	18+[h]	450	20
Lactating						+500	+20	1,200 6,000	400	15	80	600	+4	+0.5	+0.3	2.5	4.0	1200	1200	150	18	450	25

[a] Reproduced by permission of the Food and Nutrition Board, National Academy of Sciences—National Research Council. The allowances are intended to provide for individual variations among most normal persons as they live in the United States under usual environmental stresses. Diets should be based on a variety of common foods in order to provide other nutrients for which human requirements have been less well defined. See text for more detailed discussion of allowances and of nutrients not tabulated.

[b] Kilojoules (kJ) = 4.2 × kcal.

[c] Retinol equivalents.

[d] Assumed to be all as retinol in milk during the first six months of life. All subsequent intakes are assumed to be half as retinol and half as β-carotene when calculated from international units. As retinol equivalents, three fourths are as retinol and one fourth as β-carotene.

[e] Total vitamin E activity, estimated to be 80 percent as α-tocopherol and 20 percent other tocopherols.

[f] The folacin allowances refer to dietary sources as determined by Lactobacillus casei assay. Pure forms of folacin may be effective in doses less than one fourth of the recommended dietary allowance.

[g] Although allowances are expressed as niacin, it is recognized that on the average 1 mg of niacin is derived from each 60 mg of dietary tryptophan.

[h] This increased requirement cannot be met by ordinary diets; therefore, the use of supplemental iron is recommended.

normal Americans to promote good growth for children and optimum health for all. A margin of safety is incorporated in the recommendations to allow for minor variations in utilization and need of nutrients by individuals.

The MDR developed by the Food and Drug Administration have never been revised since they were issued many years ago. They are now obsolete and have been superseded by the U.S. RDA's, which were established by the Food and Drug Administration as the standard to be used for nutrition labeling (see Chapter 17).

The RDA are reevaluated and revised at approximately 5-year intervals. Revisions of the table are made to update recommendations in light of current research findings and changes in living patterns. For example, the increasingly sedentary nature of the general population has resulted in a downward revision of the recommendation for calories during the decades spanned by the use of the tables. In 1968 the revisions of the table were extensive: recommended amounts of vitamin E, folacin, vitamin B_{12}, pyridoxine, phosphorus, iodine, and magnesium were included for the first time; the recommended amount of vitamin C was reduced; and the value of iron recommended for adolescent and adult women was increased. In 1974 further revisions were made, including the addition of zinc.

By keeping an accurate record of the amounts of food eaten and calculating the nutrient content of each item (see tables of food composition in the Appendix), a summation of the total nutrient intake can be obtained. When the daily figures for several days are averaged, the average values can be compared with the recommended dietary allowances to review the nutritional adequacy of the diet pattern. Of course, disease and metabolic abnormalities may intervene in specific individuals. In such instances, application of the RDA may not present a true picture of the adequacy of nutrient intake.

Other nations and the Food and Agricultural Organization of the United Nations have also developed recommended dietary standards. Each of these is somewhat different from the others. Differences are explained partially by the rationale underlying the various standards recommended. Some are based on the minimum level considered necessary for good health. Others include a calculated margin of safety so that the recommendations are keyed to provide maximum nutritional health for a very large segment of the population. Specific information is contained in the appropriate references listed at the end of this chapter.

Summary

Nutrition, the science of food and its relation to health, is a vital concern to the individual and to all peoples of the world. Numerous scientific studies have elucidated many functions of nutrients and have provided the basis for establishing recommended intakes of the various nutrients needed by man. However, much remains to be done to extend the field of knowledge. A still greater challenge is presented in the application of this nutrition information to achieve better health.

For optimum health, man requires a diet that regularly includes carbohydrates, fats, proteins, minerals, vitamins, and water—and the last is not least! Carbohydrates are organic compounds that provide energy for the body. Fats also contribute energy, but serve the additional functions of providing the essential fatty acid (linoleic acid) and carrying the fat-soluble vitamins (A, D, E, and K) into the body. Proteins are composed of amino acids, the nitrogen-containing compounds needed by the body for building and repairing tissue and synthesizing hormones, enzymes, and antibodies. Additional functions of protein include helping to maintain proper osmotic pressure, regulating the body at essentially a neutral balance between acidity and alkalinity, and providing energy. Minerals are needed in the diet in rather small quantities to provide the building materials needed for the structure of bones and teeth. They also help to maintain a balance between acids and alkaline substances in the body and function in regulating fluid concentrations in the blood as well as in cells and in intercellular areas. Specific minerals help to regulate body processes by acting as catalysts for chemical reactions and by serving as structural parts of some hormones and enzymes. Vitamins are the organic compounds required in extremely small amounts in the diet. All water-soluble and fat-soluble vitamins are important in promoting growth and maintaining life. Many of the vitamins serve as components of enzyme systems that function in releasing energy from food. (Current knowledge of the specific roles of the various vitamins and other nutrients are discussed in detail in Chapters 6 through 11.) Water is essential for many body functions. Fiber (cellulose) is necessary for proper functioning of the large bowel.

The Basic Four is a food guide consisting of four food groups. Diets planned to conform to this useful and practical guide will include the protein, carbohydrate, vitamins, and minerals needed by the average man. Additional servings are needed to supply the extra energy required by active people. This guide can be used to gain a quick approximation of the adequacy of a diet. More accurate dietary analysis can be accomplished by comparing the nutrients in the food consumed (derived by using tables detailing food composition) with the recommended dietary allowances of nutrients established by the Food and Nutrition Board of the National Research Council.

Variety in foods consumed among the Basic Four Food Groups and within each group is the key to good nutrition and a balanced diet, with serving sizes adjusted to reach and maintain proper weight.

Selected References

Bogert, L. J., G. M. Briggs, and D. H. Calloway. *Nutrition and Physical Fitness.* 9th ed. Saunders. Philadelphia. 1973.

Chaney, M. S. and M. L. Ross. *Nutrition.* 8th ed. Houghton Mifflin. Boston. 1972.

Fleck, H. C. *Introduction to Nutrition.* 2nd ed. Macmillan. New York. 1971.

Food and Agricultural Organization. Calcium requirements, FAO Nutrition Meeting Report Series No. 30. 1962.

Food and Agricultural Organization. Calorie requirements. *FAO Nutri. Stud.* No. 15. 1957.

Food and Agricultural Organization. Protein requirements. Report of Joint FAO/WHO Expert Group. WHO Technical Report Series No. 301. 1965.

Food and Agricultural Organization. FAO requirements for vitamin A, thiamin, riboflavin, and niacin. 1967 FAO Nutritional Meeting Report Series No. 41. Rome, Italy. 1967.

Food and Agricultural Organization. FAO requirements of ascorbic acid, vitamin D, vitamin B_{12}, folate, and iron. WHO Technical Report Series No. 452. 1970.

Food and Nutrition Board, National Research Council. Recommended dietary allowances. Washington, D.C. 1974.

Guthrie, H. A. *Introductory Nutrition.* 3rd ed. Mosby. St. Louis. 1975.

Hayes, O., M. F. Trulson, and F. J. Stare. Suggested revision of the Basic 7. *J. Am. Diet. Assoc. 31:*1103. 1955.

Hegsted, D. M. Establishment of nutritional requirements in man. *Borden Rev. Nutr. Res. 20:*13. 1959.

Mitchell, H. S., et al. *Cooper's Nutrition in Health and Disease.* 15th ed. Lippincott. Philadelphia. 1968.

Report of Committee on Nutrition. Brit. Med. Assoc. London. 1950.

Roberts, L. J. Beginnings of the recommended dietary allowances. *J. Am. Diet. Assoc. 34:*903. 1958.

Robinson, C. H. *Fundamentals of Normal Nutrition.* 2nd ed. Macmillan. New York. 1973.

Stare, F. and M. McWilliams. *Nutrition for Good Health.* Plycon Press. Fullerton, Calif. 1974.

Todhunter, E. N. Historical landmarks in nutrition. *Present Knowledge of Nutrition.* 4th ed. Nutrition Foundation. New York. 1976.

Watts, B., and A. Merrill. Composition of foods—raw, processed and prepared. *U.S. Dept. Agriculture Handbook No. 8.* U.S.D.A. Washington, D.C. 1963.

SOCIOPSYCHOLOGICAL ASPECTS OF NUTRITION

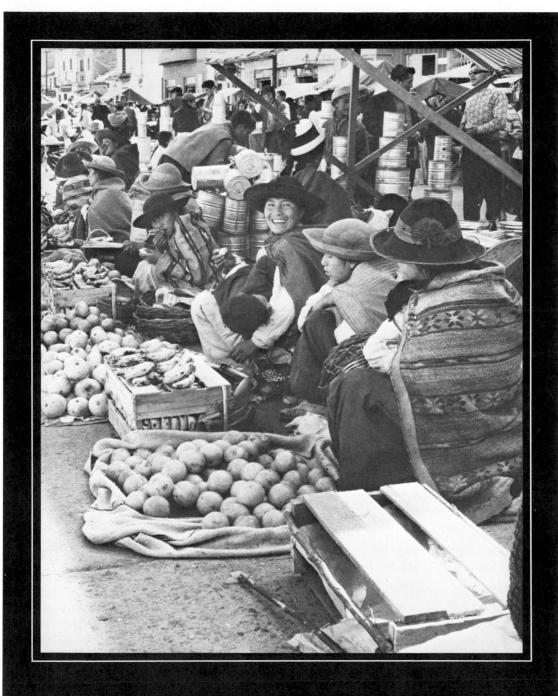

Chapter 2

Nutrition— A Worldwide Concern

The achievement of adequate nutrition for all is a complex problem of global scope. Progress toward solving this problem successfully is dependent upon meeting the challenges of such diverse, yet related problems as:

1. Population control.
2. Economic development that enables all healthy people to work for a living wage.
3. Increasing food production.
4. Development of more effective food distribution systems.
5. Understanding and appreciation of the cultural and psychological factors determining food acceptance on an individual and group basis.
6. Effective nutrition education for all people, particularly young children.
7. Stability of family life so that individuals can be well nourished throughout all stages of the life cycle.

Dr. Margaret Mead has realistically summarized the importance of nutrition to all peoples of the world:[1]

"We live in a world today where the state of nutrition in each country is relevant and important to each other country, and where the state of nutrition in the wealthy industrialized countries like the United States has profound significance for the role that such countries can play in eliminating famine and providing for adequate nutrition throughout the world. In a world in which each half knows what the other half does, we cannot live with hunger and malnutrition in one part of the world while people in another part are not only well nourished, but over-nourished. Any talk of one world, of brotherhood, rings hollow to those who have come face to face on the television screen with the emaciation of starving children and to the

[1] Margaret Mead. The changing significance of food. *American Scientist.* 58:176. 1970.

people whose children are starving as they pore over month-old issues of glossy American and European magazines, where full color prints show people glowing with health, their plates piled high with food that glistens to match the shining textures of their clothes. Peoples who have resolutely tightened their belts and put up with going to bed hungry, people who have seen their children die because they did not have the strength to resist disease, and called it fate or the will of God, can no longer do so in the vivid visual realization of the amount and quality of food eaten—and wasted—by others."

Nutrition problems on a worldwide scope are not suddenly emerging difficulties of the decade of the 1970s. Man has always needed food, and the procurement of adequate food has occupied much of his time and effort. The significance of the current concern for nutrition is that interest has shifted from involvement on a personal or family basis to a global awareness and commitment to feeding all people adequately. To achieve such a goal will require tremendous efforts not only from nutritionists, but also from sociologists, psychologists, agriculturists, economists, physicians, public health workers, teachers, and politicians. The task is not an easy one, and yet surely the opportunities for developing optimal individuals and promoting world peace are sufficient motivations for all people.

The current situation can be interpreted more accurately if the factors that contributed to the development of these nutrition problems are understood. Geographical, cultural, political, and economic factors all have had their impact on feeding the world, and their influence will continue to be of significance as people the world over cope with the nutrition problem. The enormity of these factors and their resistance to change retard and restrict efforts to seek practical solutions to worldwide nutrition problems.

Geographical Factors

Geographical factors have molded man's diet and food preferences throughout history. Even with the present remarkable technological achievements, food production and distribution are limited by geography. As research leads to improved techniques and materials, some of these limitations will be reduced, but the physical restrictions of climate and land will always place a finite limitation on world food production. It is estimated that there are 1.1 billion hectares of cultivable land in the world. By 1985, 53 percent (600 million hectares) are predicted to be in production. Much of the land presently not being utilized for agriculture is very difficult to farm at a profit. However, man's efforts to combat geographical limits on food production can be seen throughout the world today.

The role of food supplies in the history of man has been traced as archaeologists and historians have unfolded the past. Early man was dependent upon the food naturally available from the land, but people living at the eastern end of the Mediterranean Sea were raising lambs for food by 9000 B.C. Cultivation of crops appears to have been a regular pattern of life for many population groups at widely scattered points around the world by 2000 B.C. Archaeologists have studied the artifacts that provide evidence of farming in the Middle East and Central America during this period. Although the crops were quite different (wheat, lentils, peas, and barley, plus the herding of sheep and goats in the Middle East, and squash, avocados, and peppers in Central America), the cultivation of crops in both regions enabled people to live in one place rather than necessitating a nomadic existence for food. Gradually such important crops as corn, beans, tomatoes, rice, fruits of many types, coffee, tea, and the numerous other foods known today were brought under cultivation. Animal husbandry was expanded beyond sheep and goats to include cattle, pork, and poultry.

Regional patterns of temperature and rainfall dictated, in large measure, the crops that were raised, just as they still do today. In tropical regions with abundant rainfall, fruits flourished and have occupied a prominent place in the diet for a long time. Cereals indigenous to a region have continued to be the dietary backbone of some cultures throughout many centuries. The climate of Southeast Asia is well suited to the production of rice, which has been the staple food of most people throughout the world's "Rice Bowl." In comparison, corn is widely used in Central America and South America, where this important cereal originated. In Europe and the North American continent, wheat grows well and is the grain most widely used in the diet.

Sufficient water, either by irrigation or by natural rainfall, and an adequate growing season are essential for raising crops that provide a profitable yield per acre. In many areas in the temperate zone, the seasons permit the raising of only one crop per year. As the equator is approached, the growing season becomes longer, and frequently two or even more crops can be raised annually. This fact enhances the attractiveness of crop farming. Fortunately, crops also can be raised most years in several regions far from the equator if the crop is planted as early as the ground can possibly be worked. Although the growing season covers only a small portion of the calendar in northern and southern regions remote from the equator, growth during the middle of the warm season is rapid as a result of the long hours of daylight.

A nation's dietary pattern is determined not only by climate, but also by such geographical features as proximity to the sea and topography. One has only to partake of a Scandina-vian smorgasbord to appreciate how the sea and terrain have influenced the diets of Nordic populations. Since the land is extremely rugged and access to the sea does not present a problem, there has been strong reliance on the ocean for food. Similar observations can be made about the traditional dietary patterns in Japan. The very precipitous nature of the islands of Japan has certainly encouraged the development of food industries focusing on the sea. However, the pressure for food created by a crowded population has led to rather remarkable utilization of terracing techniques to retrieve land that is considered untillable by traditional standards of agricultural production. Earlier in history, the Incas in the Andes of South America used terraces effectively.

Although the quality of soil has only a limited effect on the nutritive value of foods, fertile soil rich in nutrients is essential for maximum crop yield. As the land has been farmed in some regions, the soil has been depleted of important nutrients by leaching and erosion of top soil. The loss of plant nutrients from the soil is significant because total productivity becomes restricted and less food is then available from the same land area. The addition of fertilizers to the soil replaces lost nutrients such as nitrogen, phosphorus, and potassium. With correct fertilizer treatments, the soil is enriched and productivity of the land is maximized.

The soil in some areas of the world is low in the mineral nutrient, iodide. In Ceylon, where the rainfall is extremely high in some regions, the iodide levels in the soil have become minimal as a result of the leaching action of the rain over innumerable centuries. In other regions of the world (Switzerland, Austria, the Himalayan Belt, and the Great Plains of the United States), the soil is also low in iodide. The consequence of this deficiency is that fruits and vegetables raised on such soil will be extremely low in iodide content. People eating diets comprised principally of foods raised in these areas are likely to have an inadequate intake of iodide, unless it is added as a supplement (in iodized salt). A deficiency of iodide causes endemic

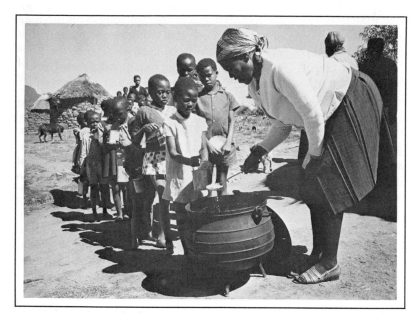

International agencies have expended considerable amounts of time and money in efforts to relieve the famine conditions created by droughts, crop failures, and wars. This program in Lesotho concentrated on providing food for school children and high-risk groups, such as pregnant and lactating women and preschoolers.

goiter, a condition common in areas where iodide levels in the soil are very low and where iodization of salt is not common. Iodized salt, one of the most significant technological achievements of applied nutrition in improving public health, provides a practical way of meeting the body's need for iodide.

Another nutritional problem related to geographic location is that of obtaining adequate vitamin D. Vitamin D is an unusual vitamin that can be produced in the body by exposing the skin to direct sunlight. In locations in the tropical zone and lower temperate regions, a reasonable amount of sunlight reaches the skin of most people throughout the year unless they are shielded unduly from the sun by clothing, housing, or air pollution. In countries closer to either of the polar regions, sunlight is available in adequate amounts only during a limited portion of the year. Skies that frequently are cloudy limit the amount of sunlight in some areas to the point where the vitamin D formed in the skin is not sufficient to meet the body's

needs. The increasing smog problem in many urban areas also limits the formation of vitamin D because of the filtering effect of the polluted atmosphere. The result in any of these circumstances may be an inadequate amount of vitamin D in the body. Such factors heighten the importance of including vitamin D in the diet so that poor calcium absorption, retarded growth, and poor bone development due to vitamin D deficiency can be avoided.

There is a common saying that everyone talks about the weather, but nobody ever does anything about it. Doubtless this saying had its origin in an agricultural environment, because weather is so crucial to optimum crop production. The unpredictability of the weather can create significant nutritional problems for a country. Some of the more fortunate nations have been able to stockpile a reserve of food to meet the emergencies created by a bad crop year. However, the increasing population of the world is rapidly eliminating (some reporters say the people already have consumed) even these reserve cushions against malnutrition. Development of irrigation systems has done much to not only increase the area of productive land, but also to insure successful crops from farmlands where rainfall is somewhat uncertain. In some places, tiles in fields have aided farmers in draining the land to avoid loss of time early in the growing season when fields may be flooded by late spring thaws or heavy rains. These are some of the advances used to promote successful crop production. However, man's crops are still largely at the mercy of nature.

Yet another geographical factor influencing dietary patterns and nutrition is the effect of location and the distribution problems resulting from location. Proportionately few people today rely exclusively on food produced within or very close to the community in which they live. A very large percentage of the food consumed today has gone through a distribution network. This network may be as un-complicated as a farmer bringing in his produce and selling it in a stall in the marketplace. However, the route from the producer to the consumer frequently is much longer and more complicated. Produce to be shipped to another part of the country has to be harvested while it is sufficiently immature to withstand the rigors of transportation. The shipping needs to be done under controlled conditions, frequently involving refrigeration, to insure reasonable quality at the end of the line. Shipping must be sufficiently rapid to deliver fresh produce before it spoils. This implies that adequate trucking, rail facilities, or air transportation are available, that loaders and drivers are working, and that a market exists at the end of the line. In the case of less perishable foods, moisture-controlled storage facilities free of insects must be available to accommodate peak production periods. Trained inspectors for meats and other inspected and graded food items must be available at production and processing facilities.

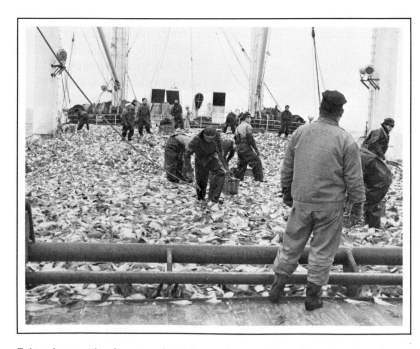

Fishing boats with adequate refrigeration and processing equipment on board are a vital link in transporting large catches from the sea to the ultimate consumer.

At the receiving end, an efficient distribution method is needed to reach the ultimate consumer. In many instances, this means the operation of a high-quality grocery store in the United States. In other cirmumstances, the picture at the end of the line may be that of a poorly run grocery store charging relatively high prices for food of less than top quality in a low-income area. Rounding out the picture for some consumers are the complicated channels of welfare and the use of food stamps. Obviously, the distribution of food in the United States is highly complex and is dependent upon cooperation from many people, beginning with production and continuing until the food ultimately reaches the consumer. In view of the numerous possibilities for poor nutrition of the consumer as food passes through the distribution network, much credit is due the total food industry that contributes so much to the nutritional status of consumers.

Other countries with similar levels of economic development have distribution problems similar to those existing in the United States. The distribution problems in small countries with less varied climates and agricultural conditions may be even more complex. Under such circumstances, large quantities of many different food products may need to be imported if adequate amounts and sufficiently varied foods are to be available to all the people in the country. A practical illustration of this circumstance is the need for the British to import citrus fruits because their climate is not suitable for growing citrus. Interestingly enough, less conventional sources of a specific nutrient sometimes can be found when import problems become overwhelming, as may be the case in wartime. The English were able to utilize rose hips (the bulblike formation that develops after roses bloom and begin to fade) as a source of vitamin C during World War II when importation of citrus fruits was not feasible.

Cultural Implications

The answer to achieving adequate nutrition for the world's people will not be found simply by producing enough food to provide the total amounts of protein and other nutrients needed for optimum growth and health. The nutrients must be contained in foods that are acceptable to the individual consumer. For nutrition programs to be successful, these individual food acceptance factors must be assessed and utilized in all phases of governmental and private nutrition programs.

Everyone has individual food preferences that have developed as a result of several factors, including:

1. The food available in the locale.
2. The foods preferred by members of his family, especially by his parents.
3. The foods purchased and prepared for him (reflecting parental and cultural attitudes as well as family income).
4. Foods permitted by religious or cultural dicta.
5. Foods that have particular taste, texture, or color appeal for the individual.

An adult's food preferences can be traced from earliest childhood. Clearly, these preferences are based on cultural and environmental factors far more than they are founded on a person's recognition of his specific nutritional needs. Cultural food patterns around the world can be traced far into antiquity, and many are influenced greatly by religion. The religious overtones are perhaps most clearly seen by reviewing the types of meats eaten by various groups.

Religious influences

Pork avoidance

The avoidance of pork by both Moslems and Jews is a familiar taboo dictated by religion. However, the status of pigs as a source of food has changed from time to time throughout history. Early Egyptians ate some pork, although the swineherds occupied such a low social position that they were not allowed in the temples. Apparently pigs were used by Egyptians then primarily as a sacrificial meat in religious ceremonies.

There is some indication that early Jews ate pork, but by 150 BC pork was viewed as an unacceptable food by followers of the Jewish faith. Several reasons for this prohibition have been suggested: (1) the pig is a possible carrier of disease because of his fondness for rolling in mud; (2) trichinosis, a prolonged parasitic infection, may result from eating undercooked pork; (3) pork spoils quickly without refrigeration; and (4) the pig does not herd well in comparison with other animals used as sources of meat. No single reason has been agreed upon, and arguments can be formulated for and against each of these points.

The Moslems, too, have ingrained feelings against swine and swine products. One theory is that Mohammed may have abolished pork from Islamic diets as a significant means of distinguishing Mohammedans from Christians. However, there is some weakening of the prejudice against pork in the Islamic world today, and the wild boar is used in Morocco for some medicinal purposes. The Moslems living in China continue to follow the practice of avoiding pork despite the fact that other Chinese find pork a highly acceptable meat.

Additional support for the pork-banning groups is found in India, where the Hindus reject pork both because of the value they place on life and the objection to the filth of pigs. Yet another factor influencing food prejudices is found among the Hindus. Traditionally, the untouchables have kept pigs and eaten pork. In an attempt to raise their social status, some of the subcastes have given up these practices and have emulated the higher castes, thus expanding the circle of those who routinely avoid pork.

In contrast, the Hindus in Southeast Asia view pigs as sacrificial animals as well as a source of food. The Buddhists in this region also eat pork, but both Hindus and Buddhists relegate the keeping and slaughtering of the animals to others. Not surprisingly, Moslem influences in this region tend to discourage the use of pork.

Attitudes toward beef

The primary focal point of beef avoidance is India. The reverence with which the Hindus view cattle in India is legendary and has led to not only a proliferation of cattle in the country, but also to a multiplication of problems in a country where good nutrition for all seems to be an all but impossible goal. To many observers, the practice of allowing "sacred cows" to consume food instead of being a source of food for hungry people is becoming a moral issue that may supersede religious dictates. In addition to not serving as a source of food, the "wandering cows" do considerable damage to vegetation. Another important negative effect on the food supply is that there is no effort to improve breeding practices with the "sacred cows" for improved milk production.

As with pork, beef is eaten by some of the low-caste Hindus, but this practice is being abandoned as higher social status is sought. Moslems in India take a broader view toward using cattle as food, although the slaughtering is done discreetly to avoid trouble. Buddhists in Southeast Asia have gradually accepted beef as a food, a transition that appears to have been hastened by the spread of Mohammedanism in that area.

In the southern, eastern, and southwestern parts of Africa, cattle are accepted widely as a symbol of culture and prosperity. A bride can even be bought with cattle. Some African

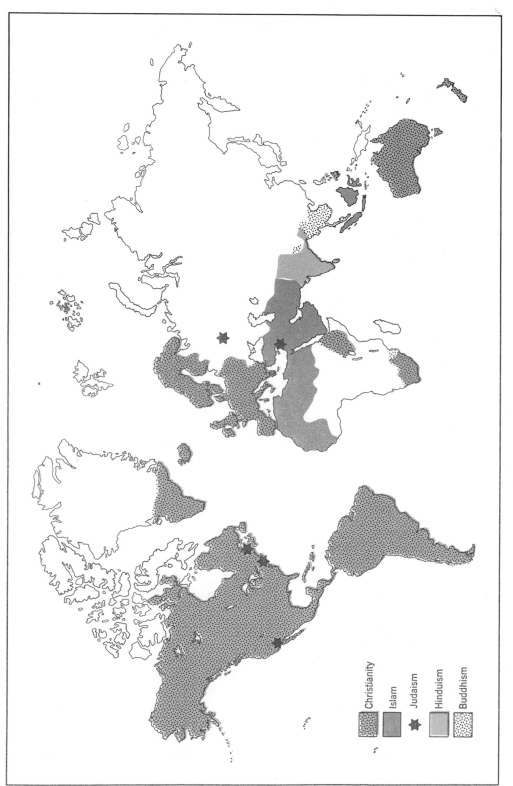

Map of religions of the world—one of the factors governing food preferences.

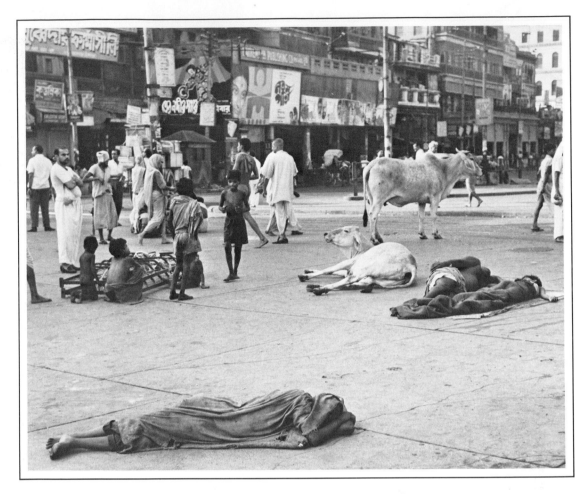

Religious beliefs provide protection and food for sacred cows in India while people suffer from lack of food.

groups view cattle as sacred. As a result, there has been greater concern with breeding for size and color of the animal than for the meat qualities or the quantity of milk produced. When cattle are slaughtered for a particular ceremonial occasion or when they die a natural death, they generally are used for meat. The Masai of Kenya are famous for their practice of bleeding cattle periodically. The blood is consumed mixed with milk to make a highly nourishing food, albeit a beverage that generally would be considered far less palatable or acceptable in this country.

Acceptance of poultry and eggs

The attitude toward chickens and eggs also varies from country to country. The Karen in Burma, believing the chicken has divine powers, revere this fowl because of the prophetic qualities attributed to the bones. However, this respect does not deter some people from cleaning the bones for prophesying tasks by eating the meat first. This attitude of the Burmese is in sharp contrast to that of Southeast Asians who use chickens as combatants in cock fights prior to assuming the role of primary

Table 2.1 *Meats Avoided by Religious Groups in Various Locations*

Food Avoided	Location	Religious Group, If Any
Pork	Worldwide	Moslems
	Worldwide	Jews
	India	Hindus
Beef	India	Hindus
	Africa[a]	
Poultry and eggs	Burma[b]	
	India[c]	Hindus

[a] Eaten when the cattle die a natural death or are killed for a ceremonial occasion.

[b] Will eat the flesh of the chicken before using the bones for prophesies.

[c] The Hindu feeling against eggs is less strong and less widespread than against eating cows.

ingredient in a curry. Eggs are completely rejected in many parts of Africa.

Various explanations of the Hindu rejection of both chicken and eggs have been offered. The primary reason may be a combination of the Hindu vegetarian practices and a feeling that chickens are unclean because they forage for food. Yet another reason for the Hindu rejection may be based on the desire to be different from the Moslems and from the primitive tribes who used chickens to appease the gods. The Buddhists have such widely varying practices that no generalizations can be made regarding their attitudes toward either chickens or eggs. Table 2.1 summarizes the avoidance of meats and poultry products practiced by various groups.

Societal pressures

Attitudes toward animals

Pork, beef, and poultry are only three of the possible flesh foods used in various cultures of the world. Of course, these are widely used in this country, and consequently the prohibition of these common meats in other cultures seems

a bit strange to many people; but consider now the cultural attitudes that are commonly ingrained in this country. There is a general feeling of repugnance at the idea of eating locusts or other insects in the United States. Such rejection may be due to the textural characteristics of insects, but the attitude more likely is the result of the mental set established from earliest childhood. Despite the fact that insects are not banned from the diet for religious reasons, they provide little temptation as a food in the United States. And yet, insects of various types are quite popular in some cultures of the world. Part of this acceptance doubtless is influenced by the somewhat limited availability of other foods in the area. Also, cultural attitudes encouraging acceptance of insects are basic to a few groups. Actually, insects can be an important source of protein and many other nutrients.

The horse is another excellent illustration of cultural attitudes and their influence upon food acceptance. Most people in this country consider the horse totally removed from the realm of food for the table. At best, they consider horse meat as an acceptable food for their pets. The thought of horseflesh for human consumption is totally foreign and unacceptable.

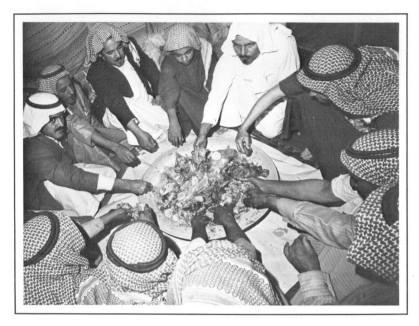

Cultural practices, such as feeding men first until they are sated, may result in malnutrition of women and children in times of economic trouble or insufficient food supply.

The view of the horse as an object leading to quick fortunes at the racetrack or as the cherished pet of the financially secure is far more acceptable to the general public than the idea of the horse as an animal to be husbanded for its meat.

In our dog- and cat-loving society, the eating of these animals is totally unacceptable and would probably be second only in revulsion to the practice of cannibalism. And yet both dogs and cats are considered a suitable food in other cultures. Indeed, even human flesh is considered a food by a small number of people in remote regions. These are only a few of the illustrations that exist to show that cultural pressures and indoctrination by society do structure an individual's dietary practices.

Status symbols

In a few cultures of the world, various beliefs have developed regarding the use of specific foods for special population groups. In some instances, the most highly revered persons in a community receive preferential treatment. The chiefs and priests may keep the best food for themselves, with the rest of the group eating whatever may be left. Some of the dietary patterns of aborigines in Australia result in the elders eating an abundance of the best food and the other members of the tribe receiving less. The underlying selfish motivation in such practices is apparent, but has been perpetuated through innumerable generations.

From a nutritional viewpoint, one of the significant concerns is the distinction made between men and women in some cultures. Some groups follow the practice of having the men eat first until they are full. The women and children receive the remaining food. If food is plentiful this does not create problems, but if food is short, nutritional needs of the women and children, particularly the young children, will not be met.

Occasionally the food preferences of a group, subtly influenced by desires for higher social status, may create serious nutritional problems. An illustration of this is the general lack of interest in vitamin A-rich plant foods in Malaysia. Sweet potatoes and various greens, notably rich in provitamin A, thrive there and also in Indonesia. Despite the availability of these foods, blindness caused by a vitamin A deficiency occurs in many Malaysian and Indonesian children. This vitamin deficiency develops because the vitamin A rich food sources are not considered a part of the cultural food pattern.

A similar situation has existed in the Philippines and many other regions where rice occupies a prominent place in the diet. Polished rice gradually replaced unpolished brown rice in the diet as social status became attached to the white rice. Unfortunately, important B vitamins are removed when rice is polished, which means that nutritional deficiencies (principally beriberi, the potentially fatal disease due to lack of thiamin) are likely to develop when white rice replaces brown rice in a predominantly rice diet. This is a classic illustration of the nutritional problems that cultural, socially motivated food patterns can create.

The breast feeding of infants has also been influenced by social pressures and desire for status. In some parts of the world, the practice of breast feeding was spurned by many women when formula feeding became possible. They viewed formula feeding as more sophisticated and an indication of social status. This developing attitude caused a significant shift toward bottle feeding in spite of the fact that adequate sanitation and a safe milk supply were not always available to replace human milk. The nutrition and health of some infants suffered because of the social prestige attached to bottle feeding (see Chapter 13). This trend is being reversed today in the United States because breast feeding is becoming the choice for a number of women in upper-class families.

Even among children the social significance of food is evidenced. Teachers in elementary schools sometimes report that a child will go without lunch rather than have other children

see that the lunch he brought from home has different foods than those brought by the others. The teasing that may begin when the other children see his food is too much for him. It is easier to go hungry. Other children may view soft drinks or diluted fruit punches as evidence of social distinction at break time in school. If the student leaders select soft drinks, the followers are not likely to elect to drink milk. The opinion of others clearly influences individual choice of foods, and food advertisers have used this fact to advantage.

Superstitions

Cultural beliefs have led to such practices as the avoidance of both eggs and chicken by women in some parts of Africa and Southeast Asia because it is thought that the consumption of these foods will result in infertility. The converse of the stigma of infertility attributed to eating eggs can be found in other parts of Africa where women avoid eating eggs to escape the aphrodisiacal qualities they believe are found in eggs. To avoid having children who look like pigs, young Zulu women do not eat pork. In Malaysia, the designation of "hot" foods excludes some nutritionally significant foods from the diets of pregnant and lactating women. In this context, "hot" designates foods considered to be dangerous to the health of the mother and the nursing infant. Because of this indoctrination, Malaysian mothers are denied meats at a time when protein intake is particularly important.

A similar attitude is found among some teen-age girls in the United States. Their preoccupation with being thin has led to the development of an almost superstitious attitude toward some foods. Some girls are persuaded that they will become fat if they drink milk. Others are sure they will be fat if they eat breakfast. Among adults in this country, the sale of vitamin E capsules apparently is spurred by people seeking greater virility. Vitamin C pills are eagerly swallowed by others seeking relief from the common cold. No matter how sophisticated the group, some element of superstition is likely to influence consumption patterns. The notions that one population group has may seem ludicrous to another group. At the same time, people have difficulty recognizing the superstitious attitudes they themselves have.

Political Factors

The impact of politics on nutrition can be enormous, particularly in time of war. Perhaps the most publicized and horrible illustrations of nutritional deficiencies caused in large measure by political maneuvers are the civil war in Biafra and the strife that resulted in the creation of Bangladesh. In both cases there was a severe shortage of food for the general population, particularly the young children. Numerous other incidents of dietary deficiencies due to the impact of war on the normal production and distribution of food are well documented in the literature. Shortages as severe as were found in Holland late in World War II caused a significant reduction in the live births reported and resulted in well-documented health problems caused by grossly inadequate nutrition.

Today various aspects of nutrition have achieved notable if not enviable prominence in the news media. Feeding people has been the major concern of food-related industries for a long time, but it has taken political ventures (including the World Food Conference in Rome in 1974, the 1969 White House Conference on Food, Nutrition, and Health and hearings before various Congressional committees) to arouse the public to some important issues involved in achieving good nutrition.

The problems inherent in providing nutritionally adequate diets even in the United States are the material from which news headlines and political careers are constructed. There is much emotional and political mileage to be won by highlighting pockets of malnutrition and leveling charges regarding the safety of substances being used to increase crop yields or prolong shelf life of processed foods. Graphic examples of the interaction between politics and nutrition frequently are top stories of the day for newspapers and telecasts. The debate between the factions favoring the use of chemicals to increase crop yield and those who champion a natural environment (with its decreased food production) provides a good opportunity for observing the impact of politics. For many years chemical fertilizers and insecticides have been employed by farmers to enable them to produce larger crop yields free of imperfections in the harvested food. In view of the need for more food to feed the world's swelling population, such practices appear to be highly advantageous. However, the ever-growing public concern with the ecological imbalances and the environmental pollution that may be associated with these agricultural tools has caused many people to question the use of DDT and other chemicals and has resulted in regulatory legislation. Clearly there is no unambiguous solution to the fertilizer-pesticide controversy. Verbal battles will continue while actual practice follows a compromise route. Societal pressures obviously greatly influence governmental agencies in the regulation of many nutrition-related matters.

Another illustration of the pressures created by society and regulated by government (not always to the public's best interests) is the controversy over fluoridation in city water supplies. Despite proof of the value of fluorides in reducing dental caries in children, an indication of the benefits in maintaining bone strength in the aging, and its total and complete safety, the arguments have raged. Special interest groups have developed sufficient societal pressure on the governments in numerous cities to prevent implementation of programs for adding fluoride to the water supply (see Chapter 10).

As recently as 1975, a referendum vote on fluoridation in the city of Los Angeles failed by a wide margin due largely to a pressure group generating undocumented publicity on the "possible link between fluoridation and cancer."

Governmental programs of various types have influenced the nutrition of many people of the world. Large-scale irrigation programs that require immense dams and extensive distribution networks cannot be undertaken by individuals or most corporations due to lack of capital. The tremendous scope and financial burden of the Aswan Dam in Egypt and other large developmental projects can only be undertaken as public works with governmental, and frequently international financing. Such land irrigation and reclamation projects have converted nonproductive land to agriculturally profitable regions, thus increasing available food supplies.

Ecological problems are closely related to governmental programs to increase food production. For example, the Aswan Dam has provided water for crops, but the spread of the snail parasite in Egypt seems to be a side product that causes some to view the dam as a mixed blessing. The negative influence of polluted streams on fish populations has been felt by commercial salmon operations and by individual fisherman. Governments have the power to implement programs that will regulate the environment. They also have broad powers that could be used to complicate ecological balance still more than has happened to date.

Economic Aspects

Economic development in the United States and other countries possessing scientific, technological, and manufacturing skills has derived considerable strength from the growth in the consumer market that resulted from the population explosion. Business flourished, more agricultural land was put into production, and food surpluses accumulated for a while in this country. Although the business climate was highly favorable, partially as a result of increasing consumer demands in the 1950s, the picture changed abruptly in the mid-1960s as it became apparent that the world's birth rate was creating a host of new problems that reversed the optimism of the preceding decade. Suddenly, the knowledge that the time for doubling the world's population had decreased from 1000 years around the time of Christ to approximately 37 years at the present time became a matter of grave concern. The fact that the developing countries in Latin America, Africa, and Asia were doubling their populations even more quickly than the industrialized nations only served to compound the concern.

To adequately feed the 75 million additional people in the world each year would require a 4 percent annual increase in food production.

Population control has become one of the key concerns of the entire world today, for clearly the physical limitations of this planet make it impossible to maintain an infinite number of people. In fact, it is highly dubious that the imminent predicted doubling of population from the 3.5 billion people in mid-1969 to around 7 billion people by 2000 A.D., can be fed and maintained at even reasonable living standards. Already the once-immense food reserves in the United States have been eliminated; roughly only one nation in 14 is able to produce more food than it consumes at the present time. In 1975 only Australia and North America exported significant quantities of grain, and exports of wheat, in 1974 and 1975 in particular, led to large increases in cost. This situation makes it still more difficult for Third World nations to buy the food they need in the world marketplace. Hopcraft (1968) reports an incidence of malnutrition ranging between 30 and 50 percent of Tanzanian children under the age of five, an infant mortality rate of 12.5 percent in the Indian village of Ajarpura, and 100 infants in Colombia dying each day from malnutrition, examples of the enormity of the world's nutrition problem, and this with only the present population. Concerned individuals throughout the world are charged with the responsibility of using all their knowledge and skills to close the gap between the human population and its physical, psychological, social, and economic needs.

Population is a fluctuating figure determined both by birth rate and death rate. Industrialized nations have been undergoing a transition period from high birth and mortality rates to lower values for each. The result is a slowly growing population, a situation that required approximately two centuries to develop. In contrast, developing countries around the world have experienced a sharp decrease in mortality rates in the last 30 years, without an accompanying drop in birth rates. This change means that the number of dependent children in these countries has increased as a result of reduced infant mortality rates. At the other end of the spectrum, more adults are living through their reproductive span of life, thus providing the potential for more children to be born. Figure 2.1 depicts the Agency for International Development's projections for the world's population in each decade to 2020 A.D. Of particular interest is the significantly larger rate of increase for the less developed countries (2.5 percent) compared with the lesser rate (0.9 percent) for the developed countries. If these projections prove to be correct, the challenge of feeding the world is almost overwhelming.

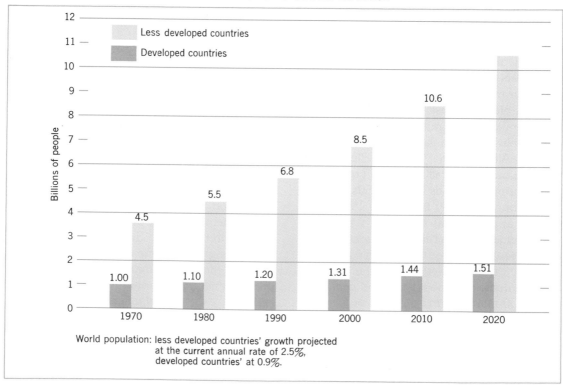

Figure 2.1   Prediction of the world population explosion from 1970 to 2020.

The productivity of a country is influenced by these demographic changes. DeFleur et al. (1971, p. 251) summarized the economic aspects of the current population trends in the developing countries:

"Whereas only 20 to 30 percent of the populations of the industrialized countries are under fifteen years of age, in the developing nations the proportion reaches nearly 50 percent. These children are essentially consumers rather than producers, and the task of providing them with education, housing, clothing, and other basic necessities puts an unusually heavy drain on the economy. Unless birth rates decline, the burden of child dependency will become greater with each generation."

Another facet of the population problem is the trend toward urbanization in the developing countries. The basic problems of food supply, housing, and education are overwhelming because of the large numbers of people migrating to the cities. The limitations on health and education that are placed on people in these circumstances initiate a circular pattern that is extremely difficult to break. Poor nutrition and health among children lead to limited success in school. In addition, poor performance in school develops a sense of failure and limits personal ambition and expectation of achievements in life. In such an environment, upward mobility through job training is unlikely. A labor force made up primarily of unskilled labor does not produce the products needed for a better life. Most of the money earned must go for food, and people become enmeshed in a lifestyle that cannot lead to change.

To state that the world's nutrition problems are due to an expanding population alone is a gross oversimplification of the situation. The factors that influence the achievement of good nutrition for the world's people are obviously varied and closely interwoven. Yet the problem of population is certainly one requiring prime consideration. If some of the ideas being proposed at the present time come to fruition, governments around the world may take a more active part in controlling overpopulation. Social pressures may lead governments to implement programs directed toward the goal of regulating the birth rate. The world's resources are more likely to be sufficient to feed all people adequately if fewer people are born to be fed. The earth has a finite capacity not only for feeding its people, but also for "living space," and this capacity will be inadequate unless the present trend in population growth is reversed.

Approaches to Improving World Nutrition

The challenge

Malnutrition appears in various forms in different parts of the world, but no country is without its problems. The obvious malnutrition of very young children (0.5 to 5 years of age) starving to death in overpopulated developing countries is perhaps the most compelling problem requiring solution. Of quite a different nature is the problem of overnutrition seen in some of the industrial nations. The specific nutritional deficiency conditions that develop from various inadequacies in the diet are considered in detail in subsequent chapters. However, there are two closely related basic deficiency conditions that are of critical significance at this time—protein and calories.

Protein is the nutrient that holds the key to preventing and curing the nutrition problems of many preschool children in the developing countries. Children must have adequate amounts of protein—protein of high quality that provides the balance of amino acids required for optimum growth and mental development. Kwashiorkor, the condition resulting from a protein deficiency, is all too familiar to physicians treating children in areas where little protein is available, where ignorance of the importance of protein and protein foods is prevalent, and where incomes are too low to buy the needed foods.

The other critical condition today is lack of calories, particularly in the presence of inadequate protein. The protein-calorie malnutrition (PCM) that results is a deficiency condition related to kwashiorkor. PCM develops when both protein and total calorie intakes are too limited in the diet over a period of time. Lechtig, et al. (1975) found that even sugar supplements, when added to the calorie-deficient diets of pregnant Guatemalan women of low socioeconomic status, were effective in reducing the incidence of low-birth-weight infants. In short, more food (particularly protein

food) needs to be produced and distributed to overcome malnutrition throughout the world. The crying need for food to contribute the energy, protein, and other nutrients that are so limited in many people's diets is not a trivial need. Already many people are dying because of the lack of workable solutions.

Cultural and social implications

For the greatest success in meeting world nutrition problems, cultural and social factors as well as the changes that may be accomplished through technological progress must be considered. The population problem is closely tied to cultural factors. For example, Moslems are devoted to the tradition of early marriage and polygyny. The religion encourages fertility and high birth rates. The concept of birth control is foreign to the basic beliefs and, therefore, is not generally accepted. Other illustrations of

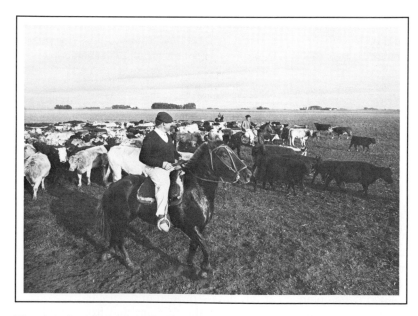

The relatively inefficient use of land for production of animal protein is a matter of growing significance as the world's people increase in number and in their need for even a subsistence level of protein.

the incompatibility of planned parenthood and religion are also familiar. If birth control is to be one of the avenues for solving the problem of feeding the world, progress in uniting these opposing viewpoints must be made.

Other approaches within the social and cultural realm that hold some prospect of success may be developed. People in the upper social strata may hold the key to one manner of coping with the problem of food prejudices. If the upper social classes begin to improve their diets in ways that can be emulated by those

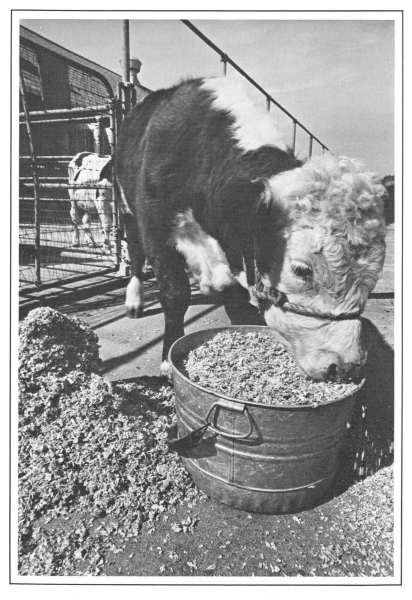

A mixture consisting of one part ground newspaper and nine parts of concentrate, such as molasses, soybean meal, and cracked corn, is an illustration of research studies being conducted to increase food production from nonconventional sources.

with far less income, food patterns can gradually be changed. In the United States, the practice of drinking milk with meals could be encouraged in this way. Soft drinks are for between-meal refreshments.

These are just two facets of the complexities of working to modify nutrition patterns. For each of the problems contributing to malnutrition throughout the world, solutions must be found. Preliminary explorations into the social, economic, and political problems are being made. However, the enormous complexities of large social systems and the inherent resistance of individuals to change have an almost antagonistic, rather than a synergistic effect on attempts to deal with the sociological aspects of malnutrition. On an individual basis, it may be easier to appreciate the human inertia involved in modifying food preferences if one considers whether he is prepared to begin eating appreciably more plant food and less meat. That choice strikes at the core of the typical American's high consumption of meat (and thus saturated fat). And yet, if one looks at maximum land utilization, there is considerable loss of potential energy for man from food as food moves along the food chain from plant, through animals, and finally to man. More succinctly, about 10 times more protein from an acre of land is available to man when he consumes the protein in the form of plant protein rather than feeding the plant food to an animal to produce animal protein. Unless population growth is drastically curtailed, such choices may become necessary for survival!

Technological and scientific contributions

Significant progress has already been made in increasing the supply of food and in improving the nutritive value of a number of products. Agricultural research, new products, fortification of existing foods, and expanded use of unconventional food sources hold promise for assisting in meeting the world food

needs. Although these approaches cannot solve the total problem (particularly the very special problem of the young child in the weaning period), they can do much to supplement and strengthen the efforts being made in the realm of the social sciences. Various aspects of these technological and scientific contributions are considered in the remainder of this chapter.

New products

Universities, the Food and Agriculture Organization, and the World Health Organization of the United Nations have all been interested in research programs to develop protein sources for use in areas where protein presently is inadequate in the diet. Incaparina and Multi-Purpose Food are two illustrations of improved protein foods developed from plant sources through extensive research. Incaparina, named for the Institute of Nutrition in Central America and Panama (INCAP) where it was developed, is a powdered blend containing maize and sorghum as the base, with cottonseed flour, calcium carbonate, torula yeast, vitamin A, and the essential amino acid lysine added. This food is mixed with water to make a gruellike beverage similar to atole, the accepted beverage of Central America. Multi-Purpose Food was developed by Dr. Henry Borsook of the California Institute of Technology; MPF has a soy protein base to which calcium carbonate, sodium ascorbate, vitamin E (as tocopherol acetate), vitamin A palmitate, niacinamide, cyanocobalamin (vitamin B_{12}), pyridoxine hydrochloride (vitamin B_6), riboflavin, vitamin D, and potassium iodide have been added. This food supplement is designed as an additive to such foods as ground meat, cereals, soups, and casseroles.

Another approach to supplying adequate protein has been the development of fish flour, a powdered product made from fish. Fish flour, also called fish protein concentrate, contains as much as 85 percent protein of high quality and can be added to various foods in much the

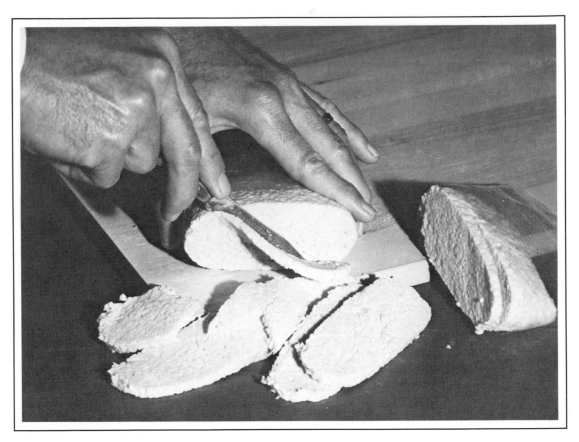

Tempeh is a popular soybean product in Oriental cuisines. This food, a concentrated source of vegetable protein, is produced by fermenting cooked soybeans with a mold. This sample is sliced before being fried in deep fat. This represents but one use of the versatile and nutritious soybean.

same way that Multi-Purpose Food is used. One serious limitation in fish flour has been the need for deodorizing and defatting the product to minimize the fishiness of the flavor and odor and to extend the shelf life. This processing raises the cost of the flour above the reach of many potential consumers who would benefit from the fish flour protein. To utilize fish flour to its greatest potential would require more consumer education, a suitable distribution network, and greater purchasing power among persons needing this food as a supplement. Fish protein concentrate has other drawbacks including an unreliable source of fish. Fish migrate and cannot always be found.

Seeds from some plants are rich in oil; soybeans, peanuts, cotton, corn, sunflower, and sesame seeds routinely are used as commercial sources of edible oils. When these seeds are pressed and the oils are extruded, a seed cake or meal containing approximately 50 percent protein remains. High-quality protein supplements can be produced at relatively low cost by mixing this meal with granular cereals. Processing problems to eliminate any toxic substances, such as gossypol in cotton-seed meal, have been overcome without increasing the cost of production significantly. The use of such products is promising.

The protein from soybeans has been used in

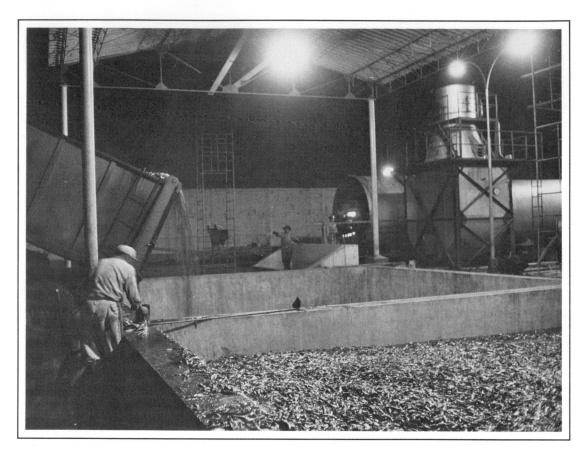

A fish meal plant in Peru where anchovetas (variety of anchovy) are ground and extracted to yield a product containing 80 percent protein.

many research projects because of its rather unique characteristics and excellent amino acid content. Researchers have developed techniques that make the spinning of fibers from soy protein commercially feasible (spun protein). These fibers are then made into simulated meat products. Some of these products are already on the market. Consumer acceptance may be expected to grow as flavor shortcomings are corrected.

Agricultural research

Under the auspices of the Rockefeller and Ford Foundations, the International Rice Research Institute in the Philippines has actively pursued research directed toward developing highly productive rice varieties resistant to diseases that commonly infest rice in the Rice Bowl of the world. The Rice Research Institute also has an educational component. Agriculturists from rice-dependent nations receive technical training and the preparation needed to continue developmental and experimental work in their home countries. Programs of this type hold considerable promise for improving production of any crop that guarantees significant economic or nutritional rewards in any country. The Rockefeller Foundation has long carried out important research studies on corn and wheat in Mexico and Colombia in South America. Recently, the Rockefeller Foundation

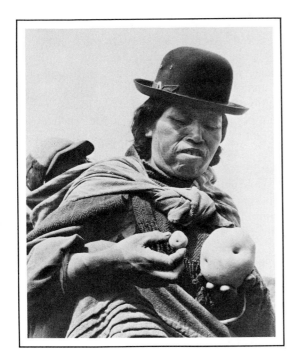

Agricultural research studies have been effective in improving crops and increasing yields from available farm lands.

and the Ford Foundation organized a center for agricultural research at the University of Ibadan in Nigeria, Africa.

The development of new strains and varieties of existing staple foods opens new avenues for improving nutrition through modification of the amino acid content of plant proteins. Geneticists have bred corn (Opaque-2, developed at Purdue University) to increase the content of two essential amino acids, lysine and tryptophan. Opaque-2 contains somewhat less total protein, but it has a balance of amino acids that makes this corn variety nutritionally superior to other traditional types. Triticale, a cross between wheat and rye, is another illustration of agricultural progress in developing excellent sources of protein from cereals.

Unconventional food sources

The sea as a source of food is a relatively untapped resource that may eventually be made to produce significantly greater quantities of food for man in the future. Opinions of the po-

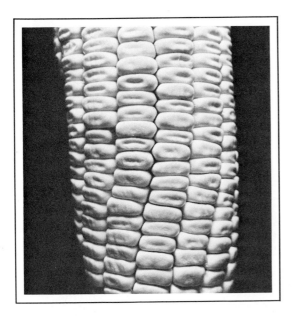
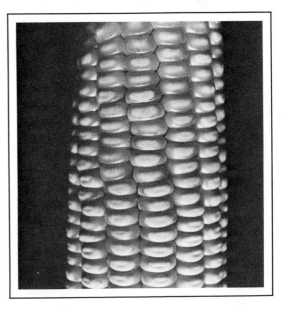

Through selective breeding, high-lysine corn (left) has been developed to help provide protein of higher nutritional quality than is contained in corn with a normal balance of amino acids (right). The high-lysine corn has a kernel with a modified shape, and the endosperm portion is more opaque and floury than that normally found in corn.

tential of the sea as one of the means of solving world malnutrition range from little expectation of increased food from the sea to optimistic statements that the sea can eventually be farmed to provide tremendous increases in food production.

Other unconventional protein sources offer promise for helping to alleviate the world protein shortage. An interest has even developed in possible protein sources from algae. At the present time, this does not appear too promising as a direct source of protein for humans, but there is a possibility of feeding algae to pigs and chickens, which ultimately can be used to provide protein for humans. Protein from leaves, commonly referred to simply as leaf protein, has also been the subject of some research. Although the protein obtained from this source is of some nutritional value, the grasslike flavor has proven to be a serious objection to introducing this product on a commercial basis. Like algae, the leaf protein is viewed as a possible feed for animals being raised for human consumption.

Certain microorganisms that grow on petroleum, cellulose, or natural gas substrates are potential sources of protein for humans. At the present time these "single-cell proteins" are of interest in the laboratory. However, many technical problems must be solved before microorganisms can seriously be considered as a solution to the protein shortage of man.

Fortification

Much of the interest in new products is directed toward improving the biological value of plant proteins. The proteins naturally occurring in plants are of somewhat less nutritional value than animal proteins because the plant proteins are limited in their content of one or more of the amino acids that man must eat to maintain his health. Since various plants have different amino acid limitations, protein from diverse plants can be blended to obtain a higher quality protein food, such as Incaparina. As noted previously, plants also can be bred se-

lectively to produce a better amino acid balance in the protein of the plant itself.

A practical approach to improving protein quality is to supplement the food with synthetic or man-made amino acids to improve the amino acid composition of plant foods. Since most populations around the world rely heavily on plant proteins, particularly rice, wheat, and corn, as their major source of amino acids, fortification of these foods with appropriate amino acids offers the opportunity to improve nutrition significantly without modifying traditional dietary practices (Table 2.2). Supplementation with the limiting amino acids—lysine and threonine to rice, lysine to wheat, lysine and tryptophan to corn, lysine to cottonseed, and methionine to soybean products—is technically possible now. Synthetic amino acids can now be produced at low cost; in fact, they may offer the most economical way of improving plant and cereal proteins. Since these do not affect

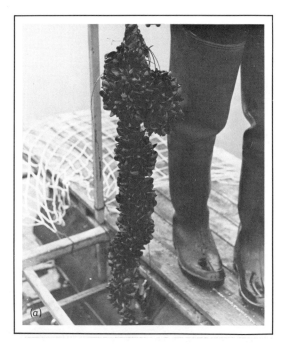

Experiments of many types including (a) growing mussels on ropes, (b) oysters seeded with strings of scallop shells and oyster spats, and (c) oysters by rack-and-stick cultivation, may lead the way toward greater productivity of food from the sea.

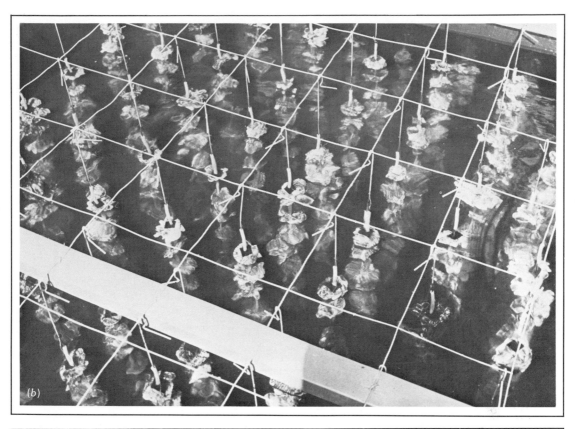

(b)

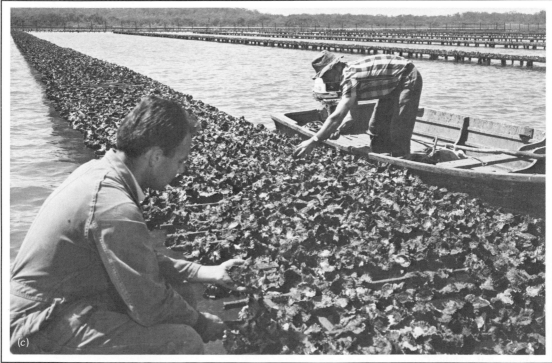

(c)

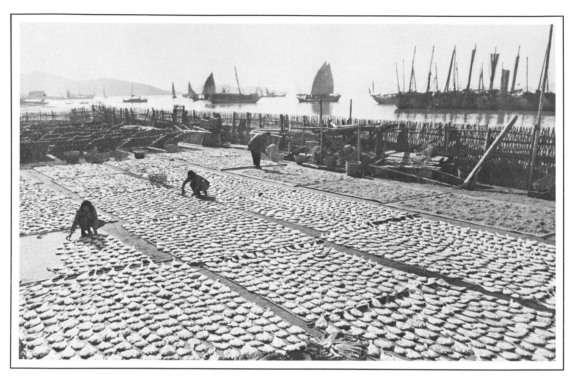

Food from the sea, such as these yellow croakers being dried in China, contributes to meeting the world's need for food. However, the sea cannot be expected to solve the dilemma of the world's food shortage.

taste, texture, color, or flavor, amino acid fortification offers the great advantage of not having to change individual food habits. It is apparent that amino acid supplementation of grain, legume, and oilseed food products is potentially an important method for improving the protein nutrition of many people in the world whose low protein intakes need to be utilized within the body as effectively as possible. The problems of protein quality and utilization of plant proteins are considered in Chapter 8.

Education and the need for changing behavior

The high incidence of mortality for children in developing countries occurs in the so-called "weaning" period—from 6 to around 24 months. These children receive breast milk and very little other food during this period, even though the supply of milk declines gradually and the child's food needs are increasing. During this critical period the undernourished child is exposed to repeated sicknesses and often succumbs.

The reasons for this negative practice of withholding solid food are lost in tradition, but undoubtedly they have something to do with the mother's fear of diarrhea and dysentery and the reduced availability of animal milk in countries where the population pressure on land has mushroomed in the last two generations. Studies made in India demonstrate that a significant improvement in child health will result from a supplement of only 50 to 100 grams of wheat or rice per day. Since such a quantity represents only a small part of the total family's daily intake, this negative behavior pattern

Table 2.2 Protein Supplies per Capita by Major Food Groups and Region[a]

Protein Source	Per Capita Protein Supply (g/day) in:		
	Europe, North America, Australia, New Zealand, Argentina, Paraguay, Uruguay	Far East, Near East, Africa, Latin America[b]	World
Vegetable protein			
Grains	33.4	33.2	33.4
Starchy roots	5.2	2.3	3.2
Pulses, oil-seeds, nuts	3.8	11.6	9.0
Vegetables and fruits	3.6	1.8	2.4
Animal protein			
Meat and poultry	19.8	3.8	8.8
Eggs	3.3	0.4	1.2
Fish	2.4	1.9	2.3
Milk and milk products	18.5	2.9	7.7
Total protein	90	58	68

[a] Adapted from J. C. Abbott. World protein resources. In **Advances in Chemistry,** 57: 3. American Chemical Society. Washington, D.C. 1966.

[b] Excluding Argentina, Paraguay, and Uruguay.

clearly is more the result of tradition than of poverty. Some Indian experts also make the point that, in this particular age period, the child's protein needs are reasonably provided by breast milk and that the significant lack is one of calories.

A related problem develops in the unborn child. In many developing countries, because of taboo and tradition, the pregnant woman eats very sparingly in the critical last trimester. As a result, the child is born with a reduced birth weight and inadequate nutrient stores. Health authorities in developing countries are well aware of the need for changed and improved practices affecting unborn and very young children, and the problem is viewed essentially as one of education.

The high mortality of very young children also has implications for family planning programs. The parents' desire for a large family is related to the experience of child survival and the need for enough children, particularly sons, so that the loss of some children can be accepted.

Education contributes also by training the rural worker to be a better food producer. Increased utilization of high yielding varieties of cereals and better agricultural practices not only increase the output of these foods, but also permit greater agricultural diversification. As cereal production becomes adequate, or almost adequate—and this is happening in many countries—some land can be released for other crops such as legumes, feed and fodder for dairy animals, and vegetables. Agricultural education also shows farmers how to realize additional crops each year from the same land through more sophisticated use of fertilizers and irrigation.

Despite the impressive array of high-protein supplemental foods that are technically feasible, the mechanism has not been found to distribute them in sufficient quantities over vast and remote areas in poor countries. Such foods can, of course, serve very usefully in demonstration and education projects. For most of the villages of the world, a great part of the needed foodstuffs must be produced locally out of local resources assisted by education and technology.

Nutrition education programs provide the opportunity of helping people learn about the nutrients they need, the food sources of these nutrients, and the consumerism that can result in more economical purchasing and better preparation of food. Mass media provide avenues for teaching nutrition to vast numbers of people. Other nutrition education takes place on a one-to-one basis. Improved communica-tion about food, through all avenues, helps to increase the range of foods accepted and utilized in the diet. Broader food tastes are essential to improving the nutritional status of populations. As people develop more cosmopolitan tastes, it becomes easier to gain acceptance of new foods. Consumption of a wide variety of foods helps to insure an adequate nutrient intake. People who eat only a very narrow segment of foods may be receiving inadequate levels of specific nutrients.

In the United States, nutrition education is included in the public schools through the school lunch programs. It is a part of some preschool programs. The extension service and some adult education programs also provide nutrition education. The vehicles for nutrition education are available in this country. More effective approaches will result in better nutrition education for all people here. In other countries, more extensive programs reaching broader segments of the population will need to be developed. Ways of accomplishing behavioral modifications in eating patterns are needed for people all around the world.

Summary

The inherent problems of feeding the world in the future are a challenge to politicians and health and social scientists alike. Geographical limitations, cultural biases, religious influences, educational deficiencies, political ramifications, and problems of agriculture and food technology are all aspects of the world's nutrition problem which are made ever more difficult by the explosive growth of world population.

The approach toward accepting the challenge of feeding the world's people in the future can be summarized by outlining four steps that appear to be absolutely essential if the crisis is to be met. These are:

1. Population control, particularly in areas of Central and South America, Asia, and Africa where over-population has already created severe nutritional problems.
2. Expanded production of food, including better utilization of land, development of better distribution and processing, effective use of

fertilizers and pesticides without upsetting the ecological balance, and reduced losses by spoilage and waste.

3. Improved protein quantity and quality in the diet, presumably to be accomplished by amino acid fortification, by genetic improvements of cereals and legumes, by diversification of agriculture, and by development of new food products.

4. More effective and broader nutrition education programs directed toward modifying basic behavior, improving food attitudes, and increasing consumer knowledge.

Selected References

Abbott, J. D. World protein resources. *Advances in Chemistry.* 57:3. 1966.

Bosley, B., and R. L. Huenemann. Nutritional problems and educational progress in Latin America. *J. Am. Diet. Assoc.* 53:99. 1968.

Curtis, B. C., and D. R. Johnston. Hybrid wheat. *Scientific American. 220,* No. 5:21. 1969.

DeFleur, M. L., et al. *Sociology: Man in Society.* Scott, Foresman. Glenview, Ill. 1971.

Devadas, R. P. Social and cultural factors influencing malnutrition. *J. Home Econ. 62:*164. 1970.

Dressler, D. *Sociology: The Study of Human Interaction.* Knopf. New York. 1969.

Ehrlich, P. R. *The Population Bomb.* Ballantine. New York. 1968.

El Lozy, M., et al. Amino acid composition of diet in region of southern Tunisia. *Am. J. Clin. Nutr.* 1975.

Goldsmith, G. A. Where are we in the race against starvation? *Am. J. Public Health. 61:*1478. 1971.

Gopalan, C. Major nutritional problems of India and Southeast Asia. Proc. 7th International Congress on Nutrition, Hamburg. *3:*320. 1966.

Harpstead, D. D. High-lysine corn. *Scientific American. 225,* No. 2:34. 1971.

Hoff, J. E. and J. Janick. *Food.* Freeman. San Francisco. 1973.

Hopcraft, A. *Born to Hunger.* Houghton Mifflin. Boston. 1968.

Jenner, A. Social, emotional and cultural influences as related to eating patterns and malnutrition. *Can. Nutr. Notes. 24:*37. 1968.

King, C. G. Contribution of nutrition research to world health problems. Proc. 6th International Congress on Nutrition, Edinburgh. 1963.

King, K. W., et al. Food patterns from dietary surveys in rural Haiti. *J. Am. Diet. Assoc. 53:*114. 1968.

Lechtig, A., et al. Maternal nutrition and fetal growth in developing countries. *Am. J. Dis. Child. 129:*553. 1975.

Lowenberg, M. E., et al. *Food and Man.* 2nd ed. Wiley. New York. 1974.

Mata, L. Nutrition and infection. In *Present Knowledge of Nutrition.* 4th ed. Nutrition Foundation. New York. 1970.

Mateles, R. I., and S. R. Tannenbaum. *Single Cell Protein.* MIT Press. Cambridge, Mass. 1968.

Mazess, R. B. Hot-cold food beliefs among Andean peasants. *J. Am. Diet. Assoc. 53:*109. 1968.

McDivitt, M. E., and S. R. Mudambi. *Human Nutrition: Principles and Applications in India.* Prentice-Hall. Bombay. 1969.

McFarlane, H. Nutrition and immunity. *Present Knowledge of Nutrition.* 4th ed. Nutrition Foundation. New York. 1976.

McWilliams, M. Food supply and world population. *Home Economics and Family Planning.* American Home Economics Assoc. Washington, D.C. P. 37. 1974.

Mead, M. The changing significance of food. *American Scientist. 58:*176. 1970.

Pinchot, G. B. Marine farming. *Scientific American. 223,* No. 6:15, 1970.

Reitz, L. P. New wheats and social progress. *Science. 169:*952. 1970.

Roderuck, C. E. Nutrition and the need for family planning. *Home Economics and Family Planning.* American Home Economics Assoc. Washington, D.C. P. 44. 1974.

Sai, F. T. Drastic change in food habits in relation to sociocultural change. Proc. 7th International Congress on Nutrition, Hamburg. Vol 2. 1966

Scrimshaw, N. S. Meeting future food needs. *J. Can. Diet. Assoc. 32* (September):117. 1971.

Scrimshaw, N. S. Nature of protein requirements. *J. Am. Diet. Assoc. 54:*94. 1969.

Scrimshaw, N. S. Malnutrition and health of children. *J. Am. Diet. Assoc. 42:*303. 1963.

Sebrell, W. H., Jr., and J. J. Haggerty. *Food and Nutrition.* Time, Inc. New York. 1967.

Simoons, F. J. *Eat Not This Flesh.* University of Wisconsin Press. Madison. 1961.

Stare, F. J. Improving nutrition for world's population. *Participant Journal.* P. 30. December, 1969.

Tesi, G., et al. Economic aspects of food, protein, and energy consumption in a region of southern Tunisia. *Ecology of Food and Nutrition. 4:*5. 1975.

Yudkin, J., and J. C. McKinrie. *Changing Food Habits.* Macmillan. London. 1964.

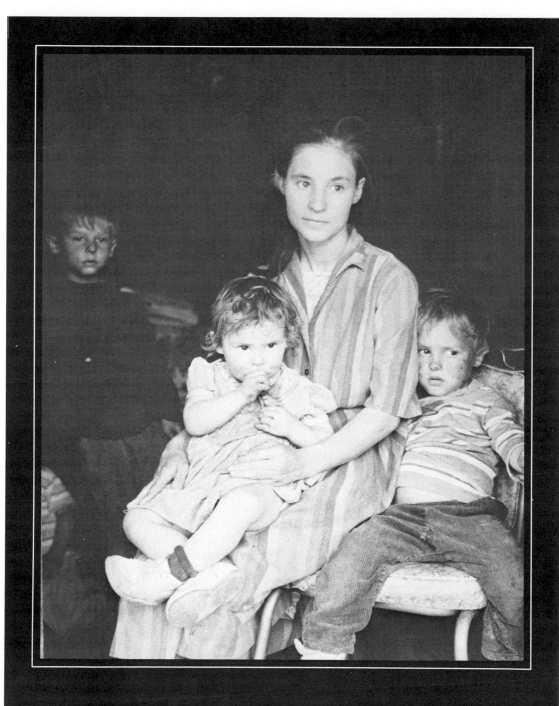

Chapter 3

Factors in American Nutrition

The United States has long been called "The Land of Plenty." Efficient farmers have utilized the technology developed by agricultural researchers to produce abundant crops on their rich farmlands. A food supply of high quality is readily available for the consumer's selection. And the most remarkable fact of all is that this abundant and varied diet is available for the smallest fraction of the consumer's income ever known. In 1969, the average American consumer spent somewhat less than 20 percent of his income after taxes for food—a truly remarkable achievement of modern food production and distribution! Innovations in farm production during the last few years enabled farmers to produce two to three times more food per hour of labor in 1969 than in 1954. Such figures clearly demonstrate that the food industry in the United States is a fast-moving, highly creative facet of the American economy.

With such a remarkable food supply, it is not surprising that obesity is a concern of many Americans. However, it is difficult to rationalize the fact that malnutrition, both undernutrition and outright starvation, also exists in this country today. The United States has the capacity to produce the food necessary to feed all its citizens adequately. The potential is even there to aid in feeding many people in other parts of the world as well.

The discrepancy between the capacity to meet the nutritional needs of all people in the United States and actual fact is closely related to sociological and economic factors in the United States. Nutritional status and dietary patterns are influenced by a wide variety of factors, including:

1. The value placed upon individual development.
2. Income of the consuming unit.
3. Stability of the family.
4. Education.

5. Cultural integration.
6. Social status.

The discussion of the social forces that influ-ence dietary patterns is most meaningful in the context of evolving changes in nutritional status. The results of nutritional surveys are presented in the following section.

Nutritional Status of Americans

Historical perspective

Public awareness of the nutritional status of people in the United States reached new di-mensions in late 1969 when the White House Conference on Food, Nutrition, and Health convened. Through the meetings of the United States Senate's Poverty Subcommittee and the Select Committee on Nutrition and Human Needs, assisted by the broad coverage of na-tional television, the picture of poor nutrition for those living in poverty was brought into focus. The publicity of these politically-based hearings was directed toward arousing public concern for the nutritional problems of low-income families, a group that nutritionists had long recognized as an important target popula-tion for receiving more food, nutritionally better food, and education about nutrition. The public furor in the United States has centered around the malnourished living on public assis-tance, and yet broad nutrition surveys have shown that good nutrition is a goal still to be reached by many others at adequate income levels, too.

The first broadly based concern with the nu-tritional status of the American people was voiced by President Franklin D. Roosevelt, who announced that one-third of the nation was poorly fed. The 1936 national food con-sumption survey, the first such nationwide as-sessment of nutritional intake in the United States, bore out the validity of President Roo-sevelt's concern and generated three significant actions at the national level:

1. Enrichment of refined wheat flour and other cereal products with three of the B vitamins (thiamin, riboflavin, and niacin) and the mineral, iron.
2. A program of nutrition education sponsored primarily by the United States Department of Agriculture.
3. The National School Lunch Program, also a responsibility of the Department of Agricul-ture.

Subsequently, less comprehensive studies of food consumption were conducted in 1942 and 1948, and the results indicated that the na-tion's dietary status was improving (Hiemstra, 1969). Progress toward adequate nutrition, based on food consumption data, was again noted in the 1955 survey.

Surveys in the 1960s

In the 1965 United States Department of Agriculture's Household Food Consumption Survey, the broadest of any of the surveys, data on food consumption in 15,000 house-holds throughout the country were collected. Information was gathered on the intake of indi-viduals as well as the foods available for con-sumption by the family as a group. The results (Table 3.1), were distinctly discouraging; the data showed that the nation had slipped back-ward in its nutritional status during the interval between the 1955 and the 1965 surveys. In the 1965 survey only 50 percent of the families

Table 3.1 Nutrients Less Than the Recommended Dietary Allowances[a]

Sex	Age (years)	Protein	Calcium	Iron	Vitamin A Value	Thiamin	Riboflavin	Ascorbic Acid
Male and Female	under 1			•••				
	1-2			•••				
	3-5							
	6-8			•				
Male	9-11							
	12-14		•			•		
	15-17		•	•				
	18-19		•					
	20-24		•					
	35-54		•					
	55-64		•					
	65-74		•					
	75 and over		••		•		••	•
Female	9-11		•	•••		•		
	12-14		••	•••	•	•		
	15-17		••	•••		•		
	18-19		••	•••	•	••		
	20-34		••	•••		•	•	
	35-54		••	••		•	•	
	55-64		••	•				
	65-74		••	•	•	•	•	
	75 and over		••	•	••	••	••	

Legend: • 1 to 10%   •• 11 to 20%   ••• 21 to 29%   •••• 30% or more

[a] NAS–NRC, 1968. *U.S. Diets of Men, Women, and Children, 1 day in Spring, 1965.* U.S. Department of Agriculture.

surveyed met or exceeded the recommendations for a good diet, in comparison with the 60 percent with a good diet in 1955. (A good diet was defined as providing the protein, calcium, iron, vitamin A, thiamin, riboflavin, and ascorbic acid recommended.) A drop of 10 percent in 10 years was indeed discouraging! To compound the discouragement, 21 percent of the families in 1965 ate diets rated as poor (providing less than two-thirds of the recommended amount of one or more of the following nutrients: protein, calcium, iron, vitamin A, thiamin, riboflavin, and ascorbic acid), compared with only 15 percent in 1955.

The summation of the 1965 survey, when reviewed in light of the 1968 revision of recommended dietary allowances (Table 3.1) revealed that calcium and iron were the two nutrients most likely to be deficient in the diet. However, since the recommended daily dietary allowances include a margin of safety to allow for individual differences, failure to completely meet the recommendations does not necessarily mean that malnutrition automatically exists. The diets of women were perpetually deficient in thiamin from the age of nine, riboflavin levels for the diets of women were inadequate from age 20 throughout life and for men after age 75. Vitamin A deficiency was sporadic in the diets for teen-age girls, and the intake of this vitamin was inadequate in diets among women after age 65 and in men after age 75. The only dietary deficiency in ascorbic acid (based on the reduced values recommended in 1968) was reported for men 75 and over. Although a specific value for fat intake is not established, the intake of approximately 45 percent of the calories from fat in the diets of men ages 20 to 64 is considered by nutritionists to be somewhat too high for optimum health (30 to 35 percent is preferred).

Although this survey was conducted more than 10 years ago, some generalizations can be drawn from the results that may well serve for people in the United States today:

1. An adequate income increases the likelihood of good nutrition, but does not assure an adequate diet.

2. Females above the age of 9 are less likely to be well fed than are males of comparable age.

3. Older people are less likely to be well fed than are younger people, a trend that apparently is influenced by a number of factors including reduced income in the retirement years.

4. Protein intake is adequate for most persons of any age or either sex, and fat intake could well be reduced in the American diet.

5. Calcium and iron intake merit special consideration in menu planning.

The national nutrition survey

Figures from the surveys of food consumption in the United States were valuable for the information they provided on the eating practices of the nation. At this point, however, additional information regarding the actual nutritional status of individuals was essential for a true assessment of the problems associated with achieving optimum nutrition for all. Averages do not reveal food consumption of a specific individual, and food consumption data must be accompanied by a physical examination and various laboratory studies to evaluate nutritional status accurately. To provide detailed current information, the National Nutrition Survey was organized as a comprehensive study designed to determine the nutritional status of people in selected locations throughout the country. Included in the experimental design were: clinical examinations, biochemical measurements, dietary assessment, dental examinations, and such nutrition-related information as income, education, and food sources.

The initial sampling for the National Nutrition Survey was limited to 10 states: California, Kentucky, Louisiana, Massachusetts, Michigan, New York (with a special survey in New York City), South Carolina, Texas, Washington, and West Virginia. Participants in the survey were randomly selected from the 1960 Census, but the districts from which these random selections were made were districts where many families lived on low incomes, the majority with less than $3000 per year. Few families had incomes above $5000 annually. One may conclude that the most critical need for improved nutrition exists in the lower-income brackets such as those surveyed in this study. However, the true picture of nutritional status in all segments of the population can only be determined when the survey is extended to all areas of the country and people from all income levels.

Although the preliminary survey drew heav-

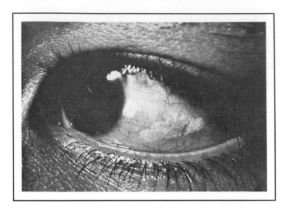

Bitot's spot, the lesion shown on the conjunctiva, is a possible indication of a vitamin A deficiency (Chapter 11).

ily from low income populations, the results shocked many well-fed and complacent citizens. Dr. Arnold E. Schaefer[1] reported the following clinical, dental, growth, biochemical, and dietary findings in December, 1969:[2]

- *"Nearly 4 percent of the 0 to 6 year old subjects show evidence of vitamin D deficiency. Several cases of rickets have been diagnosed."*
- *"Four to 5 percent of the subjects show winged scapula,[3] pot-belly or both. These symptoms are associated with protein-calorie malnutrition."*
- *"Five percent of the subjects show an enlarged thyroid gland. (This level is classified by the World Health Organization as having endemic goiter.[4])"*
- *"Several cases of Bitot's spots have been confirmed. This symptom is a dull, foamy, superficial lesion of the conjunctiva,[5] and is*

frequently attributed to vitamin A deficiency."
- *"Changes in hair, skin and lips have been noted. These may be indicative of poor nutrition."*

*   *   *

- *"Eighteen percent of all subjects aged 10 and over reported difficulty and pain in biting and chewing food."*
- *"Ninety-six percent of the sample had an average of 10 teeth either decayed, missing or filled. Five of these needed immediate attention."*
- *"The adults examined had six times as many decayed, unfilled teeth as the national average."*

*   *   *

- *"In the sample we have studied so far, the height of children 1 to 3 years falls below the average height reported for children in the U.S.A."*
- *"Three times the expected number of children fell below the sixteenth growth percentile."*
- *"A number of this group were more than 10 percent below the average height for their age."*

*   *   *

- *"One-third of the children under 6 had blood hemoglobin levels in an unacceptable range. A large number in the older age groups had levels generally associated with poor nutrition."*
- *"One-third of the children under 6 had serum vitamin A levels that were unacceptable."*
- *"Serum vitamin C levels were less than acceptable in 12 to 16 percent of all age groups. Four percent of the total age group had scorbutic gums."*

"About 16 percent of the overall population had serum protein levels that were less than acceptable. Seventeen per-

---

[1] Formerly Chief, Nutrition Program, Control Disease Center, United States Public Health Service, Atlanta, Georgia, Department of Health, Education and Welfare.
[2] A. E. Schaefer. Malnutrition in the USA? *Nutrition News.* 32, No. 4:13–16. December, 1969.
[3] Shoulder blade having a prominent vertebral border.
[4] A low number of cases of swollen thyroid gland are always present in the population.
[5] The membrane covering the surface of the eyeball in front.

cent had unacceptable levels of serum albumin."

- "Levels of riboflavin and thiamine were unacceptable in 9 to 19 percent of the sample studied."

*　　*　　*

- "In this segment, there are a relatively large number of individuals in age groups 0 to 36 months, 10 to 16 years and 60 years and older, who consumed 50 percent or less than the levels considered adequate for calories, iron, vitamin A and vitamin C."
- "Iron intake was low in over 60 percent of

the young children. Almost 40 percent of the adolescent and older age groups consumed less than half the desired amount of vitamin A."

From this quotation, the end result of nutritional patterns in the United States can be seen. Nutritionally speaking, all is not well within the United States. To better understand how this can be the case in a nation that has the resources to feed itself well, a brief exploration of the sociological aspects of American life that contribute to nutrition patterns is helpful.

Impact of Sociological Changes

The shifting pattern of American life from rural to urban setting is a change directly related to the advent of machines. Whereas 64 percent of the nation's families lived on farms in 1890, that figure had dropped to 5 percent by the 1970s. Such a transition created several changes in family life that ultimately have influenced dietary patterns and food intake. Less than 100 years ago, the United States was typically agrarian. Families lived close to the father's work, all family members could easily be home for meals, and much of the food available was raised by the family itself. Most jobs required considerable physical work, and large quantities of food were eaten to provide the necessary energy.

The move to the city has resulted in changing values and goals for family life. These values and goals are still being modified, but some trends that may influence dietary patterns can be identified at the present time:

1. Increasing value on the individual and his achievement of self identity and individual goals (as illustrated by the women's liberation movement).

2. Adjustment of family living patterns to meet the demands of the job.
3. Greater concern about increasing family income and financial security often achieved by mothers becoming the second wage earner in families.
4. Job insecurities and relatively high rates of unemployment.
5. Small increase in the frequency of families in crisis.
6. Acculturation of minorities, accompanied by a paradoxical increased interest in cultural heritage.
7. Awareness and concern for providing the basic needs for all people.
8. Alarm over ecological imbalances and a trend toward the natural and away from the world of technology and science.

Self-realization

The realization of full individual potential can mean changes in family patterns that will have a distinct influence on the dietary patterns of at least some of the family members. In families strongly committed to this goal, a regular meal with all members present is something to be remembered and treasured, but is an event that rarely happens. Invariably, active families have someone who has a late meeting in the afternoon or a session early in the evening. In the mornings, school buses may be scheduled at times that conflict with the breakfast schedule of the adults. For families with a member who works the swing shift or the very early morning production shift, an organized family breakfast is almost impossible to serve. In other families, the mother may be realizing some of her personal goals through volunteer work in the community or pursuit of individual creative projects. Such activities reduce the amount of time available for preparing meals on a regular basis.

The reasons for hasty and disorganized family meals are numerous and highly varied from one family to another. The apparent conclusion is that the pattern of family meals together three times a day is a vanishing one, even on weekends. Unless families place a high value on the tradition of family meals (at least at breakfast and dinner), many families will no longer follow the established meal patterns of earlier years. The nutritional concern resulting from this changing pattern is that "catch-as-catch-can" meals frequently are lacking in one or more of the nutrients needed for good health. An adequate diet for all family members is difficult to insure when they are eating different meals at different times.

Employment demands

The social status attached to persons in high-level positions has appeal for many Americans. To progress through a career viewed as successful and prestigious by one's family and society may require some readjustment of family living patterns. For families responding to the lure of a higher social position, there may be a significant decrease in the father's partici-

pation in the family. He may commute long distances to work daily so that his family may live in a neighborhood that the family considers compatible with its social position. Extensive travel may be required in the move up the corporation ladder. The need to entertain clients at dinner can frequently interfere with the family dinner since such occasions commonly require both parents, leaving the children to eat a special meal at home. All of these demands upon the person who is the chief source of income for the family may mean significant alterations in family meal patterns. In their early years, some children eat, at the most, only one meal a day with their father. When children eat alone, the menu may not be as valuable in either nutritive content or educational merit as when the meal is being prepared for the entire family. However, frequently the only practical solution to the family facing long commuting distances and other job pressures is to feed the children on a schedule that fits their needs. Loss of family sociability at meals is often the price exacted for prestigious positions.

The pressures in a position may influence the physical condition of a person. A heavy work load not only places a considerable amount of tension and stress on competitive executives, but also limits the time available for physical conditioning and relaxation. If the body is unable to withstand such a routine, modifications in the diet may be necessary in treating ulcers or other conditions. Reduced caloric intake may be required to offset the gradual development of overweight that frequently happens in a sedentary job. The following descriptions of typical luncheon menus[6] illustrates the problems.

Hoi Polloi. Clam chowder, frankfurter and beans, roll and butter, raisin pie a la mode, two cups of coffee.

Eager Beavers. Tomato juice, chicken cro-

[6] Adapted from M. Weinberg and O. E. Shabat. *Society and Man.* Prentice-Hall. P. 150. 1956.

quettes, mashed potatoes, peas, bread, chocolate cream pie, coffee.

No. 2. Orange juice, minute steak, french fries, salad, fruit cup, coffee.

Brass. Fruit cup, spinach, lamb chops, peas, ice cream, tea.

V.I.P.s. Cream of celery soup, chicken sandwich (white meat), milk.

Top Dogs. Cream cheese on whole wheat, buttermilk, indigestion tablets.

Increasing family income

The seemingly insatiable American appetite for a higher standard of living has led to a highly significant change in family patterns. At the beginning of this century, the traditional pattern for about half of the women in this country was that of a homemaker and mother—work outside the home was not a part of the picture. About 70 percent of the women who did work were single; widows and a few women from families with very limited income joined the work force. The picture today is remarkably different. About one fourth of the married women in this country worked in 1950. In just 20 years, the figure had increased to about 4 in every 10 married women. One of the chief motivations, although certainly not the only one, is the desire to increase the family income to provide a few of the luxury items that the husband's income alone cannot buy.

Many women are working to help insure family financial security. Broadly interpreted, this security includes supplementing the family income to buy a home, college education for the children, and other items considered essential by middle-income families. The extra income may be valued because upward social mobility from lower status into the middle class can be accomplished by families with two wage earners. In families where neither parent possesses special skills, both husband and wife may need to work just to provide the basic essentials for their children. The value of two

wage earners in a family has been demonstrated graphically among families at all income levels during the aerospace depression in such areas as Seattle and southern California. Although modifications in the standard of living must be made, families with two wage earners generally have been able to remain economically independent when one person loses his job. Security obviously is one important factor in women seeking jobs outside the home.

A number of women, particularly those whose children either have already left or are about to leave home, have chosen to join the work force as a means of self-expression and professional advancement. There is ample time for further education and a career between the time her children reach semi-independence and a woman reaches retirement age. The increasing emphasis on removing employment inequities on the basis of sex is enabling women to set career goals with expectations of success. When a homemaker works outside the home (especially if she also still has children to care for), definite modifications in the dietary patterns of the family are likely to emerge as a result of the homemaker's employment.

With more income and less time for meal preparation, there is a distinct tendency for many families with working mothers to eat in restaurants more frequently than they would if the mother were not employed. This practice need not be a detriment to good nutrition, but it can be when the restaurant selected specializes in fried foods and gives less attention to the fruit and vegetable and milk categories. Soft drinks instead of milk are more likely to be a part of a meal eaten at a drive-in than at a meal served at home. Although specific figures are not available, the rapid increase in drive-ins featuring hamburgers and french fries would seem to be proof that most families who eat meals away from home are more likely to have a narrower range of foods in a meal than persons eating in more expensive restaurants that specialize in complete meals or than families eating at home. Hamburgers and french fries can both be part of a nutritious meal, but

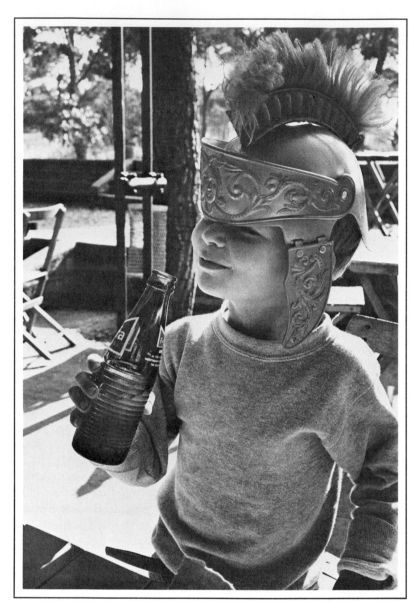

Increasing income may be accompanied by increased snacking, a pattern that can be contrary to achieving optimum nutrition unless nourishing snacks are selected.

by themselves several times a week they do not provide adequate nutrients. (They are particularly limited in calcium, vitamin D, vitamin A, and folic acid.)

Children in urban families with working mothers may tend to snack fairly extensively because dinner is likely to be rather late to accommodate the mother's work schedule or the father's late return. On the positive side, the additional income provided by two incomes in the family may enable them to buy a better diet. In some families, there are other benefits nutritionally. Frequently mothers who work have assistance from others in the family. When children are participants in meal preparation, they may gain a wider range of food likes and also improve their ability to provide nutritionally sound meals for themselves. Such benefits are largely dependent upon the skill of the mother in teaching nutrition and meal preparation to her children.

Unemployment

The problems evolving out of the increasing rate of unemployment found in 1974 and 1975 also have nutritional overtones. The reduced income sharply limits the money available for buying food. This in itself places greater demands upon the family to eat for good health while often needing to modify dietary patterns to meet a stressful situation. Although it is possible to feed a family adequately for even less money than is suggested for the low-cost food plan prepared by the U.S. Department of Agriculture (see Chapter 17), not many consumers have the knowledge and practical abilities needed to accomplish this very difficult task. Instead, the overall result may well be reduced quality of dietary intake.

Loss of a job poses problems of identity and ego satisfactions as well as creating immediate financial concerns. When the world suddenly seems remote and unfeeling, self doubt and personal hurt may become all too real. Basic uncertainty and worry can be translated into modified food patterns, some of which may be detrimental to good nutrition. If a person suddenly is around home all day, overeating may prove to be a real solace. Special treats such as candy may be selected to help one forget that there will not be so much meat on the table now. The variations are many, but the use of foods as therapy is one viable option used by some, and the dietary patterns of a life-time may be modified.

Families in crisis

Although the actual rate of divorce in the United States has shown only a rather small increase since 1920 (eight divorces per year per 1000 married women over age 15 in 1920, a little over 11 by the end of the 1960s),[7] more than 20 people per 1000 total population face the problem each year. Duvall[8] suggests that divorces are more frequent:

Among city families.

In states with lenient divorce laws.

In interfaith marriages.

In Protestant marriages.

Among working-class families.

Among less-educated people.

Among teenage marriages.

In first years of marriage.

In childless marriages.

Families in crisis may be faced by nutritional problems generated as a result of the emotional turmoil experienced by all members of the family. Persons in families confronted with problems in interpersonal relationships within the family, serious illness, alcoholism, drug abuse, unemployment, or other types of individual family crises frequently have little interest in the food they eat. The problem itself can be so all-enveloping that there simply is little interest or energy available for such seemingly unimportant matters as keeping the body well nourished.

Some people react by eating constantly, while others may be totally disinterested in food and eat very little. Still others may develop physical complications, such as diar-

[7] Monthly Vital Statistics Report 18. No. 1, supp. (April 16, 1969): 1. U.S. Dept. Health, Education, and Welfare. Public Health Service.

[8] E. M. Duvall. Family Development. 4th ed. Lippincott. Philadelphia. P. 59. 1971.

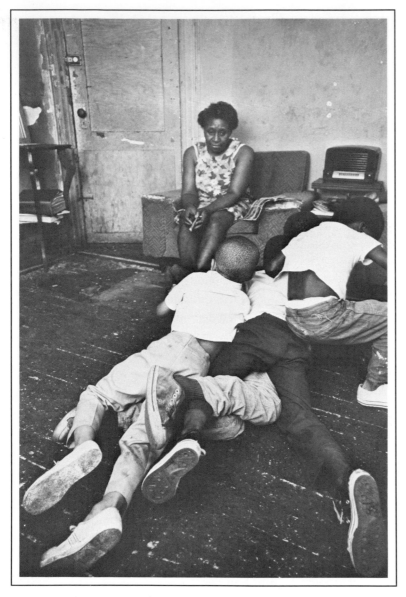

Divorce and other family crises may create financial and emotional problems that supersede the normal family meal patterns which help to insure good nutrition.

rhea or ulcers, and thus not be able to maintain themselves satisfactorily on their usual diet pattern. When meals are prepared indifferently and arguments or worries occupy the most prominent place in mealtime conversations, all family members risk the possibility of being poorly nourished. Unfortunately, this response to crisis, while very human, simply adds more fuel to the problem. Few families improve as poor nutrition decreases physical attractiveness and increases irritability.

Cultural anonymity

The loss of cultural identity is to be expected as communications networks tend to shrink the world. The United States has long been called the "melting pot" because its inhabitants, migrating from so many different countries, have brought diverse cultures to this country. This integration of cultures generally is viewed with approval by nutritionists because this cultural diffusion has tended to expand the breadth of the diet from the "meat and potatoes" mold to embrace numerous recipes from other countries. The introduction of stir-fried vegetables, pizza, tacos, papayas, macadamia nuts, and scores of other foods from other parts of the world has greatly increased the range of possibilities for meals in this country, and a broader range of food preferences increases the likelihood that individuals will be well nourished.

The actual changes in the diets of immigrants are influenced by the locale in which the people settle. In the United States there are "cultural pockets" where many people from the same part of Europe (or other parts of the world) may tend to settle. One Midwesterner described the Germanic diet in a small Illinois town as "Pork, and more pork (mostly salted), a dearth of fresh vegetables during the winter, except for the root vegetables and sauerkraut. Starch and more starch—potatoes and home baked breads and rich goodies." This diet has gradually given way to menus that include less pork, starch, and rich foods and more variety of fruits and vegetables.

Markets in Los Angeles and San Francisco provide the ingredients needed for preparing the dishes familiar to Chinese and Japanese immigrants. When families can afford to buy these foods, many of which are imported, the diet may rely heavily on their traditional menus. However, the diet frequently is augmented by including milk and fruits and vegetables produced locally.

The study by Wenkam and Wolff (1970), documenting the transition in dietary practices among the Japanese in Hawaii, provides a useful illustration of the adaptations that can be made in cultural dietary patterns over an extended period of time. The historical aspect of the study revealed the strong role that family heritage and group values played among Japanese families late in the nineteenth century. These values are a direct contrast to the individualism espoused by the present second generation of Japanese being educated in Hawaii. Among the Japanese who migrated to Hawaii, there has been a slow transition from the original diet, which consisted largely of rice, barley, soybeans, soybean products, a small quantity of vegetables, some fish, and very limited amounts of animal foods. The first change in the traditional diet of the Japanese in Hawaii was more use of polished rice (since this carried social status) and a decline in the sweet potatoes, wheat, and millet that had figured prominently in the diet. While use of polished rice was quite general among the Japanese in Hawaii, there was also a gradual shift toward more use of wheat flour products, and some of the dishes such as Hawaiian poi began to appear regularly in their diets. Breakfast became a typically American meal, occasionally eaten with the addition of rice. During World War II, the Japanese in Hawaii adopted the dietary practices of the Hawaiian and mainland segments of the population quite rapidly.

At the present time, there are essentially three different dietary patterns among the Japanese in Hawaii: the traditionalists who eat basically the expected Japanese diet augmented with a few American dishes with appropriate cultural adaptation; a middle group that eats a cosmopolitan diet clearly reflecting Japanese heritage but including many other food tastes as well; and a small group that has essentially dissociated itself from the Japanese heritage and abandoned the expected dietary pattern. This pattern appears to be relatively typical of the acculturation that has occurred throughout the United States as immigrants from different cultures have become integrated into the American scene.

Reasons cited by Wenkam and Wolff (1970)

for the dietary changes observed among the Japanese in Hawaii included a desire for higher status, disorganization of the traditional family, modified economic goals, availability of foods from other ethnic groups, and public education. Although the changes in American dietary patterns may be more subtle than those Wenkam and Wolff noted, these same motivational factors can be observed to be molding the dietary patterns of many Americans.

As is to be anticipated, dietary changes can result in some measurable physical changes. The life expectancy for the Japanese male in Hawaii in 1920 was 49.5 years, and in 1960 was 72.3. In Hawaii, the last death reported from beriberi (a thiamin deficiency condition that can result from eating a diet composed principally of polished rice) was in 1953. This is a dramatic contrast to previous years—with 96 Japanese dying from beriberi in 1922 alone. Japanese males in Hawaii who were full grown in 1961 were 7 centimeters (2.75 inches) taller and 3.5 kilograms (7.7 pounds) heavier than their fathers. Daughters full grown in 1961 were 5.7 centimeters (2.25 inches) taller than their mothers, but 3.5 kilograms (7.7 pounds) lighter. Of concern is the increasing incidence of coronary heart disease among the Japanese in the United States (10 times greater than the rate among Japanese remaining in their native country). The study conducted by Harvard's Department of Nutrition[9] to compare Irish brothers in Massachusetts and Ireland raised a similar concern. The role of diet in modifying the incidence of coronary heart disease has been discussed extensively (see Chapter 16).

In the past few years, a growing appreciation of one's cultural heritage has had a rather weak, yet a modifying influence upon the acculturation of minority food preference patterns. Sayings such as "Black is beautiful!" have given a new importance to retaining the things one likes from his early years. Greens and grits are being eaten by those who relish them rather than being shunned because of the imagined stigma these popular foods assumed for some. School lunch menus are gradually including tacos and tamales and other suitable selections popular with various minority groups.

Ecological and subcultural influences

The current interest in preserving the environment has brought together two distinctly different groups, the "New Vegetarians" and the ecologists, precariously united in a common interest. Many persons from all levels of society have rallied behind the banner of ecology to promote the restoration of a balance with nature and preservation of the country's resources. As orange groves have been sacrificed for housing tracts and industries have been generously dumping their wastes in the skies and streams, the concern for the environment has been growing. Sensitive analytical equipment can detect contaminants such as mercury, lead, and cadmium, and the news media quickly spread the word. The result has been a wave of almost irrational claims, out of which is emerging a rational approach toward protecting the food supply and other facets of the environment as well.

At about the same time that middle-class America was becoming concerned about environmental problems, the "New Vegetarian" subculture was embracing dietary ideas based on the concept of naturalness. The "organically grown" foods sought by these groups were actually rather similar to the quest of some other Americans who were seeking to minimize man's assault on his environment. The vague definition of organically grown foods did not trouble the spokesmen for either movement. The result has been some exploitation of these

[9] M. F. Trulson, et al. Comparison of siblings in Boston and Ireland. *J.A.D.A. 45*: 225. 1964.

consumers by persons marketing produce identified as "organically grown." Various legislative proposals have been drafted to clarify the definition and standards, but none has been passed at the time of this revision.

One fruitful outcome of this emotional and rather confused scene has been a greater public awareness of the importance of nutrition. On the negative side is the wealth of information on food that is both misleading and inaccurate. The average consumer is confronted with the need to discriminate between factual and fanciful information (see Chapter 5). Although consumer legislation is being developed at both the state and national levels, the full spectrum of ecological influences on the nation's food supply and dietary patterns cannot yet be seen.

The contemporary social scene

The growing awareness and public concern for adequate food for all people is yet another aspect of the sociological forces that are shaping governmental policies as well as individual action. This social force is of particular importance for improving the nutritional status of low-income families.

The difficulties of achieving adequate nutrition on a low income have been brought into sharp focus. The sharp rise in the price of various foods from 1967 to 1975 is revealed in the following figures from the consumer price index as shown for May, 1975 in the "Survey of Current Business:"

Even families with high incomes are confronted with food budget problems, and the management of the small amount of money that low-income families have available to cover the absolute minimal needs for a healthy life is a difficult assignment—one that probably could be done with only limited success by many people who are accustomed to managing a home on a less stringent budget.

One major concern is the frequently large difference in the cost and quality of food available to the middle- and upper-income shopper compared with that in the markets in low-income neighbors. Stores in low-income areas frequently are poorly maintained, and the quality of the foods stocked may be low in comparison with the price of many items in neighborhoods that have a higher average income. Captain and McIntire (1969) found that hamburger and fresh produce were the items most subject to variation in quality and price in poverty versus nonpoverty area grocery stores. Neighborhood stores, whether in poverty or nonpoverty areas, generally are more expensive than chain markets. Unfortunately, some low-income families must shop at their neighborhood market because they lack transportation to other markets. Others may be forced to shop in small markets that will sell to them on a charge account because cash is not always readily at hand.

Market managers in some of the low-income areas can readily attest to the reasons for marketing and pricing policies of their stores. They hasten to point out the higher costs of operation and the insurance problems of maintaining a store in what is considered to be a high-risk neighborhood. Clearly there are arguments on

	1974[a]	May, 1975
Food	161.7	171.8
Meats, poultry, fish	163.9	168.2
Dairy products	151.9	153.6
Fruits and vegetables	165.8	169.0

[a] Price compared with 1967, where 1967 = 100%.

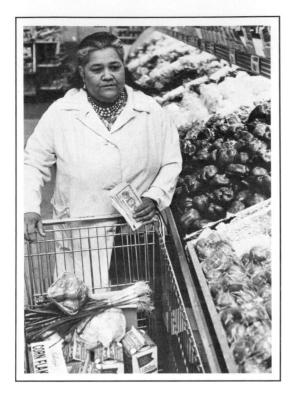

Through the use of food stamps, many disadvantaged people, including this shopper, have been able to increase their purchasing power so that they can be better fed.

quired by the government as a by-product of the price support programs, to low-income families. Although the early commodity donation program provided some foods of high nutritional value, there was no attempt to include the variety of foods needed for an adequate intake of all nutrients. In 1961, the food commodities were increased in quantity and variety, with particular emphasis being given to the protein-containing foods.

The Food Stamp Program has been another means of making food more available to those with limited incomes. This program, which is federally supported, is based on the sale of stamps to persons who are qualified to purchase food stamps because of their limited income. The face (redemption) value of these stamps is greater than the original purchase price. This enables the buyer to obtain far more food in the market than he could if he were shopping with cash. One advantage of this approach is that individuals have more choice in the selection of their food than they have in the commodity donation program. Although this governmental program appears utopian on the surface, some families wishing to participate have encountered difficulties in garnering the minimal amounts of money needed to buy stamps. Others cannot overcome the obstacles of the required governmental forms and travel to the agency selling the stamps.

Continuing modifications in the Food Stamp Act of 1964 and in the food commodities program have been implemented to make the programs more effective in meeting the nutritional needs of as many low-income families as possible. Even with concerted governmental efforts, there were still more than 400 counties prior to the 1969 White House Conference on Food, Nutrition, and Health that did not make either of these food programs available to eligible people. The furor of public concern for feeding the nation's hungry was nurtured by the White House Nutrition Conference into a concerted force that quickly caused many nonparticipating counties to utilize one of these two programs. During March 1970, 3,900,000

both sides of the issues, but the fact remains that the opportunities for purchasing high-quality food at a minimal price vary significantly, and not all people are able to shop advantageously. This single aspect of food distribution can be a major influence on a family's nutritional status.

Governmental social programs designed to increase employment or to distribute food to low-income families (and particularly pregnant and lactating women and young children) have been of some value in providing the food needed for good health. To a limited extent, the surplus commodities distributed free in the United States have had some influence in structuring adequate diets for those persons eligible to receive the food. Originally, the commodity donation program of the late 1930s was implemented to distribute surplus foods, ac-

people received donated foods, an increase of 8 percent over the previous month! By 1974, all but one eligible county in the United States had made available one of these programs, with most electing the Food Stamp Program. Participants in food stamps in 1974 numbered approximately 14 million.

The task of feeding a family a nutritious diet is much greater when ample money is not available. Special knowledge of the nutritional content of foods well suited to managing on a tight budget, imagination, and the skill required to prepare these foods so they are attractive and tempting are assets not always possessed by those who need them most. All too often, people with limited money for food will be well aware of the importance of getting the nutrients they need, but will be persuaded to buy expensive supplements or special foods, thinking that these are the way to good health. To help homemakers avoid such unnecessary expenses, interested women in some communi-

ties have been selected from low-income areas and trained as nutrition aides. These women help the homemakers learn about effective ways of feeding their families for less money. The use of paraprofessionals who are indigenous to the neighborhoods being served has proven to be an effective means of communicating practical, basic information to many families. Home economists and nutrition specialists in the Agricultural Extension Service have provided the professional training component of the program.

Education is a strong component of the federal food distribution programs. Pre-schoolers and their families receive some nutrition education through Head Start classes. School-age children, including teen-agers and young adults, are reached through the Expanded Food and Nutrition Education Program (EFNEP). This program also reaches the families of the children. The flexibility of this program has stimulated workers to develop nu-

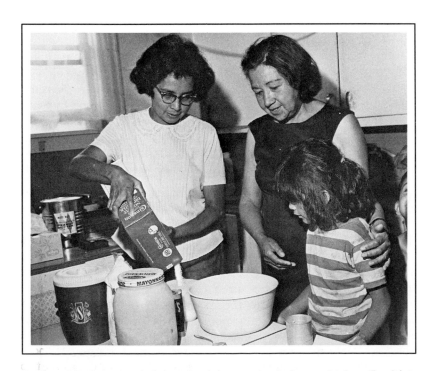

An extension program aide helps a family learn ways of using nonfat dry milk solids to improve nutrition economically.

merous imaginative ways of teaching nutrition as a viable part of living. Approaches have ranged from helping adolescents with clothing problems to figure control, budgeting, and gourmet cooking, depending upon the special interests of the group.

Public education and the National School Lunch Act have been an important combination in helping to meet the challenge of adequate nutrition on a low income. Schools have been serving lunches to some school-age children under the National School Lunch Act since 1947. Local schools are assisted financially by federal subsidy so that a lunch providing one third of the day's nutrients may be available to every child at low cost. In fact, children from families with a low income are to be given free lunches. However, this single legislative act was not sufficient to meet the needs of children in many places. Consequently, the special milk program was implemented in 1954, and the Child Nutrition Act was passed in 1966, authorizing pilot school breakfast programs as well. Practically all organized children's groups can now be fed under provisions of the 1968 legislation. That same year the breakfast program moved from the pilot stage into actual operation. Unfortunately, many schools have yet to take advantage of the recent legislation. Utilization of the program by schools is largely the responsibility and decision of the local leaders.

Federally funded programs also are operating to help improve the nutrition of special population groups. The Women, Infants, and Children Program (WIC) is a result of the 1972 modification of the Child Nutrition Act of 1966. This program, operated under the auspices of the U.S. Department of Agriculture, provides foods specifically selected to meet predicted dietary deficiencies in infants and children to age 4 and in pregnant and lactating women from specified low-income families. Emphasis is directed to meeting the need for ascorbic acid, vitamin A, protein, calcium, and iron; infants receive iron-fortified formula and cereals plus ascorbic acid-rich fruit juice and young children and pregnant and lactating women receive cheese and eggs, vitamin D-fortified milk, and a source of ascorbic acid.

Programs for the elderly include Meals-on-Wheels and Congregate Meals Programs. These projects have the ultimate goal of improving the nutrition of the elderly, but they move toward this goal by recognizing the special and associated needs of this population group. Meals-on-Wheels brings prepared meals directly to the home, and, in many instances, provides a little sociability for the person who is unable to care for himself at home. The Congregate Meals Programs fulfill the social need of the physically active elderly by providing a nourishing meal in a pleasing and sociable setting to feed the whole person as well as the body. These programs vary in their success in meeting established goals, but the need for them is apparent and many have done an excellent job of improving the status of the elderly.

The Next Steps

Despite the recent impetus and support given to nutrition education, much remains to be done if adequate nutrition for all is to be a realistic and achievable goal in the United States. Parrish[10] concludes that ". . . only a massive program of nutrition education and perhaps food fortification and enrichment for the entire population can hope to have any overall effect in raising the quality of diets and restoring the former nutrient balance." This opinion was based on the 10 keys to change in average household food habits identified by Parrish (1971).

[10] J. B. Parrish. Implications of changing food habits for nutrition educators. *J. of Nutr. Educ.* P. 144. Spring 1971.

1. Decline in wide-variety, home food production.
2. Decline in wide-variety, home-prepared foods.
3. Rise of preferred limited-variety, convenience foods.
4. Rise in percent of food consumed away from home.
5. Trend toward meal skipping—especially by teen-agers.
6. Declining importance of food in family budgets.
7. Adverse effects of differential price changes on consumption of selected items.
8. Increasing popularity of diet and health fad foods.
9. Declining availability of selected nutrients.
10. The nature of food preferences of an affluent, urbanized, mobile society.

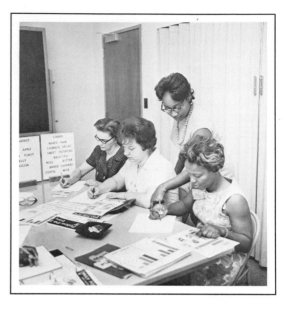

Effective nutrition education programs for all people are the key to improving the nutritional status of the nation.

The socioeconomic and cultural influences that figure so prominently in the selection of individual diet patterns provide the framework for establishing stimulating and meaningful nutrition education programs. Greater efforts by nutrition educators, in conjunction with legislative and fiscal support from state and federal governments, can make adequate nutrition for all a meaningful goal. All persons in a society need to have a working knowledge of practical nutrition; medical personnel, social workers, preschool and elementary school teachers, physical education teachers and coaches, science teachers, and home economics teachers need the training necessary to provide a strong foundation in nutrition. Only through adequate training of these key personnel can sound nutrition education programs for patients, clients, students, and parents be accomplished.

The importance of nutrition education coupled with government food programs is highlighted by studies such as the one conducted by Larkin and Sandretto (1970) to determine the use of commodity foods by Potawatami Indians living in Michigan's Upper Peninsula.

These workers found that the Indians used a large proportion of foods high in carbohydrate and fat, but did not use the dried milk powder, prunes, and scrambled egg mix that were available to them. Greater use of fruits, vegetables, milk, and protein foods would add significantly to the nutritive quality of their diets, modifications that can be encouraged by training nutrition aides to help the Potawatami homemakers. These aides, with some help from nutritionists, show the Indian women how to make easily prepared recipes from the commodity foods, using the equipment commonly available in the homes.

It is also possible to extend nutrition knowledge by working through the school lunch program and the home economics teachers to teach the students, who will then carry the information back to their homes. This seems a practical approach in view of the results of Larkin and Sandretto's survey, which showed that the children consumed a diet higher in fruits, vegetables, and milk during the school year than during the summer, indicating that some acceptance of these foods can be anticipated when they are adequately and imaginatively introduced.

A team approach to improving the country's nutritional status is becoming an increasingly appropriate way of helping people. Well-qualified social workers, doctors, and nutritionists need to work together as teams, cooperating rather than competing. The high cost of such personnel immediately emphasizes the importance of providing appropriate training to carefully selected individuals—allied health personnel—who will assist the professionals of the health team as they work in the community. Aside from the economic aspects, the use of aides is highly valuable because persons indigenous to the community understand its people and their problems and frequently can communicate more effectively than many professionals, even though the professional worker may be highly motivated and anxious to help.

One of the prevalent nutritional problems in the United States is obesity. The socioeconomic and cultural factors discussed in this chapter are related, in part, to this problem. One important factor that should be stressed is the decline in physical activity resulting from a combination of changes including greater use of the car and extensive television viewing. Programs geared toward improving nutritional status in this country must take note of this change in activity patterns. One very effective way of improving nutritional status in the United States is to encourage a great deal more physical activity and exercise on a daily basis, not just on weekends.

Additives

Some comments about food additives might well be included as the closing section of this chapter.

Additives quite logically are substances that are added to foods and these range from sugar and salt to traces of delicate spices and flavors. Salt and nitrates, among the first substances added to foods thousands of years ago, were utilized for the purpose of preserving them. Sugar has been used not only as a preservative, primarily for fruits, but also it is a food providing energy and as such makes up about 15 to 20 percent of the total calories of typical American diets.

It is often forgotten that most of our foods, for example all of those in the Basic Four food groups, are perishable or semiperishable, and must either be consumed shortly after they are harvested or preserved. This preservation is by drying, canning, freezing, or by the use of appropriate additives. Food additives not only help in the processing of foods, they make foods more convenient to prepare in the home, and they make foods more pleasant to taste, see, and smell. After all, eating is one of the pleasures of life.

There are some 2000 substances currently used as food additives, and excluding those that are used in large amounts such as sugars and salt, it has been estimated that the average American consumes about nine pounds of additives per year. They serve a great variety of useful purposes such as retarding the growth of microorganisms as, for example, mold growth on breads, slowing oxidation of fats and other components of foods that cause unacceptable flavors and odors, providing smooth textures in manufactured foods such as ice cream by means of emulsifiers and, of course, providing the many subtle flavors and colors that make foods more enjoyable.

In addition to these non-nutritive additives that provide foods with a longer shelf life and more desirable physical qualities, we also have nutritive additives. These are various nutrients that are added to some of our foods to restore or improve nutritive quality. For example, the addition of iodide to salt has essentially elimi-

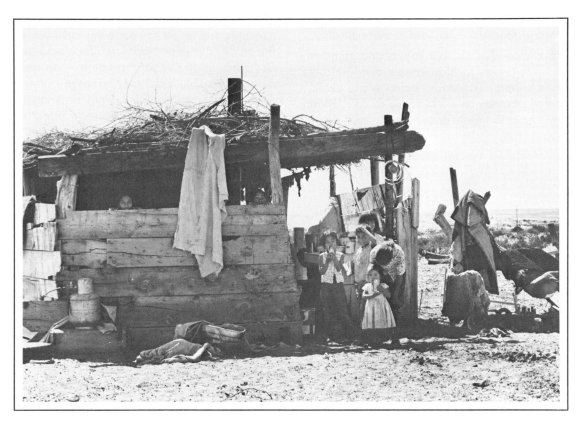

A broad-based effort involving social workers, health professionals, educators, and agriculturalists in all phases of food production and distribution is needed to overcome the problem of malnutrition for disadvantaged families throughout the nation.

nated the common goiter, not only in this country but in many other parts of the world. Fluoride added to water reduces tooth decay by more than half in those who drink fluoridated water from birth to adulthood. Vitamins A and D are added to margarines and most skimmed milks. Three of the B vitamins and the mineral iron are added to most wheat flour these days. Vitamin C is currently added to many noncitrus juices.

Additives, both the non-nutritive and the nutritive ones, play a very important role in feeding not only Americans but the other peoples of the world. Without the use of them, food wastes would be higher, costs would be appreciably higher, and our foods would be lower in nutritional quality and taste satisfac-

tion. Additives are safe in the quantities they are consumed as used in our foods today.

Reviewing the subject of food additives, Dr. Richard L. Hall, a recognized authority in this field, wrote as follows:[11]

"The use of additives everywhere is controlled in a number of ways, in fact, far more carefully than nature controls the toxins she places in foods. They must, in the judgment of competent experts, clearly be harmless under the intended condition for use. And even then, they may not be used indiscriminately, but only with the greatest restraint, and when their use assists

[11] Hall, R. L., Food additives. *Nutrition Today.* 8: 20–28, 1973.

in achieving improved palatability, convenience, reduced costs, and nutritional value.

"It is clear that microbiological and nutritional hazards are by far the greatest dangers to our food supply. These two points alone deserve the most attention because, by and large, they are hazards that each of us can control individually.

"Collectively we can attempt to do something about environmental pollutants and natural toxicants, just as we can be vigilant in seeing to the proper use of pesticides and food additives. But additives are as safe as science can make them. They play a vital role and we must not let their use be restricted by whim or imagined danger lest we seriously adversely affect the quality, safety, and cost of the food we eat."

Summary

The United States, despite and because of its tremendous agricultural resources, still has many citizens who are not well nourished, some being undernourished and some overnourished. In fact, recent surveys have indicated a regression rather than an improvement in nutritional status. This modification in dietary patterns has been influenced by many social changes, including increasing value on the individual and achievement of self identity and individual goals; adjustment of family living patterns to meet the demands of the job; greater concern about increasing family income; problems arising from unemployment; a small increase in the frequency of families in crisis; acculturation of minorities and a heightened pride in cultural heritage; awareness and concern for providing the basic needs of all people; and alarm over ecological imbalances.

Federal programs have been implemented to provide (1) food for children in group situations, (2) commodity foods or food stamps to families, (3) food for special groups (WIC and programs for the elderly), and (4) nutrition information for all citizens. Still greater efforts must be made by personnel in the health professions, educators, and appropriate government officials to make this a well-fed nation. Increased physical activity is an important adjunct in improving the nutritional status of the overnourished.

Selected References

Adams, B. N. The American Family. Markham Publishing. Chicago. 1971.

Agricultural Research Service. What Americans eat—why it is important to know. Toward the New. Washington, D.C. April, 1970.

Anonymous. Families Then and Now. Family Economics Review. P. 3. March 1968.

Briggs, G. M. The need for nutrition education. *J. Nutr. Education.* Prototype issue. P. 7. Fall 1968.

Brown, M. L., et al. Diet and nutriture of preschool children in Honolulu. *J. Am. Diet. Assoc. 57,* No. 6:22. 1970.

Bruhn, C. M., and R. M. Pangborn. Food habits of migrant farm workers in California. *J. Am. Diet. Assoc. 59*:347. 1971.

Burk, M. C. Food economic behavior in systems terms. *J. Home Econ. 62*:319. 1970.

Captain, O. B., and M. S. McIntire. Cost and quality of food in poverty and non-poverty urban areas. *J. Am. Diet. Assoc. 55,* No. 6:569. 1969.

Clark, F. A scorecard on how we Americans are eating. In *Food for Us All.* U.S. Dept. of Agriculture. Washington, D.C. P. 266. 1969.

DeFleur, M. L., et al. *Sociology: Man in Society.* Scott, Foresman. Glenview, Ill. 1971.

Dressler, D. *Sociology: The Study of Human Interaction.* Knopf. New York. 1969.

Duvall, E. M. *Family Development.* 4th ed. Lippincott. Philadelphia. 1971.

Enloe, C. H. Hitched to everything in the universe. *Nutrition Today. 4,* No. 4:2. Winter 1969–1970.

Fincher, L. J., and M. E. Rauschert. Diets of men, women, and children in the United States. *Nutrition Program News.* P. 1. September–October 1969.

Goode, W. J. *The Family.* Prentice-Hall. Englewood Cliffs, N.J. 1964.

Hiemstra, S. J. Telescoping 20 years of change in the food we eat. In *Food for Us All.* U.S. Dept. of Agriculture. Washington, D.C. P. 51. 1969.

Kight, M. A., et al. Nutritional influences of Mexican-American foods in Arizona. *J. Am. Diet. Assoc. 55,* No. 4:557. 1969.

Larkin, F. A., and A. M. Sandretto. Dietary patterns and the use of commodity foods in a Potawatami Indian community. *J. Home Econ. 62*:385. 1970.

Manufacturing Chemists' Assoc. *Food Additives.* M.C.A. 1825 Connecticut Ave., N.W., Washington, D.C. 1974.

Mayer, J. Priorities in nutrition. *Food and Nutrition News. 41,* No. 1:1. 1969.

Mayer, J. Report from the White House Conference. *Nutrition News. 33,* No. 2:5. 1970.

Meyers, T. The extra cost of being poor. *J. Home Econ. 62,* No. 6:379. 1970.

Moore, M. C., et al. Why the boys? *J. Home Econ. 62,* No. 5:338. 1970.

Morgan, A. F. *Nutritional Status U.S.A.* Calif. Ag. Exp. Sta. Bull. 769. 1959.

National Manpower Council. *Womanpower.* Columbia University Press. New York. 1957.

Parrish, J. B. Implications of changing food habits for nutrition educators. *J. Nutr. Educ.* P. 140. Spring 1971.

Schaefer, A. E. Are we well fed? The search for the answer. *Nutrition Today. 4,* No. 1:2. 1969.

Schaefer, A. E. Malnutrition in the USA? *Nutrition News. 32,* No. 4:13. 1969.

Taylor, E. F. 100 million times a day, Americans eat out. In *Food for Us All.* U.S. Dept. of Agriculture. Washington, D.C. P. 62. 1969.

Todhunter, E. N. Approaches to nutrition education. *J. Nutr. Educ.* P. 8. Fall 1968.

U.S. Bureau of the Census. *Statistical Abstract of the United States, 1969.* U.S. Govt. Printing Office. Washington. 1969. P. 220.

U.S. Dept. of Agriculture. *A Good Life for More People, the Yearbook of Agriculture.* U.S.D.A. Washington, D.C. 1971.

U.S. Dept. of Agriculture. *Shopper's Guide, the Yearbook of Agriculture.* U.S.D.A. Washington, D.C. 1974.

U.S. Dept. of Agriculture. Economic Research Service. *National Food Situation.* ERS Bulletin 132. Washington, D.C. May 1970.

Vanneman, S. C. School lunch to food stamp; America cares for its hungry. In *Food for Us All.* U.S. Dept. of Agriculture. Washington, D.C. P. 69. 1969.

Wenkam, N. S., and R. J. Wolff. A half century of changing food habits among Japanese in Hawaii. *J. Am. Diet. Assoc. 57,* No. 6:29. 1970.

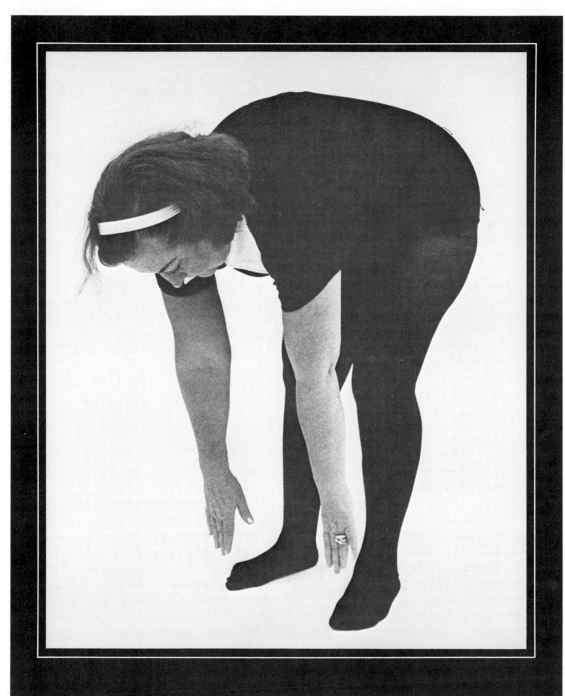

Chapter 4

Weight Control and Energy Needs

Concerns with weight and ways of losing excess pounds are problems eagerly discussed throughout the United States today. Rarely does a day pass without such subjects being brought into one's hearing. At parties there is little prospect of the occasion passing without at least one reference to a diet being brought into the conversation. Many people talk about losing weight—some even succeed!

In some cultures throughout history, the positive appreciation of well-rounded to plump figures could be attributed largely to two reasons. Social status was conveyed subtly by plumpness, which was associated with affluence (i.e., the portly banker image). Second, plumpness was interpreted to be a symbol of good health because people with tuberculosis or other serious, yet all-too-common illnesses were generally thin. In today's world the taste in figures seems to have swung almost to the opposite extreme, as typified by the gaunt fashion model's figure. From a health, if not from a fashion viewpoint, moderation appears to be the best approach.

The degree of body fatness is important from the standpoint of health, beauty, and social acceptance—actually exerting an influence on virtually all aspects of one's life. Success or failure, happiness or misery may hinge upon achieving and maintaining a figure that appears to fall within a normal range. Food and exercise are the keys, and weight control basically is a matter of balancing energy input and expenditure. The achievement of the correct degree of body fatness is analogous to balancing a budget. However, the process is a bit more complex than this may sound. The factors influencing food consumption and metabolism of the nutrients are quite complex.

Factors Influencing Weight

Physiological

The food consumption pattern of an individual represents an integration of the diverse physiological, psychological, and environmental forces that have impinged upon his life until the present moment. Some forces, such as the hunger experienced just before a meal, are temporal in nature. The enduring nature of such powerful forces as the familial food preferences established in early childhood means that some influences may mold food consumption over one's lifespan. Additional insight into the factors that shape individual food intake can be gained through the discussion contained in the following section.

Genetic factors

Experimental animals have been used to demonstrate genetic and metabolic variations that can lead to obesity. Experimentalists have long known that some strains of mice exhibit a tendency to become fat, and Aberdeen-Angus cattle fatten more readily than do the milk-producing Jersey cows. Although comparable and conclusive proof cannot be cited for humans, some people probably have an inherited tendency toward obesity.

Sheldon, a medical specialist in human constitution, conducted extensive research in which

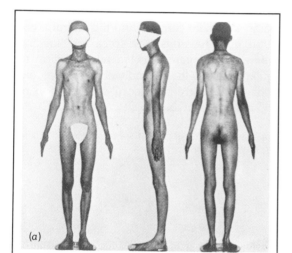

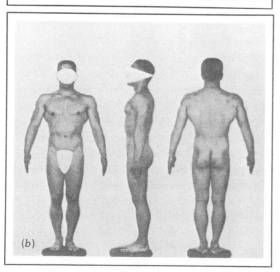

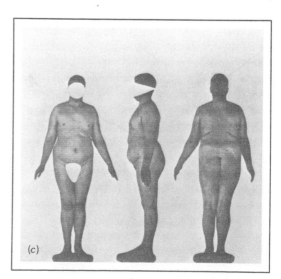

Examples of Sheldon's somatotypes: (a) ectomorph, (b) mesomorph, and (c) endomorph.

he categorized body types, also called somato-types, into ectomorphs, mesomorphs, and en-domorphs. Ectomorphs are depicted as slight in frame, with relatively long arms and legs and fine bones. Mesomorphs are pictured as possessing the ideal masculine build, heavy in bone and muscle, and athletic in appearance, with limbs of moderate length. The endomorph is characterized by roundness and softness of the body, particularly in the abdominal region. These descriptions represent the pure classifications, although people, in reality, are a blending of the three types and can be individually classified according to the combination of the individual strengths of each of the three somatotype components. According to Sheldon, the basic somatotype is a hereditary characteristic. Of course, the dietary pattern and life style of each individual may combine to camouflage some of the basic hereditary structure. On the whole, there is compelling evidence that genetic factors are important in the development of obesity.

Hunger mechanism

Hunger is an all-encompassing term that immediately directs one's thoughts to food. Hunger may be defined as the drive that motivates people to eat until they are satiated. The physiological mechanisms that prompt people to eat and to cease eating are certainly an intimate part of the total picture determining food intake.

The hypothalamus of the brain has been found to function as a control system for the ingestion of food. Dr. Jean Mayer and co-workers at Harvard's Department of Nutrition have shown that the ventromedial areas (functioning as satiety centers) and the lateral areas of the hypothalamus (the so-called "feeding centers") are interconnected and function to regulate satiety in the individual. Mayer explains his "glucostatic theory of regulation of food intake" as follows:[1]

[1] J. Mayer. *Overweight*. Prentice-Hall. Englewood Cliffs, N.J., P. 20–21. 1968.

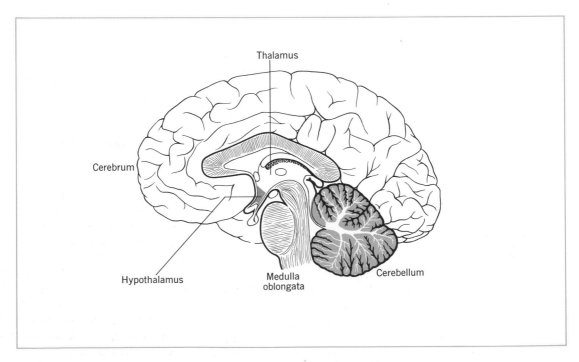

The hypothalamus of the brain exercises a regulatory role in the regulation of hunger.

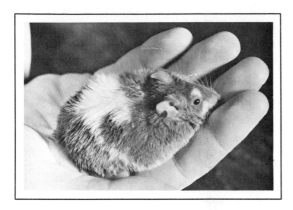

A mouse that is obese due to a hereditary obese-hyperglycemic gene.

". . . there are in the hypothalamus receptors with a special affinity for glucose, which are activated by this blood component in the measure that they utilize it. The concept was based at the start on the fact that glucose is the almost exclusive fuel of the central nervous system. Its availability in turn determines the rate at which fat and protein are utilized: it therefore plays a central role in the economy of the body. It is stored (as glycogen) in small amounts and the stores are depleted within a few hours, faster in the cold or when the subject is exercised. The utilization is influenced by various hormones, and is drastically decreased when insulin is lacking as in diabetics."

The hypothesis included the postulate that the hypothalamic receptors, unlike the rest of the brain, would be found to be influenced by the concentration of insulin.

That the satiety center in the hypothalamus does indeed control the stomach contractions of a hungry animal was demonstrated by Mayer. By injecting glucagon, the pancreatic hormone that releases glucose from stores in the liver, he found that the blood glucose level was raised and the stomach contractions of hunger ceased. However, when the satiety center in the hypothalamus was destroyed, the injection of glucagon did not cause the contractions to cease. Without the appetite control exercised by the satiety centers in the hypothalamus, experimental animals lose their ability to know when to stop eating. This theory provides a plausible explanation for obesity when the hypothalamus has been injured.

Metabolic disturbances

Occasionally, regulatory and metabolic irregularities can lead to obesity in individual cases. However, despite the fact that many fat people would prefer to consider that their weight problem is strictly a glandular error, this is *rarely* the explicit cause, and, even in those few rare cases, the ultimate treatment (or prevention) of obesity is to eat fewer calories and expend more calories through physical activity. Although relatively uncommon, an imbalance of one or more of the hormones from the endocrine glands can create a physiological need for a modified food intake if weight is to be controlled. The hormones that may be involved include thyroxine, insulin, adrenaline, glucagon, and sex hormones. Hormone imbalances may be characterized either by (1) limitations in the ability to metabolize fat (use fat for energy) or (2) rapid resynthesis (rebuilding) of fat in the tissues. To illustrate, a slight increase above normal insulin levels or a slight decrease in adrenaline can cause some fat to accumulate over a period of time.

Perhaps the most familiar hormonal problem is that of the improperly functioning thyroid gland. In hypothyroidism, the decreased level of thyroxine (the hormone secreted by the thyroid gland) is accompanied by slower metabolism and a tendency to accumulate fat. The reverse situation is found in hyperthyroidism because of the excess of thyroxine.

Psychological

Each individual's food consumption patterns are shaped partly by the variety of pressures to which he is constantly subjected, beginning from the time he is born and continuing

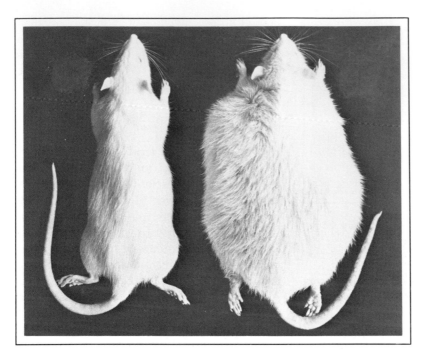

A rat with obesity resulting from a surgical lesion of the hypothalamus and a normal rat.

throughout life. Even within the same family, each child's intake patterns may be modified from those of his siblings and parents as a result of his unique interactions with others in the family.

Despite the fact that eating is a normal function that must be maintained if life is to be sustained, there are seemingly innumerable influences, beginning at birth, that mold the dietary patterns and attitudes of each person. One of the earliest satisfactions experienced by each infant is being fed until he is satiated. Even this natural act engenders the beginning of individual attitudes toward food. For infants with inattentive or resentful mothers, anxiety or frustration toward the act of eating may develop. Anxious mothers, overly concerned for the welfare of their infants and greatly in need of reassurance as to their competence in their new role as mothers, may measure their success by the rate at which their babies gain weight. This attitude may gradually generate in the infant the habit of eating until overly full or may cause

the infant to swing to the other extreme, thus creating a reluctant eater. These situations are representative of the early development of attitudes that subsequently lead to weight control difficulties. Maintenance of an appropriate weight is important from early childhood, because adults who have been overweight from childhood have more difficulty bringing their weight into the desired range and maintaining it there than people who have gained extra weight only as adults (Bruch, 1957).

Throughout a person's childhood, parental attitudes toward food exert a strong influence in the development of the child's attitudes, creating habits that can last a lifetime. Sometimes food is used as a reward, a practice that not surprisingly leads to a dependence on food as a source of comfort and may ultimately lead to overweight. Parents may give obvious approval and praise to children who clean their plates at a meal. The desire to please may cause children to eat more food than they actually need to meet their physical requirements.

Constant overeating then develops a habit of eating until the stomach feels very full. In one day, a few extra calories will have no significant effect, but over a period of years, the few extra calories a day add up to many unwanted pounds. Remember, each 3500 kilocalories that are consumed without being expended in the form of energy accumulates to deposit one pound of fat whether eaten in few or many sittings. To some people, this additive function may appear to operate exponentially!

Everyone has a self-image, that is, an inner picture of how he looks to others. A large part of this self-image is directly related to dietary habits. The person who is overweight may picture himself as being a bit heavier than the average person, at least he does if he is at all honest with himself. Unless this picture is totally unpalatable to him, it is likely that he will continue to eat the same type of diet that caused him to be too heavy. He begins to think of himself as a fat man and behaves in the world as fat people are expected to act. Often there is a facade that protects inner feelings from being exposed to the world.

Some people maintain their protective fat as a shield against threatening aspects of their lives. A person who is fat can always explain failure to get or keep a job as due to discrimination against him because his employer objected to his weight. Indeed, this may even be the case. In California in 1969, there was widespread publicity regarding the instance of a physical education teacher who was dismissed, ostensibly because she was so heavy that she did not exemplify good health to her students. (This action later was invalidated by a court ruling.)

Theorists also have suggested that some people who view social contacts as threatening, particularly those with the opposite sex, may deliberately eat themselves into an unattractive, obese state to provide an alibi for remaining aloof from intimate friendships. Overeating is a very common outlet for frustrations and anxieties. Other underlying psychological reasons for obesity certainly exist, but

these are some that are commonly observed.

Obviously, not all overweight people have deep-seated emotional problems causing their obesity. Some people have been overweight for a long period of time, often since childhood, and are psychologically well adjusted. This situation can change to a less satisfactory adjustment if pressure is put upon them to reduce and the dieting efforts are too difficult for them to maintain; even more important is the frustration some people experience if the reduction campaign fails to be effective soon after it is begun.

Bruch (1958) makes a distinction between developmental obesity and reactive obesity. Developmental obesity is characterized as psychological in cause, stemming from parental pressures during childhood that cause a child to become overweight early in life as a result of overeating. These parents may continue to compound the problem by rejecting the obese child and constantly nagging him about his weight.

In contrast, reactive obesity is triggered by some deeply emotional experience, such as a death in the family. In such cases, the individual salves his feelings with food, often cutting down on physical activity at the very time when caloric intake is increased. Some students experience a very minor demonstration of this psychological type of obesity during final examination periods. Fortunately, the pressure ceases as soon as the last examination is completed, and the dietary habits usually return to normal before being overweight becomes an established pattern.

Environmental

Family dietary patterns can lead to excessive weight when followed over a long period of time. Families that consistently eat poorly planned meals, often excessively high in meats, starchy foods, and fats, and relatively low in fruits and vegetables, may exhibit a tendency toward being too heavy. When foods are consistently prepared with a large amount of fat, as occurs when fried foods are frequently served, overweight is likely to be a problem. Obesity may be a problem in families that specialize in large servings at each meal followed with a tempting dessert that must be eaten to avoid offending the mother. The size of the servings is obviously a most important factor in determining the calories consumed. When all family members have a great propensity for food, the enthusiasm and praise heaped upon the cook may serve to spur her on to still greater endeavors in the kitchen, ultimately increasing the weight problem in the family.

As a nation, another environmental influence is leading toward weight problems. In the past, America could be described as a country of physically hard-working people carving a living out of the wilderness. Obviously, this picture no longer applies. Much of our work today is done by machines, and, while American technology and mental effort have produced the machines and other labor-saving devices, the net result is much less physical activity. As the cities have grown, so has the transportation system. With the advent of the automobile (and multiple-car families), riding is substituted for walking. Today, urbanization has reached the point where many children live so far from schools that they have to be driven instead of walking or riding a bicycle to school. To compound the problem, the hectic pace in many people's lives leaves them feeling physically tired at the end of the day, even when they have had virtually no exercise. The natural impulse under such conditions is to collapse into the softest easy chair to watch television most of the evening rather than pursuing an activity that requires some physical exercise. About the only exercise some people get is the exercise of racing to the kitchen for a snack during the television commercials, an exercise not exactly guaranteed to expend much energy.

Still other people have occupations that might be termed hazardous from the standpoint of weight control. To some waitresses, chefs, and others whose work requires them to be around food constantly, the temptation to have a little taste of this and a bite of that is simply too much, and they quickly nibble themselves into an ongoing weight control problem. In the world of business and politics, special clients may need to be entertained several times a week. Cocktail parties, heavy lunches, and elaborate dinners quickly add pounds to the unwary diner, particularly if these excess calories cannot be used up by increased physical activity.

Recent studies with rats by Dr. Jules Hirsch and his colleagues at the Rockefeller University have suggested that environmental factors early in life (overfeeding) may drastically influence body weight later in life. They showed in rats that obesity may be influenced by the number of fat cells as well as by their size. The size of fat cells is determined by the amount of fat each one contains. Dr. Hirsch found that the number of cells in fat tissues in the normal rat increases from birth up to about 15 weeks of age. Subsequently the increase in fat tissues occurs primarily through an increase in the size of the fat cells, not in their number. With rats, underfeeding during the first 15 weeks of life led to a reduction in all aspects of growth and development *including* the number of fat cells. Both the number and size of fat cells remained low despite generous refeeding after this early period.

These studies with rats indicate that the number of fat cells may be permanently modified only early in life, with overfeeding increasing the number and under-feeding leading to a reduced number of cells. Both patterns persist during the remainder of life. Thus, nutritional influences early in life may be extremely important as to whether obesity develops later in life.

If the results of Hirsch obtained with rats apply to man, a somewhat underfed infant with somewhat slower growth and development is less likely to develop obesity later in life because he may have fewer fat cells to fill with fat. This suggests to parents and physicians the potential harm in allowing infants to gain weight in excess of that appropriate for their height.

Problems of being underweight

Persons who control their weight within the recommended range throughout life have taken a very important step toward optimizing their physiological and psychological well-being. Although the problem of underweight is less common than obesity, too low a weight in relation to height may not be desirable for optimum health. Resistance to disease may be reduced by being underweight; incidence of tuberculosis is higher among the underweight than among those of normal or even excess weight. These conditions are less important today than a generation ago because of the development of effective antibiotics and various chemotherapeutic agents. Persons who are beneath the recommended weight by 10 percent or more should see a doctor to determine if there is any physical problem causing the weight deficiency and to gain advice for modifying the diet to achieve a more desirable weight.

Concerns of the overfat

Excess fat is frequently a contributor to less than optimum physical and mental health. Just the fact that obesity is viewed as being unattractive in this country today is sufficient to make many people feel uncomfortable about their rotund appearance. Fashionable styles lose much of their flair when expanded to fit the stout figure. These problems may be sufficient to motivate some people to regain their normal and desirable weight. However, for anyone who is truly obese, there are also compelling physical reasons to attempt to bring body weight to a more nearly normal level and to maintain it there.

One of the annoying and sometimes hazardous complications of overweight is the difficulty in breathing. Obese people experience difficulty in exercising, due both to their awkward bodies and the buildup of carbon dioxide in the blood resulting from decreased respiratory capacity. Obese adults run a greater risk of developing diabetes, gall bladder disorders, and appendicitis. In fact, the frequency of most diseases is higher in obese than non-obese people, and the mortality rate from other diseases is also higher in the obese. Overweight during pregnancy can be a hazard to mother and fetus. Physically inactive people who are also overweight due to excessive fatty deposits are prime candidates for heart disease, particularly if they also smoke cigarettes, have some degree of hypertension (increased blood pressure), and have an elevated level of cholesterol and fat in their blood (see Chapter 16).

Table 4.1 provides a comparison between anticipated and actual deaths of overweight men and women between the ages of 25 and 74, as predicted and reported by the Metropolitan Life Insurance Company. Evidence does not support the conclusion that obesity by itself causes specific conditions that result in death, but it is clear from statistics such as those in Table 4.1 that obesity complicates most diseases, particularly cardiovascular-renal diseases such as coronary heart disease, cerebral hemorrhage, and chronic nephritis, and also complicates surgery.

The figures for deaths attributed to diabetes, cirrhosis of the liver, appendicitis, and biliary calculi are of interest because of the significant increase over the expected death rate; however, the cardiovascular statistics are of even greater concern because of the proportionately large number of deaths compared with deaths from other causes. Lest the record appear to be one-sided, the other side of the coin shows that

	Men		Women	
		Per Cent Actual of Expected		Per Cent Actual of Expected
Cause of Death	Deaths	Deaths	Deaths	Deaths
Principal cardiovascular-renal diseases	1867	149	1103	177
Organic heart disease, diseases of the coronary arteries and angina pectoris	1377	142	697	175
Organic heart disease	748	a	515	a
Coronary disease and angina pectoris	629	a	182	a
Cerebral hemorrhage	247	159	226	162
Chronic nephritis	243	191	180	212
Cancer, all forms	385	97	476	100
Stomach	62	85	34	86
Liver and gall bladder	33	168	46	211
Peritoneum, intestines and rectum	103	115	93	104
Pancreas	19	93	21	149
Respiratory organs	39	78[b]	—	—
Breast	—	—	81	69
Genital organs	—	—	132	107
Uterus	—	—	103	121
Leukemia and Hodgkins disease	26	100	23	110
Diabetes	205	383	235	372
Tuberculosis, all forms	24	21	20	35
Pneumonia, all forms	98	102	78	129
Cirrhosis of the liver	96	249	32	147
Appendicitis	76	293	41	195
Hernia and intestinal obstruction	39	154[b]	31	141[b]
Biliary calculi and other gall bladder diseases	32	152[b]	30	188[b]
Biliary calculi	19	206	50	284
Ulcer of stomach and duodenum	30	67	—	—
Puerperal conditions	—	—	43	162
Suicide	63	78	23	73
Accidents, total	177	111	74	135
Auto	76	131	27	120
Falls	32	131	—	—

[a] Satisfactory basis for comparison not available.
[b] Based on mortality rates on Standard risks for 1935–1939.
NOTE: Percentages which have been underlined indicate statistically significant deviations from experience on Standard risks.

the actual rate compared with the predicted rate of deaths from tuberculosis, suicide, and ulcers was significantly smaller than anticipated.

Although the health hazard from being overweight is significant from the standpoint of physical well-being, there are additional reasons for controlling weight. The greater happiness that one can experience as a result of being within the normal range is difficult to measure, but many formerly fat people are highly vocal regarding their increased self-confidence, reduced fatigue, pleasure in their appearance, and improved ease of physical movement. These benefits for living are sufficiently strong motivations to help some people adhere successfully to a weight reduction and control program.

Identifying Overweight

A clear appreciation of the problem of excessive body fat can be gained by visiting any public beach, although perhaps a cross section with a different bias could be viewed at most restaurants. Estimates for the incidence of excess weight in the United States vary widely, with 25 to 30 percent being a rough average. This approximation includes people classified as overweight (up to 20 percent heavier than the desirable weight) and obese (more than 20 percent heavier than the desirable figure). The exact proportion of people with excess weight is impossible to determine with conviction because the several different methods for measuring fatness give somewhat different results.

Body composition

Body composition is an important consideration in determining whether a person is too fat. Muscular men who have long been active in strenuous athletics frequently are overweight according to height-weight tables, and yet they

are not, in fact, overly fat. The extra weight is due to the disproportionately high amount of muscle tissue compared with the average body composition. However, overweight due to excess fat rather than an unusual amount of muscular development is the common nutritional problem. Unfortunately, athletes may form food patterns that provide more energy than needed when they become less active, and muscle tissue slowly is replaced with fat.

Densitometry

One reliable but distinctly cumbersome method of determining the lean body mass is by densitometry. Densitometry is done by immersing the subject in water. This method is based upon the fact that fat has a specific gravity of 0.92, a value somewhat less than that of water (1.0). In contrast, muscle tissue and bone together have a specific gravity of 1.1. The fat of the body, with its low specific gravity, contributes to the buoyancy of people in water; bones and muscle, being heavier than water, tend to sink. Thus a person with a large percentage of body fat will have a specific gravity value approaching 0.92. A very muscular individual with little fat will have a specific gravity close to 1.1.

Hydrometry

Hydrometry is another laboratory method for determining the relative fatness of a person indirectly. This measurement is accomplished by injecting deuterium oxide into the body. After the substance has had time to be distributed throughout the body, a blood sample is taken. By measuring the dilution of the deuterium oxide in the blood, a series of calculations can be made to determine the amount of fat in the body.

Potassium[40]

Another indirect means of calculating body composition is counting the gamma rays that

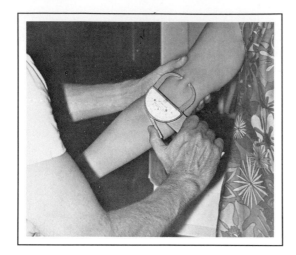

Calipers provide an accurate assessment of body fatness.

the triceps (at the midpoint of the back of the upper arm with the arm hanging freely) and subscapular (at bottom of the angle of the right scapula with the shoulder and arm relaxed) skinfolds are generally the preferred measure-

Table 4.2 *Obesity Standards for Caucasian Americans*[a]

Age (years)	Skinfold Measurements[b]	
	Males	Females
5	12	14
6	12	15
7	13	16
8	14	17
9	15	18
10	16	20
11	17	21
12	18	22
13	18	23
14	17	23
15	16	24
16	15	25
17	14	26
18	15	27
19	15	27
20	16	28
21	17	28
22	18	28
23	18	28
24	19	28
25	20	29
26	20	29
27	21	29
28	22	29
29	23	29
30-50	23	30

[a] In M. C. Latham, et al. **Scope Manual on Nutrition.** Upjohn Co. Kalamazoo, Mich. 1970. Appendix D. (Adapted from C. C. Seltzer and J. Mayer. A simple criterion of obesity. **Postgrad. Med. 38:** 101–107. 1965.)

[b] Minimum triceps skinfold thickness in millimeters indicating obesity. (Figures represent the logarithmic means of the frequency distributions plus one standard deviation.)

are constantly given off by the potassium[40] naturally present in the body. The measurement provides information on the amount of potassium in relation to body size. Interpretation of the body composition is based on the fact that fat contains essentially no potassium. Thus, a high potassium count in relation to total body size is indicative of little fat tissue; a low value characterizes obesity.

Anthropometric measurements

Anthropometric measurements are made with varying degrees of sophistication. The simplest, that of using a flexible steel tape to measure circumference of the chest, abdomen, and buttocks, and other areas, is used infrequently for surveys. Occasionally, X rays are used to study bone, fatty deposits, and muscle diameter. Although a simple pinch test[2] can be done by individuals any time, more accurate assessment of fatty deposits is made using special calipers that exert 10 grams pressure per square millimeter of any skinfold, regardless of the thickness. Although several sites can be used,

[2] Lift skin and fat away from the body by pinching with the thumb and index finger at back of upper arm, beneath the shoulder blade, or over the abdomen. Measure the thickness of the skinfold. (Normal values are between ½ and 1 inch.)

ments. Such measurements are quick to do and provide a more direct and accurate assessment of overfatness than weighing (Table 4.2).

Two methods have long been available to individuals evaluating their weight status. Much can be determined simply by looking in the mirror when stripped. Height-weight tables are less precise than anthropometric measures, but they are useful in making a rough determination of whether a person's weight is within the desirable range for his body build (see Table 4.3). The differentiation on the basis of frame is

Table 4.3   Desirable Weights for Men and Women of Age 25 and Over[a]

| | Height (in Shoes) | Weight in Pounds (in Indoor Clothing) | | |
		Small Frame	Medium Frame	Large Frame
Men	5′ 2″	112-120	118-129	126-141
	3″	115-123	121-133	129-144
	4″	118-126	124-136	132-148
	5″	121-129	127-139	135-152
	6″	124-133	130-143	138-156
	7″	128-137	134-147	142-161
	8″	132-141	138-152	147-166
	9″	136-145	142-156	151-170
	10″	140-150	146-160	155-174
	11″	144-154	150-165	159-179
	6′ 0″	148-158	154-170	164-184
	1″	152-162	158-175	168-189
	2″	156-167	162-180	173-194
	3″	160-171	167-185	178-199
	4″	164-175	172-190	182-204
Women	4′ 10″	92- 98	96-107	104-119
	11″	94-101	98-110	106-122
	5′ 0″	96-104	101-113	109-125
	1″	99-107	104-116	112-128
	2″	102-110	107-119	115-131
	3″	105-113	110-122	118-134
	4″	108-116	113-126	121-138
	5″	111-119	116-130	125-142
	6″	114-123	120-135	129-146
	7″	118-127	124-139	133-150
	8″	122-131	128-143	137-154
	9″	126-135	132-147	141-158
	10″	130-140	136-151	145-163
	11″	134-144	140-155	149-168
	6′ 0″	138-148	144-159	153-173

[a] Reproduced by permission of the Metropolitan Life Insurance Company. Data are based on weights associated with lowest mortality. To obtain weight for adults younger than 25, subtract one pound for each year under 25.

helpful because of the variation in bone structure, but similar adjustments for musculature are not available. Even the variations based on frame size have their limitations since there are no definitions of frame size. The desire to be classified as being within the appropriate weight range has prompted more than one basically honest individual to classify his small or medium frame as a large one, thus gaining an important increase in approved weight. The weights listed in Table 4.3 are desirable weights, as developed by insurance actuaries. Actually, the average weight for people in the categories listed would be appreciably higher than these values.

Energy

Measuring energy

The word "Calorie" is sprinkled generously into innumerable conversations across the country, but its actual definition is rather vague to the average person. As the term is used in nutrition work, Calorie is defined as the amount of heat energy needed to raise the temperature of 1 kilogram of water 1 Celsius degree. Although "Calorie" is most commonly used as the term to denote the heat energy available in a food, a more accurate expression (and one gaining increasing acceptance and usage) is to call this unit a kilocalorie because it is 1000 times as large as the calorie unit used by physical scientists (heat energy required to raise the temperature of 1 gram of water 1 Celsius degree).[3]

In the past, the usual way used by nutritionists to denote this "large Calorie" was to spell the word with a capital C; and this usage and even calories with a small "c" still are used by many. When reading nutrition literature, calories, Calories, and kilocalories are considered to be synonymous with the common definition given earlier in this section.

The value of kilocalories becomes somewhat clearer with illustrations of the energy available from some foods when they are burned: 1 tablespoon of jelly provides sufficient kilocalories

to raise the temperature of 1 kilogram (a little over 4 cups) of water 29 Celsius degrees; the kilocalories in 1 teaspoon ($\frac{1}{3}$ tablespoon) of butter or margarine are sufficient to raise the temperature of the same amount of water 33 Celsius degrees; and the white of one egg provides sufficient kilocalories to raise the temperature of 1 kilogram of water 15 Celsius degrees.

In today's calorie-conscious society, the energy value of foods is of considerable interest. These values have been ascertained for many foods commonly eaten in this country. Total caloric intake can be determined on a daily basis by keeping an accurate record of amounts of all foods eaten and then adding the kilocalories, as indicated in the Appendix (Food Composition Tables).

Direct calorimetry

The bomb calorimeter is an instrument for direct calorimetry that is widely used for ascertaining the caloric content of foods. Basically, the bomb calorimeter is simply a device in which a dried food sample is burned in oxygen and the amount of energy released by the burning is measured. To accomplish this, the bomb calorimeter is designed as a very well-insulated cube containing a known volume of water surrounding a small chamber or bomb containing the food sample, oxygen, and an electric ignition device. By burning the dried

[3] Recently there has been a suggestion to use the joule rather than the calorie. One kilocalorie = 4180 joules.

food sample completely and measuring the change in the temperature of the water surrounding the bomb, calculations of the energy value of the food can be made.

The values obtained by use of the bomb calorimeter are a measure of the energy available from the food itself. Specifically, an average of 4.1 kilocalories is released from each gram of pure carbohydrate, 9.45 kilocalories from a gram of pure fat, and 5.65 kilocalories per gram of protein. For practical application to humans, these figures can be converted into the values that represent the energy that is actually available to the body after digestion and metabolism of the material.

The coefficient of digestibility (the percent of food actually used by the body) obviously is another factor that must be considered in determining the physiological fuel value (energy actually available to the body from food). For carbohydrate, the coefficient of digestibility is 98 percent; for fat, it is 95 percent; and for protein, it is 92 percent. After these factors are incorporated, the average amount of energy available to the body from each gram of pure substance is approximately 4 kilocalories for carbohydrate, 9 kilocalories for fat, and 4 kilocalories for protein. For an approximation of caloric content, the energy from carbohydrate is obtained by multiplying as follows: $4 \times$ grams of carbohydrate eaten = kilocalories from carbohydrate. Similarly, fat is calculated for approximate energy value: $9 \times$ grams of fat eaten = kilocalories from fat. Protein uses the same factor as carbohydrate, namely: $4 \times$ grams of protein eaten = kilocalories from protein.

Indirect calorimetry

The oxycalorimeter is an indirect means of determining the heat energy available from foods. The oxygen consumed and the carbon dioxide formed are measured by this instrument as the food is burned. This method is seldom used.

Energy requirements

Basal metabolism and calorie needs

To compute the total number of kilocalories an individual should eat each day to maintain his weight, it is necessary to determine kilocalorie requirements for three different components of life: basal metabolism, activity, and specific dynamic effect. Basal metabolism is the amount of energy required to maintain the body functions, exclusive of activity and digestive processes. Maintenance functions for which the body requires energy include the functioning of vital organs and glands, breathing, metabolism in the cells, blood circulation, and maintenance of body temperature. Each individual has his own unique basal metabolism and thus requires an amount of energy for maintaining his body that may vary from the amount needed by someone else. The speed at which his body operates and requires energy is termed his basal metabolic rate.

Measuring basal metabolism

The technique commonly used by physicians and researchers to determine basal metabolic needs is an indirect calorimetric method. The Benedict-Roth respiration instrument measures the oxygen consumed by the subject as he breathes for a definite length of time in a closed system designed to remove the carbon dioxide and water generated during the experiment. A second indirect method is designed to permit the subject to breathe air and to measure the carbon dioxide exhaled. In either of these methods, the subject must be well rested, in a postabsorptive state (no food for at least 12 hours prior to the test), free from anxiety, and lying awake in a room that is a comfortable temperature.

Direct calorimetric measurements of basal metabolism can be made by placing the subject in a chamber that, similar to the bomb calorimeter, is well insulated. The temperature change

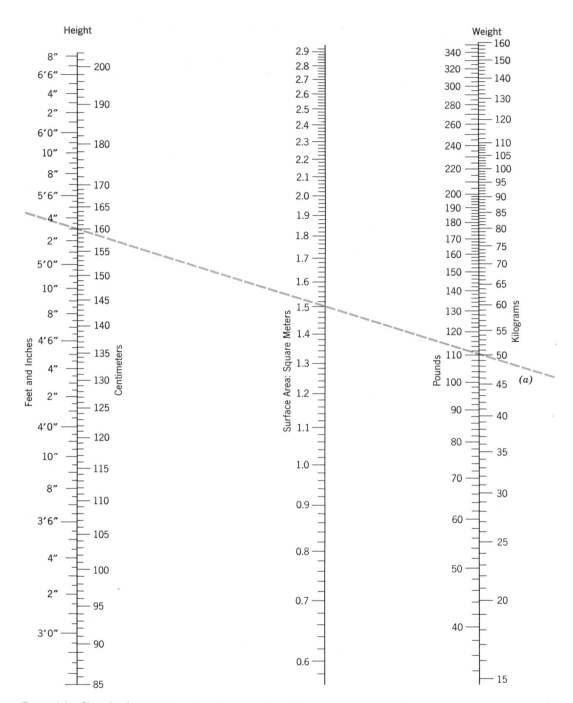

Figure 4.1   Chart for determination of surface area. Dotted line (a) represents the line that would be drawn to determine the value of 1.5 square meters used in the sample calculation in the text. (From Boothby, Berkson, and Dunn in "Studies of the Energy Metabolism of Normal Individuals, a Standard for Basal Metabolism, with a Nomogram for Clinical Application," *American Journal of Physiology, 116:* 468—484, 1936. Courtesy of the authors and publishers.)

in a known volume of water circulating in pipes at the top of the chamber is measured to determine basal metabolism of the subject.

A blood test for determining the amount of protein-bound iodine is a far more convenient and accurate laboratory test for basal metabolic rate. This laboratory test measures the amount of iodine that is chemically bound to protein in the plasma. A value within the range of 3.5 to 7.5 milligrams per milliliter of serum indicates a normal rate.

A rough estimate of the energy needed by normal individuals for basal metabolism may be calculated by using Figure 4.1 and Table 4.4. The first step is to draw a line between a person's exact height (left column, Figure 4.1) and his weight (right column, Figure 4.1) to derive the surface area. The number of square meters of surface area is then multiplied by the correct caloric value from Table 4.4 to determine hourly caloric needs for basal metabolism and then multiplied by 24 to calculate the daily need. A sample calculation is presented in the table below.

The sample calculation represents the total energy needed by the subject for basal metabolism in 24 hours. Note that body size is of significance in the calculation. Thus a young child will have a smaller amount of surface area and thus a smaller total energy need for basal metabolism than will an adult man despite the fact that the child has a higher basal metabolic *rate* than the man.

Factors influencing basal metabolic rate

A person's basal metabolic rate is not a value that remains constant throughout his life (Table 4.4). At birth the rate is relatively high, but rises still higher until approximately the age of two. From that point on, the normal individual undergoes a very slow reduction in rate throughout life. Women experience a drop in basal metabolic rate during the early stage of pregnancy; this is followed by an increase to a value almost one fifth greater than normal during the last stages of pregnancy and continuing into lactation.

The change in metabolic rate is of special interest in adulthood. The National Research Council, in comparing subsequent values for basal metabolism with that at age 25, suggests a decline of 2.5 percent in each 10-year period between ages 20 and 40; 5 percent drop between 40 and 50; 7.5 percent between 50 and 60; 10 percent between 60 and 70; and 12.5 percent after 70 years of age. Note that there is a significantly greater decline as one moves beyond the age of 40. This drop in basal metabolic rate means that the individual needs less energy to maintain vital body functions than he did earlier in his adult life. If the tendency to eat the same amount of food as in early adulthood is followed, a gradual weight gain will result from the mere reduction of basal metabolic rate. The increased incidence of overweight among the middle aged compared

---

Sample Calculation of Basal Metabolism

Surface area of person 5 feet 3 inches tall, weighing 110 pounds	**= 1.5 square meters**
Basal metabolism standard for female— age 18	**= 35.8 kilocalories/square meter/hour**
Hours in day	**= 24**
35.8 × 1.5	**= 53.70 = hourly caloric need**
53.70 × 24	**= 1288.80 kilocalories needed daily for basal metabolism**

Table 4.4 Basal Metabolism Standards: Man[a]

Age (yr)	Males (cal per sq m per hr)	Females (cal per sq m per hr)	Age (yr)	Males (cal per sq m per hr)	Females (cal per sq m per hr)
3	60.1	54.5	26	38.2	35.0
4	57.9	53.9	27	38.0	35.0
5	56.3	53.0			
6	54.0	51.2	28	37.8	35.0
7	52.3	49.7	29	37.7	35.0
			30	37.6	35.0
8	50.8	48.0	31	37.4	35.0
9	49.5	46.2	32	37.2	34.9
10	47.7	44.9			
11	46.5	43.5	33	37.1	34.9
12	45.3	42.0	34	37.0	34.9
			35	36.9	34.8
13	44.5	40.5	36	36.8	34.7
14	43.8	39.2	37	36.7	34.6
15	42.9	38.3			
16	42.0	37.2	38	36.7	34.5
17	41.5	36.4	39	36.6	34.4
			40-44	36.4	34.1
18	40.8	35.8	45-49	36.2	33.8
19	40.5	35.4	50-54	35.8	33.1
20	39.9	35.3			
21	39.5	35.2	55-59	35.1	32.8
22	39.2	35.2	60-64	34.5	32.0
			65-69	33.5	31.6
23	39.0	35.2	70-74	32.7	31.1
24	38.7	35.1	75+	31.8	
25	38.4	35.1			

[a] From Boothby, in **Handbook of Biological Data,** 1956. W. S. Spector, editor. Reprinted courtesy W. B. Saunders Co., Philadelphia. These values are smoothed means of basal calories per sq. m. per hr. from the three largest and most authoritative sets of standards. The British standards (Robertson and Reid) are based on 987 males and 1323 females; the Mayo Foundation standards (Boothby, Berkson, and Dunn) are based on 639 males and 828 females; the Carnegie Nutrition Laboratory standards (Harris and Benedict) are based on 136 males and 103 females.

with the young is attributable, in large measure, to slower basal metabolism and less physical activity.

Body composition also influences basal metabolic needs. More energy is needed for the metabolic activities in muscle and glandular tissues than in fatty tissues. This means that active people who have developed an abundance of muscle tissue and minimized their fatty deposits normally will have a faster metabolic rate than obese, sedentary individuals. Consistent with this observation is the fact that women, as a group, have a somewhat slower basal metabolic rate than men because of the characteristic male musculature and lean body in comparison with the somewhat less muscular, more rounded female physique.

Two endocrine glands, the adrenal and the thyroid, secrete hormones that have important influences on the basal metabolic rate. The adrenal gland secretes adrenaline, which is released during periods of high emotion, causing an acceleration in basal metabolic rate (BMR) for as long as 2 or 3 hours. Although this alteration of BMR is of interest, the effect of adrenaline is not of long enough duration to have lasting influence upon bodily caloric needs.

Thyroxine, an iodine-containing hormone, has a highly significant effect on basal metabolic rate. When thyroxine is secreted at a normal rate, most individuals will require approximately 1 kilocalorie per kilogram body weight per hour to meet basal metabolic needs. On that basis a 50-kilogram (110-pound) woman would need 1200 kilocalories per day for basal metabolism, compared with 1920 kilocalories for a man weighing 80 kilograms (176 pounds). This requirement may vary as much as 10 percent in either direction and still be considered normal. However, when the thyroid gland malfunctions and secretes an abnormal amount of thyroxine, basal metabolic rates may vary significantly from the average value. When the thyroxine production is reduced, the condition is known as hypothyroidism and is accompanied by a definite reduction or slowing of basal metabolic rate. This condition can result in weight gain because fewer calories are needed for basal metabolism, and yet the diet is likely to include approximately as much food as would be eaten if the thyroxine level were normal. Hypothyroidism is treated successfully by administering carefully controlled amounts of thyroid extract under a doctor's advice and care. The converse situation, that of too much thyroxine, results in hyperthyroidism, a condition marked by an accelerated basal metabolic rate. As would be predicted, the body's need for calories for basal metabolism is greatly increased in hyperthyroidism. Some success in treating hyperthyroidism is usually achieved by surgery to reduce the size of the thyroid gland.

Small influences on basal metabolic rate have been noted under varying conditions. During periods of starvation, the body exercises optimum utilization of calories ingested by slightly reducing the basal metabolic rate. The effect of sleep is not fully agreed upon by all, since the calories needed are influenced not only by the slowing of body processes during sleep, but also by the relatively strenuous activities of some sleepers. When a person is ill and has a fever, the basal metabolic rate increases sharply. This is in contrast to the minimal metabolic variations that occur as a result of environmental temperature changes.

Activity and calorie requirements

In addition to the energy required to maintain basal metabolism, energy is required for all physical activity. The actual number of calories expended in activity in a day is dependent on one's body weight, the vigorousness of the activity, and the duration of the work performed. Table 4.5 indicates the difference in caloric requirements for a heavy person and a light person to perform the same task. The point may be clarified still more by comparing the 1500 foot-pounds of work required to raise a 100-pound body 15 feet and the 3000 foot-pounds needed to raise a 200-pound body 15 feet.

Simply by watching children playing on the school grounds, one can easily see that some people are very vigorous in their motions and that they are active a far larger fraction of the time than other individuals who are seemingly content to play quietly or sit and watch the world go by. An interesting comparison of energy expenditure in relation to rate or vigorousness of activity is provided by Taylor and

McLeod[4] who reported that the expenditure in kilocalories per kilogram per hour for playing music by Mendelssohn on the piano was 0.8; for playing Beethoven's "Appassionata Sonata" it was 1.4; and for playing Liszt's "Tarantella" it was 2.0. Music lovers who have heard these works performed by musicians of varying competence will quickly recognize that these figures are standardized on the basis of the average performer, for certainly some players perform with considerably more flourish and physical abandonment than others.

The duration of various physical activities is greatly influenced by the occupation of the individual. Students often are disconcerted to find that their sedentary yet demanding tasks of

[4] C. M. Taylor, and G. McLeod. *Rose's Laboratory Handbook for Dietetics*. 5th ed. P. 18. Macmillan. New York. 1949.

studying, reading, and writing expend only 0.4 kilocalories per kilogram per hour, while walking at the rate of 3 miles per hour expends 2.0 kilocalories per kilogram per hour. With today's values on intellectual accomplishments, one might regret that the brain can operate so efficiently on so little energy.

Tables listing energy requirements for various activities are of two general types: those listing energy for activity only and those with figures that include basal metabolic energy needs plus those for activity. Table 4.5 includes the kilocalories required for basal metabolism, and Table 4.6 is an example of the type that does not include basal needs.

Several examples of energy expenditures for activities are listed in Table 4.6. Note that the figures are in kilocalories per kilogram per pound. This table represents a somewhat dif-

Table 4.5 *Energy Used for Some Routine Daily Activities*

Activity	Calories per lb per hour[b]	Weight (lb)[a]					
		120	140	160	180	200	220
		Calories Used per Hour					
Sleeping	0.4	48	56	64	72	80	88
Awake, lying still	0.5	60	70	80	90	100	110
Sitting quietly (TV)	0.6	72	84	96	108	120	132
Eating	0.7	84	98	112	126	140	154
Writing	0.7	84	98	112	126	140	154
Standing relaxed	0.8	96	112	128	144	160	176
Dressing and undressing	0.9	108	126	144	162	180	198
Driving automobile	1.0	120	140	160	180	200	220
Dishwashing	1.0	120	140	160	180	200	220
Ironing	1.0	120	140	160	180	200	220
Typing rapidly	1.0	120	140	160	180	200	220
Light laundry	1.1	132	154	176	198	220	242
Walking (3 mph)	1.5	180	210	240	270	300	330
Sweeping with vacuum cleaner	1.9	228	266	304	342	380	418

[a] For those of different weights than those listed, multiply actual weight in pounds by the calories per pound per hour for each activity (e.g., 154 lb × 0.4 = 62 calories per hour for sleeping). This chart may be used to calculate approximate daily caloric expenditure if approximate amounts of time for each activity are tabulated for an average 24-hour day.

[b] Calculated to include basal metabolic needs.

Table 4.6   *Energy Used for Some Routine Daily Activities (excluding basal metabolism and influence of food)*[a]

Activity	cal. per kg per hr	Activity	cal. per kg per hr
Bicycling (century run)	7.6	Piano playing (Beethoven's *Appassionata*)	1.4
Bicycling (moderate speed)	2.5	Piano playing (Liszt's *Tarantella*)	2.0
Bookbinding	0.8	Reading aloud	0.4
Boxing	11.4	Rowing in race	16.0
Carpentry (heavy)	2.3	Running	7.0
Cello playing	1.3	Sawing wood	5.7
Crocheting	0.4	Sewing, hand	0.4
Dancing, foxtrot	3.8	Sewing, motor driven machine	0.4
Dancing, waltz	3.0	Shoemaking	1.0
Dishwashing	1.0	Singing in loud voice	0.8
Dressing and undressing	0.7	Sitting quietly	0.4
Driving automobile	0.9	Skating	3.5
Eating	0.4	Skiing (moderate speed)	10.3
Exercise		Standing relaxed	0.5
Very light	0.9	Stone masonry	4.7
Light	1.4	Sweeping with broom, bare floor	1.4
Moderate	3.1	Sweeping with carpet sweeper	1.6
Severe	5.4	Sweeping with vacuum sweeper	2.7
Very severe	7.6	Swimming (2 mph)	7.9
Fencing	7.3	Tailoring	0.9
Horseback riding, walk	1.4	Typewriting rapidly	
Horseback riding, trot	4.3	(standard typewriter)	1.0
Horseback riding, gallop	6.7	(electric typewriter)	0.5
Ironing (5 lb iron)	1.0	Violin playing	0.6
Knitting sweater	0.7	Walking (3 mph)	2.0
Laundry, light	1.3	Walking rapidly (4 mph)	3.4
Lying still, awake	0.1	Walking at high speed (5.3 mph)	8.3
Organ playing (1/3 hand work)	1.5	Walking down stairs	b
Painting furniture	1.5	Walking up stairs	c
Paring potatoes	0.6	Washing floors	1.2
Playing ping pong	4.4	Writing	0.4
Piano playing (Mendelssohn's *Song without Words*)	0.8		

[a] Adapted with permission of The Macmillan Company from *Foundations of Nutrition,* 6th ed., by Taylor and Pye. © The Macmillan Company, 1967.

[b] Allow 0.012 calorie per kilogram for an ordinary staircase with 15 steps, without regard to time.

[c] Allow 0.036 calorie per kilogram for an ordinary staircase with 15 steps, without regard to time.

ferent calculation than that found in Table 4.5, in which the values are kilocalories per pound per hour and have been calculated to include basal metabolic needs during the hour as well as the activity requirement.

Specific dynamic action

Energy is required to convert and transport food from the form in which it is eaten to the many individual nutrients needed by cells throughout the body. This utilization of food is referred to as specific dynamic action, and the energy costs need to be included in computing total caloric expenditure. An exact figure to allow for the specific dynamic action of food is not possible, because a mixed diet varies in protein, carbohydrate, and fat composition from day to day. Pure protein requires about 30 percent of its potential energy simply for the body to utilize it, carbohydrate requires about 6 percent, and fat is intermediate. The specific dynamic action of food is observed by individuals when they become slightly warm after eating a large meal. This effect is somewhat more distinct for persons on a high-protein diet, due to the higher specific dynamic action of

Table 4.7 *Estimated Daily Calorie Requirement for a Female 18 Years Old (body surface = 1.5 square meters, wt. 50 kilograms)*

Calculations					kcal (24 hr)
Basal metabolism					
35.8 × 1.5 × 24 = 1289 kcal					
kcal/sq m/hr age 18 female = 35.8[a]					1289
Surface area (5′3″) = 1.5[b]					
Hours = 24					
Activity					
	Time (hr)	kcal/hr[c]	(kg)	kcal[d]	
Dressing	1	× 0.7	× 50 =	35	
Eating	1	× 0.4	× 50 =	20	
Driving	2	× 0.9	× 50 =	90	
Studying	8	× 0.4	× 50 =	160	
Walking	2	× 2.0	× 50 =	200	
Watching TV	2	× 0.4	× 50 =	40	
Sleeping	8			—	
	24			545 kcal	545
Specific dynamic action					
Basal metabolism	1289				
Activity	545				
	1834 kcal				
1834 × 10% = 183					183
			Total		2017

[a] From Table 4.4.
[b] From Figure 4.1.
[c] From Table 4.6.
[d] Time × kcal/hr × (kg) = kcal required.

Table 4.8 *Estimated Daily Caloric Requirement Using Figures That Include Basal Needs in the Activity Value*[a]

Activity	kcal/lb/hr[b]	Hr spent	kcal
Dressing/undressing	0.9	1	110
Walking (3 mph)	1.5	2	330
Eating	0.7	1	77
Studying and class	0.7	8	616
Driving car	1.0	2	220
Sitting quietly	0.6	2	132
Sleeping	0.4	8	352
Total		24	1837

Specific dynamic action = 1837 × 10% = 184 kcal
Total needs for day = 1837 + 184 = 2021 kcal

[a] Subject used is 110 lb (50 kg) girl.
[b] Data from Table 4.5.

protein. On mixed diets, such as those typically consumed, the energy allowance for the specific dynamic action of food is approximately 10 percent or less of the calories needed for basal metabolism and activity. Diets high in protein foods are not more effective in weight reduction because of the higher specific dynamic action of protein. Such diets are also usually high in fat and thus tend to lower the specific dynamic action of protein.

Total energy requirements

A quick approximation of the energy needs of a normal individual can be obtained simply by finding the appropriate age and sex category in Table 1.8. This figure is general and does not indicate the differences in caloric ex-penditures for persons with wide variations from the activity or weight of the average person. More precise calculations of individual needs are made by adding together the calories needed for (1) basal metabolism, (2) physical activity, and (3) specific dynamic effect. Calculations for basal metabolic needs are derived using Figure 4.1 and Table 4.4. Energy needs for activity are calculated from Table 4.6. The estimate of energy for specific dynamic action is obtained by adding the number of kilocalories for basal metabolism and physical activity and multiplying this figure by 10 percent. Table 4.7 illustrates the calculation.

Calculations that utilize figures from tables for activity in which basal metabolic needs are already incorporated with the energy for activity are somewhat simpler. The use of such figures is illustrated in Table 4.8.

Controlling Body Fatness

The final step in presenting the picture of the effect of diet on weight control is the comparison of the actual caloric intake with the expenditure of calories for activity, basal metabolism, and specific dynamic action over a 24-hour period. If the calories expended equal those consumed, the net result for the individual is maintenance of weight with neither a loss nor a gain for the day. However, if the intake is greater than the expenditure, weight is gained. When this happens, the individual is said to be in positive caloric balance. Conversely, a calorie intake that provides less energy than the body requires, known as negative caloric balance, results in weight loss.

Positive caloric balance is desirable during growth and pregnancy, but gradually leads to obesity during other periods of life. Negative caloric balance is the desired and necessary condition when weight is to be lost. Weight reduction diets are based on plans that provide fewer calories than needed for the total operation of the body during the day. In times of negative caloric balance, the body's reserves are drawn upon for the remainder of energy needed, but not supplied by the diet. On the other hand, persons of desirable weight who are not pregnant, growing, or recuperating from illness will need to eat food containing just the number of calories required to maintain the state of caloric equilibrium. Obviously, caloric intake will vary somewhat from day to day. The effect of caloric intake on body weight actually needs to be considered over an extended period of time to gain a realistic picture of weight control.

Diagnosing the problem

Weight control can best be accomplished by a continuing, but not a neurotic interest in remaining at the recommended weight in relation to height. Weight problems are far easier to correct when they begin to develop than when one has accumulated an excess of many pounds. A simple bathroom scale is sufficient to monitor weight. Preferably the measurement is made weekly on the same scales at the same time of day and with the same amount of clothing or in the nude, so that variables and excuses are minimized. If a person is as much as 10 percent or 10 pounds above or below his

recommended weight for his height, there is wisdom in considering a sensible weight control program. For extremes much beyond this, a physician should be consulted. Lesser variations can generally be corrected by following the general guidelines given in the remainder of this chapter.

If weight needs to be altered for improved appearance and general health, the next step is to determine what caused the problem to develop. Frequently, extra weight is the result of a very gradual accumulation caused by a combination of reduced activity and lowered basal metabolic rate during adulthood without a concurrent reduction in food intake. In some situations, the weight problem can be traced directly to an emotional problem that needs to be understood. Family pressures may have molded an environment that has led directly to obesity. The reasons for persons overeating are numerous and quite individualized, but weight control is most likely to be successful when the causative agent is determined and corrected while the dietary and activity habits are being modified.

Ingredients of successful weight control

Weight control programs can only be viewed as successful if they enable individuals not only to achieve the desired weight, but then also to maintain themselves at this level instead of gradually regaining weight. To accomplish the long-range goal of continued weight maintenance requires a modification in both dietary *and* activity patterns, since these are factors that caused the original weight problem to develop. It is apparent then that successful diet programs have a twofold concern: (1) adjustment of total caloric intake to provide for an encouraging rate of weight change that results in achieving the recommended weight, and (2) retraining of dietary habits to a pattern sufficiently pleasing to the individual to enable him to follow the new pattern in preference to the earlier one.

The rate at which weight should or can be gained or lost is influenced by the patience of the individual and by the amount of change needed. In extreme cases where 50 or more pounds need to be lost, weight loss may be quite rapid at first. For most people, a goal of 1 pound per week is achievable and sufficiently rapid to encourage continuing the diet. The elimination of approximately 3500 kilocalories each week (500 kilocalories per day) is needed to accomplish this objective. Another alternative is to undertake enough physical activity (beyond that done normally) to expend 500 additional kilocalories each day while leaving the food intake constant. A practical solution is a moderate increase in physical activity and some reduction in caloric intake.

The dieter must recognize that change in fluid balance, either loss or retention of fluid, will cause a change in weight. These changes can be gradual or sudden. Water retention doubtless contributes to the discouragement some people experience early in their weight control attempts. They may find their weight remaining high despite decreased caloric intake and more activity. Actually, fatty deposits are being depleted, but body weight will not reflect this until the osmotic imbalance is adjusted and water excreted. Studies of the manner in which fat is gained and lost from adipose tissues have revealed that adults do not develop additional fat cells when they gain weight. Instead, the additional fat storage is accomplished by increasing the size of these cells. The reverse situation is found in weight reduction studies, that is, adipose cells decrease in size, but not in number (Salans, et al., 1971).

To be successful, reducing diets need to be followed carefully, a practice generally achieved only by people who are convinced that they need to lose weight. There must be a strong internal motivation (usually either a desire to improve appearance or to reduce a health threat) that enables people to resist their former habits and strive to maintain the new

diet pattern. Most people stray badly from their diets when they are being nagged by someone else who feels the diet is important. Many people are helped when they have either a doctor or a friend, usually not a family member, who is interested and encouraging, but such a boost is effective only when the dieter himself is a determined and willing participant.

Additional physical activity beyond that which has previously been a part of the regular routine is a boon to weight reduction. Ideally, the exercise will be in the form of a sport or other activity enjoyed by the dieter. The benefits are threefold: (1) some calories are expended in the activity, (2) muscle tone is improved, and (3) doing something enjoyable helps to divert the mind from thoughts of food. The exercise need not be extremely taxing to accomplish some progress toward the desired weight loss. A program of sports participation or exercise on a daily basis is necessary if much is to be accomplished. An hourly session once a week is of limited value to the dieter compared with a schedule of moderately increased activity every day. If the weight problem resulted from constant nibbling because of a lack of anything interesting to do, the dieter may find it far easier to stay on his diet if he acquires some new interest or hobby that keeps his mind occupied and also increases his physical activity.

Of course, one of the most crucial parts of a weight control plan is the diet itself. There seems to be a never-ending array of diet plans bombarding the public today. Many of these are quite inappropriate for persons needing to lose weight because they are based on unusual diet plans designed more to catch the eye of the public than to provide the basis for retraining dietary habits. A good weight reducing diet is based on the Basic Four but is planned for smaller portions and uses few energy-rich foods. A diet based on this broad nutritional foundation is recommended strongly because the variety of foods is interesting to eat on a continuing basis and supplies the nutrients needed for good health. Many people will

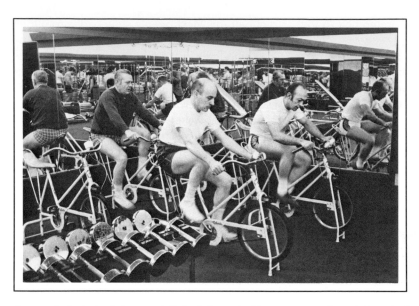

Increased physical activity on a daily basis is a valuable component of a weight control program.

experience satisfactory weight losses by reducing caloric intake by approximately 500 kilocalories per day. Individuals who have been eating a diet that contributes significantly more energy than is needed for maintenance may need to reduce caloric intake much more sharply to begin to actually lose weight. If the dieter is already following the Basic Four Food Group Plan, but is eating just a little too much, the diet can simply be a reduction in the size and number of servings eaten in a day. The direction of the dieter's thoughts should be toward concern for reducing the waist rather than reducing the waste! The simple act of preparing and serving smaller quantities of food can take care of the surpluses that formerly were eaten by the dieter.

Where more control is required for satisfactory weight loss, the elimination of desserts, smaller servings of meats and fat-containing foods, and larger servings of fruits and vegetables are useful changes.

Another consideration in developing a diet plan that is acceptable to a person and also reasonably satisfying is the frequency of eating. Young et al., 1971, tested the effects of varying meal frequencies in weight reduction. In their study, which tested three meal patterns (six meals, three, or one meal daily), subjects considered six meals a day a bother. This group favored three meals daily, and few liked having one meal only. Based on these findings, dieters may wish to divide their total intake for the day into the number of meals they prefer. For those who enjoy frequent meals or snacks, six small meals may be a pleasing way to diet. If others find it difficult to stop eating at a meal, but do not mind spacing their meals at longer intervals, three meals or even less might be a more satisfactory routine.

For some people, a few psychological crutches may be helpful in staying on a diet. The small act of putting a sign on the refrigerator stating "Taste makes waist" is sufficient to help halt the nibbling dieter who really wants to lose weight. By avoiding buying unnecessary food items such as candy and potato chips, considerable temptation is removed. Others may gain strength from maintaining a chart of their weight loss from week to week. The group therapy that is accomplished when several dieters talk about their problems together may help some people face dieting with fortitude and success. Some people gain the necessary motivation by buying a new outfit one size smaller than the size that fits at the beginning of the diet. The motivations vary in their effectiveness with different people, but a little ingenuity may enable one to discover a suitable device for helping the dieter stay on his plan instead of yielding to temptation. A reducing diet can be very difficult for some individuals, particularly those who are trying to modify the dietary patterns of a lifetime; psychological aids may be of great value to them and, indeed may be a critical key to success.

A good reducing diet provides variety. Diets that are monotonous readily tempt a person to eat other foods simply to relieve the boredom. In addition, diets (such as the grapefruit diet) that are limited in variety will be lacking in some of the essential nutrients. Simply reducing the amount of fat in the diet, substituting nonfat milk for whole milk, taking smaller helpings, and refusing second servings will provide a reasonable starting point for planning a satisfying and successful diet. The inclusion of foods that are favorites and adding some new foods makes the diet interesting.

Guidelines for successful dieting

1. Adjust serving size to meet the dieter's needs, so that the total caloric intake from all the food eaten during the day is at least 500 kilocalories less than previously eaten. Meat portions, which traditionally are larger than nutritionally necessary in the United States, can be reduced to 3-ounce servings. Pats of butter or margarine can be cut in half (or the whipped products can be used) so that less fat and fewer calories are included in the diet from these sources.

2. The standard half-cup servings of vegetables can be maintained, or even increased occasionally, to help the dieter achieve a satisfied feeling at the table without consuming a large number of calories. Some dieters have better success in controlling portion sizes if they measure them until they become familiar with the appearance of servings of the desired size. Calories in snacks can mount up quickly. If snacks are essential, foods low in calories are best. Coffee, tea, Sanka, bouillon, pickles, raw vegetables, or a little raw fruit will add a minimal amount of calories to the day's intake.

3. Zest can be added to meals by using spices and herbs imaginatively and using much less salt.

4. Sugar, honey, syrup, fruits canned in heavy syrup, and other sweets, flour, and cornstarch should be used sparingly.

5. Reduce fat intake by such devices as carefully trimming fat from meat, avoiding frequent use of fried foods, nuts, sauces, gravies, and salad dressings, and using diet margarines or reducing the quantity of fats and oils used.

6. All beverages, with the exception of water, plain tea, black coffee, and low-calorie soft drinks, contribute to the day's caloric intake and must be included in calculating the total caloric intake. Alcoholic beverages, depending on the amount of alcohol, are generous in calories. Pure alcohol contributes 7 kilocalories per gram. Table 4.9 lists the kilocalories contained in a variety of beverages.

7. The art of chewing slowly can be developed to its fullest when a person is dieting. This practice contributes to a satisfied feeling and may not allow time for second helpings.

8. A large glass of water consumed at the beginning of a meal helps lessen the desire for food at that meal.

9. Meals should be eaten with some regularity. Skipping meals is poor practice, leading to fatigue, excessive nibbling, temptation

Table 4.9 *Caloric Content of Selected Beverages in Amounts Commonly Served*[a]

	Measure	kcal
Milk type		
Whole milk	1 cup	160
Skim milk	1 cup	90
Fortified low-fat milk	1 cup	145
Buttermilk	1 cup	90
Eggnog (nonalcoholic)	1 cup	235
Malted milkshake	1 cup	330
Fruit juice type		
Orange juice	1/2 cup	60
Lemonade	1 cup	100
Carbonated		
Colas	8 oz	96
Ginger ale	8 oz	70
Sodas, fruit flavored	8 oz	112
Alcoholic		
Beer	12 oz	151
Wine, table	3 1/2 oz	85
Daiquiri	3 1/2 oz	120
Manhattan	3 1/2 oz	165
Martini	3 1/2 oz	220
Whiskey (86 proof)	2 oz	140
Gin (90 proof)	2 oz	150
Coffee, black	5 oz	2-5
Tea, unsweetened	5 oz	2

[a] Data compiled and adapted from *Composition of Foods—Raw, Processed, Prepared.* Agriculture Handbook No. 8, U.S.D.A., 1963; *Nutritive Value of American Foods,* Agriculture Handbook No. 456, U.S.D.A., 1975.

to overeat at the next meal, and haphazard nutrition.

10. A weekly instead of daily-assessment of progress using a scale and tape measure is of value. Although fast weight loss accomplished by rigid restriction may be spectacular, the weight loss seldom is permanent. A gradual weight loss can lead to permanent maintenance at the desired weight because the reducing period provides the time needed for retraining dietary patterns. An additional advantage is that gradual weight loss does not require a punishing and monotonous diet.

A look at popular approaches to dieting

Weight reduction diets are very popular fare in many magazines and paperback books on the newsstands. There is a diet suggestion to suit just about anyone's food preferences. Suggestions range from such catchy titles as "The Drinking Man's Diet," "The Grapefruit Diet," and "The Low Carbohydrate Diet" to the obvious gimmick of "Diet of the Month." The gist of these assorted approaches to weight loss is that the diet offers an *easy* way to lose weight. Promises of "all you can eat" and beautiful word pictures of lobster dripping with butter or ice cream generously bedecked with a large cloud of whipped cream are used to lure the would-be dieter into trying this new approach to losing weight.

From the previous discussion in this chapter, it is clear that there is a close relationship between the calories available from the foods eaten and the use of these calories by the body. Excess caloric intake will lead to excess body weight; a negative caloric balance will result in weight loss. Yet, despite this straightforward logic, the fantasy of easy weight loss keeps leading dieters onward. Some of these diets are so restrictive in their menus that few people are able to stay on them for more than a few days. Some will cause rapid weight loss at the beginning due to the excessive loss of water. These diets appeal to some people because the immediate loss is so dramatic.

Despite the seeming advantages of some of these drastic diets, there are potential health hazards which should be noted when a diet is selected veering significantly from the pattern of the Basic Four. For example, the Dr. Atkins' Diet provides an imbalance, being basically a diet high in both protein and fat and distinctly

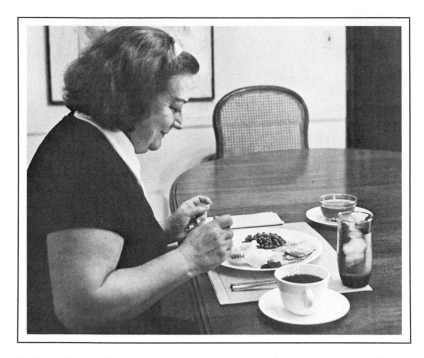

Reducing diets need to provide interesting variety for the dieter's satisfaction as well as for satisfying nutritional requirements.

low in carbohydrate. This balance of nutrients leads to an accumulation of ketone bodies because there is insufficient carbohydrate to metabolize the fat normally. This condition leads to excessive loss of water and sodium from the body. High-fat diets also are subject to challenge on the basis of the relationship between intake of saturated fat and elevated blood levels of cholesterol and occasionally also triglycerides, both identified as risk factors in atherosclerosis and coronary heart disease. Diets incorporating low levels of carbohydrate clearly present potential hazards for persons electing to follow them for more than a very brief period of time. Since weight control, to be effective, needs to modify dietary patterns on a long-range basis, the use of these crash or spectacular diets is not recommended. Indeed, they have proven to be particularly dangerous to persons with heart, liver, or kidney problems, and also may be an unnecessary hazard for pregnant women because of the indirect risk to the fetus.

These crash diets strike a common chord among overweight people, but there are other ways of approaching the common concern of weight loss. The use of group techniques will vary in effectiveness from one individual to another. The value of a group in supporting a dieter during weight reduction has been recognized by psychologists and other behaviorists. The practical application of this principle has been the development of groups such as TOPS and Weight Watchers. The diet plan in such groups focuses around a generally well-balanced diet, with emphasis on portion control and group reinforcement of achievement on a regular and frequent basis. The usual loss under these conditions is not dramatic, but it is fast enough to provide encouragement for continuing on the regimen. The diet period ordinarily is long enough to be beneficial in beginning to retrain dietary habits. The use of a leveling-off period also provides a gradual transition to the nondieting state. For some people, such a program can result in a permanent solution to their weight problem; for others there will be a periodic need for reinforcement and occasional weight reduction regimens to correct gradual weight gain.

A recent development in the weight reducing field is the use of behavior modification. Psychologists are teaming with dietitians and nutritionists to aid in reshaping people's attitudes toward food and in modifying food habits. The use of this method requires a careful examination of one's reasons for eating and then development of a plan or contract for modifying eating habits enough to achieve the desired weight loss. This approach to weight control is virtually in its infancy at the present time. There has not been sufficient time to determine how effective this method may be in achieving permanent modification.

Summary

Overweight is not, by itself, a satisfactory measure of excess fatness or obesity. A measurement of skinfold thickness, using calipers, provides a practical means of differentiating between overweight due to a well-developed muscular physique and overweight due to overfatness. Obesity, the condition in which there is a true excess of fat (adiposity), is recognized as a health hazard contributing to other physical problems such as hypertension, hyperlipidemia, and diabetes. Although obesity is a problem for some children, the incidence increases among the adult population, due at least partially to the gradual reduction in the basal metabolic rate with age. Permanent weight reduction to a desired weight range is beneficial and results in increased life expectancy.

In realistic and practical terms, obesity or overfatness is accumulated fat resulting from consuming too many calories from food and beverages and expending too few calories in physical activity. This basic fact underlines the necessity for individuals to learn that obesity is not a problem of "fattening" or "slimming" foods, but is simply a matter of *just too many calories,* and that continual consumption of calories over and above those used in any 24-hour period produces excess pounds of fat over a period of time. However, there are genetic, environmental, and psychological factors that greatly influence body weight and consumption patterns. If the specific factors underlying an individual's excess intake can be identified and subsequently modified or eliminated, weight control may be accomplished more effectively and permanently.

Exercise is of decided value as a reducing agent and moderate, daily exercise need not increase food intake. Obese persons are frequently sedentary in their habits, and their level of physical activity should be increased for successful weight control.

Total energy needs are a summation of the calories needed for basal metabolism, activity, and the specific dynamic action of food. In the typically somewhat sedentary living pattern of today, the need for energy for physical activity has decreased to the point where, in many instances, the calories for basal metabolism are greater than those required for activity.

Diets to achieve weight control are most successful in accomplishing weight change and maintaining the desired weight when they are based on the Basic Four Food Group Plan and are geared to the food preferences of the individual. And most important, persons seeking to lose weight need to reduce serving sizes and rely on vegetables and fruits instead of desserts for achieving a satisfied feeling at meals. A varied diet is important to the dieter for psychological as well as nutritional needs. For optimum health, weight control should be established from childhood, and dietary modifications plus increased physical activity should be made when small deviations from the desired weight are noted. Crash diets or fad diets may be hazardous to one's health. Diet groups and use of behavior modification have been of value to some dieters.

Selected References

Anonymous. Cellularity of rat adipose tissue in relation to growth, starvation, and obesity. *Nutrition Reviews. 27:*147. 1969.

Barnes, R. H. Calories. *Present Knowledge of Nutrition.* 4th ed. Nutrition Foundation. New York. 1976.

Bjorntorp, P., and L. Sjöström. Number and size of adipose tissue fat cells in relation to metabolism in human obesity. *Metabolism. 20:*703. 1971.

Bruch, H. Psychological aspects of obesity in adolescence. *Am. J. Pub. Health. 48:*1349. 1958.

Bruch, H. *Importance of Overweight.* Norton. New York. 1957.

Bullen, B. A., et al. Attitudes toward physical activity, food and family in obese and non-obese adolescent girls. *Am. J. Clin. Nutr. 12:*1–11. 1963.

Consolazio, C. F., and H. L. Johnson. Measurement of energy cost in humans. *Fed. Proc. 30:*1444. 1971.

Council on Foods and Nutrition. Critique of low carbohydrate, ketogenic weight reduction regimens. *J. Am. Med. Assoc. 224:*1415. 1973.

Danowski, T. S., et al. Obesity. *World Rev. Nutr. Diet. 22:*270. 1975.

Dwyer, J. T., and J. Mayer. Potential dieters: who are they? *J. Am. Diet. Assoc. 56:*510–514. 1970.

Egorov, M. F., et al. Course and treatment of obesity. *Am. J. Clin. Nutr. 7:*295–301. 1959.

Heald, F. P. History and physiological basis of adolescent obesity. *Nutr. News. 28,* No. 4:13–14. December 1965.

Konishi, F. *Exercise Equivalents of Foods.* Southern Illinois University Press. Carbondale, Ill. 1974.

Lesser, G. T., et al. Use of independent measurement of body fat to evaluate overweight and underweight. *Metabolism. 20:*792. 1971.

Maxfield, E., and F. Konishi. Patterns of food intake and physical activity in obesity. *J. Am. Diet. Assoc. 49:*406–408. 1966.

Mayer, J. *Overweight: Causes, Cost, and Control.* Prentice-Hall, Englewood Cliffs, N.J. 1968.

Mayer, J. Some aspects of the problem of the regulation of food intake and obesity. *New Eng. J. Med. 274:*610, 662, 722, 1966.

Mayer, J. Obesity: physiological consideration. *Am. J. Clin. Nutr. 9:*530–537. 1961.

Mayer, J. The physiological basis of obesity and leanness. Part I. *Nutr. Abstr. Rev. 25:*597–611. 1955.

Mayer, J. The physiological basis of obesity and leanness. Part II. *Nutr. Abstr. Rev. 25:*871–883. 1955.

Mayer, J. Genetic, traumatic, and environmental factors in the etiology of obesity. *Physiol. Rev. 33:*472–508, 1953.

Montoye, H. J. Estimation of habitual physical activity by questionnaire and interview. *Am. J. Clin. Nutr. 24:*1113. 1971.

Moore, M. E., et al. Obesity, social class and mental illness. *J. Am. Med. Assoc. 181:*926–966. 1962.

Moore, T. Calorie versus the joule. *J. Am. Diet. Assoc. 59:*327. 1971.

Prugh, D. E. Some psychologic considerations concerned with the problem of overnutrition. *Am. J. Clin. Nutr. 9:*538–547. 1961.

Rauh, J. L., and D. A. Schumsky. Relative accuracy of visual assessment of juvenile obesity. *J. Am. Diet. Assoc. 55:*459–464. 1969.

Salans, L. B., et al. Experimental obesity in man: cellular character of the adipose tissue. *J. Clin. Investigation 50:*986. 1971.

Seltzer, C. C., and J. Mayer. Body build (somatotype) distinctiveness in obese women. *J. Am. Diet. Assoc. 55:*454–458. 1969.

Seltzer, C. C., and J. Mayer. A simple criterion of obesity. *Postgrad. Med. 38:*A101. 1965.

Sheldon, W. H., et al. *Varieties of Human Physique.* Harper. New York. 1940.

Shutter, Z., and D. C. Garell. Obesity in children and adolescents. *J. School Health. 36:*273. 1966.

Stare, F. J. Overnutrition. *Am. J. Pub. Health. 53:*1175. 1963.

Weisenberg, M., and E. Fray. What's missing in behavior modification for obesity. *J. Am. Diet. Assoc. 65:*410. 1974.

West, K. Diabetes mellitus. *Present Knowledge of Nutrition.* 4th ed. Nutrition Foundation. New York. 1976.

Widdowson, E. Obesity. *Present Knowledge of Nutrition.* 4th ed. Nutrition Foundation. New York. 1976.

Wilson, R. H. L., and N. L. Wilson. Obesity and respiratory stress. *J. Am. Diet. Assoc. 55:*465–469. 1969.

Wyden, P., and L. Libien. *The All-in-one Diet Annual.* Bantam. New York. 1970.

Young, C. M., et al. Frequency of feeding, weight reduction, and nutrient utilization. *J. Am. Diet. Assoc. 59:*473. 1971.

Young, C. M. The prevention of obesity. *Med. Clin. N. Am. 48,* No. 5:1317–1333. 1964.

Young, C. M. Some comments on the obesities. *J. Am. Diet. Assoc. 45:*134–138. 1964.

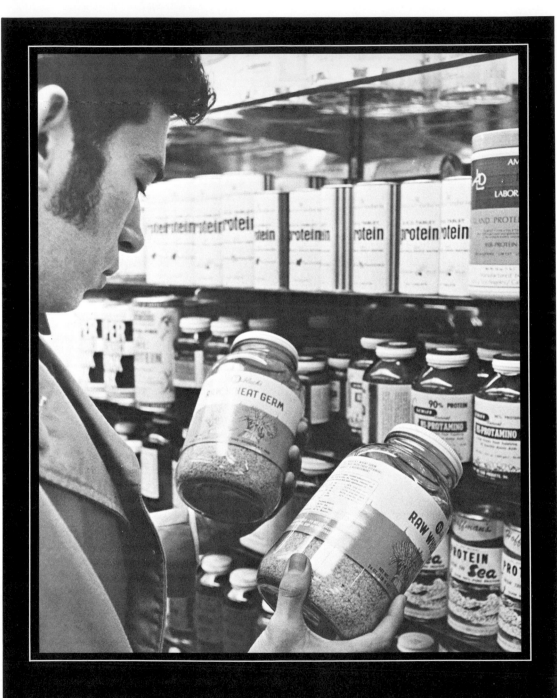

Chapter 5

Health Foods?

In a highly developed and industrialized country such as the United States, there are numerous options available to consumers when they begin to consider how to best meet their nutritional needs. For some the decision may mean that many meals will be eaten in restaurants and other commercial food operations. For others the decision may be to buy basic ingredients in the grocery store and to prepare virtually all foods at home. Another option is to grow fresh produce in a garden; still others may elect to purchase a variety of nutritive supplements in addition to their groceries. The diet each person consumes is a very personal matter and needs to be one providing psychological comfort and pleasure as well as meeting actual physiological needs. The choices made by each consumer should be ones that satisfy him and should be made with full knowledge of nutritional needs for good health and the contributions the various products make toward meeting these requirements.

There are the factors of food safety, nutritive value, food preferences, and cost—all of which influence food buying decisions. With so many factors operating, intelligent decision making is difficult, and the problem is compounded by advertising claims and articles which appear in the news media. Most consumers have a genuine concern for feeding themselves and their families in a healthful way. The problem is to determine the best way to accomplish this task. Food prices will fluctuate too much for it to be practical to list them in this book. Also, discussion of individual food items is impractical because so many are selected frequently on the basis of widely varying personal preferences. However, there are several topics of broad consumer interest which are pertinent to food-buying decisions. Some of these are discussed in this chapter.

The purpose of this discussion is to help the consumer gain an understanding of the ways in which food fads and various health food products are promoted and to evaluate the validity of claims. Each consumer certainly has the privilege of selecting where and how he will spend the food budget. Products in health food stores may be the choice of some shoppers, while others will elect to shop at the local supermarket. Some will purchase food supplements; others will buy all of their nutrition in the form of food rather than powders or capsules. Good nutrition is available whether one shops entirely at a supermarket, entirely at a health food store, or at both types of stores. The variety of foods may be somewhat different in health food stores than the fare available at the supermarket. The cost of the foods is likely to be quite different. Although prices do vary widely, comparison shopping usually reveals that shopping in a health food store is significantly more expensive than the same amount of nutrition would be in a supermarket. This is particularly true if vitamin capsules, protein supplements, and other "health" items are purchased. However, these choices are the option of the individual consumer. In short, the choice is his to make. The important point is that the consumer is entitled to a full discussion of the products so that the decision made will be the best one for each individual.

An accurate census of the self-styled nutrition "experts" in the United States has never been accomplished, but the number apparently is somewhere in the millions in this country alone. Some of these "experts" are content to practice their trade on their families and may confine their activities to the disbursement of vitamin E and wheat germ to their immediate family members. Others disseminate authoritative-sounding lectures to friends and local club members on the virtues of such items as "organically grown" fruits and vegetables and the wonders of raw milk. Yet another group, frequently costumed in white laboratory coats, willingly provides the many special foods that more than 10 million people in the United States feel they must buy if they are to stave off malnutrition and achieve glowing health, eternal youth, and retain sexual potency forever.

The business of supplying so-called "health foods" to the public is a burgeoning one that provides its owners with an income estimated at more than a billion dollars annually. From the financial viewpoint, this is undoubtedly a healthy business enterprise. From the consumer's vantage point, it is an expensive business. From the point of view of the professional nutritionist and the physician, the health food industry provides the consumer with (1) confusing, even harmful information and (2) a wide range of products that generally are more costly than comparable foods in any good supermarket.

A Backward Look

For many centuries, people have attributed special characteristics to certain foods. Garlic was long touted as an essential food for physical strength, cabbage was thought by some to have mystical powers to cure illness, truffles were generally agreed to assure great sexual potency, *ad infinitum.* These early food prejudices and practices have continued over the years, sometimes with slight modifications, sometimes unchanged, but never completely dropping out of the cultural heritage.

The mystique of food quackery slowly began to develop. During the Middle Ages, at various points around the world special foods were being recommended for curing some diseases. Apparently, some people felt that the more unpalatable the food or its source, the more it would accomplish toward curing the problem. This general philosophy culminated in such delectables as ground coffee beans blended with fat! There is still an unstated but apparent attitude today among food faddists that the general appeal of the food is far less important than the wonderful things it will do for your health.

The United States, like most other countries, has had its share of quacks and faddists. Among the most famous hucksters of earlier generations may be counted Sylvester Graham (of Graham cracker fame), Horace Fletcher (the widely followed exponent of the virtues of chewing each bite 32 times, one chew for each tooth), and finally the late Bernarr Macfadden (self-acclaimed king of the physical culturists). These noteworthy businessmen and women acquired a distinguished following over the years. Louisa May Alcott, Henry Ford, John D. Rockefeller, and George Bernard Shaw are but a few of the famous who followed the gospel of the quacks and food faddists. An equally prominent list of contemporary individuals could readily be given who follow today's quacks, including those few physicians who dispense nutrition nonsense for fancy fees. Some people have made fortunes selling pseudonutrition, many have paid considerable cash to follow the dictates of these leaders, many have paid with poor health, and some have died as a result of following the golden rainbow to health through pseudonutrition as prescribed by quacks and charlatans.

The idea that there have always been people seeking good health through food is not surprising. It is not even too amazing that some unusual and highly restrictive diets were tried as late as the nineteenth century. However, the fact that many people today still believe in virtually magical powers in some foods to the exclusion of a normal diet is difficult to accept. With the remarkable progress in understanding the role of food and the significant discoveries resulting from the dynamic development of nutrition as a science, it is truly amazing that so many people in the twentieth century still select their diets on the bases of emotion and mysticism of food instead of on scientific fact.

The Health Food Bonanza

There are several reasons why food faddism and quackery continue to flourish. Certainly the scientific knowledge of nutrition is ample to enable the normal individual to be well fed. The difficulty begins to develop at the point of transmission of that knowledge from the scientific nutrition laboratory to the training of physicians, allied health workers, and ultimately to the individual consumer. Until all people have some accurate and practical nutrition information regularly included as a part of their general education, beginning with the earliest experiences in family life and school, there will be large numbers of people who lack the knowledge required to sift through the barrage of nutrition misinformation being circulated so widely today.

The natural human desire for an easy solution to a problem sets the stage for promoting all sorts of pills and diets for effortless weight loss. Hypochondriacal tendencies are fertile territory for breeding health worries that can be allayed by eating or drinking a special food preparation. The gullible nature of some people who will subscribe to any theory with a scientific sound brings still others into the world of the faddist. These psychological undertones provide the foundation for healthy business enterprise, thus attracting imaginative and enthusiastic, if not altogether altruistic entrepreneurs. Any business so closely attuned to the public's concern for health and long life and so intimately tied to John Q. Public's wallet is virtually assured of continued success, at least until nutrition education becomes far more effective than it is at present.

A visit to a health food store is an important part of studying this aspect of nutrition. For the

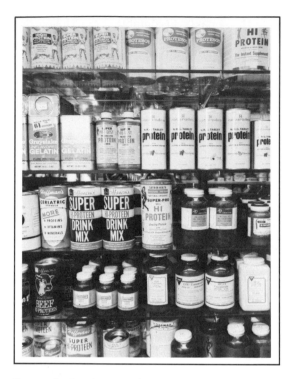

Despite the fact that most Americans are consuming meat at an all-time high, health food stores loudly and successfully promote protein supplements as well as other costly supplements of vitamins and minerals.

person who has never journeyed over the threshold of such an establishment, a new experience awaits. Some of the more plush stores boast a juice and nutrition counter featuring such delectables as celery juice. The fresh produce section houses fruits and vegetables (frequently scarred with worm holes and other indications of insect interest) that would be hard pressed to attract a buyer in a regular grocery store, but that will sell to the food faddist because it is clearly marked "organically grown." A prominent display of vitamin and mineral capsules is almost a certainty, for these are high-profit items. Various elixers, herbs, oils, sweeteners, and other fascinating food products await the interested customer. No visit would be complete without a careful survey of the literature available in the store. The choices range from leaflets extolling the amazing return to youth one can experience by drinking a tea

brewed with desert weeds to books assuring the reader that he can lose weight while eating all that he wants. Such a store is directly keyed to arouse people's concern over their health and then to capitalize on this apprehension by offering the solution to a problem that the buyer might not even have thought of before entering the store—incidentally, a solution that costs more than the customer may be able to afford.

A comparison of prices between a chain store supermarket and a health food store quickly reveals that many of the items in the health food store carry higher price tags than those in the supermarket, despite the fact that the quality may not be as good. The extra expense for health foods does not stop there. Health food store patrons are constantly cajoled to buy dietary supplements and tonics. Such items usually are fairly expensive, an expense that need not be incurred at all if one is in normal health and follows the Basic Four Food Group Plan.

All the foods needed to provide ample quantities of all the nutrients required by man are readily available in regular supermarkets at competitive prices. In fact, no vitamin or mineral supplement is needed by normal, healthy people who are eating a balanced diet of varied foods.

Aside from the extra expense of eating foods from the health food store, there is also the fact that food faddism can present a health hazard. Persons with physical ailments that need immediate medical attention may delay seeking medical help while they try to treat themselves with a special diet or product from a health food store. Such postponement of needed medical attention may introduce unnecessary complications and hazards.

There is another side to the coin that also must be presented. Many foods available in health food stores are highly nourishing and do provide considerable interest and flavor appeal to a menu. Bread made with stone-ground whole wheat flour, for example, is a food to be enjoyed by all. To condemn foods simply be-

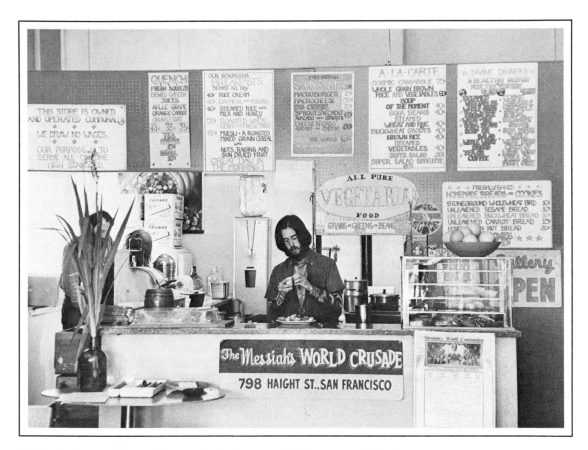

Health food stores offer a wide range of foods, some of which are unavailable elsewhere.

cause they are highly touted by food faddists is narrow minded. Many foods embraced by the faddists add an additional flair to meals and are enjoyable, despite the fact that they are not the panacea to cure all ills. Nourishing foods can be purchased in grocery stores and health food shops. If the shopper in a health food store buys some foods there because he likes their taste and texture and wants them as a part of a well-rounded diet, with price not being of any particular concern to him, obviously the purchase options are his to make.

Promoters and Proctors

Successful promotion of expensive products that people really do not need requires considerable imagination and skill. There may even be, on occasion, some small disregard of the truth. Basically, there are two approaches that have been used with great effectiveness in promoting food fads. Seemingly very little effort is required to shift people from a state of contented equilibrium to an uncomfortable premonition of trouble. Such a small thing as raising the question in someone's mind that he may feel more tired and draggy than he should is sufficient to begin thoughts that may lead toward purchase of a special tonic advertised to correct such a condition. When the "right" product is being taken to combat an imaginary ailment, a cure is almost certainly forthcoming. Surely it is only fair to share the news of such a wonderful treatment with one's friends—and so on it goes.

Other examples of attempting to increase sales by creating a concern or scaring the individual with the consequences of not taking the advertised product can readily be found by reading the advertising blurbs for health foods. Threats of diminished sexual potency or general loss of vigorous youth are frequent vehicles for frightening people into buying. Other advertising approaches emphasize the need for a sufficient supply of enzymes and maintenance of the correct stomach acidity for good digestion.

In addition to the scare approach, many advertising campaigns are keyed to appeal to a person's vanity. Anything that claims to make skin more youthful, figure and hair more beautiful, or mind and memory sharper is certain to find a large audience in need of its benefits and more than willing to pay the price. Of course, the market is far greater when the only effort required of the customer is to pay the price and eat the product. The words may be different, but the basic idea is that the consumer's problem can and will be corrected if he will just become an unquestioning user of the item.

Not all of this activity is conducted with total immunity from review and regulation. In 1962 the enforcement laws strengthened the hand of the government's Food and Drug Administration (FDA) in its prosecution of quacks and its efforts to prohibit fraudulent practices. The Food and Drug Administration is the primary governmental agency for monitoring foods, drugs, and cosmetics in the marketplace. This organization reviews products to detect misleading labeling and inadequate information on labels. Under the Federal Food, Drug, and Cosmetic Act, the FDA has the authority to prosecute companies marketing improperly labeled items and to have the offending items re-

moved from the market. Although several cases are tried annually, there are still many instances where a casual reading of a label may be misleading, but the actual wording does not violate the law. Under such circumstances, the item in question is permitted to remain on the market. The consumer then must assume responsibility for determining the value of the product in his own life. With only a relatively small staff available, the FDA is faced with the almost impossible task of trying to keep abreast of the numerous new entries on the market. An increase in the work force of the FDA would provide important policing action of the merchandise being marketed. The Environmental Protection Agency, formed in 1970, coordinates the governmental departments concerned with pollution, including pollutants in production and distribution of food.

Two other federal agencies assist in combating the spread of misinformation about nutrition. Both the Post Office Department and the Federal Trade Commission are empowered to halt false advertising claims. The American Medical Association maintains a Bureau of Investigation, which serves as a monitoring agency to determine the facts in instances where there appear to be promotion and distribution of products that may be harmful to individuals. The National Better Business Bureau and its affiliated groups do likewise.

The focus and work of these public and private agencies are directed toward restricting harmful products and misleading advertising so that the public will not be placed in physical danger. The agencies are not able to move beyond the point of obvious hazard to health. The purchase of health foods, bizarre combinations of vitamins, books on fad diets, and other related items is strictly at the discretion of the buying public. As in other facets of life in the United States, the selection and purchasing of food for good health are the responsibility of the educated consumer. The remaining concern is helping the consumer to become knowledgeable about nutrition and other matters of importance to each individual.

Myths and Misinformation

Paul Bunyan tales and fairy stories are frequently repeated to dazzle and amaze the gullible young; and the repetition of some of the folklore about food is just about as accurate as some of the amazing feats attributed to Paul's Babe, the Big Blue Ox. The credibility gap between some of the nutrition statements commonly circulating today and the actual truth is remarkable! To list all the nutrition misconceptions that are circulating today is impossible, and to attempt to predict what the new inventions regarding the magical qualities of foods will be is even less feasible. The following illustrations will serve as a guide to help the reader know what types of information are bombarding the public.

For some inexplicable reason, vinegar and honey have enjoyed a reputation for remarkable curative powers. Even before the end of the eighteenth century, Americans were informed of the wonders effected by using vinegar. The claim was even made, although quickly disproved, that vinegar was a cure for yellow fever. Lest the reader scoff at such foolishness on the part of the founding fathers of the United States, the realist must note that the book *Folk Medicine, A Vermont Doctor's Guide to Good Health,* by Dr. D. C. Jarvis was a best seller in the 1960s. Dr. Jarvis became a famous figure for his pronouncements on the efficacy of honey and vinegar in curing an amazing array of ills, ranging from arthritis to the common cold and digestive problems. He even came forth with the astounding information that a couple of teaspoons of cider vinegar in a glass of water, when taken at each meal, make it possible for the body to burn instead of store fat. Despite the fact that he claimed numerous experiments to substantiate his various statements on the curative powers of honey and vinegar, no documentation of the research was ever published to be evaluated by his peers. We know of no medical scientist who agreed with Dr. Jarvis.

Certainly, there is no indication that vinegar has any unusual influence on the metabolism of fat. Despite the inaccuracies of the basic tenets of Jarvis's book, many people came under the spell of this book, earning the author and the publishers a handsome fee. The faith in the truth of the printed word that the reading public exhibits is truly sobering.

Arthritis and the common cold have been of interest for years because they afflict so many people. To date, no food has been found to be effective in alleviating the pain of arthritis and no food or nutrient has been found to cure the common cold once it has been contracted, although an adequate diet is of value in optimizing resistance to the malady.

A book[1] by a great American chemist, Professor Linus Pauling, a two-time Nobel Prize winning scientist, extols the benefits of large doses of vitamin C in preventing and treating the common cold. The doses recommended are really astronomical—10,000 to 15,000 milligrams per day, in comparison with the 45 milligrams per day recommended for adults by the National Research Council as a daily intake. Although Pauling's theory has captured the public's interest, there have been several reasonably well-controlled studies that did not substantiate his theory. The most recent reports at the time of this writing gave little support to the Pauling hypothesis[2].

One of the more popular gambits of the food faddists over the years has been the promotion of bottled seawater. The general argument for the consumption of this item is that all life once came from the sea, and this necessarily means that our dietary needs are intimately linked with the ocean and its water. A nip of seawater is supposed to cleanse the system and lead to prolonged youth. From the distributor's view-

[1] L. Pauling. *Vitamin C and the Common Cold.* Freeman. San Francisco. 1970.
[2] Dykes, M. H. M. and P. Meier. Ascorbic acid and the common cold. Evaluation of its efficacy and toxicity. *J. Am. Med. Assoc. 231:*1073. 1975.

point, ocean water is an ideal merchandising item. The raw material is virtually limitless, albeit somewhat contaminated along the coast, and the cost of manufacture is basically that of the bottle to package it. What could possibly provide a better margin of profit? Although ocean water does contain some minerals that are needed by the human body, these minerals also are present in the variety of foods eaten in a normal diet. The money for seawater can better be kept by the consumer rather than pocketed by the huckster.

Unfortunately, the consumer no longer needs to go to the health food stores for "helpful" information these days. The mail provides an entry into all homes today. Take, for example, the interesting bit of information that arrived, unsolicited.

"It has been said that goitre is caused by certain constituents of water, but the fact that not all persons drinking from the same source do develop this condition, proves that there is something else involved. That something is a lack of normal nerve function at the point where the nerves supplying the thyroid gland emit through the spinal column.

"Most forms of goitre respond readily to Chiropractic adjustments. Cases are on record where the condition has entirely disappeared after a short course of adjustments and any case, even of long standing, may reasonably expect considerable relief from Chiropractic."

From
The Health Builder
52, No. 2:1. 1970.

The first statement in this quotation is typical of the literature prepared for food faddists. There is absolutely no indication of the source of the remark, and the "certain constituents" are so vague as to defy identity. Upon analysis, the statement says nothing meaningful, but it is highly effective in stirring up vague concerns in people's minds. Note that there is no mention of the fact that simply eating iodized salt is effective in the prevention of endemic goiter.

Additional "helps" are readily available to the alert individual who carefully reads want ads and other advertisements to keep abreast of the latest developments in health maintenance. From such want ads, here is an example of nutrition information that seemingly has become known to the quacks, but not to qualified nutritionists:

"ANTI-GRAY VITAMINS—if you are graying because of vitamin deficiencies—our anti-gray course which tells you how to correct these deficiencies may be your exact remedy."

Unfortunately, this valuable information cannot be shared with the reader in this volume because no nutrition research studies, to date, have demonstrated that vitamin deficiencies and graying of hair in humans have any relationship to each other.

Another favorite of the health food empire is the importance of the natural state of foods. Raw or unrefined sugar has been a food of continuing interest for the food faddist. Just what the nutritional merits of brown sugar are is somewhat vague, being generally described as good for maintaining vigor. Also, there possibly may be some snob appeal attributed to brown sugar because it is significantly more expensive than the refined white sugar that is in common use. Analysis of brown sugar versus white sugar reveals that there is, indeed, slightly more nutritive value in brown sugar than in white sugar. One tablespoon of brown sugar contains $\frac{1}{24}$th as much calcium as one glass of milk, or to extend this useful bit of information, an adult needs only 3 cups of brown sugar a day to provide his body with sufficient calcium. There is need to point out to those with a weight problem that these 3 cups of brown sugar would provide 2400 kilocalories, more than enough to cause a weight gain for sedentary adults. Of course, there would still be the problem of providing the necessary protein, fat, vitamins, and other minerals needed for good health.

Aside from the calcium in brown sugar, there

is also some iron. By computation, adult women can meet their daily requirement of iron by eating only 3⅔ cups of brown sugar. These figures show clearly that brown sugar, despite the presence of a speck more calcium and iron than is found in white sugar, is not of nutritional importance other than as a source of carbohydrate. And what about the vitamins contained in brown sugar? Vitamins A and C are totally absent, and so little of the B vitamins is present that merely a trace can be found.

Much has been said about the impact of the practice of refining wheat on the health of the American public. Faddists have described the loss of nutrients when wheat is refined and have loudly acclaimed the wonders of whole wheat and stone-ground flours. It is true that some vitamins and minerals are lost when the bran and germ are removed from flour. What the faddists fail to point out is that most flour today is fortified with thiamin, riboflavin, niacin, and iron. The other nutrients lost in the refining of flour are present in such small amounts and are available in so many other foods in the diet that there is little reason to include them in the fortification. As used in today's varied diets, enriched and whole wheat flours provide essentially the same nutritive value. Consequently, the consumer makes a nutritionally appropriate choice when he selects the type of bread he prefers—as long as the flour in refined products has been enriched. True, there are traces of other nutrients that may be lost in the refining of flour, but these nutrients will be obtained from other foods. Fiber may be the most desirable constituent of whole wheat products.

The merits of raw milk are touted by the food faddists who claim that drinking pasteurized milk is unnatural. They stress use of raw milk without mentioning the fact that raw milk can contain microorganisms that can cause undulant fever and tuberculosis. Although the supervision and standards of cleanliness for the production of certified raw milk are reasonably rigorous, the possibility still exists that the certified product can contain pathogens. Pasteurization is a heat processing of milk to kill many of

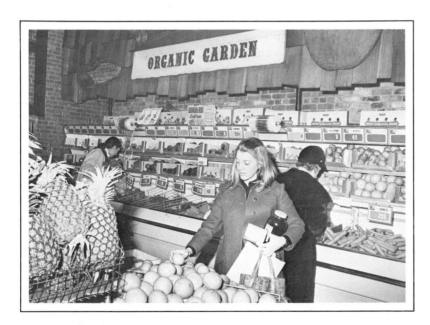

Produce marketed as "organic" may have been grown without the use of chemical fertilizers or pesticides, but this does not influence its nutritive value. Freshness is the important factor in selecting nourishing produce.

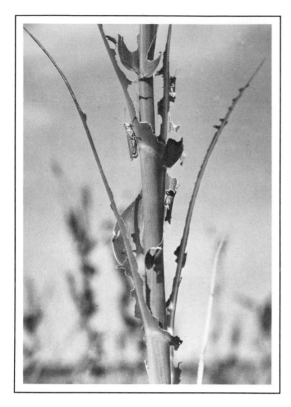

When food is grown without the use of pesticides, serious loss in production may be the result.

milk. If contamination occurs, the microorganisms will still be viable throughout the distribution process since raw milk is not heat treated.

Yet another aspect of the natural foods cult is the promotion of "organically grown" fruits and vegetables. Faddists claim that only natural fertilizers should be used to grow nutritious fruits and vegetables and that the use of chemical fertilizers is detrimental to the nutritive value of the crop. Actually, the chemical fertilizers are important because they are abundantly available and can be used to produce larger yields and profits per acre. Except for certain minerals, nutrient composition of fruits, vegetables, and cereals is not influenced by the use of natural fertilizers as compared with chemical fertilizers. Seemingly, plants are less influenced by emotional appeals than faddists would like. Fertilizers are most important to increase crop yields, but they do not affect the nutritive value—calories, protein, fat, carbohydrate, or vitamins—of the crops. Fresh produce that is marketed as being "organically grown" theoretically has been produced without any use of chemical fertilizers or pesticides. However, the absence of a legal definition of this term makes it possible to label any fresh produce as "organically grown" and collect a higher price from those who have been led to believe that such products are nutritionally superior.

Of course, it is not fair to pass this way without also directing the reader's attention to such wonders as alfalfa preparations, organic honey, squaw grass tea, and fertile eggs. The choices are seemingly endless. Unfortunately, illustrations of their wondrous cures are hard to find.

the microorganisms that are present. By legal definition, milk that is sold under the designation of "certified" must meet more rigid bacterial count specifications than milk that will be pasteurized, but pasteurization kills these microorganisms. Despite the fact that certified milk is produced under carefully controlled and inspected conditions, the possibility still exists that harmful microorganisms can get into the

The Dieter's Dilemma

In addition to the group that is captured by the wondrous values of special foods, there is yet another segment of the population that attracts the interest of the food promoter, namely the diet crowd. The fascination with weight re-

duction in this country appears to be without end. The seemingly insatiable appetites of some people for food is matched with their appetite for get-thin-quick ideas. The avenues to fad diets for weight reduction generally are paved with two ingredients—the special virtues of a particular food to be eaten in quantity and the appeal of lack of effort or will power on the part of the dieter. The following advertisement is typical of the wondrous attributes of such a diet.

LOSE 10 LBS.
IN 10 DAYS ON
GRAPEFRUIT DIET

HOLLYWOOD, CALIF. (Special)—This is the revolutionary grapefruit diet that everyone is suddenly talking about. It has made people slim, attractive and feel young again. Literally thousands upon thousands of copies have been passed from hand to hand in factories and offices throughout the U.S.

Word of its success has spread like wildfire. This is the diet that really works. No pills or drugs. We have testimonials in our files reporting on its success. If you follow it exactly, you should lose 10 pounds in 10 days. There will be no weight loss in the first 4 days, but you will suddenly drop 5 pounds on the 5th day. Thereafter you will lose one pound a day until the 10th day. Then you will lose $1\frac{1}{2}$ pounds every two days until you get down to your proper weight. Best of all, there will be no hunger pangs. Now revised and enlarged, this new diet plan lets you partake of foods formerly "forbidden" such as big juicy steaks, roast or fried chicken, rich gravies, spareribs, mayonnaise, lobster swimming in butter, bacon, sausages and scrambled eggs. You can eat until you are full and still lose 10 pounds in the first 10 days plus $1\frac{1}{2}$ pounds every two days thereafter. The secret behind this new "quick weight loss" diet is simple. Fat does not form fat. The grapefruit acts as a catalyst (the "trigger") to start the fat burning process. You eat as much as you want of the permitted foods listed in the diet plan, and still lose unsightly fat and excess body fluids. When the fat and bloat are gone your weight will remain constant. A copy of this very successful diet plan including suggested menus can be obtained by sending $2 to Grapefruit Diet. MONEY BACK GUARANTEE. If after dil-igently trying the diet plan you have not lost 7 pounds in the first 7 days and $1\frac{1}{2}$ pounds every two days thereafter, simply return the diet plan and your $2 will be refunded promptly and without argument. Fill out the coupon, mail it today and you will receive your diet rush via first class mail. Decide now to regain the trim, attractive figure of your youth, while enjoying hearty breakfasts, lunches and dinners.

In this advertisement the mere mention of such gastronomic delights as juicy steaks and lobster swimming in butter is sufficient to catch the interest of just about any would-be dieter, for these are the magic words to which he gravitates. The advertisement instills a feeling of confidence in a successful outcome while virtually guaranteeing him carte blanche to eat the delights he knows are usually deleted from a reducing diet. What more could a dieter ask? As the frosting on the cake, the ad copy begins to sound a bit sophisticated and scientific when it employs such impressive words as "catalyst" and "fat burning process." Surely such a vocabulary will add impact to the discussion of one's diet at the next social gathering!

This fascination with diets is fed by the popular magazine trade. One could safely wager that he seldom can go to a newsstand and not find at least one magazine highlighting a fad diet. In fact, one national magazine has even gone so far as to feature a diet of the month, a concept that immediately accents the probability that the diet will not be one that can be used as a continuing dietary pattern for a person.

On the other hand, some special diets are intended to be ongoing dietary patterns and are presented on the basis of emotional appeal and faith. Such diets have serious health implications when followed over a period of time, and can even be fatal. Of these, probably the most notorious recent example is the Zen Macrobiotic diet, which purportedly offers spiritual enlightenment through a combination of pseudopsychology and ascetic eating habits. With its roots tenuously planted in Oriental wisdom and mysticism, this diet has an enormous ap-

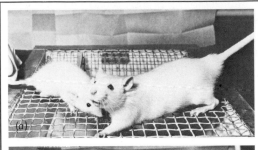

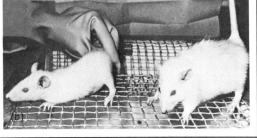

(a) Rat fed six weeks on typical macrobiotic diet (left) and typical vegetarian diet (right). (b) Rat on left was fed diet typical of foods available in a "Drive-In" for six weeks while rat on right was fed a diet based on the Basic Four.

peal to followers of the occult as well as to novice and pioneer food experimenters. Among its precepts is the notion that brown rice contains healing qualities that guarantee freedom from age, tension, and illness. Unfortunately, brown rice lacks these magical qualities.

Only a few years ago, tragedy first brought this stark macrobiotic diet to the attention of the public and the medical profession with the shocking news that a young woman had starved to death on a rigorous diet of brown rice in an effort to reach satori, a phase of enlightenment on the ladder she was convinced stretched toward nirvana. Evidence at the inquest following the girl's death revealed that similar fatalities had occurred as a result of devotees' unshakable confidence in the hypnotic theories of the then new "philosophy medicine."

Certainly this Oriental import is one of the most "screwball" diets ever to have caught the public fancy. This diet is the creation of the late George Ohsawa, a Japanese author known to his admirers as both scientist and philosopher. Anyone can comprehend Ohsawa's statement that "macrobiotic medicine is in reality a kind of Aladdin's Lamp, a Flying Carpet with which you can realize your fondest dreams." Equally persuasive are claims that macrobiotic dishes can "cure all illnesses (present or future)" and that this food results in "improvement of memory, judgement, and consequently an expansion of freedom and thinking."

With so much so alluring to so many, it is little wonder that the Macrobiotic Diet has tempted people from Cambridge to California. Despite the documented examples of fatal and near-fatal consequences and despite restraints on the combined sale of food and literature imposed by governmental action, interest continues. Ohsawa proposed a series of numbered dietary regimes that comprise ever-increasing proportions of cereals with gradual elimination of animal foods, fruits, salads, desserts and finally even of vegetables, so that the "highest, Diet 7" consists solely of one cereal—brown rice. "If you are not getting better, try Diet Number 7 for one or two weeks or even months" was the admonition that cost the lives of the diet's faithful adherents. Every mouthful of food must be chewed at least 50 times (150 is better), fluid intake must be strictly limited, and a whole list of regulations—the elimination of sugar, coffee, most spices, yeast, and fruits and vegetables—must be carefully followed. Animal foods must be avoided, because "too much animal protein results in thrombosis, cruelty, violence, etc."

The miraculous sounding Diet Number 7 is so completely deficient in many essential food constituents that it is bound to be harmful. Even some of Ohsawa's more liberal diets bearing lower numbers will eventually be damaging to health. Rice, other cereals, and vegetables are a part of good diets, but they do not contain all the known nutrients; there is no substitute for a variety of foods, and a limited food intake will inevitably spell trouble, just as a restricted fluid intake is predictably hazardous.

The gratitude with which the usual faddist

receives accurate nutrition information such as this is typified by the following letter:

Dear Dr. Stare:

I just read the reprint of an article you had published in the March issue of Today's Health about the Macrobiotic Diet. I beg to tell you that you are misinformed about the principles and precepts of George Ohsawa and do a dis-service to your students, doctors and the general public by dismissing out-of-hand this and other dietary regimens without thorough investigation and experimentation.

I have been on the Macrobiotic Diet for a year and the improvement in my physical and mental condition has been remarkable—my body cured itself of schizophrenia and bleeding gums. I was able to quit smoking and cut my eating costs by three-quarters. Many people in Austin, Texas are eating Macrobiotically. All proclaim the great value of vegetables and cereals which have historically constituted the main food for all civilizations except this one.

Human beings are animals—they should need no doctors, no hospitals, no schools . . . surely this is the goal, you, I, George Ohsawa and every other dedicated person aim for—human freedom for all men—freedom of expression and meditation; freedom from boredom and disease.

God bless you

Vegetarian diets have long been praised by many faddists, but there is no general agreement on a single vegetarian diet and composition varies. Most permit the use of dairy products and eggs (lacto-ovo-vegetarians) thus insuring good sources of complete proteins. At the opposite end of the vegetarian spectrum is the British dietary group known as the "vegans." The vegans, who eat nothing of animal origin, provide classic examples of deficiency of vitamin B_{12} as manifested by stunted growth of children and by irritability and other indications of abnormal nerve function.

Other diet crazes that surge and fade periodically include the Drinking Man's Diet, the Air Force Diet (not used by the Air Force), the Mayo Diet (not developed, used, or recommended by the Mayo Clinic), and the 60-gram Low Carbohydrate Diet.

In recent years a craze developed for "rainbow pills," so called because of their vari-colored appearance. They provide unfortunate evidence of the harm done to the public by promoters. The popular rainbow pills contained a thiazide diuretic, a vegetable-type laxative, amphetamines or amphetamine-barbiturate combinations, thyroid extract and digitalis, ovarian hormones, and hormones from the pituitary. A number of deaths have been reported due to prolonged use of the rainbow pills for weight reduction. One careful investigation by Dr. R. C. Henry, Chief Medical Investigator for the Oregon State Board of Health, established that the prolonged use of rainbow pills caused increased loss of potassium due to their diuretic and laxative effect. At the same time, the intake of potassium was reduced because of the reduced appetite resulting from the ingestion of the amphetamines. The increased excretion and decreased intake, ultimately produced a serious potassium deficiency in the body. This potassium deficiency favored digitalis intoxication and the result was dangerous and potentially fatal.

Megavitamin Therapy

Megavitamin therapy is today a concept and term which is loosely defined, but it was in use for several years before Professor Pauling promoted its use for the treatment and prevention of the common cold. Professor Roger Williams had thought it useful in the treatment of alcoholism and other diseases, and 25 years ago it was offered as a part of the treatment of schizophrenia.

Megavitamin therapy today consists of the

use of massive doses of many of the water-soluble vitamins, although originally only of one of them, nicotinic acid or niacin, was utilized. Advocates of megavitamin therapy received substantial support in 1968 when so prestigious a figure as Linus Pauling presented a theoretical paper supporting the concept that some forms of mental illness might be due to vitamin deficiencies which occurred even on diets thought by nutritionists to be well balanced and more than adequate nutritionally. Pauling termed the use of megavitamin therapy in various mental diseases as orthomolecular therapy.

A special task force on vitamin therapy in psychiatry was set up by the American Psychiatric Association to examine these concepts and their conclusions were completely negative. The task force concluded that they consider "the massive publicity . . . via radio, the lay press and popular books, using catch phrases which are really misnomers like 'megavitamin therapy' and 'orthomolecular treatment' to be deplorable."

Megavitamin therapy is another tool, or sales pitch, for the nutritional quacks and charlatans.

Summary

The public today is constantly confronted with a vast array of nutrition half-truths and misinformation that causes many consumers to be enticed into buying many food products, books, and related items that they really do not need for good health. Some of the better-known writers in the health food field have generated such strong ties with their reading audiences that it is extremely difficult to reach beyond the reader's emotions to provide even the basics of accurate nutrition information.

In addition to the abundance of books written by food faddists, there are magazines dedicated to spreading the gospel of health foods. In a quick thumbing of one recent issue a variety of amazing tidbits emerged: vitamin E wafers are an after-dinner treat of nutritional importance; lecithin must be eaten every day to nourish the sex organs and to enable the nervous system to generate nerve electricity; water is a universal fluid of death that brings on premature death; on one page yogurt was described as an essential food for good health and on another page the increased incidence of cataracts among people eating large quantities of yogurt was noted; cucumber tonic for a beautiful skin was offered for $2.75. Nine pages were devoted to listing the addresses of health food stores, with one third of the space being required just for those in California.

Although the Food and Drug Administration, the Post Office Department, the Federal Trade Commission, and the Bureau of Investigation of the American Medical Association, and many Better Business Bureaus are all working to protect consumers from fraudulent claims and harmful products, there is need for improved nutrition education to enable the individual consumer to be more knowledgeable in

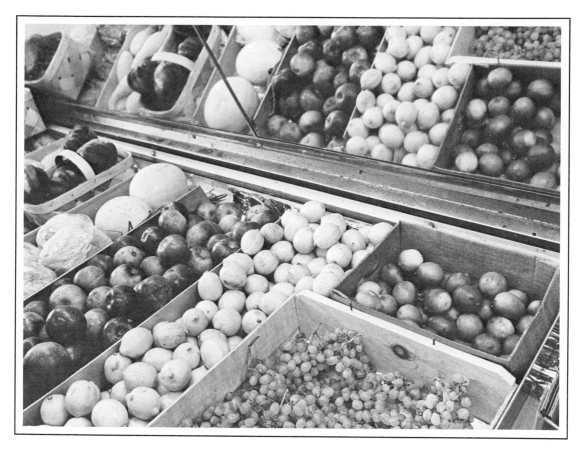

Today's supermarkets offer a remarkable array of highly nourishing and tempting foods at competitive prices.

selecting his diet. Sufficient groundwork needs to be laid so that individuals can sort through the maze of nutrition information and misinformation to determine what will provide him a good diet at a price he can afford to pay.

The weight watcher would do well to be leery of diets emphasizing: (1) single magical foods rather than a well-rounded diet, (2) promises of unusually rapid weight loss, (3) eating all the food desired, including foods high in kilocalories that are particularly tempting to overweight people, and (4) calories are unimportant and have essentially nothing to do with weight gain or loss. Others who tend to expect too much simply from the foods they eat would be well advised to be somewhat suspicious of claims that a particular food will restore one's youth or will increase virility. Words such as "natural," "poisons," and "organic" are a signal to beware. Also remember that arthritis, rheumatism, cancer, and frigidity are not cured by diet. "Miracle" cures of these ailments are not accomplished by food or anything else.

A good guideline is to remember that all the nutrients needed by man are provided simply by eating according to the Basic Four Food Group Plan. Nutrition supplements generally are not needed if this guideline is followed. Good nutrition is as close as the nearest supermarket. The choice ultimately rests with the consumer.

Selected References

American Medical Association. *Nutrients in Processed Foods—Vitamins and Minerals.* Publishing Sciences Group. Acton, Mass. 1974.

Beeuwkes, A. M. Characteristics of the self-styled scientists. *J. Am. Diet. Assoc. 32:*627. 1956.

Beeuwkes, A. M. Food faddism and consumer. *Fed. Proc. 13:*785. 1954.

Bernard, V. W. Why people become the victims of medical quackery. *Am. J. Pub. Health. 55:*1142. 1965.

Coon, M. J. Natural food toxicants—a perspective. *Present Knowledge of Nutrition.* 4th ed. Nutrition Foundation. New York. 1976.

Committee on Food Protection. *Toxicants Occurring Naturally in Foods.* 2nd ed. National Academy of Sciences. Washington, D.C. 1973.

Council on Foods and Nutrition. Zen macrobiotic diets. *J. Am. Med. Assoc. 218:*397. 1971.

Deutsch, R. M. *The Nuts among the Berries.* Ballantine. New York. 1961.

Dwyer, J. T., et al. New vegetarians. *J. Am. Diet. Assoc. 64:*376. 1974.

Erhard, Darla. The new vegetarians. *Nutrition Today 8,* No. 5:4. 1973.

Henry, R. C. The fatal interaction. *Nutrition Today 3,* No. 1:18–19. 1968.

Jalso, S. B., et al. Nutritional beliefs and practices. *J. Am. Diet. Assoc. 47:*263. 1965.

Leverton, R. Distorting facts into fads. *J. Am. Diet. Assoc. 33:*793. 1957.

Maynard, L. A. Effect of fertilizers on the nutritional value of foods. *J. Am. Med. Assoc. 161:*1478. 1956.

Mitchell, H. S. Food fads—what protection have we? *J. Home Econ. 53:*100. 1961.

Nagy, M. Yogurt-induced cataracts . . . in rats. *J. Am. Med. Assoc. 217:*1113. 1971.

Nutrition Foundation. Nutrition misinformation and food faddism. *Nutrition Reviews.* Special Supplement. July, 1974.

Sebrell, W. H., Jr., and J. J. Haggerty. *Food and Nutrition.* Life Science Library. New York. Pp. 148–157. 1967.

Sipple, H. L. Combating nutrition misinformation through coordinated programs. *Am. J. Pub. Health. 54:*823. 1964.

Smith, Ralph Lee. "Health" books: reader beware. *Today's Health.* April 1969.

Smith, Ralph Lee. "Crusade" that can hurt your health. *Today's Health.* October 1966.

Stare, F. J. Sense and nonsense about nutrition. *Harpers Magazine.* October 1964.

Stare, F. J., et al. Health foods: definitions and nutrient values. *J. Nutrition Ed.* 4:44. 1972.

Strong, F. Natural toxicants in foods. *Present Knowledge of Nutrition.* 4th ed. Nutrition Foundation. New York. 1976.

Young, James Irving. *The Medical Messiahs.* Princeton University Press. 1967.

NUTRITION FROM THE PHYSIOLOGICAL VIEWPOINT

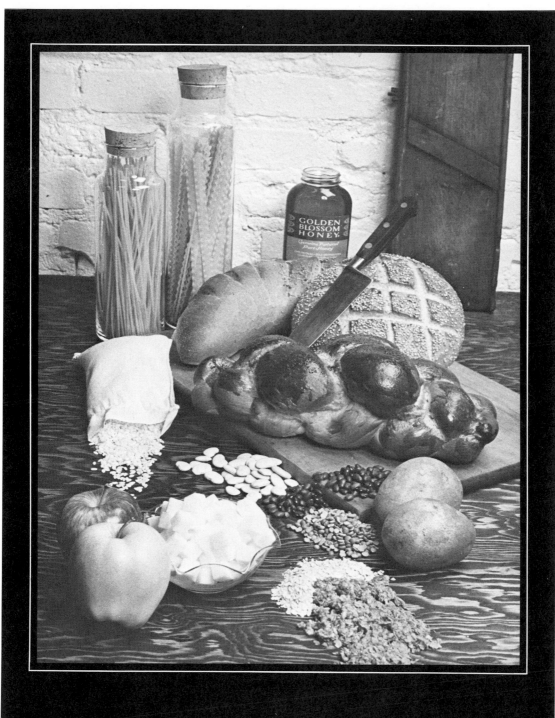

Chapter 6

Carbohydrates are a class of organic substances of significance in human nutrition. These compounds range in complexity from simple, small molecules to large, branched structures.

The formation of carbohydrates in plants is a very important chain of reactions in nature. Carbon dioxide in the air and water, through photosynthesis, are transformed in the plant into carbohydrate molecules, thus providing a utilizable storage form for solar energy. The term "carbohydrate" is the general name for a class of chemical compounds, containing carbon, hydrogen, and oxygen, that is widespread in nature and commonly used by animals and man for food. The name was derived by combining "carbo-" from the carbon in each molecule with "hydrate," indicating that the ratio of hydrogen to oxygen is the same as is found in water, that is, two to one.

Carbohydrate is suitable as the group name for all substances in this general category because all of the compounds are similar in their chemical structure. For each carbon atom in a simple carbohydrate compound, there are 2 atoms of hydrogen and 1 atom of oxygen. This formula for simple carbohydrates (monosaccharides) can be written in its empirical form: $C_n(H_2O)_n$. When these simple carbohydrate molecules are linked together, they form much larger molecules with a slightly different empirical formula: $C_n(H_2O)_{n-1}$. The close relationship between the various carbohydrates of importance in food will be explained in the next section.

Classification and Structure

Hexoses and pentoses

Carbohydrates are classified according to the number of carbon atoms in a single unit and also by the number of these basic monosaccharide units joined together to form the molecule. Although carbohydrates containing fewer than 6 carbon atoms occasionally exist in foods, the most common number of carbon atoms in monosaccharides used as food is six.

Carbohydrates containing 6 carbon atoms in their basic structure are classified as hexoses. The prefix, of course, indicates 6 carbon atoms; the suffix "-ose" is used to denote that the compound is a carbohydrate. The 5-carbon monosaccharide molecules are called pentoses.

Hexose   Pentose

Monosaccharides

Carbohydrates are also categorized on the basis of the number of monosaccharide units that are joined together into a single molecule. Chemical compounds consisting of a single monosaccharide unit, such as the hexose and pentose just shown, are called monosaccharides because each molecule consists of only one basic unit. Three of these monosaccharides, or simple sugars, are of particular interest in nutrition: glucose (also called dextrose), fructose (fruit sugar or levulose), and galactose. The chemical structures of these and other common carbohydrates are shown in Figure 6.1.

Disaccharides

Disaccharides are carbohydrates whose molecules consist of two monosaccharides joined together with the loss of a molecule of water. The simple sugars comprising the two parts of a disaccharide may be either two different monosaccharides or two molecules of the same monosaccharide linked together. Thus, lactose (also referred to as milk sugar) is composed of a molecule of glucose and one of galactose linked together with a loss of a molecule of water; sucrose, the ordinary granulated or confectioner's sugar, is a condensation of a molecule of glucose and one of fructose, again with the release of a molecule of water; and maltose is simply a union of 2 molecules of glucose with the formation of a molecule of water. These three disaccharides are commonly found in the diet.

Oligosaccharides

Next in complexity in the classification of carbohydrates is the category of oligosaccharides. Compounds belonging in this group contain between 3 and 10 monosaccharide units. These compounds are formed as intermediates in the breakdown of more complex carbohydrates, such as are formed in cooking, but are not found in abundance in nature. Therefore, these substances are not important in the diet.

Polysaccharides

Polysaccharides are complex carbohydrate molecules containing more than 10 monosaccharide units joined together. Actually, most polysaccharides in foods contain several hundred units joined together to form a single molecule. Starch is a polysaccharide polymer[1] of glucose. More precisely, starch is a mixture of amylose and amylopectin, both of which are glucose polymers. Amylose is typified as a straight chain of approximately 600 glucose units linked together to form a molecule of this starch fraction. Amylopectin is a somewhat more complicated, branched structure of as many as 1500 glucose units joined together. Although the composition of starch varies from

[1] A polymer is a large chemical molecule composed of many units of one or more simple compounds, linked together in repeating fashion.

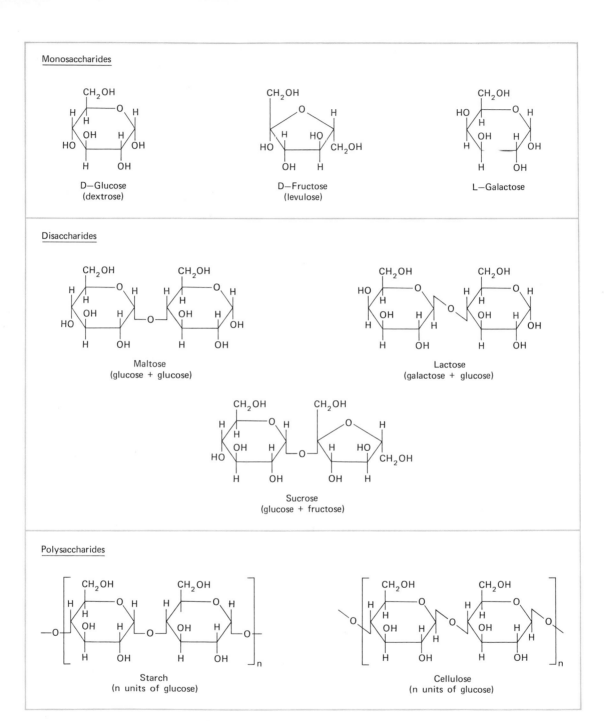

Figure 6.1 Examples of carbohydrate molecules.

one source to another, the common food starches are approximately 80 percent amylopectin and 20 percent amylose. Dextrins, since they are degradation products of starch, vary greatly in molecular size, depending upon the extent of breakdown.

Cellulose, like starch, is made up of glucose units, but the difference in linkage between the glucose units imparts a very different character to this carbohydrate. This carbohydrate is not digestible in the human intestinal tract and comprises most of the bulk or crude fiber in foods. Other constituents of the fiber portion of foods (only of vegetables, fruits, and grains) include hemicelluloses, mucilages, pectins, gums, and the noncarbohydrate lignin.

As is true with starch, pectic substances also are classified as polysaccharides. However, the basic structural unit in all pectic substances is galacturonic acid, a derivative of the monosaccharide galactose.

The previously mentioned polysaccharides are all found in foods of plant origin. Glycogen, occasionally called "animal starch," is a polysaccharide of animal origin. This compound is a very large polysaccharide which, in comparison with starch, is very highly branched and of greater complexity because of the far more numerous glucose units in a single molecule. In fact, glycogen molecules may be as much as 200 times larger than a molecule of amylopectin.

The physical qualities of carbohydrates vary with their molecular size. Monosaccharides represent the smallest molecular size in the broad spectrum of carbohydrate compounds. These small molecules of monosaccharides and disaccharides are characterized by their sweet taste, ready solubility in water, and lack of thickening power when heated. At the other end of the spectrum, polysaccharides do not possess a sweet taste nor are they easily dissolved in water. Starch, a polysaccharide of great nutritional significance, has a characteristic flavor that is distinctly lacking in sweetness. When heated in water, starch is an effective thickening agent used in food preparation.

Cellulose and other dietary fibers are not absorbed but have important roles in promoting intestinal motility and influencing the character of the intestinal flora. While crude fiber is occasionally included in food tables, it is not the same as dietary fiber. The former is defined as the insoluble material remaining after rather severe acid and base hydrolysis. Dietary fiber is really a generic term that includes those plant constituents which are resistant to digestion by the human gastrointestinal system. Thus, dietary fiber is not synonymous with crude fiber since some of the dietary fiber has been removed from crude fiber by rigorous chemical treatment. Since there are no tables for dietary fiber, the only information presently available is the crude fiber content of foods.

Food Sources

Plants

By far the largest fraction of sugars consumed in the United States is derived from plant sources. Sugar beets and sugarcane are the plants from which sucrose is extracted. Sucrose is also found in the sap of the sugar maple tree, but its far greater cost in comparison with that of sugar beets and cane limits the use of the sugar maple to the production of maple syrup. Sucrose is marketed as granulated sugar, brown sugar (less refined), powdered or confectioner's sugar, and the relatively new, globular, frosting sugar. Another sweetener, corn syrup, is a mixture of glucose, maltose, and slightly larger glucose polymers. It is manufactured by breaking down the starch obtained from corn. This hydrolysis is stopped when most of the carbohydrate has been converted to monosaccharides and disaccharides. Fruits and immature vegetables, although less concentrated sources of carbohydrate than previously named products, are also useful nutritionally for their sugars.

Starch is found in abundance in the endosperm of cereal grains. Economically and practically, cereals are polished to remove the outer bran portion and the germ or embryo of cereals, leaving the endosperm, which is an important source of starch. Starch can be separated from the protein, which is also found in the endosperm. These plant starches are used as a thickening agent in soups, sauces, and gravies. Cereal starches commonly used in food preparation include those from corn, wheat, and rice.

A wide variety of cereal products is manufactured using corn, wheat, rice, barley, rye, and oats singly or in various combinations. These foods are rich in starch content. Flour from wheat, and to a lesser extent from the other cereal grains, is used to make numerous types of baked products, including bread, pies, cakes, cookies, waffles, pancakes, doughnuts, crackers, and other similar items. Again, these are good sources of carbohydrate because they usually contain not only the starch in the flour,

Table 6.1 Carbohydrate Content of Some Familiar Foods[a]

Food	Carbohydrate Percent	Average Serving	Carbohydrate Grams
Apple	15	1 medium	18
Apricot	13	1 medium	5
Beans, kidney	21	1/2 cup, cooked	26
Beans, lima	20	1/2 cup, cooked	17
Beans, green	5	1/2 cup, cooked	3
Cola, beverage	10	12 oz	37
Bread, white	50	1 slice	12
Bread, whole wheat	48	1 slice	11
Cake, angel	60	1/12 cake	32
Cake, yellow with frosting	60	1/16 cake	45
Candy, fudge	75	1 oz	21
Candy, hard	97	1 oz	28
Candy, marshmallows	80	1 oz	23
Honey	82	1 tbsp	17
Jelly	71	1 tbsp	13
Molasses	65	1 tbsp	13
Noodles	23	1 cup	37
Pie, apple	38	1/7 pie	51
Pizza	36	1/8 of 14 in.	27
Sugar, granulated	100	1 tbsp	11
Sugar, maple	90	1 piece	14

[a] Compiled and adapted from *Composition of Foods —Raw, Processed, Prepared,* Agriculture Handbook No. 8, U.S.D.A., 1963; *Nutritive Value of Foods,* Home and Garden Bulletin No. 72, U.S.D.A., 1971; *Nutritive Value of American Foods,* Agriculture Handbook, No. 456, U.S.D.A., 1975.

but frequently sugar as well. In the intense heat during baking, some starch on the surface of the product is broken to the smaller polysaccharides known as dextrins.

Starch is widely present in legumes of all types and in many other vegetables that are classified as seeds, tubers, or roots of plants. Leaf, flower, and stem vegetables are high in cellulose content, but quite limited in starch. The carbohydrate content of several common foods is given in Table 6.1.

Animals

Animal sources of carbohydrates are very limited in comparison with those from plants. Glycogen (animal starch) is stored in the liver of animals and accounts for usually no more than 5 percent of the weight of a serving of liver. Although glucose is present in the blood of animals, the amount remaining in meat as it is consumed is negligible.

The carbohydrate in milk is lactose. This unique animal sugar is distinctly less sweet and less soluble than sucrose. About 5 percent of milk is lactose. This sugar is important for its value in improving calcium utilization. Lactose intolerance, an inability to digest lactose and resulting in gastrointestinal distress, has in recent years become of increasing interest to researchers and physicians. The condition is more prevalent in blacks and Orientals, but is still infrequent.

Honey, since it is elaborated by bees from flower nectars, may be considered as a sugar of animal origin. This food is an important source of two monosaccharides: glucose and fructose.

Digestion and Absorption

Digestion

The initial phase of carbohydrate digestion is in the mouth where the food is broken into much smaller particles by chewing and concurrently mixed with saliva, which facilitates swallowing and passage through the esophagus to the stomach (Table 6.2). Contained in saliva is an enzyme[2], salivary amylase or ptyalin, which initiates the process of hydrolyzing starch to sugar. The breakdown of food accomplished by the chewing action of the teeth is mechanical, whereas the action of salivary amylase results in chemical change in the starch molecules. The extent of the chemical breakdown is determined by the length of time the food remains in the mouth, for salivary amylase is capable of producing much shorter chain dextrins and even maltose when given sufficient time for action.

From the mouth, the food mass traverses the esophagus, a distance of about 10 inches, in approximately 7 seconds. Salivary amylase continues to act upon starch as the food moves into the stomach. However, only limited breakdown of starch occurs during the brief time that usually elapses between the time the food is eaten and the food reaches the stomach.

In the stomach, the mechanical action of the stomach continues to churn the food into a somewhat softer mass called chyme. The stomach secretes gastric juice containing several substances vital to normal digestion. Hydrochloric acid in the stomach causes some sucrose to be hydrolyzed into its component monosaccharides, fructose and glucose. The acid medium in the stomach also inactivates the salivary amylase, thus no further breakdown of starch occurs until the intestine takes over the

[2] An enzyme is a protein material that enables specific chemical reactions to occur without actually being changed itself. A more extensive discussion is presented in the section on enzymes in Chapter 11.

Table 6.2 Digestion of Carbohydrates

Site	Substrate	Enzyme	Agent	Digestion Products
Mouth	Food		Teeth	Small food particles (bolus)
Mouth	Starch	Ptyalin (salivary amylase)		Shorter chain dextrins
Esophagus	Starch	Ptyalin		Shorter chain dextrins, possibly maltose
Stomach	Sucrose		Hydrochloric acid	Glucose and fructose
Small intestine	Starch and dextrins	Pancreatic amylase		Maltose
Small intestine	Maltose	Maltase		Glucose
Small intestine	Sucrose	Sucrase		Glucose and fructose
Small intestine	Lactose	Lactase[a]		Glucose and galactose

[a] This enzyme may not be present (after infancy) in some Orientals and blacks (see Chapter 14).

digestive process. Foods high in carbohydrate remain in the stomach a relatively short time and then move through the pyloric sphincter into the small intestine.

The small intestine is the principal site for digestion and absorption of carbohydrates. The carbohydrates that enter the small intestine include: monosaccharides and disaccharides present in the food consumed; small amounts of glucose and fructose resulting from the breakdown of some sucrose in the stomach; intact starch molecules that did not come in contact with salivary amylase as the food passed through the mouth to the stomach; dextrins and maltose resulting from the action of salivary amylase; and cellulose and other carbohydrates such as pectin that are not digested by humans.

When carbohydrates first reach the upper part of the small intestine, digestion to the component monosaccharides takes place. The surface of the intestinal wall is comprised of millions of tiny, finger-shaped projections, called villi, which give the intestinal wall an almost velvet-like texture. These villi along the intestinal wall are stimulated into a swaying motion in the presence of chyme. The peristaltic action of the intestine moves the chyme along while digestion is being completed.

In the small intestine, liver bile and pancreatic juice are released to modify the intestinal environment. The acidic reaction of the stomach gives way in the intestine to an alkaline medium favorable to the action of the carbohydrases (enzymes that act on carbohydrates). Pancreatic amylase completes the con-

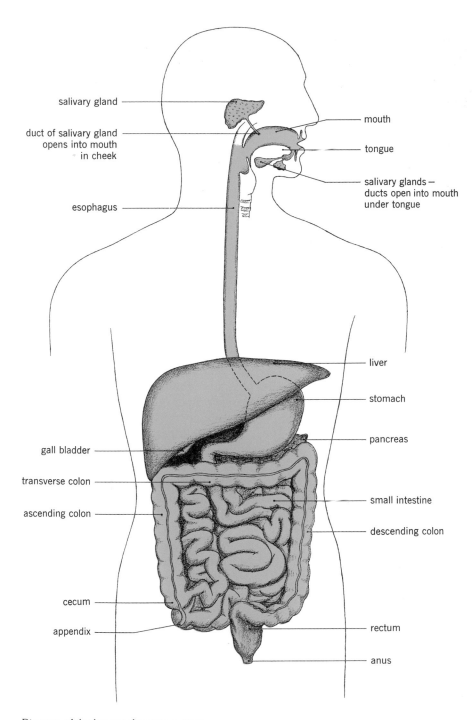

salivary gland

duct of salivary gland
opens into mouth
in cheek

esophagus

gall bladder

transverse colon

ascending colon

cecum

appendix

mouth

tongue

salivary glands —
ducts open into mouth
under tongue

liver

stomach

pancreas

small intestine

descending colon

rectum

anus

Diagram of the human digestive system.

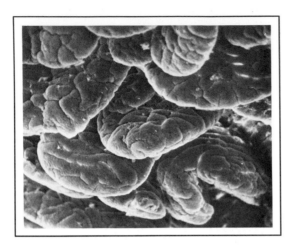

Villi in the intestine greatly increase the surface area for absorption of nutrients (Scanning electron micrograph, magnification 120×).

principal site of absorption of nutrients is the small intestine, which is uniquely designed for this extremely important function. Since each molecule must be passed through the intestinal wall before being used by the body, the amount of material that can be absorbed is influenced significantly by the surface area of that wall. The small intestine, instead of being a straight, smooth passageway, is highly convoluted, thus increasing the surface area. However, this is not the sole secret of the amazing effectiveness of the absorption mechanism. The villi lining the small intestine provide a vast area for absorption. Despite their miniature size (approximately 0.04 inches long), villi are complex in structure. The surface of their epithelial cells is covered with very tiny microvilli that increase the effective surface of the intestinal lining still more.

Absorption of monosaccharides takes place via the epithelial cells of the villi. Once within the epithelial cell, the monosaccharide molecules pass through the opposite wall of the cell and traverse a layer of connective tissue before finally entering a capillary of the bloodstream. The monosaccharides are then transported, through the portal vein, to the liver where any nonglucose monosaccharide molecules are converted to glucose.

Glucose can be utilized in at least three different ways:

1. Converted to glycogen in the liver and stored there in this form until this reserve carbohydrate is needed. The liver has a maximum capacity for storing glycogen. Glycogen is stored in muscles, too.

2. Released into the blood to be carried to all body tissues and cells. Although the level rises substantially above the minimum value after eating, glucose levels in the bloodstream are regulated in the normally healthy individual at 80 to 100 milligrams of glucose per 100 milliliters of blood or slightly higher.

3. Converted to fatty acids for ultimate storage as fat in the adipose tissues.

version of starch and dextrin molecules to the disaccharide, maltose. Specific intestinal enzymes complete the task of transforming all disaccharides into their component monosaccharides, ready for absorption. The enzyme that hydrolyzes maltose into two glucose molecules is maltase; sucrase converts sucrose into glucose and fructose; and lactase splits lactose into galactose and glucose. By the time carbohydrates reach the lower part of the upper small intestine, the monosaccharides are released from digestible carbohydrate and absorption takes place. Cellulose and other indigestible carbohydrates proceed into the large intestine and are excreted in the feces after traversing between 24 and 36 feet of digestive tract. They are important in promoting intestinal motility and influencing the character of intestinal microflora.

Absorption

After the digestible disaccharides, oligosaccharides, and polysaccharides have been transformed into their component monosaccharides, they are ready for absorption. The

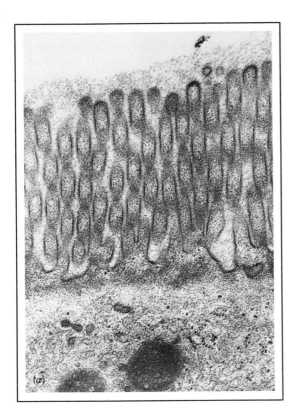

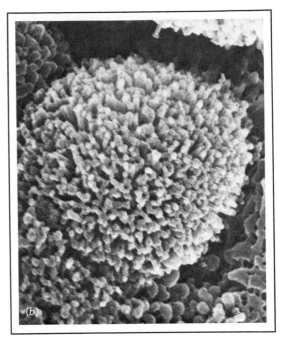

(a) *Microvilli of epithelial cell of human intestine (magnification 27,000×). (b) Single epithelial cell (scanning electron micrograph, enlarged 12,000×) on the surface of the villi is covered by microvilli.*

Metabolism

Metabolism, the utilization of food, is the total process of chemical synthesis and degradation of nutrients in the body. In some instances, there will be a chemical breakdown of organic substances into simpler molecules. This process specifically is called catabolism. The reverse of catabolism, or the formation of more complex substances in the body, is anabolism. The series of chemical changes involved in anabolism and catabolism are referred to as metabolic pathways. The tracing of these metabolic pathways has been done meticulously and with intensive research efforts. Much is known presently about the metabolism of glucose, although there are still points requiring additional clarification.

When glucose enters a cell, catabolism is ini-

tiated; ultimately, energy is released at various stages in the route to forming water and carbon dioxide from the breakdown of glucose. Much of this energy is in the form of heat. Less than half of the energy is transferred to other molecular compounds in the cells to be used as needed for operating the body. When energy is stored in compounds in the cell, it is stored in rather unstable bonds called "energy-rich bonds." Adenosine triphosphate (ATP) is a very important compound in metabolism because of its energy-storing capability. Some reactions in metabolism require energy. This energy can be provided by splitting the unstable, energy-rich bond of ATP, the net result being energy and adenosine diphosphate (ADP). This reaction is reversible, and adenosine diphosphate can be converted back to ATP when energy and phosphate become available. Some other compounds that are chemically similar to ATP and ADP can undergo comparable metabolic reactions.

In the initial phases of the breakdown of glucose, the single six-carbon molecule is split during a series of chemical reactions to form an important three-carbon substance, pyruvic acid or pyruvate. This process is called glycolysis. Adenosine triphosphate is needed to provide the energy required in this transition.

The next step in releasing energy from glucose is the transformation of pyruvate to acetate, an intermediate product containing two carbon atoms. Three of the B vitamins, niacin, thiamin, and riboflavin, are required as parts of coenzymes in the formation of acetate. Coenzymes are compounds required by enzymes (see Chapter 11) if the enzymes are to catalyze the reactions. Niacin is a part of the coenzyme nicotinamide-adenine dinucleotide (commonly called NAD); riboflavin is a part of flavin-adenine dinucleotide (FAD); thiamin is contained in thiamin pyrophosphate (TPP). The acetate formed with the aid of these coenzymes then combines with Coenzyme A (coenzyme containing pantothenic acid) to form acetyl CoA.

After the metabolism of glucose has proceeded this far, the acetyl CoA reacts with oxaloacetate to form citrate. The citrate then undergoes a series of oxidative changes, known collectively as the Krebs Cycle (sometimes called the Citric Acid Cycle or the Tricarboxylic Acid Cycle). Concomitant with the several reactions that take place in the Krebs Cycle, carbon dioxide is formed and hydrogen is released for entry into the electron transport system outlined below. As can be seen in Figure 6.2, the Krebs Cycle is ongoing, because oxaloacetate is regenerated ultimately and is once again ready to combine with a molecule of acetyl CoA to perpetuate the cyclic nature of the reactions and continue this essential cycle to ultimately release energy for the body. Four B vitamins, namely thiamin, riboflavin, niacin, and pantothenic acid (in the form of thiamin pyrophosphate, flavin-adenine dinucleotide, nicotinamide-adenine dinucleotide, and Coenzyme A, respectively) are required during the Krebs Cycle (Table 6.3).

The coenzymes that have participated in the Krebs Cycle are reoxidized by electron transport, as outlined in Figure 6.3. The cytochromes are proteins with an iron-containing porphyrin structure like that of hemoglobin. The hydrogen ions release from the reactions in the Krebs Cycle enter the electron transport system, where they ultimately combine with oxygen to form water. ATP is formed as a result of electron transport. This high-energy compound thus is available for use in the formation of

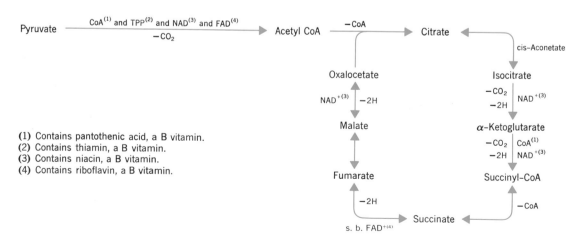

(1) Contains pantothenic acid, a B vitamin.
(2) Contains thiamin, a B vitamin.
(3) Contains niacin, a B vitamin.
(4) Contains riboflavin, a B vitamin.

Figure 6.2 Overview of the Krebs Cycle.

Table 6.3 *Some Key Catalytic Compounds Involved in Metabolism of Carbohydrates*

Compound	Catalytic Action	Components
NAD (nicotin-amide-adenine dinucleotide)	1. Glucose to pyruvate 2. Pyruvate to acetyl CoA 3. Isocitrate to α-ketoglutarate 4. α-ketoglutarate to succinyl-CoA 5. Malate to oxaloacetate	Niacin
TPP (thiamin pyrophosphate)	1. Pyruvate to acetyl CoA 2. α-ketoglutarate to succinyl CoA	Thiamin
Coenzyme A (CoA)	1. Pyruvate to acetyl CoA 2. α-ketoglutarate to succinyl CoA	Pantothenic acid
FAD (flavin-adenine dinucleotide)	1. Pyruvate to acetyl CoA 2. Succinate to fumarate	Riboflavin
Cytochromes (cytochromes a, b, and c)	1. Electron transport	Iron and copper

pyruvic acid (through glycolysis), reactions in the Krebs Cycle, muscle contraction, and other processes requiring energy.

The processes of metabolism are performed in the cell, as previously outlined. The breakdown of glucose to pyruvic acid occurs in the cytoplasm, the Krebs Cycle and electron transport in the mitochondria. The energy that is available as a result of the chemical transitions that occur when carbohydrate is metabolized may be used to meet the energy needs of various chemical syntheses. Energy is needed not only for the formation of new compounds required for body maintenance, but is used for all bodily movement and activities, including the transmission of nerve impulses. Anyone who has shivered from the cold is well aware of the need for energy to maintain the body's temperature. Another product of carbohydrate metabolism is carbon dioxide. This gaseous compound is transported from the site of glucose oxidation to the lungs, where it is simply excreted by exhaling. The third by-product of glucose utilization is water. This water, sometimes referred to as metabolic water, is excreted ultimately in the urine or through the skin and lungs.

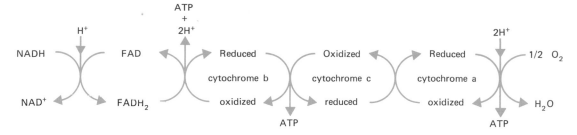

Figure 6.3 Electron transport.

Storage

Although the body stores of glycogen are limited, there is some transformation of glucose to glycogen in the liver and in muscles. The polymerization of glucose to glycogen produces a much larger carbohydrate molecule. This formation of a larger molecule from small ones is called anabolism. Such a chemical change is the body's way of storing energy for subsequent use when the energy needs of the body are not being met by the immediate supply of glucose available for oxidation. The formation of glycogen in animals is comparable to the production of starch in plants. Both are complex carbohydrates polymerized from a simple carbohydrate, glucose.

The Role of Carbohydrates

The outstanding role of carbohydrate in the diet is to provide energy for the body. Most carbohydrate foods are useful potential sources of the glucose needed by the body to yield energy for body movements, functioning of the brain, utilization of food, and maintenance of body temperature. In addition, carbohydrate in the diet is important in sparing protein and preventing the development of ketosis that occurs when fats are not metabolized normally.

Carbohydrates are the major source of energy for the vast majority of the world's population both because of the relative abundance of carbohydrate-rich foods (rice, wheat, corn, and sugar, for example) and because of the lower price of these items in comparison with either fats or protein foods. Both of these facts are true because of the tremendous productivity of the cereal grains under modern agricultural procedures. The average diet in the United States appears to derive approximately 45 to 50 percent of its calories from carbohydrates.[3] Of this total, somewhat more than half is usually provided by starch and somewhat less than half by sugar. The total caloric contribution of carbohydrates hovers in that range, although starches are used more extensively when income is limited and sugars are consumed in greater amounts when money available for food is increased. In parts of the world where financial problems are more acute for the typical family, the percentage of the day's caloric intake derived from carbohydrates rises to as high as 85 to 90 percent. As discussed in Chapter 4, pure carbohydrates provided

[3] Economy in the food budget and good health can be provided by increasing the caloric contribution of carbohydrates to between 50 and 55 percent of the total intake, with the remainder being available from protein (10 to 20 percent) and fat (30 to 35 percent).

approximately 4 kilocalories per gram when utilized in the body. Therefore, the caloric contribution of carbohydrates to the diet is calculated by multiplying the number of grams of pure carbohydrate by the factor of four.

Despite the importance of carbohydrate in the diet for energy, this nutrient also may have a negative aspect. Carbohydrate (particularly as sugar) between meals creates an environment in the mouth favorable to the growth of microorganisms that produce weak organic acids that favor the development of dental caries. These microorganisms require carbohydrate for their metabolism. In its absence, they approach the resting stage, with little production of organic acids and therefore less ability to destroy tooth substance. The situation is aggravated by carbohydrate foods that cling to the teeth for a period of time and by frequent between-meal consumption of sticky, high-carbohydrate foods. If the mouth is cleansed thoroughly by a good brushing of the teeth, the impact of carbohydrates on dental decay is reduced. However, the use of fluoridated water from birth to old age is of utmost importance if the dental enamel is to develop and maintain maximum resistance to decay. The ideal for caries prevention is the combination of fluoride incorporation during tooth development and throughout life, with restriction in consumption of sticky sugars between meals, and good dental care.

Carbohydrates, in combination with protein, form several compounds important in the body. Mucopolysaccharides (hexosamine derivatives) such as hyaluronic acid are invaluable as lubricants in the joints. Other mucopolysaccharides and mucoproteins in the body are important components of nails, bone, cartilage, and skin.

One important function of carbohydrates is to facilitate the utilization of fatty acids in the body (see the section entitled "Metabolism" in Chapter 7), thus preventing the accumulation of ketone bodies and ketosis. Carbohydrates, as metabolism proceeds through the Krebs Cycle, lead to the production of oxaloacetate.

This compound is essential if the two-carbon fragments resulting from fatty acid oxidation are to enter the Krebs Cycle for the final breakdown to carbon dioxide, water, and energy.

Sugar (sucrose), a major carbohydrate in the diet and second only to starch in the amount occurring in the diet, has in recent years come in for considerable criticism, some from nutritionists, but mostly from consumer activists and largely on an emotional basis, not a factual basis. It has been "blamed" as playing a major role in many of the common diseases—heart disease, obesity, diabetes, hypoglycemia, and others. A recent review of this subject by nine authorities in these various fields gives sugar a pretty clean bill of health when used in moderation, that is, 15 to 20 percent of total calories.

Sugar is frequently denigrated as being only "empty calories," meaning that sugar is a pure carbohydrate and provides no vitamins, minerals, protein, or other nutrients. What is generally overlooked is that most sugar is consumed as a part of other foods, actually as an additive. It is added to milk and other foods to make ice cream; to flour, shortening, and eggs to make baked goods; to fruits and vegetables to make them more palatable. Thus, while sugar contains only calories, its actual use in the diet makes more palatable many other foods that do provide the many nutrients needed for good health.

Another point in favor of sugar is that it is the most efficient source of calories in terms of land use and production costs—and in a world short of calories this is important. To produce one million kilocalories from sugar beets or cane requires only 0.15 acres of fertile land. To produce the same number of kilocalories from potatoes requires 0.4 acres; from rice, wheat or corn, approximately 1 acre; and from animal products, anywhere from 2 to 17 acres.

Fiber, although it is not actually absorbed into the body, nevertheless performs the valuable functions of promoting intestinal motility and influencing the microbiological flora of the intestine. Recognition of the significance of these roles has been increasing recently. Epidemiologic studies coming largely from Central Africa and done primarily by three British investigators—Doctors D. P. Burkitt, N. S. Painter, and H. Trowell—have suggested that lack of fiber in the diet may be of importance not only in the causation of many diseases of the lower bowel such as cancer of the colon, but also of appendicitis, coronary heart disease, obesity, and diabetes. Theoretically, an appreciable increase in the fiber content of the diet may interfere with the absorption of certain essential nutrients such as calcium and zinc, so there may be a negative aspect to increasing appreciably the fiber content of our diets. Diets which predominate in meats, dairy products, and refined cereal products are low in fiber. Those generous in fruits, vegetables, and whole grain breads and cereals have appreciably more fiber.

Summary

Carbohydrates are chemically related organic compounds that are classified as monosaccharides, disaccharides, oligosaccharides, and polysaccharides. Sugars, dextrins, starch, glycogen, cellulose, and pectic substances are familiar examples of carbohydrates. During the digestive process, monosaccharides are released. These monosaccharides are absorbed in the small intestine and then transported through the bloodstream to the liver. The glucose formed in the liver can be converted to glycogen for storage, transported to the tissues for metabolism and the release of energy, or stored as fat. Carbohydrate is metabolized in a series of reactions called glycolysis, which changes glucose to pyruvic acid. Pyruvic acid is modified to acetyl-CoA and then enters the Krebs Cycle. Coenzymes participating in the Krebs Cycle then are reoxidized by electron transport and more energy is released.

Carbohydrates are essential to the body as a source of energy. They provide a sparing action for protein in the body, because protein from the body is not needed for energy if sufficient carbohydrate is available to supply the body's needs. Carbohydrates also are needed to metabolize fat normally.

The nondigestible carbohydrates generally referred to as dietary fiber, while thought to have no nutritive value, play an important role in the elimination of body wastes through formation of feces, influence the character and quantity of the bacterial flora of the lower intestine, and may play an important role in a number of common diseases of man.

Selected References

Burkitt, D. P., et al. Dietary fiber and disease. *J. Am. Med. Assoc. 229:* 1068. 1974.

Connor, W. E. Sugar. *Present Knowledge of Nutrition.* 4th ed. Nutrition Foundation. New York. 1976.

Danowski, T. S., et al. Hypoglycemia. *World Rev. Nutr. Diet. 22:*288. 1975.

Finn, S. B., and R. B. Glass. Sugar and dental decay. *World Rev. Nutr. Diet. 22:*301. 1975.

Gustafsson, B. E. Survey of the literature on carbohydrates and dental caries. *Acta Odontologica Scandinavica. 11:*207. 1954.

Gustafsson, B. E., et al. Effect of different levels of carbohydrate intake on caries activity in 436 individuals observed for five years. *Acta Odontologica Scandinavica. 11:*232. 1954.

Hodges, R. Present knowledge of carbohydrate. *Nutrition Rev. 24:*65. 1966.

Leichter, J., and M. Lee. Lactose intolerance in Canadian West Coast Indians. *Am. J. Digestive Diseases. 16:*809. 1971.

MacDonald, I. Symposium on dietary carbohydrates in man. *Am. J. Clin. Nutr. 20:*65. 1967.

McWilliams, M. *Food Fundamentals.* 2nd ed. Wiley. New York. 1974.

Mendeloff, A. I. Fiber. *Present Knowledge of Nutrition.* 4th ed. Nutrition Foundation. New York. 1976.

Mertz, W. Glucose tolerance factor. *Present Knowledge of Nutrition.* 4th ed. Nutrition Foundation. New York. 1976.

Mitchell, H. S., et al. *Cooper's Nutrition in Health and Disease.* 15th ed. Lippincott. Philadelphia. 1968.

Reilly, R. W., and J. B. Kirsner. *Fiber Deficiency and Colonic Disorders.* Plenum Publishing. New York. 1975.

Review. Carbohydrate digestion and absorption. *Nutr. Rev. 21:*279. 1963.

Scala, J. Fiber, the forgotten nutrient. *Food Tech. 28:*34. 1974.

Schaefer, O. When the Eskimo comes to town. *Nutrition Today. 6,* No. 6:8. 1971.

Sebrell, W. H., Jr., and J. J. Haggerty. *Food and Nutrition.* Life Science Library. New York. 1967.

Stare, F. J. Role of sugar in modern nutrition. *World Rev. Nutr. Diet. 22:*239. 1975.

Woodruff, C. W. Milk intolerance. *Present Knowledge of Nutrition.* 4th ed. Nutrition Foundation. New York. 1976.

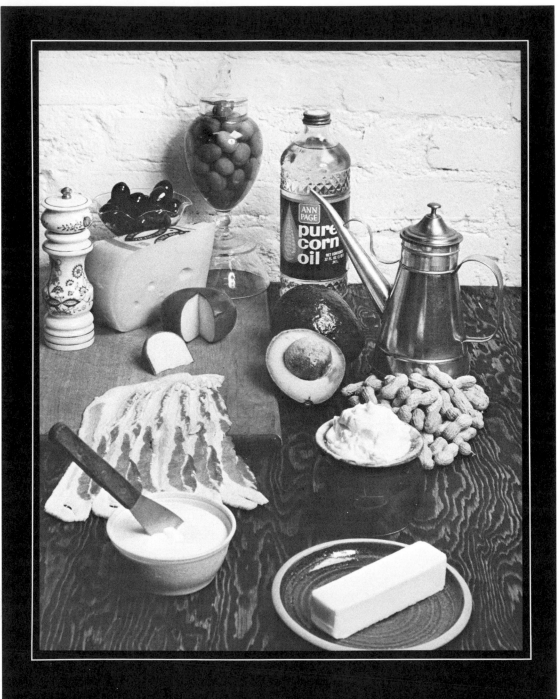

Chapter 7

The term "lipid" is a broad term used to designate several types of substances that are water insoluble and ether soluble. Under this broad term, there are three categories that are generally recognized: (1) simple lipids, (2) compound lipids, and (3) derived lipids. The first category, the simple lipids, is of particular interest in this chapter. Simple fats and oils, defined as fatty acid esters of glycerol (see the next section), are classified as simple lipids. The other class of materials designated as simple lipids is waxes. Waxes are fatty acids combined with any alcohol except glycerol. Cholesterol is a familiar example of an alcohol that may be a component of a wax.

One of the fascinating aspects of nutrition is the commonalities that can be noted when one compares some of the nutrients. For example, note the fact that carbohydrates and simple fats are composed of three common elements: carbon, hydrogen, and oxygen. Yet another similarity that may be cited is that both of these food groups are important in the diet because they are valuable sources of energy. In addition, both carbohydrates and simple fats are found in foods of animal and plant origin. With so many apparent parallels between the two groups, one might be tempted to conclude that there really is very little difference chemically between them, and yet that certainly is not the case. The chemical nature of fats, as can be seen in the following discussion, is unique and bears little resemblance to the carbohydrates described in the preceding chapter.

Glycerol

The molecules of simple fats that occur in foods consist of two types of compounds: (1) alcohol (glycerol) and (2) organic acids, known as fatty acids. Only one alcohol, glycerol, is found in the common food fats. Glycerol (also called glycerine) is of small molecular size and contains only 3 carbon atoms. The unusual and rather interesting feature of glycerol is that it contains three hydroxyl (—OH) groups, in contrast to the more usual single hydroxyl group of common alcohols such as ethanol and propanol. The three hydroxyl groups are important because these are the reactive groups by which glycerol can combine with fatty acids to form fats.

Glycerol   Ethanol   Propanol

Fatty acids

One has only to look at butter and oil to recognize that some obvious differences exist in fats. Since the glycerol portion of the molecule is the same in both solid fats and in oils, the unique characteristics of particular fats must be due to the fatty acids in the molecule.

Fatty acids are organic acids that occur, either alone or combined with glycerol, in many foods. A chain of carbon atoms, to which hydrogen atoms are attached, makes up the larger portion of the fatty acid. This fragment is attached to a carboxyl group (organic acid radical). To simplify writing the structure of a fatty

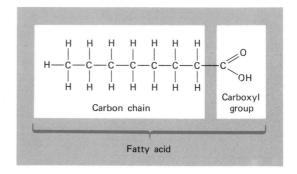

Carbon chain   Carboxyl group

Fatty acid

acid, the carbon chain portion often is designated by using R:

$$R—C\begin{smallmatrix}O\\OH\end{smallmatrix}$$

Fatty acids all have this same general type of structure, although the length of the carbon chain and the amount of hydrogen attached to the chain varies.

Length of carbon chain

The fatty acids found in foods may vary significantly in the length of the carbon chains. Some fatty acids comprised of as few as four carbon atoms are found in food. Butyric acid, the four-carbon fatty acid that is fairly abundant in butter, is an illustration of a short-chain fatty acid in food. Foods commonly contain fatty acids with chain lengths of 16 or 18 carbon atoms, and occasionally as many as 20. Furthermore, there will always be an even number of carbon atoms in the molecule (counting the carbon atom in the carboxyl group).

The length of the carbon chain in the fatty acid is important because it influences the physical characteristics of the fat. Short-chain fatty acids are fluid; long-chain fatty acids are

Table 7.1   Structures of Some Fatty Acids Found in Foods[a]

Fatty Acid	Structure	Melting Point (°C)

Butyric	<pre> H H H
	  | | | O
	H-C-C-C-C⟨
	  | | | OH
	  H H H</pre>
		−4.7

Palmitic	<pre> H H H H H H H H H H H H H H H
	  | | | | | | | | | | | | | | | O
	H-C-C-C-C-C-C-C-C-C-C-C-C-C-C-C-C⟨
	  | | | | | | | | | | | | | | | OH
	  H H H H H H H H H H H H H H H</pre>
		63

Stearic	<pre> H H H H H H H H H H H H H H H H H
	  | | | | | | | | | | | | | | | | | O
	H-C-C-C-C-C-C-C-C-C-C-C-C-C-C-C-C-C-C⟨
	  | | | | | | | | | | | | | | | | | OH
	  H H H H H H H H H H H H H H H H H</pre>
		69.6

Oleic	<pre> H H H H H H H H H H H H H H H H H
	  | | | | | | | | | | | | | | | | | O
	H-C-C-C-C-C-C-C-C-C=C-C-C-C-C-C-C-C-C⟨
	  | | | | | | | | | | | | | | | OH
	  H H H H H H H H H H H H H H H</pre>
		13.4

Linoleic	<pre> H H H H H H H H H H H H H H H H H
	  | | | | | | | | | | | | | | | | | O
	H-C-C-C-C-C-C=C-C- C=C-C-C-C-C-C-C-C-C⟨
	  | | | | | | | | | | | | | OH
	  H H H H H H H H H H H H H</pre>
		−5

Linolenic	<pre> H H H H H H H H H H H H H H H H H
	  | | | | | | | | | | | | | | | | | O
	H-C-C-C=C-C-C-C=C-C-C-C=C-C-C-C-C-C-C⟨
	  | | | | | | | | | | OH
	  H H H H H H H H H H</pre>
		−11

Arachidonic	<pre> H H H H H H H H H H H H H H H H H H H
	  | | | | | | | | | | | | | | | | | | | O
	H-C-C-C-C-C-C=C-C-C-C=C-C-C-C=C-C-C=C-C-C-C-C⟨
	  | | | | | | | | | | | OH
	  H H H H H H H H H H H</pre>
		−49.5

[a] Selected from **Biochemists' Handbook,** ed. by C. D. Long, Van Nostrand, Princeton, N.J. 1961.

quite firm at room temperature. If a short-chain fatty acid is combined with glycerol, the fat will be softer than a similar fat containing a long-chain fatty acid.

Saturated and unsaturated fatty acids

In addition to the length of the carbon chain of a fatty acid, there is another very important variable in chemical structure that influences the physical characteristics of a fatty acid. This variable is the amount of hydrogen contained in the fatty acid. Ordinarily, a carbon atom is attached to four other atoms. As can be seen in the fatty acid molecule just shown, usually all except the end carbon atoms will be attached to two carbon atoms and two hydrogen atoms. This type of structure is quite stable and will not react with hydrogen. Molecules of this type are called "saturated" fatty acids.

A review of Table 7.1 reveals that not all fatty acids are saturated with all the hydrogen they are potentially capable of containing. For example, note the structure for oleic acid. Two carbon atoms in the center of the chain are joined together by a chemical bond, called a double bond. The presence of even one double bond in a fatty acid causes the unsaturated fatty acid (containing the double bond) to be more fluid than is the saturated fatty acid of the same chain length. Note that stearic acid, a saturated fatty acid containing 18 carbon atoms, is a waxy solid at room temperature. In contrast, oleic acid, which is also an 18-carbon fatty acid, has such a low melting point that it is a liquid at room temperature. The single difference between these two fatty acids is the degree of unsaturation. The one double bond in oleic acid causes the tremendous difference in the physical characteristics. When a fatty acid has one double bond in its structure, the fatty acid is said to be monounsaturated.

A few fatty acids contain more than one double bond. Linoleic acid contains two double bonds. Linolenic acid has three double bonds, and arachidonic acid (20 carbon atoms) has four double bonds. Fatty acids with two or more double bonds in their structures are called polyunsaturated fatty acids (commonly abbreviated as PUFA).

Glycerides

Fats are classified according to the number of fatty acids esterified to the glycerol portion of the molecule. When a fat molecule contains only one fatty acid at one of the potential sites for attachment to the glycerol portion, the molecule is said to be a monoglyceride (Table 7.2). Fat molecules containing two fatty acids are classified as diglycerides; note that the molecule is a diglyceride regardless of whether the two fatty acids are arranged on the end carbons or on adjacent ones. As would be expected, the molecule formed when three fatty acids are combined with glycerol is classified as a triglyceride.

Triglycerides are of considerable interest from the nutritionist's viewpoint because much of the fat in foods is found in the form of triglycerides. However, monoglycerides and diglycerides are used extensively in the formulation of various prepared baked and processed foods to modify the behavioral characteristics of fats in specific products, such as cakes.

Each food source of fat has certain typical patterns of fatty acids that will be attached to glycerol to form the triglycerides as they naturally occur. In a few instances, a fat will have the same fatty acid attached to all three points on glycerol. Such molecules are referred to as simple triglycerides. When at least two different fatty acids are found in the fat molecule, the compound is said to be a mixed triglyceride. This type of triglyceride is far more common in foods than the simple triglyceride is.

Lecithins

These naturally occurring compounds are similar to glycerides in that they are composed of glycerol, two fatty acids, and phosphoric acid

Table 7.2 Structures of Glycerides

Classification	Chemical Structure[a]
Monoglyceride	H H | | H–C – O – C̈–R or H–C – OH | O | H–C – OH H–C – O – C̈–R | | O H–C – OH H–C – OH | | H H
Diglyceride	H H | | H–C – O – C̈–R or H–C – O – C̈–R | O | O H–C – OH H–C – O – C̈–R′ | | O H–C – O – C̈–R′ H–C – OH | O | H H
Triglyceride	H | H–C – O C̈–R | O H–C – O C̈–R′ | O H–C – O C̈–R″ | O H

[a] R, R′, and R″ are general formulas for fatty acids and thus represent carbon chains up to 19 carbon atoms in length.

attached to a nitrogenous base. They are therefore phospholipids. They are essential constituents of all cells, of mitochondria, and they function as metabolic intermediates in the transport and utilization of fatty acids in body tissues.

They are mentioned here briefly because some food faddists attach special significance to lecithins as substances with unusual health-promoting properties, particularly in helping to regulate (lower) the level of cholesterol in the blood. They have no such properties.

The general formula for lecithins is:

$$
\begin{array}{l}
\quad\quad\quad\quad\quad O \\
\quad\quad\quad\quad\quad \| \\
H_2{-}C{-}O{-}C{-}R \\
\quad\quad\quad\quad\quad O \\
\quad\quad\quad\quad\quad \| \\
H{-}C{-}O{-}C{-}R' \\
\quad\quad\quad\quad\quad O \quad\quad\quad\quad\quad CH_3 \\
\quad\quad\quad\quad\quad \| \quad\quad\quad\quad\quad\quad | \\
H_2{-}C{-}O{-}P{-}O{-}CH_2{-}CH_2{-}\overset{+}{N}{-}CH_3 \\
\quad\quad\quad\quad\quad | \quad\quad\quad\quad\quad\quad | \\
\quad\quad\quad\quad\quad O^- \quad\quad\quad\quad\quad CH_3
\end{array}
$$

Lecithins are prepared commercially from soybeans, and also from egg yolks, and are used in many food products as a smoothing or emulsifying agent. They are completely metabolized by the body and, because of the fatty acids they contain, they are generous sources of calories. Defatted lecithin is simply lecithin from which extraneous fat has been removed from a crude preparation, but the two fatty acids of the lecithin molecule still remain.

Fats in Foods

Plant and animal sources

Fats are found in many foods of animal origin and in some plant foods. Some foods are recognized by practically everyone as being good sources of fat because the fat is clearly visible. Examples of visible fats include butter, margarine, salad oil, and the fatty deposits surrounding or adjacent to the muscle in a cut of meat. These visible fats occupy a prominent position in the typical American diet. Other sources of fat are far less obvious, yet may be eaten in surprisingly large quantities, even by persons who think they are eating a relatively low-fat diet. These so-called "hidden fats" occur as marbling or small deposits of fat within the muscle of high-quality, mature meat animals such as prime and choice grades of beef. Additional illustrations are the cream in milk, cheeses (except those made with skim milk), avocados, nuts, chocolate, and desserts containing whipped cream, butter, margarine, or shortening.

Animal foods are usually good sources of fat in the diet. For example, butter is approximately 80 percent fat, pork contains between 20 and 30 percent fat, and various cuts of beef range between 15 and 30 percent fat. On the other hand, chicken is fairly low in fat, with fat levels ranging between 6 and 15 percent. Fish also are generally low in fat.

Several plants are particularly significant sources of oils. Familiar examples include oil from soybeans, cottonseed, olives, corn, coconut, peanuts, palm, sunflower, and safflower. These plant materials are the usual sources of the various edible oil products that are available to the consumer for preparing fried foods, making salad dressings, and for use in a wide variety of baked products. Margarine, which may be considered as the vegetable oil counterpart of butter, is widely used, not only in the United States, but in many other countries too.

Hydrogenation

Although there are many uses for the edible vegetable oils in their fluid form, products made by modifying these oils also are popular in the American diet. The peanut butter of today is a good example of what food technologists can do to enhance a product. As peanut butter was developed and marketed originally, it was a blend of peanut oil and solids. During the time the peanut butter sat on the shelf, there was always a distinct separation between the solids and the oil, with the oil rising to the top. The first task in preparing a peanut butter sandwich automatically became the stirring of the peanut butter in the jar. Since this mixing operation seldom was done until a homogeneous mixture was obtained, the result generally was a distinctly oily sandwich at the beginning of the jar, and such a dry product in the bottom of the jar that it was almost impossible to spread. As can be deduced from the previous discussion, peanut oil is naturally rather high in unsaturated fatty acids.

This improvement in peanut butter became possible when technologists developed a process whereby some of the unsaturated fatty acids could be changed to saturated fatty acids, to a controlled extent, by adding hydrogen at some of the double bonds. The addition of hydrogen, referred to as hydrogenation, raises the melting point of those fatty acids in peanut butter that are treated in this manner. As a result, the oil is sufficiently firm at room temperature to remain mixed with the solids. In actual practice hydrogenated soya or cottonseed oil also may be added to the peanut butter to help achieve the goal of lasting "spreadability."

Another application of the hydrogenation process is the production of shortenings and margarines from vegetable oils. A portion of the oil that is to be used in making a shortening or margarine is hydrogenated to convert the oil into a solid. This solid fat may then be blended with the natural oils that have not been hydrogenated. The final product is unlike the original oil in its physical character, yet retains a relatively large proportion of the unsaturated fatty acids needed in the human diet. In the market today, the consumer is confronted with a wide choice of margarines. Label reading is a necessary part of shopping if a particular type of margarine is desired. Ingredients on the label are listed in order of decreasing quantities, beginning with the most abundant item and ending with the substance present in the smallest quantity. Therefore, a margarine listing safflower or corn oil first will have more polyunsaturated fatty acids in the product than will one listing vegetable or hydrogenated vegetable oil first.

Digestion, Absorption, and Transport

The first step in the digestion of most fats is the physical warming of the fats that are consumed. When cold fats, such as butter or margarine are eaten, the fat is quite firm and is found in relatively large particles instead of in a highly fluid state. During the time the fat is in the mouth and traversing the esophagus to the stomach, there is a softening that begins to take place (Table 7.3). In the stomach the fat becomes very fluid. This fluidity is essential to the next stage of the digestive process when the fat passes into the small intestine.

Within the stomach, there is some digestion of fats that occur in foods in an emulsion, such as is true with the fat in egg yolks and in some salad dressings. In emulsions, fats are dispersed in very tiny droplets with a great deal of surface area exposed. This makes it possible for gastric lipase, the enzyme present in the stomach, to begin splitting off the fatty acid portions of fat molecules. Gastric lipase, however, is ineffective in digesting nonemulsified fats.

From the stomach, fat moves into the small intestine, where bile is readily available to emulsify the remaining fats. The emulsified fats now present sufficient surface area for highly effective enzyme action. Two enzymes, pancreatic lipase and intestinal lipase, split the fat molecules, producing diglycerides and monoglycerides, free fatty acids, and glycerol. These digested fragments of fat are absorbed through the intestinal wall.

Fats are efficiently digested and absorbed by normal, healthy individuals. The digestion and absorption of fat are distinctly less efficient when a person has diarrhea. With increased motility through the digestive tract, there is less time for enzyme action to take place, which inhibits normal digestion and absorption of fats. For this reason the use of mineral oil and various proprietary laxatives is detrimental to the absorption of fats (and also fat-soluble vitamins). If physical problems cause a reduction in the level of either bile or lipases (the fat-splitting enzymes), fats will be absorbed less efficiently, also. Inefficient digestion and absorp-

Table 7.3 Digestion of Fats

Site	Substrate	Enzyme	Agent	Digestion Products
Mouth and esophagus	Fats		Body heat	Warmer (more fluid) fats
Stomach	Nonemulsified fats		Body heat	Fluid fats
Stomach	Emulsified fat (present in the food)	Gastric lipase		Some diglycerides and monoglycerides, free fatty acids, and glycerol
Small intestine	Nonemulsified fats		Bile	Emulsified fats
Small intestine	Emulsified fat	Pancreatic lipase and intestinal lipase		Monoglycerides and a few diglycerides, free fatty acids, and glycerol

tion of fats result in the elimination of intact fat in the feces. This condition is called steatorrhea.

Upon absorption, two routes to body tissues are available. About one third of the free fatty acids (less than 12 carbons in length) and glycerol enter the blood for direct transport to the liver. The remaining two thirds of the absorbed free fatty acids and glycerol recombine immediately into monoglycerides, diglycerides, and triglycerides. These compounds are not readily miscible with the aqueous medium of the blood. Hence, their route of transport is somewhat different. The resynthesized fat enters ducts (the lacteals) of the lymphatic system. In turn, these glycerides are combined with a protein to form very tiny fat-protein particles called chylomicrons. These microscopic chylomicrons are carried through the lymphatic system and then enter the blood in the neck region before the blood enters the heart. Fat, in the form of chylomicrons, is more soluble in the blood than is fat that is not combined with protein. The minute chylomicrons give the blood a cloudy or milky appearance during this phase of utilization of dietary fats.

When fats are split in the liver and other tissues by lipases (fat-splitting enzymes), free fatty acids are formed. In the presence of choline, free fatty acids can be combined with protein to form lipoproteins that contain between 10 and 45 percent protein. Lipoproteins, because they contain a far greater proportion of protein than the chylomicrons, are readily transported in blood plasma to tissues where the fat can be stored or utilized for energy.

Metabolism

When fat is used for energy, the fat molecule is split into glycerol and the component fatty acids. The three-carbon glycerol fragment is metabolized through pyruvate and the Krebs Cycle described in Chapter 6. These numerous chemical reactions ultimately produce energy, carbon dioxide, and water.

The first step in the metabolism of the fatty

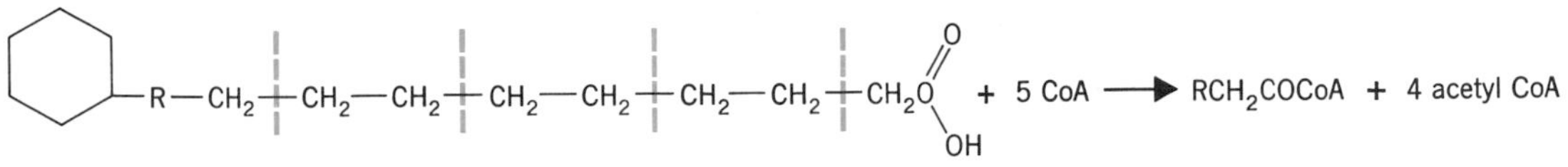

Figure 7.1   Beta oxidation of fatty acids. (Dotted lines on left side of equation show points where cleavage occurs.)

acid portions of fat molecules is a process known as beta oxidation (see Figure 7.1). Beta oxidation begins when Coenzyme A (an essential compound containing the B vitamin, pantothenic acid) replaces the hydroxyl (—OH) group of the acid. ATP provides the energy for this first step. Flavin-adenine dinucleotide (the coenzyme containing riboflavin) and nicotinamide-adenine dinucleotide (the coenzyme containing niacin) are involved in subsequent reactions of the beta oxidation process. The fatty acid chain is then split after the second carbon, hence the term "beta oxidation." The products of this cleavage are acetyl CoA and a fatty acid containing two less carbon atoms than in the original fatty acid. Coenzyme A is added to this shortened fatty acid chain, and the beta oxidation reactions are repeated until the fatty acid is metabolized completely. Reoxidation of the coenzymes reduced in beta oxidation results in the formation of ATP (via electron transport) to provide potential energy for the body.

The acetyl CoA resulting from beta oxidation can be utilized in either anabolic or catabolic reactions. The anabolic reactions may result in the formation of several different products. Some of the acetyl Coenzyme A molecules recombine to make different fatty acids. Others may be combined to synthesize such complex biochemical compounds as the sex hormones and cholesterol.

The acetyl CoA that will be catabolized for energy enters the Krebs Cycle by combining with oxaloacetate (see Figure 6.2). The participation of the acetyl CoA in the Krebs Cycle and electron transport system provides additional energy for the body.

For effective utilization of the products resulting from beta oxidation, carbohydrate must be present so that the fatty acid portion can condense with the carbohydrate derivatives and enter the Krebs Cycle. When diets are unusually high in fat and low in carbohydrate, these two-carbon units condense with each other to form "ketone bodies." An accumulation of ketone bodies results in the condition known as ketosis; this occurs in uncontrolled diabetes, leading to a possible coma and even death.

Functions of Fat

Fat serves several useful functions in the diet of man. One of its notable contributions is that it is a concentrated source of energy, and, as has been pointed out previously, the body needs energy for physical activity, basal metabolism, and in a minor way for the specific dynamic effect of food. Since fat contributes more than twice as many kilocalories per gram as either protein or carbohydrate, it is possible to consume a significant quantity of energy-containing fats without overtaxing the stomach capacity of an individual.

When fat is present in the diet, the fat contributes to the satiety value of food. Fats remain in the stomach longer than other foods (as long as 3½ hours after eating), and hence are digested rather slowly. Thus, the consumer has some feeling of satisfaction and appetite contentment. Even on weight reduction diets, fat has this satiety role to perform. Small amounts of fat can delay significantly the diner's awareness of interest in the next meal.

Fats are needed in the diet not only because of their energy value, but also because they are the source of linoleic acid, an essential nutrient which is a polyunsaturated fatty acid containing 18 carbon atoms and two double bonds (see Table 7.2). The body is capable of forming various fatty acids by normal physiological processes, but it cannot manufacture linoleic acid from other organic compounds. Linoleic acid has been demonstrated to be necessary for growth and also for the prevention of certain types of dermatitis in infants.

Two other polyunsaturated fatty acids, linolenic and arachidonic, are of limited usefulness in overcoming the problems of restricted growth and dermatitis. In experimental animals (rats), linolenic acid promotes growth, and arachidonic acid corrects the skin problem that develops in the absence of these important polyunsaturated fatty acids. Although both arachidonic and linolenic acids are of value in the body, they are not considered essential dietary factors because the body can produce both of these important polyunsaturated fatty acids from linoleic acid. The significant factor is to be certain that linoleic acid is present in sufficiently large quantities so that the other two acids can be synthesized to meet the body's need. Polyunsaturated fatty acids, notably arachidonic acid, are the precursors of prostaglandins, which are synthesized in the body. Prostaglandins are regulators or "local hormones." They may stimulate such actions as contraction of smooth muscle, lowering of blood pressure, and reduction of gastric secretion.

Fats serve yet another function in the diet, and that is as the carrier of fat-soluble vitamins —vitamins A, D, E, and K. These vitamins are miscible with the fats and oils in foods, but are not soluble in water. Thus, various fats and oils are the vehicle for ingesting and absorbing these vitamins. Even the precursors of vitamin A (see Chapter 11) require the presence of fatty substances for absorption to take place.

The gustatory value of fats also deserves to be mentioned. Most individuals find foods considerably more appealing when fat is included in the recipe. The popularity of frozen vegetables amply coated by a butter or margarine sauce is a clear testimonial to the improved consumer acceptance when fat is added to foods. Some meat markets have even gone to the extreme in packaging the more highly prized meat cuts when they place a large pat of butter or margarine prominently in the center of a steak. The practice of serving ice cream or whipped cream on desserts is yet another indication of the palatability people associate with the presence of fat in foods.

When not all the fat that is eaten is needed for energy, the excess can be deposited in the cells, and some is stored in special adipose tissue. These storage depots of fat are important for energy reserves at times when the intake of food is insufficient to meet the body's need for energy. These stores of fat help to remove the angular look of the body by providing some padding to disguise the body skeleton a bit. In cases of optimum nutrition, such deposits are considered aesthetically satisfying; in cases of obesity, they become disfiguring.

Stores of fat beneath the skin are effective insulators against a chilly environment and help to prevent uncomfortable heat loss from the body. Internal fatty deposits cushion various vital parts from jarring shocks and injury.

Fat in the Diet

Although there is no specific quantity of fat in the diet that is generally recognized as ideal for meeting human nutritional needs, the typical American diet is higher in fat than is necessary for good health. Table 7.4 outlines some of the more important dietary sources of fat. The

Table 7.4 *Dietary Sources of Fat and Relative Amounts of Saturated and Unsaturated Fatty Acids*[a]

Food	Amount	Total Fat (g)	Saturated Fat (g)	Unsaturated Fat	
				Oleic (g)	Linoleic (g)
Meats					
Sirloin steak, fat and lean, broiled	3 oz	27	13	12	1
Sirloin steak, lean, broiled	3 oz	6	3	3	Trace
Ground beef, regular, broiled	3 oz	17	8	8	Trace
Ground beef, lean, broiled	3 oz	10	5	4	Trace
Ham, fat and lean, roasted	3 oz	19	7	8	2
Lamb, leg roast, fat and lean	3 oz	16	9	6	Trace
Veal, fat and lean, roasted	3 oz	9	5	4	Trace
Chicken, white meat, broiled	3 oz	3	1	1	1
Tuna, oil packed	3 oz	7	2	1	1
Dairy					
Milk, 3.5% fat	1 cup	9	5	3	Trace
Milk, fortified low fat	1 cup	5	3	2	Trace
Cream, 12%	1 tbsp	3	2	1	Trace
Butter	1 tbsp	12	6	4	Trace
Cheese, cheddar	1 oz	9	5	3	Trace
Cheese, cream	1 oz	11	6	4	Trace
Vegetable fats					
Margarine, regular	1 tbsp	12	2	6	3
Margarine, soft	1 tbsp	11	2	4	4
Margarine, special	1 tbsp	11	2	4	4
Mayonnaise	1 tbsp	11	2	2	6
Oils: safflower	1 tbsp	14	1	2	10
corn	1 tbsp	14	1	4	7
soybean	1 tbsp	14	2	3	7
cottonseed	1 tbsp	14	4	3	7
peanut	1 tbsp	14	3	7	4
olive	1 tbsp	14	2	11	1
coconut	1 tbsp	14	12	1	Trace
Vegetable fat	1 tbsp	13	3	6	3

[a] Compiled from **Nutritive Value of Foods,** Home and Garden Bulletin No. 72, U.S.D.A., 1971.

average fat intake in the typical American diet for adults ranges between 40 and 45 percent of the day's total calorie consumption. This value is in marked contrast to some other countries of the world where fat contributes a far smaller percentage of the total caloric intake, actually as little as 2 to 3 percent of the total caloric intake. Nutritionists generally agree that a diet in which approximately 30 to 35 percent of the calories come from fat is more healthful than one with a higher proportion of the calories contributed by fat. One of the main arguments supporting the lower fat consumption is the hazard of overweight and increase in the level of serum cholesterol, which often occurs when a diet high in saturated fat is the pattern (see Chapter 16).

As a nutrient group, fats are of particular interest from a sociological viewpoint, for generally the proportion of fat in the diet of a nation is closely linked to the economic stature of the country. Where the development and technological progress of a nation are great, the proportion of kilocalories from fat usually is high in the nation's diet. Conversely, in developing countries with limited incomes and a largely agrarian economy, fat consumption tends to be lower.

Two guidelines are suitable in evaluating the fat in the diet. First, at least 1 percent of the total calories in the diet should be derived from the intake of linoleic acid. For example, the person who consumes 1800 kilocalories per day needs a minimum of about 2 grams of linoleic acid daily. This value is calculated as follows: 1 percent of 1800 kilocalories is 18 kilocalories, and 2 grams of fat (at 9 kilocalories per gram) contributes approximately 18 kilocalories. As can be seen from Table 7.4, vegetable oils generally are good sources of linoleic acid. Of course, the hydrogenation of linoleic acid causes this essential fatty acid to be transformed to oleic and stearic acids, neither of which is capable of performing the functions of linoleic acid in the body. For this reason, the nonhydrogenated polyunsaturated oils (or lightly hydrogenated) commonly are blended into more saturated fats when margarines and solid vegetable shortenings are being manufactured.

The second guideline for fat consumption is that fried foods, butter and margarine, and cream of all types should be eaten in moderation. If weight gain is a problem, this is a reasonably good indication that the amount of fat in the diet is higher than is optimum for good health. An exception to this statement is the person who consumes alcoholic beverages generously, in which case the kilocalories from alcohol may be the prime factor in overweight. For persons wishing to gain weight, an increased intake of fat may be useful.

Summary

Fats in the diet are: (1) an important source of concentrated energy, (2) the sole source of the essential fatty acid (linoleic acid), (3) carriers of vitamins A, D, E, and K, the fat-soluble vitamins, (4) helpful in increasing the satiety value of a meal, and (5) significant in their ability to improve the palatability of many foods. In the body, fatty deposits serve as reserves of energy, protectors of vital organs and the skeleton, and as insulation against the cold.

Although fats are rather widely available in animal foods, some plants are valuable sources of oils, particularly the unsaturated oils. The recommended intake of fat is 30 to 35 percent of the total intake of calories, but typical diets in the United States contain in the vicinity of 45 percent of the calories from fat. The recommended intake of linoleic acid daily is 1 percent of the day's kilocalories.

Fat is digested and absorbed relatively completely in the healthy individual. During digestion, fats are emulsified and usually broken down to fatty acids, glycerol, monoglycerides, and a few diglycerides. The absorbed molecules may be transported in the blood, but generally simple fats are reformed in the body, combined with a protein and transported as chylomicrons. Ultimately, fat is either stored in the body or used for anabolic or catabolic reactions. When fat is metabolized, glycerol is split from the fatty acids, thus becoming available for entry into the Krebs Cycle. The fatty acids are oxidized (beta oxidation) and split into acetyl CoA that can be used to make new fatty acids or complex substances such as the sex hormones. Acetyl CoA can also be utilized in the Krebs Cycle, in conjunction with carbohydrates.

Selected References

Baldwin, R. L. Metabolic functions affecting the contribution of adipose tissue to total energy expenditure. *Fed. Proc. 29:*1277. 1970.

Council of Food and Nutrition, American Medical Assoc. Regulation of dietary fat. *J. Am. Med. Assoc. 181:*441. 1962.

Hansen, A. E., et al. Role of linoleic acid in infant nutrition. *Pediatrics. 31:*171–192. 1963.

Herman, R. H., et al. Effect of diet on lipid metabolism in experimental animals and man. *Fed. Proc. 29:*1302. 1970.

Hirsch, J., and J. L. Knittle. Cellularity of obese and nonobese human adipose tissue. *Fed. Proc. 29:*1516. 1970.

Kahn, H. A. Change in serum cholesterol associated with changes in the United States civilian diet, 1909 to 1965. *Am. J. Clin. Nutr. 23:*879. 1970.

Leveille, G. H. Adipose tissue metabolism: influence of periodicity of eating and diet composition. *Fed. Proc. 29:*1294. 1970.

Mattson, F. H. Fat. *Present Knowledge of Nutrition.* 4th ed. Nutrition Foundation. New York. 1976.

Mead, J. F. Present knowledge of fat. *Nutr. Rev. 24:*33. 1966.

Murphy, E. W., L. Page, and P. O. Koons. Lipid components of Type A school lunches. *J. Am. Diet. Assoc. 56:*504. 1970.

National Academy of Sciences. *Dietary Fat and Human Health.* Publ. 1147. Washington, D.C. National Research Council. 1966.

Review. Exercise, nutrition, and caloric sources of energy. *Nutr. Rev. 28:*180. 1970.

Scott, D. F., and V. R. Potter. Metabolic oscillations in lipid metabolism in rats on controlled feeding schedules. *Fed. Proc. 29:*1553. 1970.

Tepperman, J., and H. M. Tepperman. Gluconeogenesis, lipogenesis, and the Sherrington metaphor. *Fed. Proc. 29:*1284. 1970.

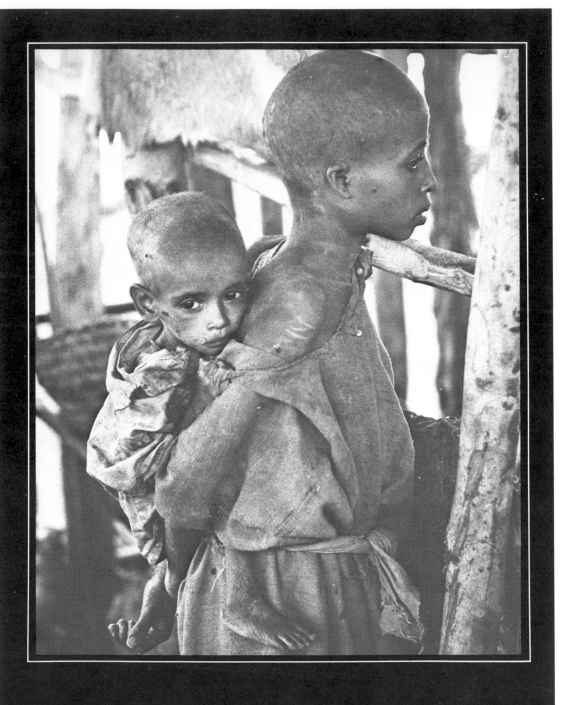

Chapter 8

Proteins

There has been extensive discussion and study of the problems centering around the world population crisis. The two prime concerns regarding the food supply are the availability of sufficient calories and an adequate amount of protein, particularly animal protein. Both calories and protein are limiting factors in feeding the growing population, particularly infants and young children. Lack of calories may be more important for the adult population.

As agricultural lands are being taxed to supply the greatest possible amount of food from the space available, the efficiencies of producing various foods are carefully scrutinized. Criteria for raising food have been and still are the profit and demand for foods that rate high in consumer preference. However, when food is viewed from the standpoint of the health of man, consideration in determining crop priorities must also be given to the nutritive qualities of the food produced. In a critical food shortage, one must question the reality of devoting vast resources of cropland to the production of animal protein when more vegetable protein can be produced far more efficiently from the same acreage. Such a statement arouses defensive feelings and antagonism in many people, and yet such decisions may need to become a practical reality before the beginning of the next century.

To more fully appreciate the critical nature of protein in man's diet, particularly in the diet of the preschool child and the pregnant or lactating woman, it is necessary to examine the nature of proteins and the roles they perform in the human body. The psychological and sociological factors that influence man's choice of protein foods have been discussed in Chapters 2 and 3. Protein is viewed in the physiological context in this chapter.

Structure

Protein molecules are large and complex organic compounds. They are, in a sense, similar to carbohydrates and fats because proteins also are composed of carbon, oxygen, and hydrogen. However, the element, nitrogen, is a structural part of all proteins, and this is the element that provides the key to protein's uniqueness in the body. These four elements are found in all protein molecules. In addition, sulfur is a significant element in some proteins, and iron, phosphorus, and iodine are found in still others.

The basic component of protein molecules is a rather small compound called an amino acid. Amino acids have the general structure

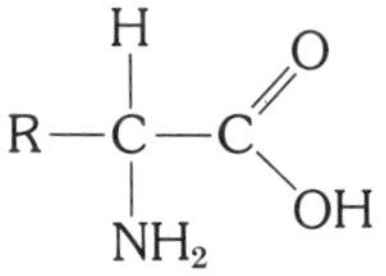

$$R-\underset{\underset{NH_2}{|}}{\overset{\overset{H}{|}}{C}}-C\underset{OH}{\overset{O}{\diagup}}$$

This molecule is composed of an amino group (—NH_2) joined to the first carbon next to the acid group $\left(-C\underset{OH}{\overset{O}{\diagup}}\right)$. Thus, amino acid molecules are named after the two characteristic groups that are always a part of their structure. The amino group is on the alpha (first carbon after the carboxyl group) carbon, which explains why these are called alpha (α) amino acids. The R that is shown as a part of the molecule represents a variety of structures that may be attached to the alpha carbon. R may simply be an atom of hydrogen, as it is in the amino acid glycine, or it may be a rather bulky arrangement such as a ring structure as in the case of histidine. The Appendix includes structures of the common amino acids in foods. The variation in the R group can be seen in these structures.

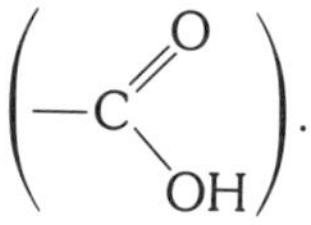

In an actual protein molecule, considerably more than 100 amino acid units are linked together by what are termed peptide linkages. These are formed by joining the nitrogen of the amino group of one amino acid to the carbon of the carboxyl group in another amino acid, with the loss of a molecule of water as shown below. When this linkage is repeated over and over again, highly complex protein molecules are formed.

There are some 22 amino acids that are contained in the numerous types of protein found in animal tissues. Each type of protein is highly specific in its composition. Each molecule of a specific protein will have exactly the same pattern of amino acids in exactly the same position along the amino acid chain that makes up the

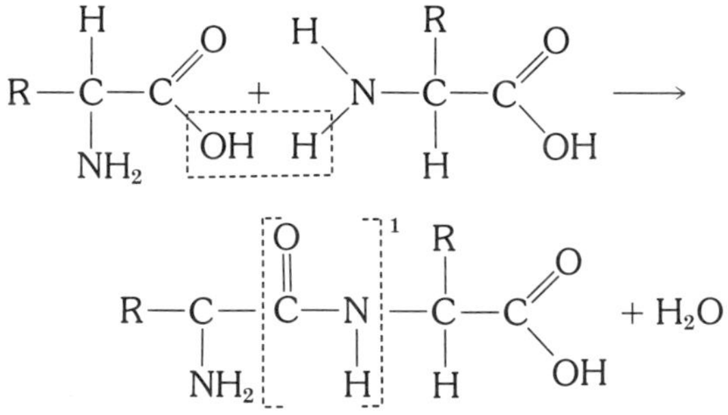

$$R-\underset{\underset{NH_2}{|}}{\overset{\overset{H}{|}}{C}}-C\overset{O}{\underset{OH}{\diagdown}} + \underset{H}{\overset{H}{\underset{|}{N}}}-\underset{\underset{H}{|}}{\overset{\overset{R}{|}}{C}}-C\overset{O}{\underset{OH}{\diagdown}} \longrightarrow$$

$$R-\underset{\underset{NH_2}{|}}{C}-\overset{\overset{O}{\|}}{C}-\underset{\underset{H}{|}}{N}-\underset{\underset{H}{|}}{\overset{\overset{R}{|}}{C}}-C\overset{O}{\underset{OH}{\diagdown}} + H_2O$$

molecule. Thus, one molecule of human hemoglobin is the same as another molecule of human hemoglobin. However, the hemoglobin protein molecule of humans is somewhat different in its structure from the hemoglobin molecule of any other species. This uniqueness of protein from one species to another is called species specificity.

In a sense, the study of protein structure is in its infancy, for while methods for identifying the sequence of amino acids in proteins are known at the present time, only a limited number of proteins has been decoded to the point where the structure has been completely elucidated. The careful study of myoglobin structure, reported in 1961, marked the beginning of the era of protein structure clarification.

$$^1 -\overset{\overset{O}{\|}}{C}-\underset{\underset{H}{|}}{N}-$$ is the region where the peptide linkage

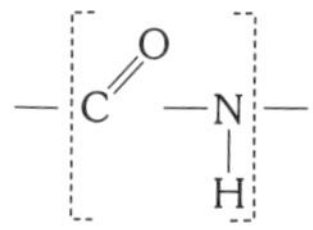

is formed between the carbon and the nitrogen atoms.

Essential Amino Acids

For the formation of each molecule of the different proteins required in the body, all of the amino acids needed to make the molecule must be available. In some cases, these amino acids will be used in the form in which they were absorbed. However, some of the amino acids that are required may not be present. Sometimes the missing amino acids can be formed from other amino acids, but some amino acids cannot be formed in sufficient quantities in the body. For these particular amino acids to be available for synthesizing proteins, they must be a component of proteins eaten in foods.

The necessity for specific amino acids has been studied with considerable care. Ten amino acids have been identified as being essential for the growth and maintenance of experimental rats. Human infants have an identified need for a dietary source of nine amino acids, and human adults need only eight. These amino acids that are needed by the body, and yet cannot be synthesized in the body from other substances, are termed "essential amino acids." For adults the essential amino acids are methionine, threonine, tryptophan, isoleucine, leucine, lysine, valine, and phenylalanine (Table 8.1). Infants need these eight essential amino acids plus histidine.

The essential amino acids must be provided by foods eaten on a daily basis. Meats and other animal proteins commonly serve as important sources of these amino acids. Foods of animal origin, with the exception of gelatin, are excellent sources of complete proteins. Gelatin is deficient in tryptophan and lysine. Protein from plant sources such as legumes and cereals

Table 8.1 *Minimum Requirements for Individual Essential Amino Acids by Adults*[a]

Essential Amino Acid	Normal Adult Requirement	
	Male (mg/day)	Female (mg/day)
Methionine	200[b]	350
Threonine	500	305
Tryptophan	250	157
Isoleucine	700	450
Leucine	1100	620
Lysine	800	500
Valine	800	650
Phenylalanine	300[c]	220

[a] Adapted from Food and Nutrition Board Committee on Amino Acids. ***Evaluation of Protein Nutrition.*** Publication 711. Washington, D.C. 1959. National Academy of Sciences—National Research Council.
[b] In presence of adequate tyrosine.
[c] In presence of adequate cystine.

also contribute valuable amounts of the essential as well as the nonessential amino acids.

Nonessential amino acids are useful in synthesizing proteins in the body. These may be available directly from dietary sources or they may be manufactured in the body. Since the body is able to synthesize these amino acids, they do not have to be eaten in precisely the same form. The amino group can be transferred to make the desired amino acid by a process known as *transamination*. Animal and plant proteins contain mixtures of essential and nonessential amino acids.

Native and denatured

There are several ways of classifying proteins. Perhaps the most basic categories are native proteins and denatured proteins. Any protein that is exactly the same as it occurs in nature is a native protein. Actually, many of the proteins man consumes belong to the group classified as denatured proteins. Denatured proteins are proteins that have undergone some change from the form in which they existed in nature. When protein is heated or agitated, the structure of the protein becomes slightly modified and the molecule behaves differently. Such a change is readily observed when an egg is cooking. The translucent char-

acter and the flow properties of egg white, for example, are grossly modified when heat is applied. Actually, the protein molecule remains the same size and continues to contain exactly the same amino acids that were present in the native protein. The different behavior that is noted is due to the fact that the protein molecule has changed its outer shape a bit. The different geometry and different R groups that are exposed modify the protein's characteristics significantly in the denatured form. From a nutritional viewpoint, some denatured proteins are important because they may be digested more readily than the native protein. Also, they often are considered to be more palatable than native protein.

Native proteins are classified according to the basic shape or spatial arrangement of the molecule. Many of the native proteins in food have a spherical shape and are referred to as globular proteins. Other native proteins, such as those in hair and connective tissue, occur as long, fibrous molecules or folded, sheetlike arrangements.

Simple and conjugated

Yet another means of categorizing proteins is on the basis of their molecular structure. Proteins containing only amino acids are called simple proteins. This caption "simple proteins" applies despite the number of different amino acids found in the molecule and irrespective of the total molecular weight of the molecule.

Many protein molecules contain not only amino acids, but also other substances. Such proteins are "conjugated proteins." Conjugated proteins are the subject of numerous elegant research projects today. Perhaps the type of conjugated protein that recently has captured the public's eye and interest more than other proteins has been the nucleopro-

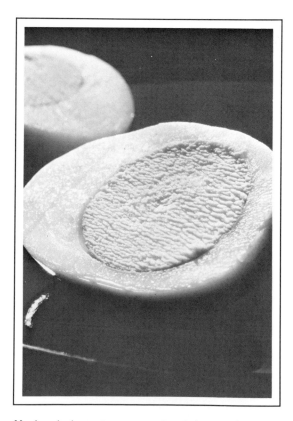

Hard-cooked egg is an example of denatured protein.

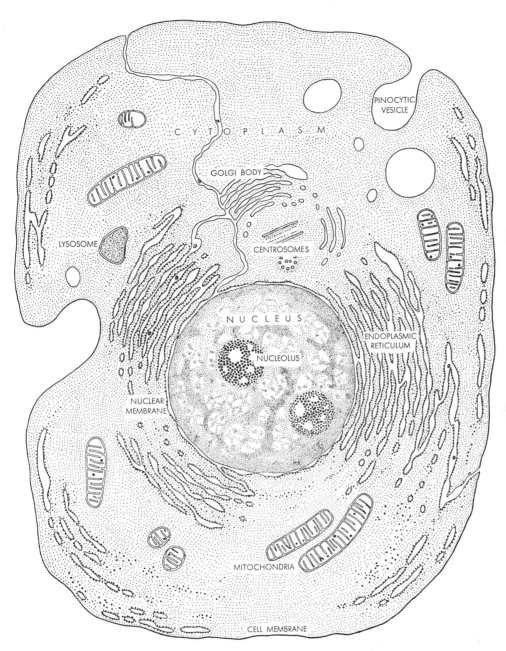

Schematic diagram of a typical cell, magnified approximately 10,000 times. Protein synthesis is accomplished when messenger RNA carries the template of a protein (provided by DNA in the nucleus) to the surface of ribosomes (the structures studding the endoplasmic reticulum). Free amino acids are utilized from the cytoplasm and arranged according to the template.

teins. Nucleoproteins are compounds containing nucleic acids and amino acids. Nucleic acids are composed of three components: phosphoric acid, a sugar containing five carbons (a pentose), and a nitrogen-containing base. Deoxyribonucleic acid (DNA) and ribonucleic acid (RNA) are both nucleic acids. They are particularly interesting because of their genetically significant roles in nature.

DNA is found in cell nuclei and contains the genetic code needed for cellular reproduction. "Messenger" RNA is credited with carrying the message or template of the arrangement of amino acids in a protein; the message is transported from the DNA in the nucleus to the surface of ribosomes in the cytoplasm of the cell. Yet another type of RNA, "transfer" RNA, collects free amino acids in the cytoplasm and orients them at the appropriate place along the surface of the messenger RNA. After the amino acids are suitably aligned, the newly formed protein molecule is freed from the messenger RNA. These nucleic acids appear to be essential for synthesizing (making) all proteins in the body, including enzymes!

Lipoproteins are also classified as conjugated proteins. As mentioned in Chapter 7, lipoproteins (molecules composed of lipid or fatty material and protein) are significant in the human body as a mode of transporting fatty materials in an aqueous medium. Hemoglobin is yet another type of conjugated protein in which protein is complexed to a metal-containing compound (heme). Conjugated proteins composed of amino acids linked to carbohydrates are termed "glycoproteins."

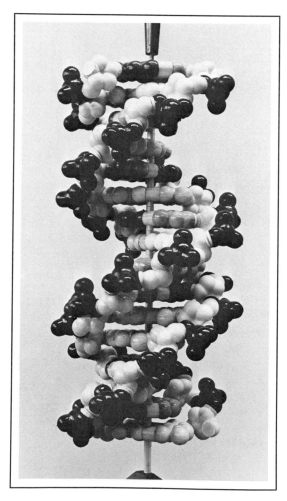

Model of a conjugated protein, DNA. DNA is a nucleic acid containing phosphoric acid, a five-carbon sugar, and a nitrogen-containing base.

Complete and incomplete

These might seem to be all the possible ways of classifying proteins, and yet the most important classification from the nutritionist's point of view has not yet been discussed. The most fundamental classification of proteins, based on nutritional significance, is that of complete or incomplete protein. Complete proteins are proteins that contain all of the 8 to 10 amino acids needed by animals, including man, for growth and maintenance of life. Complete proteins also contain many additional amino acids that contribute to meeting the body's need for protein materials. In contrast to complete proteins, incomplete proteins do not contain sufficient amounts of all of the essential amino acids even though they do contain at least some of all of the amino acids required for growth and maintenance. If a protein is inadequate in the level of even one amino acid required for life, the protein is said to be incomplete.

Functions of Protein

The ubiquitous presence of proteins in all living matter is indicative of the tremendous significance of protein for promoting growth and maintaining life. Proteins are found in all cells of the body. The specific roles of protein in the body are outlined here.

Tissue growth and maintenance

Protein is vital to the growth and maintenance of body tissues. For growth to occur in children, adequate protein must be included in the diet. In instances where not all of the essential amino acids are supplied in the diet in adequate amounts, or where total protein intake is insufficient, growth is impeded or even stopped. In adults with an inadequate intake of protein, there will be a wasting of the tissues over a period of time as body protein is broken down and the nitrogen excreted as urea.

Fluid balance

The fluid balance of cells is regulated, in part, by the presence of proteins, because proteins are too large to pass through cell membranes. Consequently, plasma proteins remain in the blood instead of penetrating the interstitial spaces with the plasma fluid. This resulting concentration of plasma proteins creates the pressure needed to draw the fluid back out of the cells and into the bloodstream, thus preventing the accumulation of fluid in the tissues. When plasma protein is at a low level (as occurs in a protein deficiency), there is insufficient pressure to remove the liquid from the tissues and edema (the accumulation of fluid outside the cells) results.

Hormone, enzyme, and antibody formation

Proteins are needed to form some hormones, enzymes, and antibodies; all of these substances are protein. Thyroxine, insulin, and adrenaline are examples of hormones, all of which are essential for regulating various fundamental body processes. A few of the enzymes in the body have already been mentioned in reference to the digestion and metabolism of carbohydrates and fats. Others are required for the utilization of proteins. Actually, the body contains greatly in excess of 1000 enzymes that catalyze innumerable specific chemical reactions in the body. At this point in scientific understanding, all enzymes are thought to be proteins.

Protein must be included in the diet if the body is to have the raw materials available that it will need to synthesize some hormones and the many enzymes needed for the body to function. Without protein, these hormones and enzymes could not be formed. However, even in times of serious food shortages, these compounds required by the brain are extremely resistant to depletion.

Antibodies, the protein materials that are a part of the body defenses to fight infection, are reduced in number by an inadequate intake of protein. With adequate ingestion of protein, these protective proteins are formed to provide maximum resistance to infectious agents. This protection applies to chemical invasion by toxic substances as well as to microorganisms.

pH maintenance[2]

Proteins are important for maintaining the body at a just slightly alkaline pH. These compounds can function in this regulating capacity because their structural composition enables them to act in the role of either an acid or a base as needed to maintain the normal pH of the body—about pH 7.2. If body fluids contain excess alkali, the proteins can function as an acid; conversely, in the presence of excess acid, the proteins function as a base. This amphoteric nature of proteins promotes the neutral medium needed for normal metabolism.

Energy source

Proteins, like carbohydrates and fats, also serve ultimately as a source of energy for the body. Protein, similar to carbohydrate, provides approximately 4 kilocalories per gram when it is metabolized for energy. From the viewpoint of the body, it is advantageous to supply sufficient energy from carbohydrate and fat in the diet so the amino acids from dietary protein can be used for the unique and essential functions mentioned above before they ultimately are metabolized to yield energy. Energy release from protein is less efficient than from either carbohydrates or fats (see Chapter 4). The use of protein for energy is expensive from the economic standpoint as well. A brief tour through even the most competitively priced supermarket will be sufficient to remind the consumer that protein foods are the most expensive foods one buys.

Food Sources

The varied and essential roles of protein in the body serve to emphasize the importance of having an adequate supply of protein in the diet. A knowledge of the numerous food sources of protein will help consumers to provide this nutrient in their diets in a practical and relatively economical way.

Meats of all types, such as beef, veal, pork, lamb, and mutton, are excellent sources of protein. Other equally useful sources of complete protein include fish, chicken, turkey, duck, goose, pheasant, and Cornish hens. Certainly no list of animal protein sources is complete without including eggs, milk, and cheese.

Plant sources are generally less expensive than the animal proteins, and yet they provide useful amounts of protein. Peas, lentils, navy

beans, kidney beans, garbanzo beans, pinto beans, and lima beans are illustrations of vegetable proteins that occupy a position of importance in many diets. Soybeans are increasing rapidly in their use as a protein source in the American diet. The protein extracted from soybeans can be spun into fibers and converted into simulated meat products that are being marketed successfully. The particular attraction of soybeans is the nutritive quality of the protein in them as well as the generous amount of protein they contain. While soybeans are not quite as good a protein source as animal foods, they generally are superior to cereals (because of a better amino acid pattern) and do have a protein content of 30 to 35 percent. Ground beef mixed with textured vegetable protein (TVP) provides a blend of amino acids that is utilized by the body as well as pure animal protein foods; this use of TVP is an economical

[2] pH is the scale used to denote relative acidity and alkalinity. Values smaller than seven are acidic; those greater than seven are alkaline.

way of providing high quality protein in the diet.

The various legumes, averaging 20 percent, are higher in protein content than are cereals. However, rice and other cereals are valuable sources of protein in diets where they are eaten in large quantities. On a dry-weight basis, rice averages 7 to 8 percent protein, corn 9 to 10 percent, and wheat 10 to 12 percent. Geneticists have recently succeeded in producing strains of cereals with higher total protein content. Limitations at present are that the nutritive quality (amino acid pattern) of these higher protein cereals is less desirable and the yield per acre may be less.

Although plant proteins are classified as incomplete proteins because they are deficient in one or more of the essential amino acids, plants are of considerable importance in supplying the world's protein needs. Despite the fact that plant proteins are incomplete, their nutritional contribution should not be downgraded. Plant proteins are an inexpensive and realistic way of providing much of the protein that people need. Simply by the addition of a small amount of animal protein or a blending of certain plant proteins, particularly the protein from the germ of cereals, the total protein becomes nutritionally adequate. Needed amino acids can be added to cereals during processing to improve the nutritive value of these products. Amino acid fortification is of particular merit in diets that are based largely on a single cereal, such as wheat, corn, or rice. Geneticists are breeding toward new strains of cereal with improved amino acid composition. Plant proteins, because of their abundance and low cost, hold the key to adequate protein nutrition for the world's people. However, they are most useful when improved nutritionally by fortification with the essential amino acids in which they are low or by genetic means.

A diet deriving most of its protein from plant sources can be improved in its quality by using a variety of grains and legumes. The use of corn and beans, such as is possible when serving corn tortillas and refried beans, provides more adequate protein than will either the corn or the beans alone. Rice and soybean curd is another useful example of complementary use of vegetable proteins.

Digestion and Absorption

As the protein molecules exist in food, there is much chemical action required before they are ready for absorption into the body. Protein molecules must be broken down to their individual amino acid components, no small task when one considers the relative immensity and complexity of these molecules. This feat is initiated in the stomach where pepsinogen, the inactive precursor of pepsin, is changed to the active enzyme, pepsin, by hydrochloric acid (Table 8.2). Pepsin is termed a "gastric protease" because it occurs in the stomach (gastric) and it is a protein-splitting (prote-) enzyme (-ase). Pepsin can align itself at various positions along the amino acid chain comprising the protein molecule and catalyze a splitting of the molecule into shorter amino acid chains. These shorter protein fragments are called polypeptides. The partially digested protein then passes into the small intestine, where the more alkaline medium inactivates the action of pepsin.

In the small intestine, proteolytic enzymes from the pancreatic juice and intestinal juice complete the breakdown of protein into its component amino acids. The main protein-splitting enzyme contributed by the pancreatic juice is trypsin, an enzyme that catalyzes the cleavage of polypeptides at any point where the acid group of either lysine or arginine is a part of the backbone amino acid chain. The action of trypsin thus results in the formation of a

Table 8.2   Digestion of Proteins

Site	Substrate	Enzymes	Digestion Product
Stomach	Protein	Pepsin (activated by hydrochloric acid)	Polypeptides
Small intestine	Polypeptides containing lysine or arginine	Trypsin (pancreatic juice)	Shorter polypeptides to dipeptides
Small intestine	Polypeptides	Carboxypeptidase and aminopeptidase (intestinal juice)	Dipeptides
Small intestine	Dipeptides	Dipeptidase (intestinal juice)	Amino acids

variety of peptides ranging from dipeptides (two amino acids linked together) to fairly short polypeptides. The intestinal juice itself contains other enzymes necessary for protein metabolism: carboxypeptidase, aminopeptidase, and dipeptidase. Carboxypeptidase effects cleavage along a polypeptide chain by acting at the end of the chain where the carboxyl group (—COOH) is the terminal formation. Aminopeptidase is comparable to carboxypeptidase in its action, with the exception that its action initiates at the amino (—NH$_2$) end of the peptide chain instead of at the carboxyl end. The splitting action continues from both ends of the chain until a dipeptide remains. The final cleavage is then effected by the action of dipeptidase, apparently reacting in the membrane in the intestinal wall.

Absorption of the individual amino acids then takes place, either as a result of diffusion into the bloodstream or by active transport. The amino acids are carried in the blood to the liver where they become part of an amino acid pool until being carried through the blood to other parts of the body.

The preceding procedure is the normal circumstance for the digestion and absorption of protein. Some individuals are unable to effect the digestion of specific proteins to their component amino acids. Instead, the protein may progress through the intestinal tract with little or no cleavage occurring. If the protein molecule succeeds in passing through the intestinal wall, the body reacts against this foreign protein. Thus, when some individuals eat eggs, chocolate, or other specific protein-containing foods, an allergic reaction will occur, because the body has not digested the protein to its component amino acids. Itching, rashes, and restricted breathing may be the symptoms triggered by the absorption of intact protein molecules. Although such a phenomenon is not the usual pathway for protein absorption, it does illustrate effectively the importance of breaking down protein to individual amino acids prior to absorption.

Protein synthesis (anabolism)

Amino acids are removed from the liver and transported throughout the body where they are needed to form specific proteins required by the cells and tissues. Both nonessential and essential amino acids are required to synthesize the numerous proteins of the body. All of the essential amino acids needed for protein synthesis must be supplied in the cell. If essential amino acids are lacking, protein synthesis cannot take place. The nonessential amino acids required for the specific protein synthesis also may be provided directly to the cell from the blood. However, if specific nonessential amino acids needed for protein synthesis are not immediately available from the blood supply, they can be formed in the cells. The formation of these nonessential amino acids is accomplished by a process known as transamination. In simplest terms, transamination is the transfer of the amino group from an amino acid to an appropriate nonnitrogenous substance to form a different amino acid. Pyridoxine, or vitamin B_6 (in the form of pyridoxal-5-phosphate), is the vitamin involved in transamination reactions.

Within the cell, protein synthesis takes place very rapidly. The assembled essential and nonessential amino acids are arranged by the transfer RNA according to the message carried by messenger RNA from DNA (see section on Classification of Proteins). However, the essential key to protein synthesis is an adequate supply of amino acids, both essential and nonessential.

Catabolism

Anabolic processes are not the only form of protein metabolism. There is also a continual catabolism of protein taking place, for there is a dynamic situation between the synthesis and degradation of proteins in the body.

Decarboxylation

In the presence of pyridoxal-5-phosphate (a coenzyme containing vitamin B_6), some amino acids are converted to amines by a decarboxylation reaction. An illustration of this type of metabolic reaction is the conversion of histidine to histamine. Histamine dilates blood capillaries.

Deamination

Some reactions form acids called "keto" acids. To perform this special type of reaction in which the amino group is removed, either nicotinamide-adenine dinucleotide or flavin-adenine dinucleotide is required. Once again the importance of the B vitamins as essential parts of coenzymes functioning in metabolic reactions comes to the fore. This removal of the —NH_2 radical is called deamination. Ultimately, the amino group undergoes transformation (through the Urea Cycle) to a chemical substance called urea. Urea is excreted in the urine.

The nonnitrogenous fragment

The remainder of the degraded amino acid is a nonnitrogenous material that can be oxidized through the metabolic cycle described for carbohydrates and fats (Krebs Cycle and electron transport system) to release energy and form carbon dioxide and water. Some amino acids readily are transformed to glucose when deaminated, and hence are termed glucogenic amino acids; others are converted to fatty acids when deaminated (ketogenic amino acids). If energy is not needed, the nonnitrogenous material can be synthesized to fat and stored in the body. Thus, carbohydrates, fats, and proteins (after deamination) are closely related in their metabolic paths. The unique aspect of protein metabolism is in relation to the various routes the amino group may follow.

Metabolic abnormalities

A few individuals have impaired amino acid metabolism. Probably not all metabolic disorders related to protein utilization are known. The most widely publicized of these abnormalities is phenylketonuria (PKU), in which the individual is unable to metabolize phenylala-nine efficiently, thus causing an accumulation of this amino acid and its derivatives. The result of this problem is severe mental retardation early in infancy. This problem can be met by very early diagnosis of the problem and a strict adherence to a diet containing just enough phenylalanine to supply the body's need for this essential amino acid.

Improper metabolism of other amino acids, including histidine, leucine, and valine, has been noted by various researchers. As more is learned about diagnosis and dietary control, reduction of the permanent damage some infants suffer as a result of being born with inadequate enzymes for utilizing protein is becoming possible.

Meeting Protein Needs

Dietary recommendations

The amount of protein that needs to be eaten daily to meet the body's demands for this nutrient is influenced by size and age as well as several other factors to be considered in the next section. Considerable study has been done in an attempt to estimate with accuracy just how much protein is needed in the diet each day. Calculations can be based upon the minimum protein intake required to achieve a normal growth rate for children or to maintain adults. Precise calculations of protein needs for an individual should include the quantity of protein required to replace the proteins lost through the urine, feces, skin, growth of nails and hair, and any additional proteins needed for growth (including pregnancy) or losses due to lactation.

For the reference man (see Table 8.3), the daily protein recommendation is 56 grams of protein and for the reference woman, it is 46 grams. Since many people are not the same weight as the reference weight used in the recommendations of the Food and Nutrition Board, the values must be adapted to individual cases. To do this, a rough estimate of protein need is obtained for adult men and women by multiplying the body weight (in kilograms) by the factor 0.8. Notice that the factor used for calculating protein recommendations for adults is significantly smaller than the factor recommended from birth to 6 months (2.2), or even from 6 months to 1 year (2.0).

The recommended level of protein can be provided readily in the diet by consuming two or more servings of meat or meat substitutes and the 2 or more glasses of milk recommended daily for individuals of various ages. To illustrate this point, Table 8.4 lists the amount of protein contained in a variety of protein sources. In the United States, many people frequently eat larger servings of meat than those indicated in the tables.

Table 8.3 *Recommended Allowance of Protein for Various Ages*[a]

Population Group	Age (years)	Weight (kg)	Protein (g)
Infants	0.0–0.5	6	kg × 2.2
	0.5–1.0	9	kg × 2.0
Children	1–3	13	23
	4–6	20	30
	7–10	30	36
Males	11–14	44	44
	15–18	61	54
	19–22	67	54
	23–50	70	56
	51+	70	56
Females	11–14	44	44
	15–16	54	48
	19–22	58	46
	23–50	58	46
	51+	58	46
Pregnancy	—	—	+30
Lactation	—	—	+20

[a] Based on *Recommended Daily Dietary Allowances,* revised 1974. Food and Nutrition Board, National Academy of Sciences—National Research Council.

Nitrogen balance studies

The recommendations for protein intake, as presented in Table 8.3, are general recommendations for normal people. Precise evaluation of the adequacy of protein intake for a specific individual can be done by determining nitrogen balance. Nitrogen balance studies are conducted by carefully determining the total amount of nitrogen that is contained in all of the food eaten each day. The excretion of nitrogen in the feces and urine must also be determined. The rationale for the use of nitrogen as the means of determining protein adequacy is based on the fact that nitrogen is contained in proteins at a relatively constant level of 16 percent. By using a thoroughly tested procedure known as the Kjeldahl method for determining

nitrogen, the amount of nitrogen contained in the food ingested and the nitrogen eliminated through the urine and feces can be measured accurately. The intake is then compared with the excretion to determine the nitrogen balance of the subject.

Adults normally will be in nitrogen equilibrium, that is, the amount of nitrogen excreted is equal to the amount ingested. Nitrogen equilibrium exists when the diet contains enough or more than enough protein to meet the body's need for protein to maintain the existing tissues and other essential nitrogen-containing compounds in the body.

Positive nitrogen balance, or the retention of more protein in the body than is being excreted, is the normal circumstance during childhood when growth is occurring. Positive nitrogen balance also is the normal state during pregnancy and lactation.

Negative nitrogen balance is indicative of an excretion rate greater than the consumption of protein. This circumstance results in wasting of body tissues and does not provide for the protein demands of the body. Negative nitrogen balance may be the result of a fever, body burns, or other wasting conditions in which protein is being lost from the body more rapidly than it is being consumed, absorbed, and retained. Negative nitrogen balance also develops when body tissue has to be used for energy because of an inadequate caloric intake. A narrowly restricted diet that provides inadequate amounts of the essential amino acids also can be the cause of negative nitrogen balance. Such a condition is distinctly undesirable and should be remedied by increasing the amount or quality of protein in the diet.

Nitrogen balance studies are indicative only of the gross protein picture in the body and do not reflect the immediate circumstance in all cases. A person may begin to consume a protein-deficient diet and yet briefly indicate nitrogen equilibrium while the labile plasma protein is being depleted to meet tissue protein requirements.

Table 8.4 *Protein Content in Selected Foods*[a]

	Amount	Protein
Meat group:		
Beef, sirloin steak, lean	3 1/2 oz	32
Beef, rump roast, lean	3 1/2 oz	29
Beef, ground beef, lean	3 1/2 oz	27
Veal, leg roast	3 1/2 oz	27
Veal, loin chop	3 1/2 oz	26
Lamb, leg roast, lean	3 1/2 oz	29
Lamb, loin chop, lean	3 1/2 oz	28
Pork shoulder roast	3 1/2 oz	29
Pork loin chop, lean	3 1/2 oz	31
Pork, center ham slice, lean	3 1/2 oz	25
Poultry:		
Chicken, white meat	3 1/2 oz	33
Egg, whole	1 medium	6
Fish and shellfish:		
Haddock, broiled	3 1/2 oz	25
Salmon, canned	3 1/2 oz	27
Tuna, canned	3 1/2 oz	29
Shrimp, cooked	3 1/2 oz	24
Crab, canned	3 1/2 oz	17
Legumes and nuts:		
Dry beans, white, cooked	1/2 cup	8
Split peas, cooked	1/2 cup	8
Peanut butter	2 tbsp	8
Mixed nuts, roasted	1 oz	5
Dairy group:		
Milk, whole 3.5% fat	1 cup	9
Milk, skim	1 cup	9
Milk, fortified low fat	1 cup	10
Cheese, creamed cottage	1/2 cup	15
Cheese, cheddar	1 oz	7
Bread — cereal group:		
Bread, enriched white	1 slice	2
Oatmeal, cooked	1 cup	5
Shredded wheat	1 biscuit	3
Rice, enriched	1 cup	4
Noodles, cooked	1 cup	7
Macaroni, cooked	1 cup	5

[a] Data compiled and adapted from **Composition of Foods—Raw, Processed, Prepared,** Agriculture Handbook No. 8, U.S.D.A., 1963; **Nutritive Value of Foods,** Home and Garden Bulletin No. 72, U.S.D.A., 1971; **Nutritive Value of American Foods,** Agriculture Handbook No. 456, U.S.D.A., 1975.

Kwashiorkor

For a variety of reasons, some individuals will develop a protein deficiency. Ignorance of dietary needs and lack of money to buy protein-containing foods are common reasons for an inadequate intake of protein. Because of the relatively great need for proteins for growth of children, adequate protein intake is a particularly serious problem in childhood, especially early in childhood during the first few months and years after weaning.

Kwashiorkor, the protein deficiency condition of early childhood, is probably the most publicized nutritional deficiency existing today.

This is a condition all too prevalent among children ages 1 to 4 in developing countries. Generally, breast-fed infants receive sufficient protein to meet their body's minimum protein needs for at least the first 6 months of nursing. However, the protein intake usually decreases dramatically when the infant is weaned unless human milk is replaced in the diet by a suitable formula or cow's milk. A safe supply of milk is often neither available nor within the economic reach of the family. The customary practice in many of the underdeveloped areas of the world is to rely heavily on thin, starchy gruels

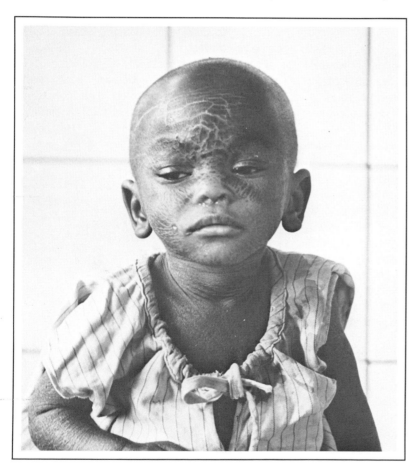

Kwashiorkor is a protein-deficiency condition that is most likely to be found in children between the ages of 1 and 4, who have had some other illness, and are from disadvantaged families.

for the infant's sustenance. The result is a serious limitation in protein intake. This protein deficiency will result in poor growth and seriously decreased resistance to infection.

In the early years, children are relatively susceptible to infections and gastroenteritis, resulting in severe diarrhea and dehydration. Lowered resistance due to inadequate protein, combined with less than ideal living conditions and sanitation, leads to almost certain illness for the child. When the protein-deficient child does contract an illness, the fever, vomiting, and diarrhea that ordinarily accompany childhood diseases serve to aggravate his protein-deficient condition. The small amount of protein he may be fed will be excreted before the body has sufficient opportunity to digest and absorb the protein.

The usual pattern is for a protein-deficient child to have a mild degree of kwashiorkor until he contracts some illness. At the time of the illness, the protein deficiency becomes more intense; advanced kwashiorkor may develop, often with fatal results.

Numerous classical symptoms occur in cases of kwashiorkor. The patient will be lackadaisical, lethargic, and irritable. The child will fail to grow or put on weight; muscles will be poorly developed and limbs will appear to be wasting. Skin will become blotchy, discolored, and scaly in places, particularly on the legs and feet. The hair may take on a flaglike appearance due to development of a reddish pigment in normally black hair. Additional symptoms include anemia, loss of appetite, enlargement of the liver, diarrhea, and vomiting. In advanced cases, edema is significant.

Kwashiorkor can be treated successfully when the diet is modified in time. The usual procedure in extreme cases is to feed nonfat milk with extra skim milk solids added until the edema disappears. Subsequently, whole milk and other protein foods of high quality are included in the diet.

Ideally, kwashiorkor should be prevented instead of being permitted to develop and require treatment. Prevention will need to be approached from various angles. If family planning can be used to extend the duration of lactation for an infant before the mother conceives again, the infant can be maintained on human milk protein for a longer length of time. An increase in the quantity of cereal gruels can be the means of providing adequate energy. The protein in the milk can be used for growth and formation of antibodies, hormones, and enzymes. Nutrition education is needed to help families understand that young children and newly weaned infants need protein and energy as well as other important nutrients. Improved sanitation and living conditions are needed to reduce the likelihood of infectious diseases. Greater food production and improved distribution, of course, are also vital if kwashiorkor is to be prevented.

Frequently the problems of a protein deficiency are further complicated by a grossly inadequate level of calories. This condition, protein-calorie-malnutrition (PCM), is particularly grave because the protein that is ingested

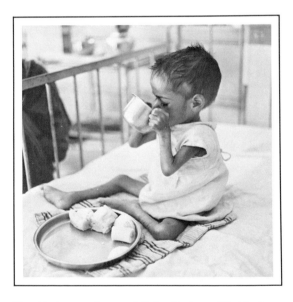

Kwashiorkor can be cured if the diet is modified in time.

is not sufficient for both providing energy and performing the various functions unique to protein. Without treatment, death is virtually a certainty, usually due to the combination of malnutrition, gastrointestinal disease, and infections.

A still more stringent diet, one particularly lacking in calories and also in most of the nutrients needed by humans, quickly leads to the condition known as marasmus. Marasmus is tantamount to starvation.

Utilization of Protein

Various factors are involved in the efficiency with which dietary protein is used in the body. The source of the protein, the amino acid balance, the digestibility of the protein, the overall composition of the diet, and the physical condition of the individual all have an influence on the actual utilization of dietary protein.

Physical condition

While people in good health utilize protein in the diet with good efficiency, sick individuals and those with various stress conditions do not utilize protein efficiently. Protein utilization during illness may also be reduced. Even when a person is kept in bed without any problems of fever or diarrhea, there is loss of body nitrogen. Fever, severe burns, or diarrhea greatly decrease the utilization of nitrogen in the diet.

Composition of the diet

Nitrogen utilization is poor when the diet is low in caloric content. Under this condition, protein is needed for energy, and protein that is used for energy is not available for its unique role in synthesis of body protein or protein compounds such as enzymes and hormones. In a diet containing sufficient energy, utilization of protein is influenced by need and protein quality.

Digestibility

The digestibility of protein has a significant influence on utilization of dietary protein. Protein from animal sources is digested with relative efficiency. Approximately 97 percent of the protein in animal foods is available for absorption. On the other hand, proteins from legumes, cereals and other plant sources vary in their digestibility from 65 to 90 percent, with legumes averaging about 78 percent. The processing of dietary protein, as well as the source, influences utilization of protein. Overheating of proteins, particularly with dry heat, frequently impairs their utilization. Moderate moist heating of soybeans and other legumes increases their usefulness, apparently by facilitating the availability of methionine, the limiting amino acid, during digestion. The proteins of rice, corn, and wheat are not appreciably affected by ordinary heating. Milk that is overheated through careless processing of dried milk undergoes some protein damage. Despite the possible impaired utilization of protein, some plant protein sources must be heated to remove the toxicity of some substances (for example, gossypol in cottonseed meal) or to inactivate enzymes. In general, moist heat usually improves protein utilization, and dry heat, if too extreme or for too long a period, impairs utilization of protein.

Biological value

Yet another factor influencing protein utilization is the balance of amino acids contained in the dietary protein. Protein is used inefficiently when essential amino acids are available in inadequate amounts. The significance of the balance between amino acids in the diet is of much less importance when total protein intake is high.

The value of the various protein sources in the human diet is due not only to the total protein present in the food, but also to the balance of amino acids contained in the food proteins. The actual merit of a protein in meeting the body's need for amino acids is sometimes expressed as its biological value (B.V.). Biological value is a measure of the body's retention of the nitrogen contained in the ingested protein and is computed as follows:

$$\text{B.V.} = \frac{\text{Dietary N} - (\text{Urinary N} + \text{Fecal N})}{\text{Dietary N} - \text{Fecal N}} \times 100$$

This value is calculated by determining the amount of nitrogen ingested in a day (dietary N), the nitrogen excreted through the urine (urinary N), and the nitrogen content that has been absorbed and utilized by the body prior to being excreted in the urine. Fecal nitrogen is the result of incomplete absorption of dietary proteins, the elimination of intestinal enzymes, and cells lost from the intestinal tract.

In effect, the biological value of a protein is a means of stating the value or efficiency of a protein in meeting the body's need for protein. Egg protein has been deemed to have the highest biological value (B.V. = 100) for man; milk with a B.V. of 93 is a reasonably close second; rice has the highest B.V. of the cereals (B.V. is 86 for rice in contrast to corn at 72, and wheat gluten at 44). Fish, beef, and casein (from milk) have a B.V. of 75. Any biological value of 70 or higher is considered sufficient for meeting the demands for protein for maintenance and growth, provided that the caloric content of the diet is adequate.

Other measures of efficiency

Other attempts at evaluating protein quality for humans include the use of the protein efficiency ratio (PER) and the net protein utilization (NPU). The protein efficiency ratio is a measure of the efficiency of weight gain per gram of nitrogen in the diet. The net protein utilization value is based both on the biological value of the protein and the digestibility or availability of nitrogen contained in dietary proteins.

Limiting amino acids

Another important facet of protein utilization is the concept of limiting amino acids. Since not all amino acids are found in any single protein in the relative proportions needed by the body, there will be at least one amino acid present in a protein in less adequate quantity than any other amino acid in meeting the body's needs. This amino acid that is found in the relatively smallest proportion in relation to physiological need is termed the "limiting" amino acid. Today's technology makes it possible to supplement cereal protein foods with the limiting amino acid, thus significantly improving the utilization of such protein by the body. For example, wheat products can be fortified with lysine to increase the value of wheat protein in the diet. The value of such fortification is questionable for populations already consuming adequate quantities of complete protein, but may be of importance when protein intake or the nutritive quality of the protein is restricted by availability or cost. However, careful research studies are required to determine the levels of fortification that are most appropriate (Kato and Muramatsu, 1971) and to ascertain whether a health benefit to the public is really obtained.

Summary

Proteins are nitrogen-containing organic compounds needed by the body to (1) promote growth and maintain tissues, (2) regulate the fluid balance in cells, (3) form hormones, enzymes, and antibodies, and (4) maintain the proper pH of the body. Protein also serves as a source of energy. A deficiency of protein in the diet leads to kwashiorkor and death.

Protein undergoes many reactions in the body. During digestion of protein, the molecules are broken apart into the component peptides and finally to amino acids, the form in which protein normally is absorbed. These absorbed amino acids are used by the body to synthesize needed proteins. Essential amino acids and nonessential amino acids are used in forming these proteins in the body. Essential amino acids must be obtained from the diet. The nonessential amino acids are obtained from the diet, but also can be formed from other substances by the process of transamination. When an amino acid is to be excreted, it is first deaminated. The amino group ultimately is removed through the urine as urea. The remainder of the molecule can be used for energy or stored as fat.

Throughout life, protein is an essential nutrient, but the greatest need in proportion to body size is for infants and young children. As individuals proceed through childhood, the requirement per kilogram of body weight diminishes gradually until the static requirement of adulthood is reached. Protein from different sources is used with varying efficiency because of such factors as differences in digestibility and the balance of amino acids. Dietary protein requirements can be met satisfactorily and with moderate cost by including milk, two or more servings of meat or meat substitutes, and various cereal products in the diet each day. An inadequate intake of protein can cause children to develop kwashiorkor, protein-calorie malnutrition, or marasmus.

Selected References

Allison, J. B. Protein malnutrition. *Tr. N.Y. Acad. Sci. 25:*293. 1963.

Allison, J. B., and W. H. Fitzpatrick. *Dietary Proteins in Health and Disease.* C. C. Thomas, Springfield, Ill. 1960.

Clause, A. S. Cereal grains as dietary protein sources. *Food Tech. 25:*63. August. 1971.

Food and Agr. Org. Human protein requirements and their fulfillment in practice. *F.A.O. Nutr. Stud.,* Series 16. Rome. 1957.

Food and Nutrition Board, National Acad. of Sciences. *Evaluation of Protein Quality.* Publication No. 1100. National Research Council. Washington, D.C. 1963.

Food and Nutrition Board, National Acad. of Science. *Meeting Protein Needs of Infants and Children.* Publication No. 943. National Research Council. Washington, D.C. 1961.

Frost, H. C., and D. Robinson. High lysine corn—what lies ahead? *J. Am. Oil Chem. Soc. 48:*407. 1971.

Harper, A. E. Some implications of amino acid supplementation. *Am. J. Clin. Nutrition. 9:*533. 1961.

Hartsook, E. W., and T. V. Hershberger. Interactions of major nutrients in whole-animal energy metabolism. *Fed. Proc. 30:*1466. 1971.

Holt, L. E., et al. *Protein and Amino Acid Requirements in Early Life.* New York University Press. New York. 1960.

Kato, J., and N. Muramatsu. Amino acid supplementation of grain. *J. Am. Oil Chem. Soc. 48:*415. 1971.

Muramatsu, K., et al. Effect of excess levels of individual amino acids on growth of rats fed casein diets. *J. Nutr. 101:*1117. 1971.

Orten, J. M., and A. U. Orten. DNA and inborn errors of metabolism. *J. Am. Diet. Assoc. 59:*331. 1971.

Sadre, M., et al. Protein food mixture for Iran. *J. Am. Diet. Assoc. 60:*131. 1972.

Scrimshaw, N. S., and A. M. Altschul. *Amino Acid Fortification of Protein Foods.* MIT Press. Cambridge, Mass. 1971.

Stillings, B. R., and G. M. Knobl, Jr. Fish protein concentrate: a new source of dietary protein. *J. Am. Oil Chem. Soc. 48:*412. 1971.

Stillings, B. R., et al. Nutritive quality of wheat flour and bread supplemented with either fish protein concentrate or lysine. *Cereal Chem. 48:*292. 1971.

Walker, D. B., et al. Engineered foods—the place for oilseed proteins. *Food Tech. 25:*55. August, 1971.

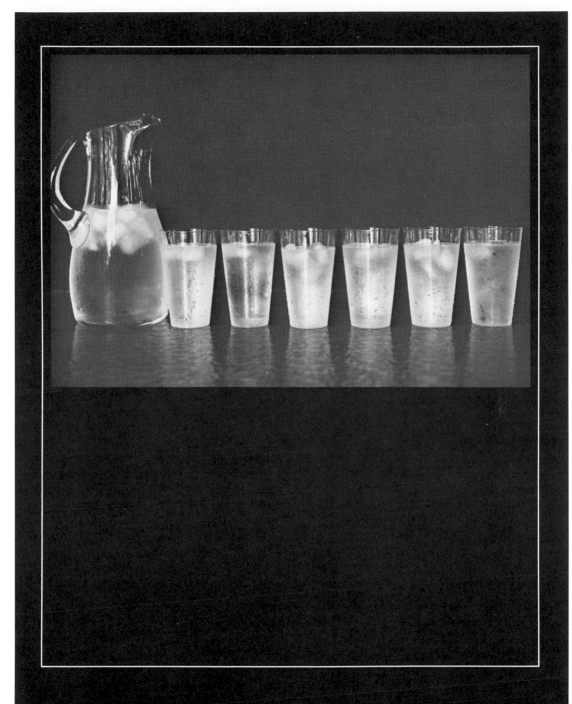

Chapter 9

If one were to question passersby on a street corner to determine what single substance is of greatest nutritional significance to man, doubtless numerous nutrients would be named. Perhaps protein or possibly vitamin C would be named most frequently; both of these seem to have captured the public's fancy at various times. Almost certainly, water would receive very few, if any, votes in an informal poll such as this. After all, water is such a common, utilitarian material that it tends to escape attention. And yet if water is removed from the diet completely, death will occur in a matter of a few days. People can survive for much longer periods of time when any other nutrient is eliminated from the diet than they can exist without water. Surely this is ample proof of the importance of water to human survival.

The fact that water accounts for between 55 and 65 percent of total body weight is additional evidence of the importance of water as a nutritional factor. Persons who have a well-developed musculature will have a higher percentage of body weight as water than will individuals who have relatively large amounts of adipose tissue. Therefore, it is not surprising that young children have a higher percentage of body weight because of water than adults do.

Water in the Body

Intracellular water

In the human adult, an amount of fluid equal to approximately 40 percent of the body weight is located within the cells. Such water is referred to as intracellular water. Cell walls are semipermeable membranes that permit the passage of water while preventing the movement of many other materials from one side of the membrane to the other. This ability of water to pass in and out of cells is of considerable significance in maintaining the total health of the individual. Conditions within the body need to be controlled so that the proper amount of water is contained in the body as intracellular water. If too much fluid is retained in individual cells, water causes the cells to swell, a condition called edema. Under reverse circumstances, too little water may be retained as intracellular water and dehydration of the cells develops.

Extracellular water

As the name implies, extracellular water is the water located outside the cells. Extracellular water accounts for approximately 15 percent of the body weight. The water that is a component of connective tissue, bone, and cartilage is one form of extracellular water. This water is held tightly and is not available to participate in various reactions.

Water that is found in the interstitial fluid of the body is of considerable importance. The interstitial water, which bathes the cells, is the mode of transport by which nutrients travel to the cells and waste products are carried away from the cell membranes. The interstitial water may be viewed as being the delivery service between the blood and the cells. Much of the interstitial (intercellular) water is drawn into the bloodstream, but the remainder is incorporated into the lymphatic system, finally being delivered into the bloodstream.

Transcellular water is extracellular water that is basically a lubricant. Examples of transcellular water include the water in spinal fluid, ocular fluid, and mucous secretions. The synovial fluid that lubricates joints also contains transcellular water.

Water is also an important component of the bloodstream. This intravascular water is found in the arteries, veins, and capillaries as an important constituent of the plasma.

Functions

Water is often referred to as the universal solvent because so many materials are soluble in it. A primary function of water in the body is to act as a solvent. Due to the efficacy of water as a solvent, water is a suitable and practical medium for transporting nutrients to the various cells of the body and for removing the cellular waste products. Without such a highly suitable and efficient transport mechanism, the nourishment of the cells would be impossible. Fortunately, water ably transports amino acids, proteins, monosaccharides, minerals, vitamins, gases (carbon dioxide and ammonia), and lipids in the form of phospholipids.

The lubricating role of water is significant in body movement. Water is not readily compressible. Because of this fact, plus its flow characteristics, water serves as a cushioning device that facilitates movement of the joints. The lubricating role of water may be viewed in yet another way. Water, as a constituent of saliva, lubricates food in the mouth and thus provides great assistance in the swallowing process. The value of water as a lubricant can be noted all along the alimentary canal. Movement of bolus and chyme would be very difficult, if not impossible, without water in the body.

Water is an essential compound in the chemical reactions of digestion. The breakdown of carbohydrates to monosaccharides, the splitting of glycerol from the fatty acids, and the cleavage of proteins to the amino acid components are all examples of hydrolytic reactions; that is, water actually participates in the chemical reaction. For digestion to occur, water must be available.

Water in the body performs the very useful function of helping to regulate the temperature of the body. Overheating of the body is prevented by the evaporation of water from the skin. This process of water secretion in the form of perspiration and subsequent evaporation is happening continually, but at varying rates that are dependent upon the environment. At room temperature, the process usually is unnoticed, but nevertheless is occurring. This is termed insensible perspiration. Of course, in a hot environment or after heavy physical exercise, perspiration is much more apparent because considerably more water is evaporating to restore the body to an equilibrium state.

One of the important functions of water is its role as a structural component of the body. The water that occurs in cells is necessary to retain the shape of the cell. With loss of water from the cell, the cell membrane begins to collapse. This role of water may be viewed in a somewhat exaggerated way by putting a leaf of lettuce in a salt water solution for several hours. This condition draws the water from the cells of the lettuce. The cells gradually lose their normal appearance and become limp and compact. A similar modification in cellular rigidity occurs in humans when the water content of cells is reduced.

Sources and Recommended Intakes of Water

The requirement for dietary sources of water is a highly individual matter and shows considerable variation from one person to another. Indeed, the need varies widely from day to day even for a given individual because of the tremendous influence of environment and physical activity on the excretion rate.

Under ordinary conditions, a reasonable recommendation of water intake for adults is 1 liter (a little more than 1 quart) for each 1000 kilocalories consumed. This would mean the recommendation for most of the adult population would range between 2 and $2\frac{1}{2}$ liters of water daily. The requirement of water per kilocalorie consumed for children may be half again as much. The consumption of water, either alone or in beverages such as tea and coffee, has the advantage of providing some mineral elements in addition to the water itself. Hard water is often a source of calcium and magnesium. Fluoridated water is the only practical dietary source of fluoride.

Water is available to the body not only simply as water that one drinks, but also in more subtle forms. All beverages are high in their water content. Even many foods that may not appear to be watery actually are good sources of water. Bread, for example, seems dry, and yet it contains approximately 35 percent water. On the other hand, the juiciness of some foods obviously suggests a much higher water content. Most fruits have a water content of 80 percent or more, and even bananas (which certainly do not seem juicy) are about 76 percent water.

It appears that the solid foods in an average diet contribute 25 to 50 percent of the water needed by the body each day. Liquids will provide slightly less than half the total water needed. The remainder of the water utilized by the body daily is provided internally as a result of the water released during metabolism. When amino acids are utilized in the synthesis of protein in the body, water is a by-product of the reaction. The formation of fats in the body is another source of this metabolic water. These are only a few of the chemical reactions that form water for the body's use.

Excretion

Despite the fact that water is vital to the body, some water still must be excreted for various reasons. Water is excreted in the urine, feces, breath, and perspiration. This is the body's means of eliminating a variety of unnecessary substances. If sufficient water is not available to eliminate waste materials in feces and urine, toxic levels of waste will build up in the body. The amount of water that is excreted in the urine and feces is determined, in part, by the total liquid intake and also by the state of motility of the digestive tract. Diarrhea greatly increases the rate of water excretion. Large intakes of water result in increased urinary volume.

Water is lost through evaporation in the lungs and on the skin. The loss of water through perspiration is variable, but ordinarily will be about one third of the day's water excretion. The moisture loss through the lungs can be demonstrated easily by simply breathing directly onto a piece of glass. The glass will be covered with a fine mist. Each exhalation carries some moisture from the body. The loss through the lungs is influenced considerably by the rate of breathing, as would be expected. On an average, slightly less water is excreted through the lungs than through the skin.

Summary

Water is vital to life. Its roles in the body are varied and include: (1) a solvent to transport nutrient materials to the cells and remove the waste products; (2) a lubricant for joints and the movement of food along the alimentary canal; (3) a chemical reactant; (4) regulation of body temperature; and (5) a structural component of the cells.

Within the body, water is distributed as intracellular and extracellular water. The extracellular water includes: (1) the bound water of connective tissue, bone, and cartilage; (2) interstitial water, which serves as a transport mechanism; (3) transcellular water, important as a lubricant; and (4) intravascular water, a constituent of the blood plasma.

Water is available to the body in beverages, in foods (particularly fruits), and from metabolism. It is excreted in urine and feces, through respiration in the lungs, and perspiration on the skin.

Selected References

McDermott, J. H., et al. Health aspects of toxic materials in drinking water. *Am. J. Public Health. 61:2269.* 1971.

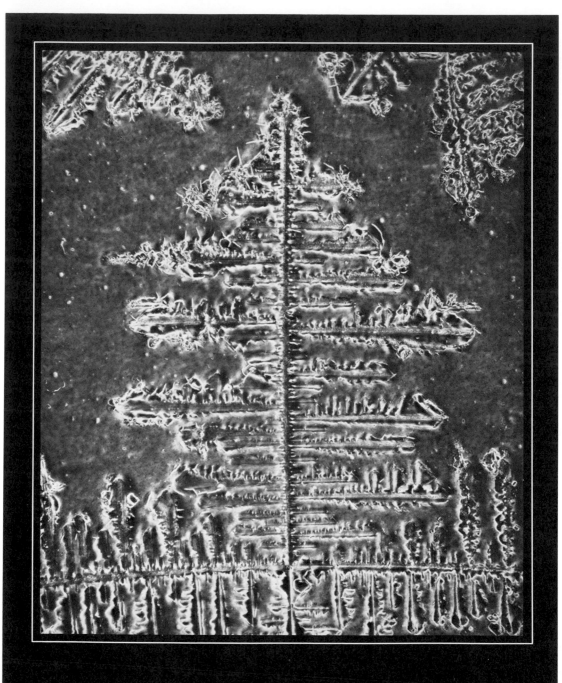

Chapter 10

The ABC's of Minerals

The importance of carbohydrates, fats, proteins, and water for optimum body functioning has been discussed in the previous chapters. These nutrients are required in quantities designated in grams or ounces. Now the discussion will focus on several inorganic substances that are extremely significant to normal body operation despite the fact that they are needed in milligram, or even microgram quantities.

Minerals may be defined as inorganic, crystalline, and homogeneous chemicals. When foods are combusted completely, there still remains a small amount of powderlike residue that is commonly referred to as ash. This ash is the mineral content of the food. Compared with the original bulk of the food, the mineral content of foods is rather miniscule. Both plants and animals contain minerals. For example, the human body is approximately 4 percent ash; the remaining 96 percent is mostly water plus fat, protein, and carbohydrate.

On the basis of a comparison of relative

Chapter opening photo: Eric V. Gravé.

amounts in the body, one might conclude that minerals are of very limited significance in the human body. Nothing could be further from the truth. As a group, minerals perform some unique and necessary roles in the body: (1) control of water balance, (2) regulation of acid-base balance, (3) structural components, (4) constituents of enzymes, hormones, and some other key compounds, and (5) catalysts for various reactions in the body. Individual minerals function in highly specific ways, such as in transmission of nerve impulses and muscular contraction.

Frequently, minerals are classified as either macronutrient or micronutrient (or trace) minerals. This designation is based on the relative amounts or weight of the various minerals in the body. On this basis, calcium, chlorine, magnesium, phosphorus, potassium, sodium, and sulfur are macronutrient minerals; chromium, cobalt, copper, fluorine, iodine, iron, manganese, molybdenum, selenium, and zinc are

Table 10.1 *Some of the Minerals in the Body*[a]

Mineral	Amount in a 60 kg Person	
	Percent	g
Macronutrient		
Calcium	1.5-2.2	900-1320
Phosphorus	0.8-1.2	480-720
Potassium	0.35	210
Sulfur	0.25	150
Sodium	0.15	90
Chloride	0.15	90
Magnesium	0.05	30
Micronutrient		
Iron	0.004	2.4
Manganese	0.0003	0.18
Copper	0.00015	0.09
Iodine	0.00004	0.024

[a] Based on data on the elementary composition of the body. H. C. Sherman. *Chemistry of Food and Nutrition.* Macmillan. New York. P. 227. 1952.

trace minerals. Table 10.1 illustrates the range of values between the macro- and micronutrient minerals. Calcium, which is the most abundant of the minerals in the body, comprises approximately 2 percent of the body's weight; iodine, an extremely important trace mineral, contributes only 0.00004 percent of the body's weight. Another way of expressing these values is to say that calcium occurs in the body at the level of 20,000 parts per million and iodine at 0.4 parts per million.

The significance of the above-named minerals has been studied by scientists, and many of their functions have been elucidated. However, many other minerals—lead, gold, and mercury, for example—also occur in body tissues. Some of these other minerals may prove to have various physiologic functions, but most are known to have harmful effects even in quite small amounts. The relationship of these various minerals to the general health, growth, and development of the body is causing increasing concern as the problems of environmental pollution multiply, and as traces of many of these heavy metals are found to be present in foods. In addition, these nutritional problems may be compounded because of the concentration of mineral elements that can occur as the mineral is moved along the food chain via consumption by larger and more complex organisms. Man appears to be standing on the threshold of a new phase of mineral research.

Obviously, there is much yet to be learned about these minerals, facts that need to be ferreted out quickly as the ecological balance is gradually altered. An illustration of the importance of these emerging interrelationships is the concern regarding levels of mercury that have recently been found in fish, primarily because of improved analytical techniques. Mercury has been found not only in fish, but also in most of our foods, although generally at lower levels than in fish. However, because Americans typically do not eat fish frequently, more total mercury probably is ingested from bread, potatoes, and meat than from fish. The levels of mercury and other heavy metals in food, including fish, are not at a level to give concern today, but control of the environment is imperative so that harmful levels are not reached in the future.

Not only is it important to consider the total amount of heavy metal that may be present in foods, but also the form in which it is found. For example, methyl and ethyl mercury, the forms in which most mercury is present in fish, are far more toxic compounds than the inorganic salts of mercury that appear to be present in most other foods. However, evidence is lacking that methyl mercury in fish—even swordfish—in the quantities normally consumed has been responsible for any ill health in man in the United States.

General Functions of Minerals

Acid-base balance

Minerals absorbed from food interact in vital ways to maintain acid-base balance in the body. The various tissues and fluids of the body need to be maintained at optimum pH values required for the innumerable metabolic reactions to take place. The pH scale of acidity and alkalinity ranges from 0 to 7 for acids and 7 to 14 for bases (alkaline materials), with 7 being exactly neutral. The blood and other tissues must be maintained within a limited range, close to neutrality but slightly alkaline, approximately pH 7.2–7.4 for blood and slightly lower in tissues and cells. To accomplish the delicate control required to maintain the pH within a variation not exceeding 0.2 on the pH scale, the body has several mechanisms in which minerals figure prominently.

Acid and base formers

Some minerals contribute toward developing a more acidic medium, while others tend to make the body more alkaline. The term "minerals," as usually used in nutrition and as used in this discussion, is not strictly correct since fluoride, chloride, sulfate, and phosphate are anions (negatively charged ions) and sodium, potassium, iron, magnesium, and calcium are cations (ions bearing a positive charge). The affinity for phosphate to act as a hydrogen ion "acceptor" accounts for the ability of phosphate to buffer excess acid loads (high hydrogen ion concentration) in the blood. Similarly, the ability of calcium to buffer weak organic acids (including beta-hydroxybutyric acid, lactic acid, and citric acid) accounts for calcium being considered as a "base" or buffer for acids. Therefore, all the most important cations and anions considered in this section,

while not strictly minerals, are classified as such.

The minerals that are acid-forming include chloride, sulfur, and phosphorus. These minerals provide the potential for forming phosphoric acid, hydrochloric acid, and sulfuric acid. As a counterbalance, calcium, iron, magnesium, potassium, and sodium contribute to the formation of a more alkaline medium (Table 10.2).

The acid-forming minerals, that is, phosphorus, chloride, and sulfur, are relatively abundant in grain and cereal products, meat, eggs, poultry, and fish. In a somewhat surprising contrast, fruits, and vegetables generally are alkaline in reaction in the body. The predominating acids in fruits are organic acids that are fully metabolized by the body and hence do not contribute to the body's total acidity. Even such noticeably acidic fruits as lemons actually are base forming in the body because,

Table 10.2 Acid and Base Formers in the Human Body

	Acid Forming	Base Forming
Minerals	Chloride Sulfur Phosphorus	Calcium Iron Magnesium Potassium Sodium
Foods	Grain and cereals products Meat Eggs Poultry Fish	Fruits Vegetables

after the metabolic breakdown of the organic acids by the body, an alkaline residue of sodium and potassium remains. Exceptions to this, because of their content of nonmetabolizable acids, are cranberries, spinach, rhubarb, chocolate, tea, and coffee. For the average individual, these exceptions are of very limited significance.

The other food group still remaining for consideration relative to minerals includes milk and dairy products. Milk contains both acid and base-forming materials; the acid-forming phosphorus and base-forming calcium essentially neutralize each other.

Normal pH controls

The average diet, containing generous quantities of meat, is slightly acidic because of phosphorus and sulfur-containing amino acids; however, the body readily compensates for this. One means of accommodation is the buffer systems. Proteins are amphoteric, that is, they can react as acids or bases. Therefore, they can help to neutralize the acid-forming minerals when they are in excess. Conversely, proteins can react with the alkaline minerals to achieve the necessary neutrality.

Carbonic acid and bicarbonate ion provide another illustration of buffering in the body. The body has the potential for using the water and carbon dioxide formed during metabolism to make carbonic acid when it is needed to neutralize excess alkali in the body. Still other examples of buffering compounds in the body are phosphates and hemoglobin. Removal of excess acid is facilitated by the expiration of carbon dioxide. Hemoglobin combines with carbon dioxide to transport carbon dioxide to the lungs, where the gas is released and exhaled.

The kidney can also contribute to the maintenance of desirable pH by producing a distinctly more acidic urine when excess acid is a problem. The urine may become as much as 1.5 pH units more acidic in extreme cases. The other contribution of the kidney toward maintenance of correct pH in the body is the formation of the ammonium ion (NH_4^+). This ion can be excreted in place of sodium and potassium ions. This reduces the loss of sodium and potassium ions so that they are available to carry more carbon dioxide as the alkaline sodium and potassium bicarbonates.

Potential problem of antacids

The body of the normal individual is well equipped to maintain the pH of the blood within the narrow range of normalcy at the slightly alkaline pH level of about 7.4. Unfortunately, innumerable advertisements have been carefully conceived to persuade the buying public that it is necessary to aid the body in maintaining this appropriate pH. Only a recluse who shuns all mass media of communication can escape the suggestion that excess stomach acidity is the common plague of modern men. After presenting the disquieting thought that excess stomach acidity can strike at any hour of the day or night, advertisers quickly offer their panacea to correct or prevent problems. The urgency of the appeal suggests that excess acidity is a never-ending problem. Such persuasions may lead normal individuals to consume antacid medications to avoid the discomforts of excess acidity. Regular use of these alkaline medications is to be discouraged since this can result in just the opposite problem—alkalosis. The normal individual will do well to avoid the use of these antacid concoctions unless they are specifically prescribed by a physician for a specific purpose.

Control of water balance

Water is found in the body within the blood vessels, within the cells, and between the cells. To move from one of these locations to another, water must pass through semipermeable membranes by a process known as osmosis. This movement is determined in direction and amount by the concentration of minerals on either side of the membrane. If the concentration of minerals is higher on one side of the membrane than on the other, water will be drawn through the membrane toward the side where the mineral concentration is greater. For proper nourishment of the cells, water must transport nutrients from the blood, through the extracellular space, and into the cells. Under ordinary circumstances, the typical diet contains an appropriate balance of mineral salts to permit this passage of water through membranes into other parts of the body. However, occasional circumstances may upset the mineral balance, leading to accumulation of fluids (edema) or to dehydration.

Sodium levels provide a useful illustration of the role of minerals in regulating osmotic pressure and, thus, the distribution of water within the body. When the level of sodium in the body drops (as happens when perspiration has been excessive), water is drawn from the cells in an attempt to equalize the electrolyte concentration within and outside the cell. This causes dehydration of the cell and may be observed as weakness and dizziness. In the reverse circumstance, the level of sodium ions in the blood builds up, and water is drawn from the extracellular spaces into the blood vessels. This increased volume of blood may be evidenced by an increase in blood pressure. In turn, some water may be withdrawn from the cells and accumulated in the interstitial fluids. This accumulation of water between the tissues causes an obvious bloating or spongy character to the tissues called edema. The edematous condition is determined readily by pressing a finger firmly into the puffed up area. A clear indentation remains for a short period of time after the finger is removed. The movement of the interstitial fluid back into the previously compressed area can be seen as the depression swells again to follow the contour of the rest of the skin in the area.

Structural components

Several minerals are structural components of the body. The concentration of such minerals as calcium, phosphate, and fluoride in the bones and teeth attests to their significance in the development of hard tissues. Optimal skeletal development is dependent upon the presence of adequate amounts of these minerals during the growing years. The maintenance of strong bones in adulthood continues to be dependent upon these minerals. Another of the minerals—potassium—is a component of soft tissue.

Constituents of compounds essential to the body

Various minerals are structural components of hormones, enzyme systems, vitamins, and other important chemical components in the body. Some of the hormones of the body require minerals for their formation. Iodine is a structural part of thyroxine, the hormone secreted by the thyroid gland. Zinc is essential for the formation of insulin in the pancreas.

Two of the vitamins contain a mineral as a structural part of the molecule. Sulfur is a structural component of thiamin, and cobalt is contained in the molecule of cobalamin (vitamin B_{12}).

The cytochrome enzyme systems contain iron and copper. Another enzyme (carbonic anhydrase) contains zinc. Carbonic anhydrase is necessary to liberate carbon dioxide from red blood cells when it is brought to the lungs so it can be exhaled as a gas. Carboxypeptidase, the proteolytic enzyme that attacks from the carboxyl end of the protein chain, also contains zinc. The rather exotic sounding mineral, molybdenum, is a structural part of xanthine oxidase, an enzyme instrumental in uric acid metabolism.

Iron, as will be seen subsequently, is a significant part of the hemoglobin in blood. Chloride is a component of hydrochloric acid, the acid of the stomach, which plays an important role in digestion.

Catalytic roles

In numerous and varied reactions in the body, individual minerals function in a catalytic capacity, either in an enzyme system or as an ion. Magnesium is required for catabolism and anabolism of carbohydrates, fats, and proteins. Additionally, copper, calcium, potassium, manganese, zinc, and several other minerals catalyze various metabolic reactions. Copper is required for hemoglobin formation although it is not actually a part of the molecule.

Absorption of nutrients is enhanced by minerals in some cases. For example, the very large vitamin B_{12} molecule passes through the intestinal wall with the assistance of calcium. Although carbohydrate molecules are much smaller, even the absorption of monosaccharides is aided by the presence of sodium and magnesium.

Nerve impulses and muscular contraction

The ionizing capability of minerals is used by the body in the performance of certain vital tasks. Take, for example, the transmission of nerve impulses. For movement and thought, it is mandatory that nerve impulses be transmitted to and from the brain. Actually, this is accomplished by passing a small electric charge along the nerve fiber to and from the brain. When a nerve is stimulated, the permeability of the affected membrane increases, making it possible to move potassium and sodium ions through the membrane of the nerve cell. This movement changes the electric charge of the membrane, which then excites the next part. Thus, the signal is passed along.

The minerals whose concentrations are related particularly closely to contraction and relaxation of various muscle tissues are calcium, potassium, magnesium, and sodium. An appropriate balance of these minerals is necessary for normally controlled contraction and relaxation of muscles. Calcium is the mineral important in muscular contraction. Counterbalancing calcium are potassium, sodium, and magnesium, which function in relaxing muscles.

Calcium

The preceding discussion has indicated that calcium is an extremely important mineral in the body. It is also the most abundant of the minerals in the body. Actually, a reasonable estimate is that the weight of calcium in adults generally ranges between 2 and 3 pounds, depending upon the size of the individual. A 110-pound woman will contain a little over 2 pounds of calcium if her health is normal and her diet has been good. A 200-pound man may have more than 3 pounds of calcium in his body. A general rule of thumb is that calcium contributes 2 percent of the body's total weight. Obviously, many variations from this figure may be found without much searching.

Calcium in the body is found primarily in the bones and teeth but about 1 percent of the total body calcium is distributed in muscle and extracellular fluid throughout the body. The calcium in the bones may be viewed as a storage reservoir that is drawn upon to meet the requirements of the cells for calcium when the intake of the mineral is inadequate. The calcium in the teeth is much less readily available to meet the top priority needs of the body for calcium.

Functions

Bone formation, maintenance, and growth

Calcium is essential for optimum ossification (sometimes referred to as mineralization) of bones to occur. As children slowly mature, the collagenous framework of the bone is strengthened by the deposition of calcium phosphate in stable hydroxyapatite crystals. The calcifying bone gradually becomes less flexible with age and more rigid and strong. This process should proceed rapidly enough for the long bones to be strong enough to support the weight of a young child when he first begins to stand and walk. Obviously, bone strength is needed if the long bones are to remain straight. With an adequate calcium intake, even the bones of young children should be strong.

The lengthening of bones occurs normally during the growth period if calcium and other mineral materials are available as needed. The average daily retention of calcium in bone during the growing years is about 165 milligrams. However, actual retention shows wide variations because calcium retention varies with the growth actually taking place at the time. Growth follows a somewhat sporadic, rather than a completely uniform pattern during childhood and puberty. The dietary recommendations for calcium show less variation than would be revealed by a longitudinal plotting of an individual's growth rate. This permits repletion of body stores of calcium that may have been reduced during a growth spurt.

A bone appears to be a solid, distinctly permanent sort of structure, and yet that appearance is deceiving. Actually, bone is a fairly dynamic tissue, with bone formation and dissolution constantly occurring. It is because of the continuing need to replace calcium which is being removed from bones that adults still have a requirement for calcium.

Tooth formation

The deposition of calcium in teeth is similar to that in bone. Again, it is the formation and precipitation of calcium phosphates in the form of strong crystals that account for much of the strength of the teeth. In dentin, the hydroxyapatite crystals are deposited in a protein matrix, similar to the collagen matrix in bone. In enamel, the protein matrix is a very insoluble mixture of proteins which are not known to occur elsewhere in the body. They have been given the name of enkeratin, largely because enamel has the same ectodermal order as skin.

In teeth, the crystals are packed densely to give great strength to the structure. This calcification process of the primary teeth begins at about the midway point in pregnancy and essentially is completed at the time the tooth breaks through the gum. Although some replacement of the calcium in the dentin may take place in childhood, the exchange and redeposition of calcium in teeth must be extremely minute when compared with the turnover of calcium in bones.

The same pattern holds true for the formation of secondary or permanent teeth, despite the fact that the total period for calcification covers a far greater span of time than is customary in the primary (deciduous) teeth. Initial calcification takes place between the ages of 3 and 36 months, while the calcification of the late-forming wisdom teeth begins around 10 years of age. The secondary teeth, like the primary teeth, undergo only very slow calcium turnover. The approximately 10 grams of calcium in a full set of secondary teeth is in sharp contrast to the approximate value of 1000 grams or more of calcium in the total adult bone structure.

The effectiveness of the mineral nutrient fluoride in lessening tooth decay is explained as follows. Some fluoride ions replace the hydroxyl ($—OH^-$) ions in the complex calcium salts that form the tooth enamel during childhood and adolescence. This fluoride-containing tooth crystal is simply more resistant to the decay-producing effects of the simple organic acids that are formed in the mouth whenever any food is eaten.

Blood clot formation

Calcium is essential to the normal formation of blood clots. Its role, as an ion in the blood, is twofold: calcium triggers the blood platelets to release a catalyst called thromboplastin. With thromboplastin thus available in the blood, prothrombin that naturally occurs in the blood is immediately modified to thrombin. In turn, thrombin causes the joining together or polymerization of fibrinogen to the large, bulky molecule of fibrin that forms the actual clot. This process also requires calcium ions (Figure 10.1).

Utilization of nutrients

Calcium ions function in several different ways to improve the utilization of various nutrients. Even before food is digested completely in the digestive tract, calcium is exerting its influence. Pancreatic lipase, one of the enzymes that splits fatty acids from glycerol when fat is digested in the small intestine, is activated by calcium. As discussed in Chapter 6, this enzyme is vital to optimum utilization of fat by the body. Also in the small intestine, calcium complexes intimately with vitamin B_{12} to effect its passage through the epithelial wall. This bulky vitamin (see Chapter 11) is needed for maintaining normal health of nerves. Within the body, calcium bound to lecithin influences cell permeability, thus influencing cell composition.

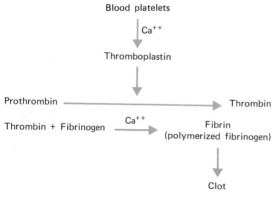

Figure 10.1   The role of calcium in blood clot formation.

Roles in nerves and muscles

Perhaps the most dramatic function of calcium is in the maintenance of the heartbeat. Regular contraction and relaxation are essential to a healthy heart. Calcium in the interstitial fluid that contacts the muscles regulates contraction of the muscle, while various other minerals also present in the fluid promote muscle relaxation that follows. Abnormally low levels of ionized calcium in muscle cells, cause uncontrolled tetanic spasms (or muscle contraction). Calcium is needed to make acetylcholine available for transmitting nerve impulses. Acetylcholine is required for the message to be passed from a nerve cell to the cell adjacent to it.

Deficiency and excess

A calcium deficiency alone is an unlikely occurrence in human nutrition but is more likely to result from one of several accompanying inadequacies. In growing children, one would expect that abnormalities of growth and of bone structure would be one clear-cut result of an inadequate calcium intake. However, the body has protective mechanisms to promote more efficient calcium utilization when the diet provides suboptimal levels of calcium. Poor growth and the deformed bones of rickets generally are more likely the result of inadequate vitamin D intake and poor absorption of calcium, rather than simply the product of a diet low in calcium. The actual contribution of inadequate calcium to the physical condition may be complicated still further by inadequate protein and ascorbic acid levels.

Inadequate calcium intake in adults, particularly women who have undergone numerous pregnancies, may lead to osteomalacia and osteoporosis in later life. Osteoporosis is a condition in which the total amount of bone is reduced. Causes of this bone resorption are varied. These include: inadequate calcium intake for years, loss because of bed confinement for long periods, too low a level of estrogens, and poor collagen matrix in the bone. Osteomalacia is found in instances where calcium levels are depleted. The bones of a person with osteomalacia are reduced in the content of calcium, but are not changed in size. The efficacy of fluoride in helping bone tissue retain calcium and, hence, avoid these demineralizing diseases is not clear but is one of the more interesting developments of the modern study of bone metabolism. The theory is that fluoride, by replacing the hydroxyl group in the bone crystals, forms a crystal that is not readily resorbed. The need for magnesium to maintain bone integrity has also been noted.

Inadequate calcium during the period of tooth formation may lead to subsequent dental problems. Soft teeth all too quickly become decayed, missing, or filled teeth. Again, the actual significance of calcium is difficult to assess because of various other dietary factors, such as fluoride and oral hygiene that influence the health of the teeth. However, the dietary intake of calcium after tooth formation is completed appears to have little significance on the integrity of the teeth because of their static nature.

One frequently hears from adults that they do not drink milk because they are afraid of developing kidney stones. Excessive milk intake does not produce elevated blood and urine calcium levels. These levels are more likely secondary to some underlying hormonal abnormality. Generally, adults need to be more concerned about consuming sufficient calcium rather than avoiding excessive quantities. A glass of milk or its equivalent in cheese is one of the best ways most adults can improve their diets.

Absorption and excretion

Calcium is absorbed, with varying efficiency, primarily in the upper part of the small intestine. The actual percentage of dietary calcium that is absorbed varies widely from person to person and, indeed, from time to time for each individual. The diverse factors related to

calcium absorption are discussed in the following paragraphs (Figure 10.2).

Both the age and nutritional status of an individual are related directly to the absorption of dietary calcium. In periods of growth, including pregnancy and lactation, the body absorbs calcium more efficiently than in periods of life in which only maintenance is involved.

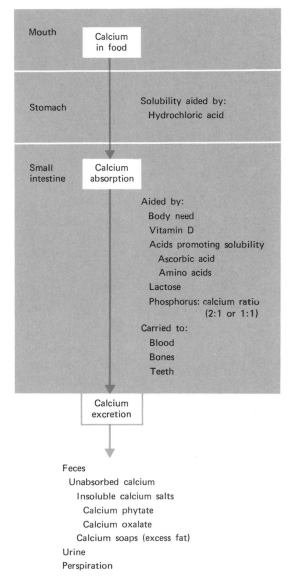

Figure 10.2 Fates of calcium ingested in food.

The body is a remarkably adaptive organism and can make adjustments to various levels of calcium intake. In diets containing very small quantities of dietary calcium, the percentage of calcium absorbed may rise to as high as 60 percent during periods of growth. This figure is in sharp contrast to the 10 percent absorption rate that is occasionally found among adults who regularly have a high dietary intake of calcium. Approximately 30 percent absorption of dietary calcium is a realistic expectation for the normal individual.

Vitamin D is instrumental in effecting calcium absorption. This vitamin facilitates passage of calcium through the intestinal wall by stimulating the production of a calcium-binding protein in the intestine. This facilitates absorption through the intestinal membrane. The fortification of milk with vitamin D is commendable because of the enhanced absorption of calcium. By adding the vitamin to a valuable food source of calcium, one can be certain that both nutrients will be available when needed.

Various acids have the capacity of increasing the absorption of calcium. One example is that of hydrochloric acid in the stomach. Since calcium is more soluble in an acidic medium, the presence of hydrochloric acid in the stomach helps liberate ionic calcium for absorption. Calcium must be soluble instead of being combined in an insoluble salt, if it is to be absorbed. Ascorbic acid is a vitamin that encourages better absorption of calcium because its acidic reaction favors solubility of calcium. Some amino acids—notably lysine—also promote the absorption of this mineral.

Calcium combines with some organic acids to form insoluble salts, thus hindering calcium absorption when these acids are a part of the food being digested. Two specific illustrations of organic acids that form insoluble precipitates with calcium are phytic acid and oxalic acid. Phytic acid, a component of the bran in cereals, is capable of tying up some of the calcium when milk is consumed along with whole-grain cereals. A similar situation occurs when foods high in oxalic acid (for example, spinach and rhubarb) are eaten. The oxalic acid and calcium combine to form calcium oxalate, an insoluble calcium salt that is not absorbed through the intestinal membrane. These illustrations are of academic interest but not of tremendous practical importance. The usual diet contains these foods in small quantities, so calcium absorption is not impaired significantly. Furthermore, these foods are rich in other nutrients and belong in the diet.

Excess fat in the diet is another factor influencing calcium absorption. Calcium will combine with fatty acids in the intestine to form calcium soaps that are insoluble, thus rendering the calcium unavailable. In sprue, where fats are not absorbed well, calcium absorption is impaired; the patient may be calcium deficient despite an adequate amount of calcium in the diet.

Lactose, the sugar occurring naturally in milk, also favors calcium absorption. Calcium and lactose form a soluble complex, thus impeding the formation of insoluble calcium salts that might otherwise be formed in the digestive tract. This favorable effect of lactose is particularly fortuitous since lactose is a normal component of milk, the richest source of calcium in the diet. Milk is the primary source of lactose in the diet.

As is true with the absorption of other nutrients, anything that accelerates the passage of food through the small intestine results in reduced absorption of calcium. When food passes through too rapidly, there simply is insufficient opportunity for foods to be digested and their nutrients passed through the intestinal membrane. Also worthy of note is the fact that individuals who are bedfast or relatively immobile for even a few days go into negative calcium balance, that is, they are excreting more calcium in the urine and feces than they are ingesting from food. This is primarily due to increased resorption of bone, which takes place during inactivity and results in an increased excretion of calcium in the urine. This phenomenon also has been noted in astronauts during space missions, perhaps because only limited

Table 10.3 *Recommended Daily Dietary Allowances for Minerals*[a]

	Age (years)	Weight (kg)	Weight (lb)	Height (cm)	Height (in.)	Calcium (mg)	Phosphorus (mg)	Iodine (µg)	Iron (mg)	Magnesium (mg)	Zinc (mg)
Infants	0–0.5	6	14	60	24	360	240	35	10	60	3
	0.5–1	9	20	71	28	540	400	45	15	70	5
	1–3	13	28	86	34	800	800	60	15	150	10
Children	4–6	20	44	110	44	800	800	80	10	200	10
	7–10	30	66	135	54	800	800	110	10	250	10
	11–14	44	97	158	63	1200	1200	130	18	350	15
	15–18	61	134	172	69	1200	1200	150	18	400	15
Males	19–22	67	147	172	69	800	800	140	10	350	15
	23–50	70	154	172	69	800	800	130	10	350	15
	51+	70	154	172	69	800	800	110	10	350	15
	11–14	44	97	155	62	1200	1200	115	18	300	15
	15–18	54	119	162	65	1200	1200	115	18	300	15
Females	19–22	58	128	162	65	800	800	100	18	300	15
	23–50	58	128	162	65	800	800	100	18	300	15
	51+	58	128	162	65	800	800	80	10	300	15
Pregnancy						1200	1200	125	18+	450	20
Lactation						1200	1200	150	18	450	25

[a] Food and Nutrition Board, National Academy of Sciences—National Research Council. *Recommended Daily Dietary Allowances*, revised 1974.

movement is possible within the confined area of the space capsule. This effect cannot be overcome simply by an increased intake of calcium.

The ratio of phosphate to calcium that occurs in the normal diet ranges between two parts of phosphate and one part of calcium (2:1) to the ratio of equal parts (1:1) of the two minerals. Although intestinal absorption of calcium is somewhat greater on the 2:1 ratio, the absorption of calcium still is excellent when the percentages are equal. In experiments in which abnormal diets with a ratio of one part phosphate to two parts calcium (1:2) were fed, calcium absorption was reduced.

Calcium that is not absorbed continues on through the intestinal tract and is excreted in the feces. The calcium that is absorbed is carried in the bloodstream. The normal value is 10 milligrams of calcium per 100 milliliters of serum. Serum calcium levels are regulated by parathyroid hormones and are remarkably stable from day to day. Parathormone is the hormone secreted by the parathyroids to stimulate resorption of calcium when serum calcium levels drop below normal values. Calcitonin, a hormone that lowers the level of blood calcium, is synthesized and secreted by the thyroid and parathyroid glands whenever the serum calcium becomes elevated to abnormally high levels. Calcitonin acts by decreasing calcium mobilization from bone. It can be seen, therefore, that the parathormone and calcitonin provide a system of checks and balances to regulate the level of calcium in the blood.

Calcium is found in the fluids that nourish the tissues. When the calcium level exceeds a critical point in the fluid contacting bone cartilage, calcium will be deposited as calcium phosphate, eventually forming a crystalline structure. The digestive secretions of the stomach and small intestine contain calcium, which can be recycled by being absorbed again through the intestinal wall.

For the most part, calcium is excreted in the urine and feces, although a small amount may be lost in sweat. Urinary excretion is approximately nine times as great as the loss in perspiration under normal conditions. However, if the individual is doing hard physical labor in a hot, humid environment, the calcium loss in perspiration will be greatly in excess of the estimated 20 milligrams of calcium excreted daily by the normal individual via this route.

Recommended allowance

The recommended dietary allowance for calcium has been a highly contested issue. The Food and Nutrition Board of the National Academy of Sciences has adopted the position of recommending a generous allowance because some individuals do not adapt as well as others to marginal or suboptimal calcium levels. It is this adaptive capacity that makes it difficult to determine what the minimal recommendation for the normal adult should be. Some people believe that an apparent calcium deficiency may actually be a problem of vitamin D adequacy. Others feel that a fairly high recommendation for calcium is important in this country because not all people can adapt to a lower level, and food supplies providing calcium are readily available. Table 10.3 lists the recommended dietary allowances for calcium, phosphorus, iodine, iron, and magnesium. Note the gradual increase to cover the needs for the growing body and the subsequent reduction for the mature, maintenance years. Sharp increases are recommended for periods of pregnancy and lactation.

Food sources

Milk is unquestionably the outstanding source of calcium. Not only is milk rich in calcium and phosphate but it also contains protein, lactose and, frequently, vitamin D is added. These nutrients enhance the utilization of the calcium present in milk. Cow's milk is approximately four times richer in calcium than

Table 10.4 *Calcium Content of Selected Foods*[a]

	Amount	Calcium (mg)
Dairy foods		
Milk, 3.5% fat	1 cup	288
Milk, skim	1 cup	295
Milk, fortified low fat	1 cup	349
Milk, chocolate	1 cup	269
Milk, buttermilk	1 cup	295
Milk, yogurt	1 cup	122
Milk, evaporated	1 cup	635
Milk, condensed	1 cup	802
Milk, eggnog	1 cup	242
Milk, "Instant" breakfast	1 cup	413
Cheese, cheddar	1 oz	213
Cheese, Swiss	1 oz	262
Cheese, blue	1 oz	89
Cheese, American process	1 oz	198
Cheese, cottage	1/2 cup	106
Ice cream	1/2 cup	88
Ice milk	1/2 cup	146
Fish and shellfish		
Salmon, pink, canned	3 1/2 oz	196
Sardines	1 medium	45
Oysters	6 medium	94
Vegetables		
Broccoli, cooked	1/2 cup	72
Spinach, cooked	1/2 cup	93
Beet or turnip greens, cooked	1/2 cup	106
Collard greens, cooked	1/2 cup	176
Dandelion or mustard greens, cooked	1/2 cup	140
Kale, cooked	1/2 cup	121
Sweet potato, baked in skin	1 large	72
Other foods		
Orange, fresh	1 medium	62
Bread, 3-4% nonfat dry, milk solids added	1 slice	19

[a] Data compiled and adapted from ***Composition of Foods—Raw, Processed, Prepared,*** Agriculture Handbook No. 8, U.S.D.A., 1963; ***Nutritive Value of Foods,*** Home and Garden Bulletin No. 72, U.S.D.A., 1971; manufacturers' information and ***Nutritive Value of American Foods,*** Agriculture Handbook No. 456, U.S.D.A., 1975.

is human milk. However, infants are able to utilize about two thirds of the calcium contained in human milk; the absorption of calcium from cow's milk ranges between 35 and 50 percent. This is a clear demonstration of the adaptability of the human in relation to meeting calcium needs. Cheeses, chocolate beverages, puddings, and custard desserts made with milk are good sources of calcium.

Although milk and its products are the outstanding sources of calcium, several other foods assume a significant role in some diets. Small fish or products made from small fish in which the bones are processed along with the meat are good sources of calcium, as are salmon when the bones are broken into fine pieces and retained in the food. Greens, either raw or cooked, are rather high in calcium. Other good vegetable sources are included in Table 10.4. In general, meats and fruits provide only a limited amount of calcium in the average diet. Cereals also make a small contribution in the typical American diet. However, cereal products may assume some importance in meeting the calcium needs when the diet contains regularly a large amount of cereal.

Chloride

Chloride, although comprising only 0.15 percent of the total body weight, is a rather ubiquitous element. One of the important functions of chloride in the body is to serve as the negative ion (anion) in hydrochloric acid in the stomach. The importance of this acid in digestion has been discussed. Since chloride is a component of hydrochloric acid, it is not surprising to find some concentration of the total chloride in the body in the digestive tract secretions.

The permeability of membranes to chloride accounts for the role chloride assumes in maintaining normal osmotic pressure in the body. Within cells, chloride is found in the form of potassium chloride and, in the extracellular fluid, it combines with sodium to form sodium chloride. The movement of chloride between red blood cells and the plasma (termed the chloride shift) is instrumental in maintaining acid-base balance in the blood while it is transporting carbon dioxide to the lungs. As one of three significant acid-forming minerals in the body, chloride is important in maintaining acid-base balance in fluids throughout the body. Diarrhea and vomiting can contribute substantially to body losses of this mineral and be instrumental in electrolyte imbalances under these circumstances.

There appears to be virtually no possibility of an inadequate chloride intake when people are healthy. Table salt is the principal source of chloride in the diet. It is estimated that persons consuming a minimal amount of salt will ingest somewhat more than the necessary amount of chloride; many individuals may be using as much as three times the amount needed to meet chloride requirements of the body. In addition to table salt, meat, milk, and eggs are sources of chloride. Chloride is excreted normally through perspiration, urine, and feces.

Chromium

Only within the last 10 years has chromium been identified as an essential nutrient, and its precise role(s) and recommended intake remain to be defined. Apparently chromium interacts with insulin to improve glucose uptake. Other roles in amino acid and lipid metabolism are being suggested. Possible deficiencies of chromium have been suggested to be linked to old age, pregnancy, and protein-calorie malnutrition. The amount of chromium in the body declines throughout life. Good sources of available chromium include meats, milk, poultry, and whole-grain cereal products.

Cobalt

Cobalt is of significance in the human body because it is a structural component of vitamin B_{12} (see Chapter 11). One atom of cobalt is included in each molecule of this important vitamin. However, vitamin B_{12}, and not atomic cobalt, is a dietary requirement. Humans do use cobalt to synthesize vitamin B_{12} in the lower intestinal tract but the site of synthesis is beyond the site of absorption in the intestine, and thus B_{12} is excreted. In rare instances, an excess of cobalt has caused problems when livestock have been fed plants grown in soil overly endowed with cobalt. Organ meats are the richest sources of dietary cobalt, muscle meats contain somewhat less cobalt, and plants generally are classified as poor sources of this mineral.

Copper

The level of copper in the normal adult ranges between 75 and 150 milligrams in the entire body. Such a small quantity might appear to indicate insignificance but copper performs some important (although presently somewhat ill-defined) roles in preventing anemia. Although copper is not a component of hemoglobin, it is necessary as a catalyst for the formation of hemoglobin. Other possible roles of copper in the prevention of anemia have been suggested. These include such suggestions as aiding in iron absorption and promoting maturation of red blood cells.

This mineral performs other functions in the body. Copper is contained in catalase and in cytochrome oxidase, thus performing an important metabolic role in the release of energy. In combination with vitamin C, copper assists in the formation of elastin, a connective tissue of importance in the heart. It also serves a role in the formation of collagen, an abundant connective tissue in the body. Copper figures in another aspect of protein metabolism. Melanin, a dark pigment in hair and skin, is formed from tyrosine by a chemical reaction. Tyrosinase, a copper-containing enzyme, is required to transform the amino acid (tyrosine) into melanin. Yet another facet of copper's role is in the formation of phospholipids. The phospholipids are essential to the myelin sheath, which serves as an insulating protection for nerve fibers.

Generally, about one-third of the copper consumed is absorbed. This absorbed copper is found in the bloodstream, either loosely bound with albumin or tightly bound with globulin. Some serum copper goes into the bone marrow for incorporation in red blood cells. Much of the copper that is absorbed ultimately is excreted in the feces. Copper can be eliminated by this avenue as a result of incorporation in biliary secretion and leaching through the intestinal membrane.

Copper is an essential mineral nutrient although a definite dietary allowance has not been established. The 2 to 5 milligrams that are available in the normal diet appear to be adequate. Cereals, nuts, legumes, liver, shellfish, and grapes are good sources of copper. Other protein foods are useful sources, and milk and vegetables other than legumes contain only small amounts of copper.

Fluoride

Fluoride is considered to be an essential mineral nutrient because it is always found in the bones and teeth and is required for maximum resistance to dental caries. The actual amount of fluoride present in the body varies widely from one individual to another, depending upon the fluoride intake in the diet over an extended period of time. Even when the fluoride intake is relatively high, the quantity of fluoride in the body will be small, with about 99 percent of this trace mineral being found in the bones and teeth.

Most minerals evoke virtually no emotional response when they are being discussed but this certainly is not true for fluoride. In numerous city council meetings and state legislatures across the country, the merits of fluoride have been the subject of very heated and emotional debates. Invariably, the debate is prompted by a proposal to fluoridate the city water supply. Some citizens sincerely feel that adding fluoride to the water supply violates a person's right to consume foods in their natural state. Others are concerned about the cost involved in adding fluoride to the water. Still other people are concerned for the health of the community because they either think fluoride in any amount is toxic, or they doubt that the level of fluoride can be maintained within the limits generally regarded as safe. Such arguments appear superficial and rather curious when one considers that chloride, an element closely related to fluoride, has been added in carefully regulated amounts without public furor for many years. The fact that dentists, physicians, and nutritionists have been advocating fluoride as an important safeguard against dental caries has little impact upon emotionally involved people who wish to block

fluoridation of the city's water. However, at this writing, ten states and the nation of Ireland require fluoridation of communal water supplies.

A review of some of the studies showing the efficacy of fluoride in reducing the incidence of dental caries will serve to provide some of the information needed to refute the claims for fluoride toxicity that may be proclaimed by opponents of fluoridation. The original observations regarding the effects of fluoride may explain, in part, the concern some people have regarding the use of fluoride in drinking water. Early in this century, a dentist in Colorado Springs investigated the brown stain he noted on the teeth of some of his patients. Despite the brown stain, the healthiness of the teeth and the freedom from decay were readily apparent to him. Although fluoride was identified as the

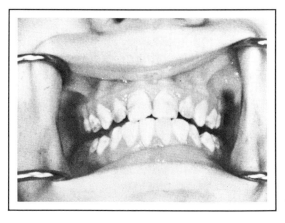

Mottling of the teeth is the result of excessively high intake of fluoride, in this case prolonged ingestion of water containing 5.5 ppm. This level of fluorides is more than five times greater than the amount recommended for optimum dental health.

culprit causing the staining, the protective role this mineral played in caries reduction quickly generated considerable interest. Further study showed that the mottled appearance of the teeth could be avoided while still getting the desired protection against caries by simply reducing the fluoride level in the water to a value below 2.5 parts per million. (This means that 2.5 milligrams of fluoride are contained in each liter of water.)

A classic study was conducted in Newburgh and Kingston, New York to determine if it was valuable to provide a water supply containing fluoride at the level of 1 part per million. The water supply of Newburgh, New York was fluoridated at the level of 1 part per million and Kingston served as the nonfluoridated control. Children who had received the fluoridated water from birth during the 10-year study had a great reduction in caries when compared with their counterparts in Kingston. The level of decayed, missing, and filled teeth had been reduced by about 65 percent. Less protection was afforded when fluoride was added in childhood than when it was present from birth but the decrease in dental caries was still highly significant. Many other studies have been conducted in widely scattered parts of the United States, and these bear out the original conclusion that fluoride at a controlled level of 1 part per million in drinking water from infancy will reduce dental caries by 60 to 70 percent. For maximum effectiveness in protecting against decay, fluoride must be available while teeth are forming. Currently somewhat more than 100 million people in about 5000 urban areas receive the appropriate amount of fluoride through their water supplies.

Modern technology clearly provides the capability for controlling the addition of fluoride within the range of safety. Furthermore, fluoridation costs only a few cents a year per person; far, far less than is spent by the average family to care for the results of dental caries. The technology also is available for the few areas having excessive fluorides in the water. For these cities, some fluoride can be removed from the water so that discoloration of the teeth will not occur. In such instances, the level is adjusted to the desired 0.8 to 1.2 part per million.

At any age, dissolved fluoride is absorbed efficiently from the intestinal tract. Consequently, most of the ingested fluoride that is excreted is found in the urine and not in the feces. Fluoride is incorporated into developing teeth in partial replacement for the hydroxyl ion in hydroxyapatite. If all hydroxyl ions (OH^-) were replaced by fluoride (F^-), the reaction would be

$$Ca_{10}(PO_4)_6(CH)_2 + 2F^- \rightarrow Ca_{10}(PO_4)_6F_2 + 2OH^-$$

Fluoride is deposited in bones as well as in the enamel of the teeth. Here again, the fluoride replaces some of the hydroxyl ion in bone mineral. The resulting fluoride-containing bone crystals are somewhat larger and more perfectly formed and thus are less readily resorbed than those crystals containing less fluoride.

The average fluoride concentration in enamel formed in any area of the United States where the water supply has a low fluoride content is about 80 ppm. Where water adjusted to the optimal for dental benefit was consumed throughout tooth development, enamel contains on the average about 130 ppm. A very thin outer layer of enamel contains 8 to 10 times as much fluoride. The latter design in nature provides a remarkable defense because the carious lesion begins at the interface between the microorganisms on the tooth surface and the external "skin" of the enamel. In any case, the actual amount of OH^- replaced by F^- is still tiny compared to the 38,000 ppm F^- which would be present if all OH^- were replaced by F^-.

One of the most common problems of aging is the development of osteoporosis. This condition is frequently a painful one in which the mass of bone diminishes, because of gradual resorption of bone crystals. One other problem of osteoporosis is the greater likelihood of fractures and collapsed vertebrae. When fluoride is ingested throughout life, there is less likelihood for an older person to develop osteoporosis than is the case when the fluoride intake is lower than the recommended levels in the water supply. Bernstein (1966) reported that, in two similar areas of North Dakota, the area with high fluoride level in the water had far fewer cases of osteoporosis than did the area in which the fluoride level in the drinking water was low. Because of its efficacy in maintaining the structural integrity of bone, high levels of fluoride (as well as calcium and vitamin D) commonly are used in the treatment of osteoporosis. Since the deposition of fluoride in the teeth is essentially nil after the teeth are formed, there is no discoloration of the teeth when therapeutic doses of fluoride are administered to adults.

The best source of fluoride is drinking water that is maintained at a level of 0.8 to 1.2 part per million fluoride. This provides an effective means for all citizens to obtain the fluoride they need. Since not all communities have fluoridated water, other sources of fluoride need to be sought until local health departments or citizens effectively demand the fluoridation of the water supply. Less desirable, but sometimes necessary, alternatives are sodium fluoride tablets, fluoride toothpastes, bottled fluoridated water, and topical application of stannous fluoride by dentists. There are drawbacks to each of these alternatives. The tablets require conscientious parents and cooperative children because it is very easy to use up a bottle of them and forget to replace them or to neglect taking them even when they are available. While fluoride toothpastes are of some value, the constant ingestion of fluoride via the water supply is far more effective. Bottled water is expensive and unfortunately is available only when children are at home. For preschool children this may not be too much of a problem, providing they can be persuaded to always drink the bottled water and not just drink the water that is available from the tap. With the increasing numbers of children in day care centers, this approach has obvious limitations. The topical applications of fluoride are far more

expensive than the 30 to 40 cents a year per person that it costs to fluoridate the city water. In addition, when fluoridated water is available, topical fluoride applications are not needed, and the dentist is freed to do other essential dental work.

Although there is no allowance recommended by the Food and Nutrition Board, a daily intake of 1 to 2 milligrams of fluoride appears to be adequate to reduce tooth decay. Under normal conditions, this amount of fluoride is consumed when water is fluoridated. None of the foods consumed in quantity contributes significant amounts of fluoride. Tea and sardines (because of the bones) are fair sources of fluoride. Of course, dehydrated foods that are reconstituted with fluoridated water become sources of this important mineral.

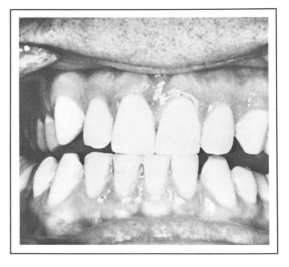

The teeth of a 44-year-old man reflect the value of consuming fluoridated water containing 1 ppm during the early years. He has no decayed, missing, or filled teeth.

In the well-nourished individual, iodine (as a salt iodide) is omnipresent in the body. Despite the fact that the iodine in the body represents only 0.00004 percent of the total weight, this mineral plays a unique and highly significant role in the body's operation. About 8 milligrams of iodine are concentrated in the thyroid gland in the neck, with the remaining iodide being scattered throughout all the cells.

Functions

The recognized role of iodide in the body is in the production of thyroxine, a hormone secreted by the thyroid gland. Since iodine is a structural component of thyroxine, this essential hormone cannot be produced if the iodine atoms are not available in the thyroid gland.

The thyroid gland, located near the base of the neck, is a two-lobed structure connected by a thin tissue called the thyroid isthmus. The thyroid manufactures two iodine-containing compounds: thyroxine (four atoms of iodine attached to the amino acid tyrosine) and tri-iodo-thyronine. These compounds are stored in the thyroid as thyroglobulin, a protein molecule. Thyroxine and the more active tri-iodo-thyronine are slowly released into the bloodstream, either as the free hormone or combined with albumin in the blood. The most obvious function of thyroxine and tri-iodo-thyronine is the regulation of the rate at which oxidation reactions take place in the body. The regulation of energy metabolism has been identified as an essential role of thyroxine for a relatively long period of time; but recent research suggests that protein synthesis, cholesterol production in the body, conversion of carotene to vitamin A, and carbohydrate absorption also are influenced by the availability of thyroxine. Excessive levels of thyroxine cause the oxidative processes (producing en-

ergy) to be accelerated. This results in excessive loss of nitrogen from the body because of the need to use proteins for energy. Excess thyroxine also is accompanied by reduced synthesis of cholesterol in the body.

Hyperthyroidism

Excessive secretion of thyroxine results in a condition known as hyperthyroidism. This is marked by a high basal metabolic rate, weight loss, accelerated heart action, and an emotional state of tension and nervousness. When accompanied by thyroidal enlargement to protrusion forward of the eyeballs, this condition is designated as exophthalmic goiter. Mild cases may be treated by antithyroid medication or radioactive iodine, while surgical removal of at least a large portion of the thyroid gland may be required sometimes.

Deficiency conditions

Simple goiter is a deformation of the thyroid gland caused by an inadequate supply of iodine in the thyroid gland. When the available iodide in the thyroid gland is insufficient to produce all the thyroxine and thyronine needed for maintaining normal metabolic rate, the thyroid-stimulating hormone (TSH) will be released to the thyroid gland from the pituitary gland in larger quantities. Increased secretion of TSH occurs when the dietary intake of iodide falls below 20 micrograms daily. TSH directs the thyroid gland toward ever greater efforts to produce the thyroxine that is needed, thus producing an enlarged thyroid or goiter.

Endemic goiter can be prevented by insuring that an adequate supply of iodide is available in the local diet. Iodide or thyroxine therapy is effective in many cases of endemic goiter. Some geographic areas are notably deficient in iodide levels in the soil, resulting in low iodide content in the locally produced foodstuffs. The likelihood of endemic goiter is significantly increased in such instances. Because of the low iodide levels in the soil of the Midwest and Great Lakes areas of the United States, this area often is referred to as the "Goiter Belt."

Other geographic regions where soil depletion presents a problem include interior regions of most of the continents. Since the sea is relatively rich in iodide, populations consuming significant quantities of ocean fish or foods grown near the sea where the soil has more iodide are far less likely to have an iodide deficiency than are people living in the interior.

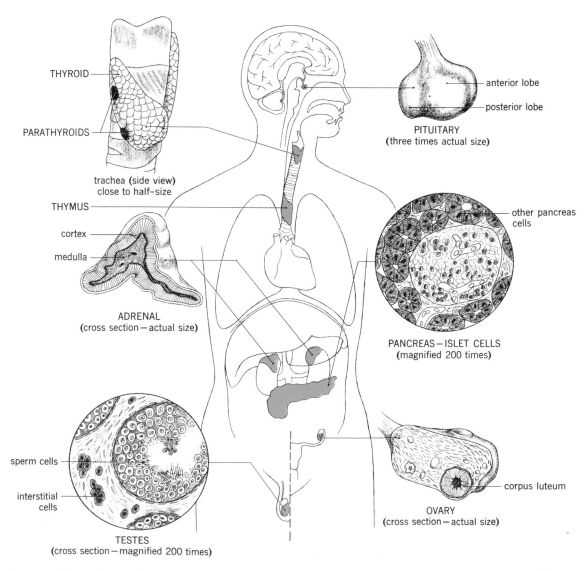

Diagram of the endocrine glands. The thyroid gland produces thyroxine, an iodine-containing hormone; the pancreas utilizes zinc in producing insulin. The parathyroids, via parathormone and calcitonin, regulate calcium levels in the blood.

The iodide needs of the fetus and of the mother during pregnancy appear to be critical. If the mother's diet is seriously inadequate in this mineral, the result may be the birth of a cretin. This may not be detectable immediately at birth but will become manifest later as the infant exhibits the characteristics of cretins: retarded growth, low mentality, thick skin, a recessed nose, thick lips, and an enlarged tongue. Early treatment after birth can correct many of the problems of cretinism.

There is a higher incidence of deaf mutes and mentally retarded children born from mothers with enlarged thyroid glands than from those with a thyroid gland of normal size. Such evidence provides compelling motivation for attempting to insure an adequate intake of iodide throughout pregnancy. Clearly, goiter in women is not to be considered a mark of aristocracy, as it was viewed in the Middle Ages in Europe. It is a condition which can and should be prevented.

Prolonged hypothyroidism (a result of inadequate iodide intake) during the growing years results in adults with the conditon known as myxedema. Symptoms include lethargy, weight gain, very dry skin, poor adaptability to cold, changes in the texture of the hair, and an unusually husky voice.

Iodide is absorbed very readily along the entire gastrointestinal tract, with the greatest amount being absorbed in the small intestine. If radioactive iodine (I^{131}) is administered, the very rapid uptake of this element into the blood can be observed. The absorbed mineral is transported to the thyroid gland, if needed, or is excreted via the kidney.

The adequacy of iodide in the diet can be assessed by testing the level of circulating thyroxine in the blood. Normal values for thyroxine range from 4 to 11 micrograms per 100 milliliters of blood. A value above 11 micrograms indicates hyperthyroidism and a value of less than 4 indicates hypothyroidism. Another useful measurement is the determination of the rate at which the thyroid gland takes up radioactive iodine. Persons with hyper-

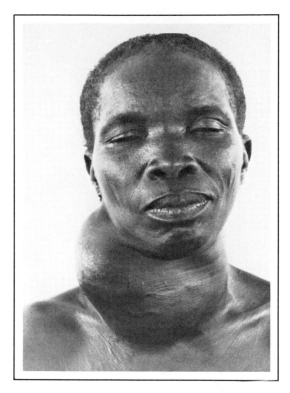

A severe case of goiter, or enlargement of the thyroid gland, resulting from an inadequate intake of iodine.

thyroidism take up iodide rapidly while the normal individual takes up iodide more gradually. As would be expected, the uptake of iodide is slow in hypothyroidism.

Some external factors influence the utilization of iodide and deserve some mention. A few foods are goitrogenic, that is, they may predispose persons on a marginal diet toward development of goiter. Members of the cabbage family are notable in this regard. They contain a substance called pregoitren, which interferes somewhat with iodide utilization when it is converted to goitren. Sulphonamides, antithyroid drugs, and a few other chemical substances also appear to have a deleterious influence on iodide utilization. When a diet contains adequate iodide, these impedances to iodide utilization are not of sufficient magnitude to cause a deficiency.

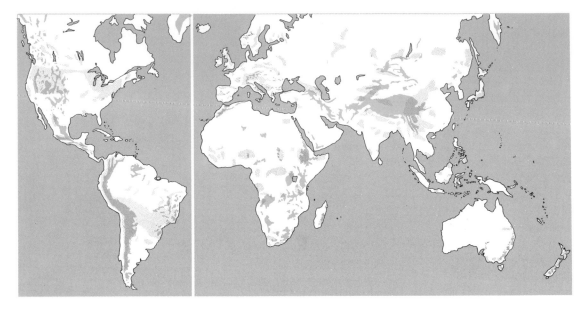

Regions of endemic goiter and the mountainous terrain with which it is often associated were mapped by the World Health Organization. Areas where iodine-deficiency goiter is endemic are indicated by the black hatching. Populations near seacoasts are seldom affected because of the iodine content of seafood. Not all inland areas are equally affected; the geology and remoteness of mountainous regions (black) make them most susceptible. (From "Endemic Goiter" by R. Bruce Gillie, June 1971. Copyright © 1971 by Scientific American, Inc. All rights reserved.)

The most effective way of insuring adequate iodine in a population's diet is by adding potassium iodide to salt. When potassium iodide is added to salt at the level of 0.01 percent, the iodide intake is sufficient to prevent endemic goiter. In the United States, the consumer is offered the alternative of buying plain or iodized salt. Either through carelessness or inadequate information regarding the advisability of using iodized salt, many consumers who really need the iodide available in the salt have neglected to purchase the iodized product. However, legislation designed to become effective in mid-1973 requires noniodized salt to state on its label, "This salt does not supply iodide, a necessary nutrient." This measure should aid in educating consumers to include iodized salt as a regular part of the diet. When iodization was initiated in the United States nearly half a century ago, the incidence of goiter dropped

sharply, but the problem has been increasing again as consumers have grown more careless in the selection of salt. As can be seen in Table 10.3, recommended dietary intake is greatest in adolescence and during pregnancy and lactation.

Yet another impediment to adequate iodide intake is developing as a result of increasing use of prepared foods, which customarily are manufactured with noniodized salt as an ingredient. The intake of iodide among consumers relying heavily on ready-to-eat commercial food products is being reduced by this modification in food consumption practices. By simply requiring that iodized salt be used in the preparation of such commercial products, the iodide level in the diet could be raised without necessitating a change in dietary patterns.

Saltwater fish and shellfish from the sea are sources of iodide. Anadromous fish such as salmon are somewhat lower in their iodide content although they still contain useful amounts. Freshwater fish contain little iodide. If the diet of lactating women and dairy animals is high in iodide, the level of iodide in the milk will be excellent.

Iron

Paradoxically, one of the nutrients receiving the greatest consideration in food enrichment programs actually constitutes only about 4 grams in the entire body of a well-nourished adult. This nutrient, which is so important to physical well being despite its miniscule quantity in the body, is iron. The American public is well aware of the importance of iron. Hucksters have attended to the education of the populace, and yet, despite the skills and ballyhoo from Madison Avenue's elite, iron deficiency still is very much a part of the contemporary scene! A close examination of the unique nature of this mineral will provide some insight into this situation.

Functions of iron

The ability of iron to aid in the transport of oxygen and to participate in oxidation and reduction reactions because of shifts between the ferrous and ferric states chemically explains much of the significance of this mineral in the body. One of the key functions of iron is in the formation of hemoglobin, the oxygen-transporting protein in the blood. One atom of iron is a structural part of each hemoglobin molecule. Hemoglobin is formed in bone marrow when the erythroblasts are maturing into red blood cells. This synthesis takes place when glycine (an amino acid) and iron, with pyridoxine acting as a catalyst, are combined to form heme. In turn, heme is joined with globin to form the rather large hemoglobin molecule. Hemoglobin becomes available for oxygen transport in the body when it enters the bloodstream as a compound contained in mature red blood cells (erythrocytes). The hemoglobin transports oxygen from the lungs to the tissues where oxygen is required for oxidation reactions. In turn, carbon dioxide formed in the cells also is transported via hemoglobin in the erythrocytes for exhalation via the lungs.

Another iron-containing protein pigment in the body is myoglobin. Myoglobin may be considered to be the heart's and muscles' version of hemoglobin since the basic structure of the iron-containing portion of the molecule is the same. Hemoglobin contains four heme groups and myoglobin contains only one. Myoglobin is the recipient of the oxygen carried by hemoglobin to the cells.

Iron is a component of enzymes that catalyze the oxidation-reduction reactions involved in the metabolism of glucose and fatty acids. The cytochromes, cytochrome oxidase, peroxidase, and catalase are effective because of the ability for iron to change reversibly between the ferrous and ferric states, thus enabling oxidation or reduction reactions to take place in the mitochondria. Energy release is dependent upon the presence of these iron-containing enzymes. Iron is also needed for myeloperoxidase, an enzyme essential for intracellular killing of bacteria (Arbeter et al., 1971).

Iron in the body

The absorption of iron by the body is definitely inefficient. When an individual is in normal health and well nourished, the absorption rate may be less than 5 percent, usually averaging between 5 and 10 percent. Only in iron depletion does the absorption rate rise and then only to 20 to 30 percent. The primary site for absorption is the upper part of the small intestine, with a very limited amount being absorbed in the stomach. Iron seems to be absorbed through the membrane by being held loosely to an organic substance such as carbohydrate, alcohol, or certain amino acids.

This bound iron enters the epithelial cells and is transferred from the carrier to apoferritin (see Figure 10.3). The complex of apoferritin and iron—called ferritin—is held in the epithelial cells until binding sites for iron are available on molecules of transferrin in the blood. Then the iron atoms are released from the ferritin, recombined with an organic carrier, and transported into the blood where the iron is released to combine with transferrin in the plasma. One molecule of transferrin can complex two iron atoms. Between 2 and 4 milligrams of iron may be transported as a transferrin-iron complex at any one time, but as much as 40 milligrams may be moved around the body in the course of a day. This iron may be carried to: (1) cells to make myoglobin or respiratory enzymes; (2) storage areas in the liver and spleen; and (3) to bone marrow where it will be used as needed in hemoglobin production. The uptake and transport of iron in the body occurs rather rapidly. Absorption takes place within 4 hours, and evidence of incorporation of iron in hemoglobin within erythroblasts in a day has been noted.

Iron is stored in two forms in the liver. Hemosiderin contains as much as one-third iron by weight; the remainder of the insoluble hemosiderin molecule is a protein. Ferritin, the soluble iron-protein complex, is the other form for iron storage. It contains less iron per molecule than hemosiderin but releases it more readily when iron is needed.

Factors influencing iron absorption

Several factors influence the actual amount of iron that an individual absorbs. Persons deficient in iron will absorb this mineral more efficiently than do persons with adequate stores of

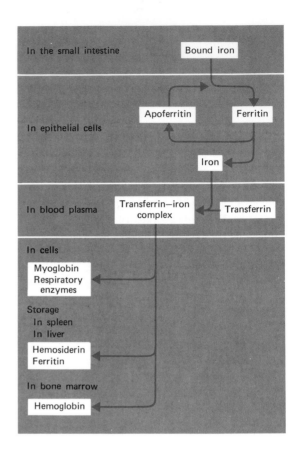

Figure 10.3   Iron distribution and forms in the body.

iron in the body. Children are considerably more efficient in absorbing iron than adults, presumably because of their somewhat higher metabolic rate and their increasing volume of blood as they grow. Pregnant women in the late stages of pregnancy have a high demand for iron as a result of transfer of iron from mother to fetus. Lactating women also may be expected to absorb iron more efficiently than they did prior to pregnancy in order to replace the small amount of iron being secreted in the milk. A similar situation—but one of more importance—exists in patients recuperating from blood losses. Also, persons living at high altitudes absorb iron more efficiently to meet their needs for the larger quantity of hemoglobin that is found in the erythrocytes of mountain dwellers.

The source and form of iron both influence the absorption rate. Divalent iron (ferrous-Fe^{++}) is absorbed more readily than its oxidized trivalent counterpart (ferric-Fe^{+++}). As a general rule, the iron from animal foods is absorbed more readily than that from plants. The presence of phytates impedes iron absorption, thus accounting, at least partially, for the rather poor absorption of the iron present in wheat. The cellulose in vegetables and fruits diminishes iron absorption. Starch in the diet tends to inhibit iron absorption, while sugar accelerates absorption. Iron salts, administered as dietary supplements, are quite available for absorption since they ordinarily are in the reduced ferrous form and are unencumbered by roughage.

Acids favor iron absorption, presumably since they are capable of reducing ferric iron to the ferrous form. Thus, the hydrochloric acid of the stomach is useful in promoting iron absorption in the portion of the small intestine adjacent to the stomach. Ascorbic acid also promotes absorption of iron. On the other hand, pancreatic secretions do not favor iron utilization and neither do antacid preparations that reduce stomach acidity. The organic acids in foods such as citrus fruits also are helpful in the reduction of iron.

Conservation

Parsimonious is the key word to describe iron usage in the body. Iron that is incorporated into an erythrocyte as hemoglobin remains in the cell until the red blood cell dies, a span of approximately four months. The dead erythrocytes leave the circulating blood when they reach the liver, spleen, or bone marrow. The now useless erythrocytes are broken down to release the iron and amino acids. The iron is transported to the bone marrow, where it is available for incorporation into another hemoglobin molecule, and the cycle begins again. Thus, it is possible for iron to be reused many times before it may be excreted.

Excretion

The only losses of absorbed iron of quantitative significance occur as a result of blood loss. Of course, erythrocytes are a component of any blood that is lost as a result of hemorrhaging, wounds, or menstruation. Small losses of iron, estimated to average less than 1 milligram per day, occur as a consequence of sweating, sloughing of cells, trimming of hair and nails, and minor excretion of red blood cells in the urine. Fecal losses are unabsorbed iron and the iron contained in cells that slough off along the gastrointestinal tract.

Recommended dietary allowances

The recommended allowances for iron clearly reflect the increased need for this mineral either as a result of growth needs or elevated excretion levels. Although there is apparently little, if any, absorption of iron by the newborn, it is recommended that the infant up to the age of 6 months ingest 10 milligrams daily. This recommendation is increased to 15 milligrams during the next 6 months and it remains at that level until age 4. In proportion to body size, the recommended intake is high to supply needs for this very rapid growth period of infancy and early childhood. When the growth rate slows and iron reserves have had an opportunity to accumulate by about age four, the recommended intake is reduced by one third. The growth spurt of the teens prompts a sharp increase in iron intake. The recommendation for boys takes cognizance of the large body size as well as the growth spurt. The level for girls is based on the adolescent growth period and on the onset of menstruation. The level remains high for women throughout the entire reproductive period to replace the iron that is lost through menstruation. During pregnancy the level still is high to insure maximum transfer of iron to the fetus.

Table 10.5 *Iron Content of Selected Foods*[a]

	Amount	Iron (mg)
Meat group		
Beef, sirloin steak, lean	3 1/2 oz	3.9
Veal loin chop	3 1/2 oz	3.2
Pork loin chop, lean	3 1/2 oz	3.9
Lamb loin chop, lean	3 1/2 oz	2.0
Calf liver, fried	3 1/2 oz	14.2
Bologna	1 slice	0.5
Poultry and eggs		
Chicken, white meat	3 1/2 oz	1.7
Egg	1 medium	1.1
Legumes and nuts		
Kidney beans, cooked	1/2 cup	2.3
Mixed nuts, oil roasted	1 oz	1.0
Peanut butter	2 tbsp	0.6
Fish and shellfish		
Swordfish, broiled	3 1/2 oz	1.3
Tuna, oil packed	3 1/2 oz	1.9
Clams	3 1/2 oz	6.1
Oysters	1/2 cup	6.6
Shrimp	3 1/2 oz	3.1

An intake of 18 milligrams during lactation is recommended to compensate for iron losses in the milk.

Food sources

Careful planning is required to insure an adequate intake of iron. This is true throughout life but may be a particular problem in infancy. Milk is notably low in iron, a fact which is not fully appreciated by many new mothers. Unless an infant is receiving supplementary foods or regular doses of iron by the age of 3 months, a deficiency of iron may start to develop because the iron store from birth will be depleted. If the infant was born with little reserve iron as a result of the mother's poor diet, dietary iron will be needed even sooner than 3 months. The very small amount of iron he received from cow's milk (approximately 0.1 milligrams per cup) is totally inadequate to meet the body's need for iron.

Meats generally are good sources of iron. Variety meats, such as heart and liver, are outstanding in their iron content. Clams, oysters, lima beans, spinach, dates, dried fruits, and nuts are rich in iron. When enriched or whole-grain cereal products are eaten in quantity, they make a substantial contribution toward meeting the iron requirement. The iron content of selected foods is given in Table 10.5. On the average, only about 10 percent of the iron in food is available (absorbed), and in some foods (egg yolks, for example) the amount may be even less. This is an important area of research under current investigation.

Table 10.5   (*continued*)

Bread and cereal group		
White bread, enriched	1 slice	0.6
Whole wheat bread	1 slice	0.5
Rye bread	1 slice	0.4
Bran flakes	1 oz	1.2
Shredded wheat	1 biscuit	1.0
Oatmeal	1 cup	1.4
Corn grits	1 cup	0.7
Rice, enriched, cooked	1 cup	1.8
Macaroni, cooked	1 cup	1.3
Vegetable and fruit group *Fruits*		
Prune juice	1/2 cup	5.1
Prunes, cooked	4 medium	1.1
Raisins	1 oz	0.6
Fig, dried	1 medium	0.6
Grapefruit	1/2 medium	0.5
Vegetables		
Spinach, cooked	1/2 cup	2.2
Beet greens, cooked	1/2 cup	1.4
Peas, cooked	1/2 cup	1.6
Lima beans, green, cooked	1/2 cup	2.1
Potato, baked	1 medium	0.7

[a] Data compiled and adapted from *Composition of Foods—Raw, Processed, Prepared,* Agriculture Handbook No. 8, U.S.D.A. 1963; *Nutritive Value of Foods,* Home and Garden Bulletin No. 72, U.S.D.A., 1971; and manufacturers' information.

The widespread incidence of iron deficiency has prompted considerable discussion about the possibility of fortifying or enriching several food products. At the present time higher levels of enrichment are still being suggested, but the problems of palatability as well as possible overdoses are not resolved and enforcement of modifying legislation appears unlikely.

Iron-deficiency anemia

The normal adult hemoglobin value for males is 14 to 15 grams of hemoglobin per 100 milliliters of blood and for females is 13 to 14 grams per 100 milliliters. However, when iron levels are too low in the body, the hemoglobin level in the blood falls below these values, and the individual develops iron-deficiency anemia. This condition can be caused either by an inadequate intake of iron (nutritional anemia) or by excessive blood loss (hemorrhagic anemia). Persons most likely to have nutritional anemia due to iron deficiency are: young infants subsisting almost solely on milk, teenage girls (particularly teenage mothers), and women who have undergone closely successive pregnancies. However, others in the population also may develop this all-too-common deficiency condition. In many parts of the world where hookworm and other parasitic infections cause blood loss, iron-deficiency anemia is common.

A lack of iron in the diet over a period of time is evidenced by erythrocytes of smaller (microcytic) than normal size and by reduced hemoglobin levels (hypochromic). The small cell size is attributable to the fact that cells do not grow to normal size without hemoglobin; and hemoglobin cannot be synthesized if sufficient iron is not available. Persons with anemia of this type are often tired and listless. Fatigue is caused by the limited ability to transport oxygen to the tissues and to remove carbon dioxide when hemoglobin values are reduced. Persons with iron-deficiency anemia have decreased pigmentation in the interior of the mouth and on the inside of the eyelids because the blood is less pigmented when the hemoglobin level decreases. Additional symptoms include soreness in the mouth, increased susceptibility to infections, and gastric distress.

Anemia can be prevented in most instances by careful attention to diet and by limiting blood donations to no greater frequency than once every 2 or 3 months. When anemia has been diagnosed, it often is advisable to administer ferrous sulfate or other iron salts in the ferrous form. An elevated intake of ascorbic acid enhances the utilization of the iron.

Nutritional anemia often is caused by an iron deficiency but a copper deficiency also can cause too little hemoglobin to be formed. A lack of ascorbic acid interferes with both iron absorption and the release of iron from the transferrin to which it is complexed while in transit to tissues. A deficiency of pyridoxine, the B vitamin which serves as a catalytic agent in heme synthesis, also impedes the formation of hemoglobin. In addition, red blood cells are destroyed at a faster rate when vitamin E, vitamin B_{12}, or ascorbic acid levels are inadequate.

Excess

Although dietary excesses of iron are virtually nonexistent in adults in the United States, they have been observed in areas where iron cooking pots are used exclusively or in individuals ingesting excessive iron supplements, as exemplified in the Bantu tribe in Africa. This condition, known as hemosiderosis, can be fatal to infants given large therapeutic iron supplements. Some adults are so zealous in their efforts to avoid the advertised hazards of an iron deficiency that they may overdose themselves gradually with iron-containing supplements and tonics. As long as one has a normal hemoglobin value, and eats a sensible, mixed diet (including breads and cereals that are either whole grain or fortified with iron), there appears to be little value in taking iron supplements.

Magnesium

Magnesium is a mineral occurring in rather small quantities in soft tissues and the skeleton. About 17 of the 25 grams of magnesium in an adult are contained in the bones, which appear to be the storage reservoirs for this mineral. Although man has known for more than 100 years that magnesium was a constituent of the human body, actual information regarding its functions in the body has only been gleaned by research during the last two decades.

The magnesium in the cells of soft tissue catalyzes virtually hundreds of metabolic reactions resulting in changes in energy states. The oxidative phosphorylation of adenosine diphosphate (ADP) to the high energy adenosine triphosphate (ATP) is effected in the presence of magnesium. Conversely, the release of energy that results when ATP is converted to ADP requires the presence of magnesium. Some of these reactions involving ATP and ADP appear to require magnesium specifically, while others require only the presence of a divalent cation. Normally, there is about seven times more magnesium in the cells than in the serum. Reserves of magnesium in bone become available for use if the level of magnesium in the blood and tissues decreases.

The catalytic role of magnesium in respiratory reactions would seem to be sufficient justification for the presence of this mineral in the body, and yet it also functions in other important ways. Magnesium in the extracellular fluid bathing nerve cells helps to conduct nerve impulses that relax muscles following contraction. Adequate magnesium appears to be valuable in promoting the retention of calcium in tooth enamel, thus increasing resistance to dental caries and loss of teeth. Magnesium, presumably through its role in releasing thyroxine, helps people adjust to a cold environment. Magnesium may also be a factor in promoting protein synthesis. The fact that people on high magnesium appear to have less predisposition to cardiovascular diseases is the cause of some speculation regarding other roles of magnesium.

Deficiency

Although examples of magnesium deficiency in man are rare, they have been observed in cases of chronic alcoholism, kwashiorkor, some neuromuscular disorders, and in surgical patients maintained on parenterally administered fluids for long periods of time. Moderate deficiencies of magnesium may lead to calcification of soft tissues and atheromatous lesions when dietary cholesterol is high. More severe magnesium deficiency causes tetany similar to that noted when calcium levels fall. Muscle tremors may build up to convulsions, as observed in severe alcoholism. Alcohol or excessive use of diuretics may foster poor absorption and excessive excretion of magnesium, culminating in a magnesium deficiency.

Recommended dietary allowances

When the Food and Nutrition Board expanded its recommendations in 1968 to include several previously unlisted nutrients, magnesium was one of three minerals added, the others being phosphorus and iodine. For this initial statement of recommended dietary magnesium levels, infant recommendations were based on the amount of magnesium contained in the milk consumed. Since cow's milk contains about 12 milligrams per 100 milliliters, it appeared reasonable that the normal infant received sufficient magnesium when he consumed between 3 and 4 cups of milk daily. Hence, the recommendation for 40 milligrams was set for the newborn, a value that was changed to 60 in 1974. Adult levels were set at 350 milligrams daily for males and 300 for women. The recommendation for pregnant and lactating women was set at 450 milligrams, although there is little evidence on which to base the recommendations for these periods in a woman's life.

Food sources

Meats and vegetables are quite variable in their magnesium content, as can be seen in Table 10.6. Fats and fruits tend to be poor sources of this mineral. Milk provides useful amounts, and whole-grain breads and cereals and potatoes may be of significance when eaten in the large quantities consumed by some people. All green vegetables contain some magnesium; this mineral is a structural component of the chlorophyll pigment, occupying the same position that iron fills in heme.

Table 10.6 *Magnesium Content of Selected Foods*[a]

	Amount	Magnesium (mg)
Meat, fish, shellfish		
Beef round, lean	3 1/2 oz	29
Lamb chop	3 1/2 oz	22
Pork loin chop	3 1/2 oz	32
Turkey	3 1/2 oz	28
Veal cutlet	3 1/2 oz	18
Flounder	3 1/2 oz	30
Haddock	3 1/2 oz	24
Salmon	3 1/2 oz	30
Crab meat	3 1/2 oz	34
Lobster	3 1/2 oz	22
Oysters	3 1/2 oz	32
Shrimp	3 1/2 oz	30
Nuts		
Almonds	1 oz	77
Brazil nuts	1 oz	64
Cashews	1 oz	76
Filberts	1 oz	52
Hickory nuts	1 oz	45
Peanuts	1 oz	50
Pecans	1 oz	40
Pistachio nuts	1 oz	42
Walnuts, black	1 oz	54
Walnuts, English	1 oz	37
Dairy products		
Milk, whole	1 cup	31
Cheese, cheddar	1 oz	13
Cereals and breads		
Bread, whole wheat	1 slice	18
Puffed oats	1 cup	28
Shredded wheat	1 biscuit	34
Fruits and vegetables		
Banana	1 medium	33
Orange	1 medium	16
Spinach, canned	1/2 cup	57
Baked beans	1/2 cup	42
Potato, whole, raw	1 medium	34

[a] Data compiled and adapted from *Composition of Foods—Raw, Processed, Prepared,* Agriculture Handbook No. 8, U.S.D.A., 1963; *Nutritive Value of Foods,* Home and Garden Bulletin No. 72, U.S.D.A., 1971; and manufacturers' information.

Manganese

Manganese is a trace mineral that is classified as an essential nutrient. It is needed for normal bone development and as a component of arginase, an enzyme system needed to form urea. Manganese also enhances thiamin storage in the body. Despite the importance of these functions plus its role in several other enzyme systems, a manganese deficiency has yet to be recognized in man. Consequently, no dietary allowance has been recommended. It appears that virtually all diets contain the necessary quantities of manganese. Cereals and legumes are good sources of manganese.

Manganese toxicity has been observed when unusual dietary modifications resulted in intakes of more than 1000 parts per million. A serious decline in hemoglobin levels, seemingly caused by impaired iron absorption, resulted. Persons who have inhaled large quantities of dust while mining manganese over a period of years have developed serious disturbances in muscular coordination and inability to control voice level and laughter. Of course, the dosage of manganese absorbed by the miners is magnified tremendously in comparison with the level contained in the usual diet. Excesses of manganese appear to be extremely unlikely, if not impossible, in the usual diet sources.

Molybdenum

Molybdenum is an exotic mineral with the dubious distinction of appearing to be virtually unpronounceable. It has been noted that molybdenum is a component of xanthine oxidase and aldehyde oxidase. These enzyme systems function in the formation of uric acid and the shifting of iron into transport transferrin when more iron is required. These are important functions but they may be performed by other pathways, too.

Since present evidence has not established the essential nature of molybdenum, a recommended allowance has not been established. Although it is not a problem in man, molybdenum toxicity occasionally has been a problem in animals grazing on plants grown in molybdenum-rich soil. Bone abnormalities may develop and hemoglobin levels drop. The problem can be corrected by increasing the copper intake.

Phosphorus

The mineral that occurs in the second greatest quantity in the human body is phosphorus in the form of phosphate. About 1 percent of an adult's total body weight is due to the presence of phosphorus. Almost 90 percent of the body's phosphorus is deposited as insoluble phosphate (in combination with calcium) in the bones and teeth. The remainder, between 65 and 100 grams, is found in the nuclei and cytoplasm of all the cells of the body, occurring in combination with a variety of organic compounds. It is concentrated primarily in the muscles, where it performs unique and important functions.

Functions

Doubtless the best known function of phosphate is as a structural component of bones and teeth (in conjunction with calcium). Such a contribution should not be minimized despite the fact that there is twice as much calcium as phosphate in bones. The truth of the situation is that both of these minerals must be present for the formation and deposition of crystalline apatite, which gives strength and rigidity to bones.

With the accelerated rate of discoveries leading to a better understanding of biochemical processes, phosphate has achieved a significant stature among nutrients. It now is known that phosphate is a structural part of both ribonucleic acid (RNA) and deoxyribonucleic acid (DNA). As was discussed in Chapter 8, these two nucleic acids have prominent roles in protein synthesis and genetic coding.

One of the unusual functions of phosphate is in controlling the release of energy. Adenosine diphosphate (ADP) contains two phosphate radicals. It is possible to add a third phosphate radical to make adenosine triphosphate (ATP). Yet another related compound, adenosine monophosphate (AMP) is also found to a more limited extent in the body. The phosphate groups are bound by high-energy phosphate bonds. ATP is converted to ADP or, less frequently, AMP by removing the phosphate group. When the phosphate group is released, energy becomes available. This reaction can be reversed if energy is supplied to add phosphate to ADP or AMP. This ability to convert from ADP to ATP or from ATP to ADP is vital to energy metabolism in the body. The high-energy phosphate group provides this avenue for controlled availability of energy (see Chapter 6). Phosphate, by virtue of its ability to combine with hydrogen ion liberated during metabolism, acts as the most important buffer for acids in the body. Excess acid can be excreted rapidly by the kidney.

The phosphate group is capable of reacting with many different organic compounds in vivo. Phosphorylation facilitates passage of some nutrients through cell membranes. Also, the replacement of a fatty acid with phosphate in triglycerides to yield phospholipids is instrumental in the transport of fatty acids via the bloodstream. Without this transport mode, fats would be quite immiscible in the aqueous medium of the blood. Phosphate, as a part of many proteins, is a component of many enzymes. Thiamin, one of the B vitamins, is complexed with phosphate in its active form. Thus, it can be seen that phosphate performs independently in the body as well as in conjunction with calcium. Although calcium and phosphate are mentioned in tandem so frequently that they seem to blend into one, these independent functions of phosphate merit identification of this mineral as an important nutrient in its own right.

Absorption and metabolism

Since only about 10 percent of the phosphorus in the diet is absorbed, this certainly cannot be considered to be a very efficient process. However, there is some exchange of phosphate between the saliva and enamel of the teeth in the mouth, a process that clearly circumvents the need for this phosphate to pass through the intestinal mucosa. Antacid preparations are consumed in quantity by some persons seeking to avoid "acid stomach" and heartburn. Large quantities of these products interfere with phosphorus absorption and can lead to a deficiency condition, with resulting bone demineralization.

Recommended dietary allowances

Examination of Table 10.3 reveals that the recommended ratio of calcium to phosphate gradually shifts from the initial 1.5:1 ratio (half again as much calcium as phosphate) to equal proportions by the age of one year, a ratio that then remains constant throughout life. The high calcium to phosphate ratio found in human milk (2:1) appears to be appropriate to prevent the occurrence of hypocalcemic tetany that can be found occasionally in the newborn when phosphate levels are disproportionately high. (The ratio of calcium to phosphorus in cow's milk is approximately $1.2:1$.) Within a period of a couple of months, the phosphate intake can begin to be increased in proportion to calcium.

Food sources

Almost all animal protein contains phosphorus which, when metabolized, forms small amounts of phosphoric acid. This is responsible for the slightly acidic nature of all diets high in animal protein. Animal sources of phosphorus include cheese, milk, meats, fish, poultry, and eggs. Plant sources are cereals and cereal products, nuts, and legumes. Carbonated beverages, when consumed with frequency, contribute greatly to phosphorus intake and may lead to a low calcium to phosphorus ratio in the body, creating an undesirable imbalance.

Potassium

Potassium, though contributing no more than half a pound to an adult's body weight, functions in several ways in the body. It plays a key role in maintaining the proper osmotic pressure of the cell. A large proportion of the body's potassium is found within the cells; only a small amount is present in the extracellular fluids under normal conditions. A second function of potassium is that of a base to aid in the control of optimum acid-base balance. Potassium helps in transmitting nerve impulses and also has a catalytic role in energy metabolism that results in making energy available from carbohydrates, fats, and proteins. Still another facet of its catalytic activity is in the formation of proteins and glycogen.

Although potassium deficiencies are uncommon, they occur on occasion, particularly when diuretics are being administered. Another possible cause is that a high sodium intake may upset the delicate hormonal balance controlling potassium and sodium excretion and absorption. Diarrhea, which is a frequent problem in childhood illnesses, can cause a potassium deficiency by hampering absorption and increasing excretion of potassium previously absorbed. This problem was noted in the use of the so-called "rainbow" reducing pills. A potassium deficiency also has been a complicating factor in the treatment of kwashiorkor. Symptoms of a potassium deficiency include cardiac abnormalities, muscular weakness, respiratory failure, and renal failure.

Good dietary sources of potassium include orange juice, bananas, dried fruits, meats, peanut butter, and potatoes. Coffee is also a reasonably good source. Numerous other fruits and vegetables contribute somewhat lesser quantities of potassium. By avoiding excessive salt intake, potassium levels in the body will be enhanced. No recommended level of intake has been stated for potassium but it appears that normal intakes, estimated to range between 0.8 and 1.5 grams per 1000 kilocalories consumed, are safely in excess of the amount that seems absolutely necessary. Persons taking diuretics may need to be careful to include foods rich in potassium in their diets.

Selenium

Selenium is a rather curious mineral. Like vitamin E, selenium has the capability of functioning as an antioxidant. Selenium protects the red blood cell membrane and also may protect against cancer growth. Growth and fertility in rats are promoted by selenium. However, when selenium is breathed or consumed at levels as high as five parts per million, it interferes with some important reactions by being used in preference to sulfur, which would be the component of choice under normal conditions. Excessive selenium content leading to toxicity is not known to be a food hazard for humans although milk from cows grazing on plants grown in soil containing high levels of selenium may contain more than six times as much selenium as human milk; such milk may not be safe for infants.

Silicon

Silicon is a mineral that has been studied more for its toxic effect than for essential roles. This element promotes calcification of bone when calcium is limited in the diets of rats and chicks. This role has not been demonstrated in humans yet.

Sodium

Sodium is a mineral that frequently tends to lose its individual identity as a nutrient because of the common consumption of sodium in the form of sodium chloride or table salt. However, the nutritional significance of sodium can be appreciated more fully when this mineral is viewed as a single, functional element in the body.

The maintenance of normal acid-base balance is essential to general well being. Sodium functions in acid-base metabolism, mainly through a kidney mechanism that enables sodium to be exchanged for hydrogen ion. Other roles of sodium include: (1) aiding in relaxing contracted muscle (in the presence of potassium), (2) facilitating the absorption of various nutrients, including glucose, and (3) transmitting nerve impulses.

Functions

Sodium plays a crucial role in the body in maintaining equilibrium between extra and intracellular fluids. Sodium, by being concentrated largely in the extracellular fluids, exerts an opposite force to that attributable to potassium within the cells. The result is the balance of fluid between the fluid compartments that is observed in the normal, healthy individual. This function alone would seem to be a significant accomplishment for only one-fourth pound of a mineral distributed throughout the entire body, and yet other roles also are performed by sodium.

Meeting dietary sodium needs

The establishment of a set figure for sodium intake would be more a matter of an exercise than one of practicality since the appropriate sodium intake varies somewhat from one individual to another and also is modified by differences in activity and environmental temperatures. In any case, sodium intake is usually much more than is needed. As most people are aware, sodium is an obvious constituent of perspiration, where it is excreted as sodium chloride. Therefore, it is not suprising that the sodium intake for persons doing hard, physical labor in a hot and humid environment needs to be greater than for sedentary workers in an air-conditioned building. In our comparatively inactive society, probably one or two grams of sodium would meet the body's requirement. The quantities of salt consumed as the consequence of routine salting of food at the table as well as in the kitchen, although obviously quite variable, usually are considerably in excess of actual need.

Much sodium is consumed as salt, but other foods also are reasonably good sources of sodium. Salted meats that have large quantities of salt added as a preservative are obviously good sources of sodium. These include such meats as ham, bacon, and dried beef. Foods of animal origin are much higher in sodium than are most plant sources. However, some plant foods, such as potato chips and olives, are rich sources of sodium due to the practice of adding large amounts of salt during processing. Milk is a good source of sodium. Salt tablets obviously are concentrated sources of sodium; however, with most of us (even athletes or others who may perspire freely) there seldom will be a situation where these are necessary or even desirable.

Excess and deficiency

The level of sodium in the body ordinarily is carefully regulated by aldosterone, a hormone originating in the adrenals. This hormone causes sodium to be excreted via the urine. If fluid intake has been restricted to the extent that urine volume is significantly reduced, the body is hampered in its attempt to remove extra sodium from the body. In such an instance, the sodium levels in the blood are elevated, apparently triggering the thirst receptors. If the signal of the thirst receptors is heeded, the person with excess sodium in his blood will alleviate the sensation of thirst by drinking liq-

uids. Then the sodium level in the body can once again be controlled by the action of aldosterone because the volume of urine will be increased.

Some individuals regularly consume very large quantities of salt, a practice which is creating some concern. In such instances, the body's regulatory mechanisms are unable to achieve normal sodium values in the extracellular fluids. There is some evidence linking these prolonged excessive intakes of sodium with the development of hypertension.

The tragic mistake that was made in the preparation of a hospital's infant dietary formula a few years ago dramatizes the concern for excess sodium in the body. In this instance, salt was substituted for sugar with fatal results. Although the quantity of salt needed to cause such problems in adults is far too much for such an error to occur, still there is good reason to consider far less use of salt in contemporary food patterns.

The body is capable of storing small amounts of sodium in the bone tissue and cartilage as a reservoir against temporary depletion of sodium in the extracellular fluids. However, this supply is too limited to meet the demands for sodium that result when heavy sweating occurs without an increase in sodium intake. These demands are readily met by the ordinary use of salt at mealtime. Gradual depletion of this reserve sodium also occurs when sodium losses are heavy due to diarrhea or vomiting. As sodium levels in the body drop, there will be some shifting of potassium from within the cell into the extracellular fluid. When this happens, muscular weakness, dizziness, and nausea generally are quickly noted. This condition requires the ingestion of both sodium and water. Since sodium is absorbed very rapidly from the stomach and the small intestine, relief generally is quick when sodium is consumed. Individuals repeatedly doing heavy physical labor in a hot environment commonly are provided with salt tablets or water with added salt that can be taken at the first sign of a sodium deficiency.

Sulfur

Sulfur, a ubiquitous mineral in the body, is a component of such crucial structures as hair, fingernails, toenails, and skin. It also is a structural part of the B vitamins: thiamin, pantothenic acid, and biotin. In proteins, sulfur is contained in these amino acids: cystine, cysteine, and methionine. In fact, these amino acids serve as dietary sources of sulfur. The ability of sulfur to form cross linkages in protein molecules is responsible for the notably rigid structure of hair and nails. It is not surprising to learn that methionine and cystine are found in relatively large concentrations in these proteins of the body.

Presently there is not a recommended dietary allowance for sulfur. The national pattern of ample consumption of protein foods negates the likelihood of problems with a sulfur deficiency.

Zinc

The total quantity of zinc in the human body is just about as short as its name—only around 2 grams in the entire body. Despite the small concentration of zinc, it does perform key functions because it activates enzymes needed in protein metabolism and also is a part of carbonic anhydrase, the enzyme that is prominent in carbon dioxide transfer. Zinc is actually involved in many enzymes as cofactors for their metabolic action and is also closely associated with insulin, the important hormone in regulating carbohydrate metabolism.

The recommended level of intake of zinc for all persons older than 10 years of age is 15 milligrams, with recommendations increasing to 20 milligrams for pregnancy and 25 milligrams for lactation. Neither is there a likelihood that the normal individual will have a zinc deficiency or a toxic excess. However, a marginal zinc deficiency (insufficient to cause dwarfism) which responds to zinc therapy has been reported in the Middle East. Symptoms have included poor wound healing and impaired sense of taste (Fox, 1971). Some individuals may not utilize zinc well. In that event, a zinc deficiency may impair thiamin utilization, thus resulting in an impedance in metabolic reactions and an ultimate retardation of growth.

Food sources high in zinc include meats, eggs, liver, and seafood; milk and whole grain cereal products are good sources. The zinc content of selected foods is presented in the Appendix. Some attention may need to be given to increasing the zinc content of the diet. Marginal to inadequate levels of this mineral may be a problem when incomes are low because of the relatively high cost of the foods rich in zinc.

Lead, Mercury, and Other Heavy Metals

Lead, mercury, and other heavy metals are mineral elements widely distributed in nature, and thus in our foods, but they have no known physiologic function. They are known in biology and medicine primarily because of toxic properties at critical levels in humans.

Lead poisoning is all too common among children living in homes with old paint that flakes off the walls and ceilings. Children pick it off the floor or walls, consume it, and can thus be poisoned from the lead in the paint. Lead has not been used in most paints in recent years so this source of lead poisoning should disappear in time. Unfortunately, lead used in the glazes of some pottery is proving to be a definite health hazard. Although pottery dishes coated with lead-containing glazes present a potential hazard whenever food is served in them, many people still are unaware that lead leaches gradually out of the glaze and into the food they eat. Fruit juices and other acidic foods, since they favor the release of lead from the glaze, should not be served in pottery dishes or cups that have a lead-containing glaze.

With the improvement of analytical techniques in recent years, mercury has been found in most of our foods, with higher levels being detected in large and old ocean fish. The chances are good it has always been in our foods, and there is no evidence that its concentration has recently increased. However, mercury is used in some industrial plants, and steps must be taken promptly to see that it is properly disposed of and not just simply dumped in our rivers, lakes, and oceans to increase the contamination of our waters.

Except for a few rather bizarre situations such as in Japan several years ago and one in New Mexico more recently, there is no evidence of ill health from mercury contamination of foods. It is most unlikely that toxic levels of mercury will ever be ingested by eating any of our ordinary foods, particularly as they are consumed in mixed and varied diets.

No doubt other heavy metals such as gold, silver, vanadium, cadmium, and tin—all natural constituents of soil and water—are also present in our foods, but, like mercury, at levels too low to cause ill health. In fact, there is some evidence that some of these metals have important physiologic roles to play in trace amounts. However, the important point is to lessen and minimize the unnecessary pollution of our environment with these heavy metals.

Summary

The importance of the various minerals in the body has been pointed out. The nutritional value of these inorganic substances far outweighs the 6 or 7 pounds of these minerals that actually occur in adults. The macronutrient minerals, that is, minerals found in the largest quantities include calcium, chloride, magnesium, phosphorus, potassium, sodium, and sulfur. Microminerals that have been discussed include cobalt, copper, fluorine, iodine, iron, manganese, molybdenum, selenium, and zinc.

Minerals, as a group, provide the important functions of maintaining acid-base balance and proper osmotic pressure in the body. Various individual minerals are components of vitamins, hormones, and enzymes. Examples of these are iodine in thyroxine, sulfur in thiamin, iron in the cytochromes, and cobalt in vitamin B_{12}. Several minerals are needed for normal functioning of the nerves and also for muscular contraction and relaxation. Calcium, phosphate, fluoride, and magnesium are structural constituents of bones and teeth. Copper and iron are necessary for hemoglobin to be maintained at normal levels in the

Table 10.7 *Overview of Minerals—Functions and Sources*

Mineral	Functions	Food Sources
Calcium	1. Bone formation, maintenance, and growth 2. Tooth formation 3. Blood clot formation 4. Activation of pancreatic lipase 5. Absorption of vitamin B_{12} 6. Contraction of muscle	Milk, cheese, puddings, custards, chocolate beverages Fish with bones, including salmon Greens Broccoli
Chloride	1. Regulate pH of stomach (as component of hydrochloric acid) 2. Maintenance of proper osmotic pressure 3. Acid-base balance	Table salt Meats Milk Eggs
Chromium	1. Improve glucose uptake in cells	Meats Poultry Milk Whole-grain cereals
Cobalt	1. Aid in maturation of red blood cells (as part of vitamin B_{12} molecule)	Organ meats Meats
Copper	1. Catalyst for hemoglobin formation 2. Formation of elastin (connective tissue) 3. Release of energy (in cytochrome oxidase and catalase) 4. Formation of melanin (pigment) 5. Formation of phospholipids for myelin sheath of nerves	Cereals Nuts Legumes Liver Shellfish Grapes Meats
Fluoride	1. Strengthen bones and teeth	Fluoridated water
Iodine	1. Aid in regulating basal metabolism (as component of thyroxine and tri-iodo-thyronine)	Iodized salt Fish (salt water and anadromous)
Iron	1. Aid in transporting oxygen and carbon dioxide (as component of hemoglobin and myoglobin) 2. Aid in releasing energy (as component of cytochromes, cytochrome oxidase, catalase, peroxidase, myeloperoxidase)	Meats Heart, liver Clams Oysters Lima beans Spinach Dates, dried fruits Nuts Enriched and whole-grain cereals

Table 10.7 (continued)

Mineral	Functions	Food Sources
Magnesium	1. Catalyze ATP $\longleftrightarrow$ ADP 2. Conduct nerve impulses 3. Retention of calcium in teeth 4. Adjust to cold environment	Milk Green vegetables Nuts Breads and cereals
Manganese	1. Bone development 2. Aid in amino acid metabolism (as component of arginase) 3. Promotes thiamin storage	Cereals Legumes
Molybdenum	1. Aid in oxidation reactions (as component of xanthine oxidase and aldehyde oxidase)	
Phosphorus	1. Bone formation, maintenance, and growth 2. Tooth formation 3. Aid in metabolic reactions (as components of DNA and RNA, ADP and ATP, and TPP) 4. Lipid transport 5. Acid-base balance	Meats Poultry Fish Milk Fruits Vegetables
Potassium	1. Maintenance of osmotic pressure 2. Acid-base balance 3. Transmission of nerve impulses 4. Catalyst in energy metabolism 5. Formation of proteins 6. Formation of glycogen	Orange juice Dried fruits Bananas Meats Potatoes Peanut butter Coffee
Selenium	1. Antioxidant	
Silicon	1. Promote calcification in chicks and rats	Milk
Sodium	1. Maintenance of osmotic pressure 2. Acid-base balance 3. Relaxation of muscles 4. Absorption of glucose 5. Transmission of nerve impulses	Table salt Salted meats Milk
Sulfur	1. Aid in metabolic reactions (as component of thiamin) 2. Structural role (as component of some proteins, such as hair, nails, skin)	Meats Milk and cheese Eggs Legumes Nuts
Zinc	1. Aid in protein metabolism (as component of carboxypeptidase) 2. Aid in carbon dioxide transfer (as component of carbonic anhydrase)	Whole-grain cereals Meats Eggs Legumes

blood. An overview of functions and food sources is presented in Table 10.7.

This summary of functions must necessarily be viewed as a potpourri rather than an all-inclusive summation. Even from this abbreviated citing of functions, the essential nature of minerals is clear. These inorganic substances are contained in a wide variety of foods, thus emphasizing again the importance of a mixed diet. The rare occurrence of poisoning from food containing heavy metals serves as a reminder that continuing rational awareness of the interaction between the environment and food supply is an important component of good nutrition.

Selected References

Al-Rashid, R. A. and J. Spangler. Neonatal copper deficiency. *New England J. Med. 285:*841. 1971.

Amine, E. K. and D. M. Hegsted. Effect of diet on iron absorption in iron deficient rats. *J. Nutr. 101:*927. 1971.

Arbeter, A., et al. Nutrition and infection. *Fed. Proc. 30:*1421. 1971.

Ash, D. B. and B. Fitzgerald. Effectiveness of water fluoridation. *J. Am. Dent. Assoc. 65:*581. 1962.

Bernstein, D. S., et al. Prevalence of osteoporosis in high- and low-fluoride areas in North Dakota. *J. Am. Med. Assoc. 198:*499. 1966.

Bing, F. C. Assaying the availability of iron. *J. Am. Diet. Assoc. 60:*114. 1972.

Breeling, J. L. Allergy to fluoridated water?—no evidence. Questions and answers. *J. Am. Med. Assoc. 217:*1399. 1971.

Burroughs, A. L. and J. J. Chan. Iron content of some Mexican American foods. *J. Am. Diet. Assoc. 60:*123. 1972.

Cartwright, G. E. and M. M. Wintrobe. Copper metabolism in normal subjects. *Am. J. Clin. Nutr. 14:*224. 1964.

Cheek, D. B. and D. E. Hill. Muscle and liver cell growth, role of hormones and nutritional factors. *Fed. Proc. 29:*1503. 1970.

Crosby, W. H. Iron-enrichment-now Bronhalia. *J. Am. Med. Assoc. 231:*1054. 1975.

Food and Nutrition Board. *Recommended Dietary Allowances.* National Research Council-National Academy of Sciences. Washington, D.C. 8th ed. 1974.

Fox, M. R. S. Essential trace elements. *FDA Papers 5* (May):8. 1971.

Goldberg, A. and A. Reshef. Vitamin A and iron in infants' diets in Israel. *J. Am. Diet. Assoc. 60:*127. 1972.

Hambidge, K. M. C. Chromium nutrition in mother and growing child. *Newer*

Trace Elements in Nutrition. Ed. by Mertz, W. and W. E. Cornatzer. Dekker, New York, P. 169. 1971.

Hambidge, K. M. C., et al. Low levels of zinc in hair, anorexia, poor growth, and hypogeusia in children. *Pediat. Res. 6:*868. 1972.

Hegsted, D. M. Osteoporosis and fluoride deficiency. Postgrad. Med. 41, No. 1. 1967.

Krehl, W. A. Selenium—the maddening mineral. *Nutrition Today. 5,* No. 4:26. 1970.

Krehl, W. A. Mercury, the slippery metal. *Nutrition Today. 7,* No. 6:4. 1972.

Lutwak, L. and G. D. Whedon. Osteoporosis—a mineral deficiency disease? *J. Am. Diet. Assoc. 44:*173. 1964.

Lutwak, L. and G. D. Whedon. Osteoporosis—a disorder of mineral metabolism. *Borden Rev. Nutr. Res.* (23) *4:*45. 1962.

Mayer, J. Zinc deficiency, a cause of growth retardation. *Postgrad. Med. 35:*206. 1964.

Mertz, W. Some aspects of nutritional trace element research. *Fed. Proc. 29:*1482. 1970.

Mills, C. F. Metabolic interrelationships in the utilization of trace elements. *Proc. Nutr. Soc. 23:*38. 1964.

Munro, H. N. and J. W. Drysdale. Role of iron in the regulation of ferritin metabolism. *Fed. Proc. 29:*1469. 1970.

Munson, P. L. and T. K. Gray. Function of thyrocalcitonin in normal physiology. *Fed. Proc. 29:*1206. 1970.

Pike, R. L. and D. S. Gursky. Further evidence of deleterious effects produced by sodium restriction during pregnancy. *Am. J. Clin. Nutr. 23:*883. 1970.

Reddy, B. S. Calcium and magnesium absorption: role of intestinal microflora. *Fed. Proc. 30:*1815. 1971.

Reinhold, J. G. High phytate content of rural Iranian bread: possible cause of human zinc deficiency. *Am. J. Clin. Nutr. 24:*1204. 1971.

Review. Endemic goiter. *Nutr. Rev. 21:*73. 1963.

Review. Absorption of dietary iron in man. *Nutr. Rev. 29:*113. 1971.

Sandstead, H. H., et al. Zinc and wound healing. *Am. J. Clin. Nutr. 23:*514. 1970.

Schwarz, K. Recent dietary trace element research exemplified by tin, fluorine, and silicon. *Fed. Proc. 33:*17. 1974.

Schwarz, K. and D. B. Milne. Growth effects of vanadium in the rat. *Science 174:*426. 1971.

Seelig, M. S. The requirement of magnesium by the normal adult. *Am. J. Clin. Nutr. 14:*342. 1964.

Stare, F. J. Fluoridation—1969. *Worcester Medical News. XXXIII,* No. 4:5. 1968.

Tyuma, I. and K. Shimizu. Effect of organic phosphates on the difference in oxygen affinity between fetal and adult human hemoglobin. *Fed. Proc. 29:*1112. 1970.

Underwood, E. J. *Trace Elements in Human and Animal Nutrition.* 3rd. ed. Academic Press. New York. 1971.

Wacker, E. C. Magnesium metabolism. *J. Am. Diet. Assoc. 44:*362. 1964.

Westerman, R. Fluid and electrolyte replacement in sweating athletes. *J. Am. Med. Assoc. 212:*1713. 1970.

WHO. *Fluorides in Human Health.* Geneva. 1970.

WHO. Technical Report Series No. 532. *Trace Elements in Human Nutrition.* Geneva. 1973.

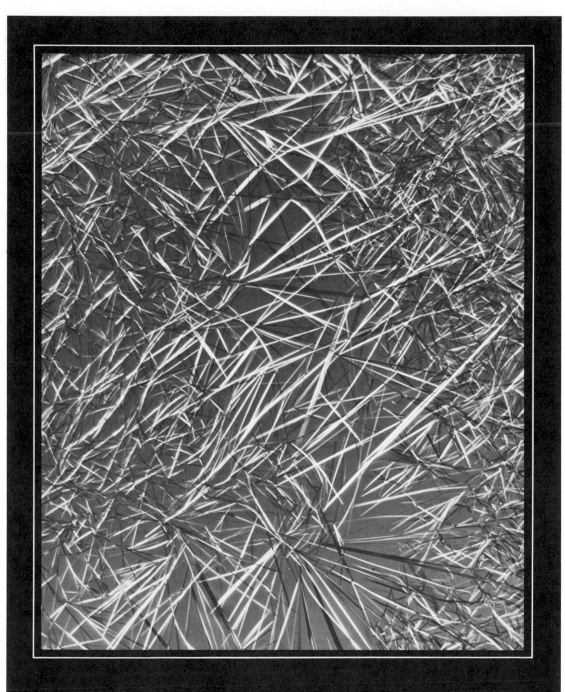

Chapter 11

Vitamins

Introduction

Historical perspective

Although nutrition had been a subject of a limited amount of research during the nineteenth century, it was not until the twentieth century that the elusive substances that are presently recognized as vitamins were studied. Even before the turn of the century, protein, minerals, and "fuel nutrients" had been shown to be insufficient in themselves to sustain life. In the first decade of the twentieth century, Sir Frederick G. Hopkins of Cambridge, England, demonstrated that a diet of pure protein, fat, carbohydrate, and all the known mineral elements was not adequate to provide good nutrition for experimental rats. He found that the addition of only a teaspoon of milk, a supplement prepared by alcoholic extraction of milk solids, or some dried vegetables greatly improved the health of the animals. When he discovered that the mineral ash from these supplements did not prevent the death of the experimental rats, he conclusively demonstrated that this elusive substance was organic in nature.

Other contemporaries of Hopkins actively pursued the study of this mysterious organic material in their laboratories. Some of the early vitamin researchers included Osborne and Mendel at Yale University; McCollum and Davis, working then at the University of Wisconsin and later at Johns Hopkins; and Casimir Funk, working at the Lister Institute in London.

It was Funk who coined the forerunner of today's term for these substances. In 1912, Funk proposed that the word "vitamine" be the word selected to designate these life-giving substances. "Vita" was a part of the word because it represented the life-promoting aspect of the materials; and because Funk thought these substances were chemical compounds called "amines," the term "amine" was appended. This nomenclature was appropriate for the substance that Funk was studying, since it did indeed contain an "amine" and was essential for life. However, it soon became evident that the life-promoting material in question actually was a group of substances. Although it was true that each of the materials was necessary for life, not all of them could be classified chemically as amines. To remove the misleading chemical implications and yet retain the euphony and popularity of the term, the final "e" was dropped and the accepted term became "vitamin."

Definition

A vitamin is an organic compound that is needed in very small quantities in the diet to promote growth and maintain life. This definition is relatively brief, yet specific. Note that the stipulation of very small quantities indicated in the definition eliminates the possibility that carbohydrates, fats, or proteins could be classified as vitamins despite the fact that they are organic and are a part of the diet. Minerals, because they are inorganic substances, cannot be confused with vitamins. By indicating that the compounds are needed in the diet, the possibility of confusing vitamins with substances, such as enzymes, that can be synthesized in the body is eliminated. The stipulation that the compound must be needed for reproduction, growth, and maintenance of life avoids the possibility that the many miscellaneous organic substances occurring in small amounts in foods could be classified as vitamins.

As research on vitamins has been conducted during this century, the fact has become clear that a substance may be classified as a vitamin for one species, yet may not be a vitamin for another species. The most familiar example of

species variation is ascorbic acid. This substance is a vitamin for humans, monkeys, and guinea pigs, yet is not a vitamin for other animals because they synthesize it.

Nomenclature

In the earliest phase of vitamin research, the tremendous divergence of substances that would be classified as vitamins was not appreciated. However, as early as 1913 at least one water soluble component and one fat soluble substance that could fit the definition of a vitamin had been recognized. Vitamins still are categorized on the basis of solubility. The fat soluble vitamins are vitamins A, D, E, and K. The water soluble vitamins include all of the B vitamins (thiamin, riboflavin, niacin, biotin, vitamin B_6, pantothenic acid, folacin, and vitamin B_{12}) and ascorbic acid (vitamin C).

The nomenclature of the individual vitamins may appear to be somewhat random and disorganized. However, naming did begin systematically, with the first substance identified receiving the appellation of vitamin A, the second vitamin B, and so forth. Up to this point, all went well. As research techniques became more sophisticated, more effective separation and purification of unknown substances became possible. Then scientists recognized that vitamin B was not a single substance. Since vitamin C was already designated as the name for a substance that was not a part of this vitamin B group, some system had to be devised for identifying the various compounds that were isolated from the collective "vitamin B." One logical way was to begin to designate these separate components of "vitamin B" under the general classification of vitamin B. This rationale explains why one hears the various B vitamins identified by a subscript, such as vitamin B_1. Particularly within the B group, there has been increasing use of names that reflect, at least in part, the chemical nature of the substance. This imparts considerably more meaning than can be attached to a compound designated only by a letter and a subscript.

The original scheme of alphabetical designation in order of discovery was further hampered by the fact that a substance might be given a letter, only to have additional research prove that it was not a vitamin by strict definition. This, of course, led to gaps in the alphabet. The ultimate departure from the alphabetical listing may be deemed a curse by students who do not have a background in chemistry, but the use of chemically based names is a boon to the researcher and student with some orientation into chemical nomenclature.

In general terms, vitamins as a group are required by the body for growth, maintenance of a healthy body, and reproduction. They play a role in the metabolism of nutrients, energy metabolism, maintenance of healthy tissues, normal operation of the digestive tract and, perhaps, resistance to infections. The specific roles of the individual vitamins will be considered in the appropriate sections of this chapter. The problems created by deficiencies of specific vitamins will be discussed also.

Enzymes

Since a large fraction of the action of vitamins is due to their ability to serve as parts of coenzymes in metabolic reactions, a brief review of enzymes and related compounds will make this chapter more meaningful. An enzyme is defined as an organic catalyst. It is a protein that is capable of altering the rate of a chemical reaction without undergoing a chemical change itself, and it does so under the mild conditions found in living cells.

Enzymes accomplish their catalytic role by providing a very specific structural conformation to which chemical compounds can be linked briefly. By such arrangements, the reactants are anchored into the close physical prox-

imity required for the reaction to occur. The active sites for such catalytic reactions are on the surface of the enzymes. This theory of enzyme action is generally referred to as the "lock and key" theory. If the surface of the enzyme changes in any way at the active site (the lock), the enzyme no longer is able to serve as a catalyst because the key (substrate) no longer fits the lock. Since the surfaces of proteins change with increases in temperature or other environmental changes, such as a modification in the acidity of the medium, enzymes easily lose their ability to effect a specific chemical reaction.

All living animal and plant tissues contain a great variety of enzymes. When these materials are harvested as foods, the enzymes are rapidly inactivated. They are completely inactivated by cooking the food. Enzymes in foods eaten raw are inactivated by the hydrochloric acid of the stomach. Thus we do not depend upon foods for any enzymes; all enzymes needed for the proper functioning of the body are made or synthesized in various body tissues and organs. Despite advertising and food enthusiasts' ardent claims, enzymes consumed in foods and special enzyme preparations will not aid in the digestive process of humans.

Apoenzyme and coenzymes

Enzymes are proteins or protein-containing complex systems in which the protein is attached to another substance. The protein portion of the enzyme system is termed the "apoenzyme." This apoenzyme then must be joined to another substance before it has enzyme activity. The group or compound to which the proteinaceous apoenzyme is attached is known as a "coenzyme." Some of the vitamins perform their functions in the body by serving as structural parts of coenzymes to catalyze important metabolic reactions. Vitamins that are incorporated in coenzymes become a part of diverse enzyme systems in the body when the coenzymes complex with different apoenzymes.

Provitamins and antivitamins

To present a full introduction to the role of vitamins in the body, the influence of provitamins and antivitamins also needs to be considered. Provitamins are chemical compounds closely related to vitamins in their structure. The body is capable of converting the inactive provitamin into the chemical structure that is the vitamin. Consequently, when this conversion is accomplished, the substance (now in the active form) performs in the same manner as the vitamin that actually was consumed in the active form. Thus, foods that contain a provitamin actually are good potential sources of the vitamin; this is true despite the fact that a food may not contain any of the actual active form of the vitamin. A good example of this would be carotene, a substance found in green and yellow vegetables. Carotene is a provitamin A, and is converted in the body into vitamin A.

Antivitamins are antagonists to the vitamins, and can replace the vitamin in chemical reactions. However, the antivitamin blocks the reaction instead of facilitating it. This blocking of vital chemical reactions is used by some researchers to produce a specific vitamin deficiency so that the functions of the vitamin may be studied. These antagonists may have a useful role in medicine as their action is studied and understood in greater detail.

Sources of vitamins

Not surprisingly, the various vitamins are widely scattered through the many foods consumed by man. No one food contains all the vitamins, but a varied diet encompassing all the food groups will provide all the vitamins in the amounts required for optimum health. For the normally healthy person, a vitamin supplement does not need to be included as a part of the diet if a wide range of food is being eaten regularly. Food includes all the vitamins needed by man; the inclusion of vitamin pills is an unnecessary expense when one is eating wisely. The use of vitamin supplements is recommended only to correct an existing deficiency due to faulty diet or improper absorption of the vitamins, to provide vitamins known to be lacking in a restricted and poorly selected diet, or to act as a therapeutic measure in the medical treatment of some illnesses. Armchair doctoring by casual inclusion of vitamin supplements may be a totally unnecessary expense, and of more importance, may delay proper diagnosis and treatment. As will be discussed later in this chapter, gigantic doses of fat-soluble vitamins A and D not only are expensive, but actually present a serious health hazard (especially to children) when taken in massive quantities over a period of time. Since water-soluble vitamins are excreted readily from the body, they do not accumulate at harmful levels in the body. However, when repeatedly consumed in extremely large amounts, as some people have been doing with vitamin C, even water-soluble vitamins may cause a variety of serious health problems.

A quick glance at a vitamin capsule is sufficient to confirm the fact that vitamins are available in a highly purified form. Clearly, the volume of a vitamin capsule is only a small fraction of the amount of food one eats in a day to supply the comparable quantity of vitamins from food sources. Vitamins in capsules are synthetic nutrients that are manufactured by man. Since these compounds have the same chemical structure as the vitamins in foods, they act in exactly the same way in the body. As far as the body is concerned, there is no difference between a synthetic vitamin and one that is present in food. Contrary to the statements of food faddists, the so-called "natural" vitamins in foods offer no special powers over those of the synthetic vitamins.

Vitamin A

Even in the early years of the scientific race in nutritional research, there were competing research teams. Vitamin A was discovered independently, and at the same time by two outstanding groups of investigators—Osborne and Mendel at Yale, and McCollum and Davis at the University of Wisconsin. Both groups share the credit for the announcement of the first vitamin known to man. This dramatic event occurred in 1912. Osborne and Mendel demonstrated an important substance in milk fat. Experimental animals that remained healthy and grew normally on a laboratory ration containing milk fat failed to thrive and eventually died following the onset of an eye disease if milk fat was omitted from the ration. McCollum and Davis obtained similar symptoms when they fed their rats a purified ration in which lard was the only fat. Symptoms were found to be reversed when butter or an ether extract of egg yolk was added to the diet. Soon cod liver oil also was found to contain this important substance, and the era of the spoonful of cod liver oil for breakfast was launched.

In 1919, Steenbock, of the University of Wisconsin, found that yellow and green vegetables contained a similar growth-promoting substance. After nine years of study, carotene, the

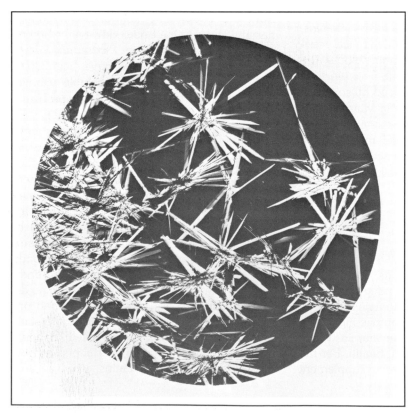

Crystals of vitamin A.

yellow pigment of these vegetables, was confirmed to be a precursor or provitamin of vitamin A.

Research on vitamin A was not confined to the United States. The chemical structure of the vitamin was elucidated in Europe in the early 1930s. Crystallization of the pure vitamin was accomplished from halibut liver oil in 1937. Synthetic vitamin A was made in 1946. Since that time, various means of synthesizing the vitamin have been explored, with the result that vitamin A now can be made so inexpensively that it costs only a little over a penny to produce 50,000 International Units of the material, a 10-day supply for the average adult man.

Chemistry of vitamin A

Vitamin A perhaps is a somewhat misleading term to many people because it sounds as if only one chemical compound has vitamin A activity. Actually, several forms of vitamin A exist, with each possessing activity to varying degrees. In fact, there are two types of vitamin A itself, which differ only by one double bond between carbon atoms. These two substances, vitamin A_1 and vitamin A_2, are equally effective in the body. Vitamin A_1, which is found as an ester (retinyl palmitate) in ocean fish oils and fats, and in liver, butter fat, and egg yolk, is biologically active as an alcohol, an aldehyde, or an acid. The alcohol (the most common form) frequently is referred to as retinol, the aldehyde as retinal, and the acid as retinoic acid. Vitamin A_2 is of limited interest since it is found only in freshwater fish and birds that eat these fish.

In addition to the actual forms of vitamin A mentioned above, related compounds, known as the carotenoids, are found in some fruits and vegetables. There are several carotenoids that contribute significantly to the body's total potential vitamin A intake. The most important are alpha, beta, and gamma carotenes, and cryptoxanthin. These compounds are responsible for the yellow to yellow-orange pigments in many fruits and vegetables. As a general rule of

thumb, the more intense the pigmentation in these foods, the higher is the provitamin A content. Green vegetables, particularly dark green and leafy ones, are rich in provitamin A. These vegetables also contain carotenoids, despite their misleading green color. The green chlorophyll masks the color of the carotenoids, but the nutritive contribution is not impaired. The yellow color of purified beta carotene is so intense that this substance is widely used as a coloring agent by the food industry. In such instances, beta carotene is valued more for its aesthetic contribution than its nutritive value, although the potential vitamin A value of the food it colors is also increased.

Vitamin A is a fat-soluble material, virtually without color, and insoluble in water. Although the esters of vitamin A are relatively stable compounds, the alcohol, aldehyde, and acid forms are rapidly destroyed by oxidation when they are exposed to air and light. Since vitamin A occurs in the stable form (the ester) in most foods, normal preparation procedures do not destroy much vitamin A activity. However, fats that undergo oxidative rancidity, can lose their vitamin A rapidly.

Functions

Vitamin A is widely recognized as the vitamin that prevents night blindness. This vitamin is an important component in the visual cycle that enables one to see in a dim light. Although this may seem to be a rather trivial role in the body, consider carefully the amount of driving that is done at night. Certainly driving is more hazardous at night as a result of the more limited visibility in comparison with the daytime hours, but the danger is increased significantly for people suffering from night blindness. Such thoughts give added importance to the need for adequate vitamin A in the diet.

The key substance in the ability to see in dim lights is rhodopsin, which also is known by the colorful name of visual purple. Rhodopsin is formed in the rods of the retina of the eyes by the union of retinal (the aldehyde, also called

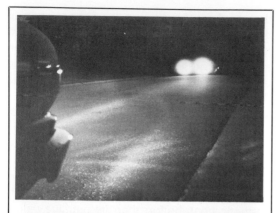

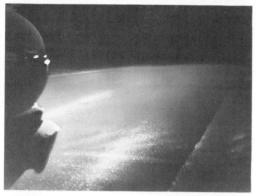

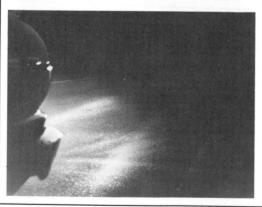

Following the approach of a car in the evening with its headlights on (top), the person with adequate vitamin A will be able to see a broad view of the road when the car passes (center). In contrast, the person suffering from night blindness due to a vitamin A deficiency will have limited ability to adapt to the change in light and be able to see only a few feet ahead (bottom).

retinene) and opsin, a protein present in the rods. When light strikes the rods, the rhodopsin (or visual purple) is bleached to retinene (or visual yellow), releasing the opsin (Figure 11.1). This reaction produces electrical energy, which is sent from the retina via the optic nerve to the brain, resulting in the communication of visual images. The protein that is released during the conversion from rhodopsin to visual yellow is now available for recombination with retinal to form rhodopsin and perpetuate the cycle. The recombination occurs in darkness, generally during sleep at night. The retinene (or retinal that is freed when visual purple is bleached) can either be reduced to the alcohol or recombined directly with opsin in darkness to provide the needed visual purple. Some vitamin A is removed from the rods, but it can be replaced by retinal that is circulating in the blood of well-nourished individuals. Because of this partial loss of vitamin A, it is necessary that a continuing supply of vitamin A be available for the formation of rhodopsin. The liver is capable of storing a supply of vitamin A for use when the diet is low in vitamin A. Such storage may provide adequate vitamin A for several months. With prolonged deficiency, the visual cells lose their rhodopsin, thus causing permanent visual impairment. Vitamin A is also necessary for the formation of the visual pigments that function in the cones of the retina. However, since the metabolism and turnover rate of the cones is much slower than that of the rods, cones are able to function much longer than rods after onset of the deficiency.

One of the significant functions of vitamin A in children is to promote optimum growth. This is accomplished by maintaining many physiological processes required for normal growth, including proper bone growth. In the vitamin A-deficient child or animal, the faulty reshaping and limited growth of bones can present a particular problem for the central nervous system. The soft tissues will grow at a faster rate than the bone, and the spinal cord and brain may be compressed. Such a situation can cause a

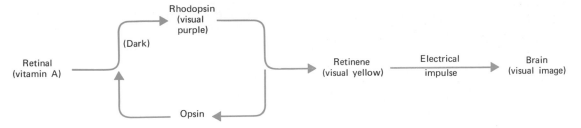

Figure 11.1   Role of vitamin A in night vision.

pinching of nerves and produce various neurological signs.

Vitamin A also functions in the reproductive processes of rats. In the male, vitamin A is essential for spermatogenesis in the testes. This vitamin is required for prevention of resorption of the fetus in the pregnant female, with fetal abnormalities occurring in other instances where vitamin A intake was inadequate.

The epithelial cells that line the body surfaces, including intestine and skin, require vitamin A for maintaining their normal levels of

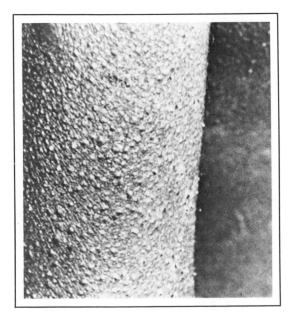

Follicular hyperkeratosis of the arm, a result of prolonged deficiency of vitamin A.

mucus secretion. Apparently, the mucopolysaccharide that is a normal carbohydrate constituent of mucus is not formed in normal amounts in the absence of vitamin A, and the outer layer of cells becomes keratinized. Over a period of time, the layers of keratinized cells build up, creating the appearance of a rough goose flesh. The little filaments or cilia, which normally project from respiratory epithelial cells, are lost. Without the protective action provided by mucus and these cilia, bacteria may be more likely to enter the body and cause infections. Here, as in bone, one cell type (keratinizing) slowly replaces a second type (mucus) as the deficiency worsens.

Related to the alterations in the epithelial tissue—and the formation of mucopolysaccharide—is the role vitamin A plays in maintaining the external health of the eye. With vitamin A present, lachrymal secretions bathe the eye regularly and the cornea is healthy. When the availability of vitamin A in the body is decreased, the cornea begins to dry up. Keratinization and an opaque appearance (Bitot's spots) develop and lead, ultimately, to a severe disease of the eye known as xerophthalmia. Blindness results if the deficiency is not promptly corrected.

In addition to these obvious changes produced by vitamin A deficiency, similar defective mechanisms produce changes in formation of tooth enamel, in carbohydrate metabolism and the synthesis of glycogen for storage of body energy, and in fat metabolism concerning the handling of cholesterol.

Utilization of vitamin A

All forms of vitamin A are absorbed through the wall of the small intestine, where they enter the lymphatic system in the form of a fatty acid ester (retinyl palmitate), and ultimately reach the bloodstream. Conversion of the various forms of provitamin A to vitamin A also occurs in the intestinal wall. After the esterified vitamin A enters the blood, it is transported to the liver. There the surplus vitamin A is removed and stored for subsequent use, thus maintaining a relatively stable level of vitamin A in the blood. When vitamin A is needed to maintain the normal value of about 130 International Units per 100 milliliters of blood, it leaves the liver in the form of retinol, complexed with a protein carrier. Failure to form this protein carrier may explain, at least in part, the low level of circulating vitamin A that has been noted during protein deficiencies.

Vitamin A excretion does occur despite the ability of the liver to store rather large quantities of this vitamin. Since vitamin A is fat soluble rather than water soluble, vitamin A is not excreted in the urine. The normal route of excretion is with the bile salts in the feces. Vitamin A also is excreted in milk during lactation. Vitamin A is poorly absorbed when an individual has impairment in the formation of bile, when protein intake is severely restricted, or when mineral oil or some disease factor inhibits the absorption of fat.

Dietary sources of vitamin A and provitamin A

Vitamin A itself is available only from animal sources. In view of the preceding discussion regarding the storage of vitamin A in the liver, it is not the least bit surprising that liver from all types of animals is a particularly rich source of this nutrient. Of course, the dietary intake of the animal will influence the level of vitamin A contained in its liver. An interesting illustration of this is that polar-bear liver, as a source of food for man, has a dangerously high concentration of vitamin A. This high concentration is

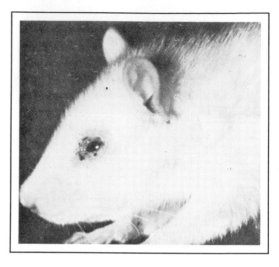

Xerophthalmia in its beginning stages is characterized by dryness of the cornea and conjunctiva. This is due to a vitamin A deficiency.

probably a reflection of the bears' practice of consuming fish, whose livers are themselves excellent sources of vitamin A. Other animal livers provide excellent sources of vitamin A, and egg yolks are also a good, albeit slightly variable source of vitamin A. The actual vitamin A content of egg yolk is influenced considerably through fortification of the ration fed the hen. The vitamin A content of milk and butterfat is of importance in the diets of many people, and is also dependent on the ration available to the cows. Summer butter and milk, when the cows have had fresh grass, contain appreciably more vitamin A than do their winter counterparts. Typical vitamin A values of animal foods are presented in Table 11.1, along with the vitamin A activity of plant foods that are sources of provitamin A. The values for animal sources should be viewed as average levels because, as previously mentioned, the actual content is influenced significantly by the diet fed the animal.

The outstanding sources of provitamin A in the fruit and vegetable category are, generally speaking, the brightly pigmented yellow and dark green foods containing carotenoids. Among those foods, the more strongly pig-

Table 11.1 *Vitamin A Value of Commonly Used Foods*[a]

	Amount	Vitamin A (I.U.)
Meat group		
Beef roast, cooked	3 1/2 oz	82
Calf liver, fried	3 1/2 oz	32,700
Halibut, broiled	3 1/2 oz	680
Swordfish, broiled	3 1/2 oz	2,050
Egg	1 whole	562
Milk group		
Milk, whole, 3.5% fat	1 cup	342
Milk, fortified low fat	1 cup	195
Milk, skim	1 cup	Trace
Cheese, cheddar	1 oz	371
Cheese, Swiss	1 oz	323
Cheese, cottage, creamed	1/2 cup	191
Cheese, cottage, uncreamed	1/2 cup	11
Cheese food	1 oz	346
Ice cream	1/2 cup	369
Ice milk	1/2 cup	196
Egg nog	1 cup	843
"Instant" breakfast	1 cup	1,400
Vegetables		
Broccoli, cooked	Medium stalk	2,500
Carrots, diced, cooked	1/2 cup	8,400
Collard greens, cooked	1/2 cup	4,590
Kale, cooked	1/2 cup	7,544
Mustard greens, cooked	1/2 cup	5,800
Pumpkin, cooked	1/2 cup	7,400
Spinach, cooked	1/2 cup	8,100
Sweet potato, baked in skin	1 medium	9,720
Tomato, ripe	1 medium	1,640
Winter squash, cooked	1/2 cup	4,270
Fruits		
Apricot, raw	1 medium	1,134
Cantaloupe	1/2 small	6,290
Mango, ripe	1/2 medium	4,800
Papaya	1/3 medium	1,750
Peach, yellow	1 medium	1,330
Other foods		
Margarine	1 tbsp	470
Butter	1 tbsp	470

[a] Data compiled and adapted from *Composition of Foods—Raw, Processed, Prepared,* Agriculture Handbook No. 8, U.S.D.A., 1963; *Nutritive Value of Foods,* Home and Garden Bulletin No. 72, U.S.D.A., 1971; and manufacturers' information.

mented the food, the greater will be its provitamin A content. Since carotenoid levels roughly parallel the intensity of chlorophyll pigmentation, the deeper-green leaves of leafy vegetables will be the highest in their vitamin A activity. Two notable exceptions to the general rule of the parallel between vitamin A activity and yellow pigmentation are the pigments lycopene and xanthophyll. Lycopene provides the reddish color of tomatoes and watermelon, and xanthophyll is the yellow pigment in yellow corn and egg yolks. Neither of these pigments can be converted to vitamin A in the body. Therefore, the intensity of their hue is not a measure of potential vitamin A in the diet. However, tomatoes and watermelon do contain provitamin A; the red of lycopene is simply masking the pigmentation of the provitamin.

Table 11.2 *Recommended Daily Dietary Allowances for the Fat-Soluble Vitamins*[a]

Age (years)	Weight (kg)	Weight (lb)	Height (cm)	Height (in)	Vitamin A Activity (RE)[b]	Vitamin A Activity (I.U.)	Vitamin D Activity (I.U.)	Vitamin E Activity (I.U.)
Infants								
0.0–0.5	6	14	60	24	420	1400	400	4
0.5–1.0	9	20	71	28	400	2000	400	5
Children								
1–3	13	28	86	34	400	2000	400	7
4–6	20	44	110	44	500	2500	400	9
7–10	30	66	135	54	700	3300	400	10
Males								
11–14	44	97	158	63	1000	5000	400	12
15–18	61	134	172	69	1000	5000	400	15
19–22	67	147	172	69	1000	5000	400	15
23–50	70	154	172	69	1000	5000	—	15
51+	70	154	172	69	1000	5000	—	15
Females								
11–14	44	97	155	62	800	4000	400	12
15–18	54	119	162	65	800	4000	400	12
19–22	58	128	162	65	800	4000	400	12
23–50	58	128	162	65	800	4000	—	12
51+	58	128	162	65	800	4000	—	12
Pregnancy					1000	5000	400	15
Lactation					1200	6000	400	15

[a] Adapted from the Food and Nutrition Board, National Academy of Sciences—National Research Council. **Recommended Daily Dietary Allowances,** revised 1974.
[b] Retinol equivalents. (Assumed to be all as retinol in milk during first six months of life. All subsequent intakes are assumed to be half as retinol and half as β-carotene when calculated from International Units. As retinol equivalents, three-fourths are as retinol and one-fourth as β-carotene.

Particularly rich sources of provitamin A include: sweet potatoes, yellow winter squash, spinach, Swiss chard, apricots, carrots, tomatoes, broccoli, papaya, and peaches.

Provitamin A is not converted to vitamin A in the body with complete efficiency. Of the various carotenoid compounds, beta-carotene is converted most efficiently. Theoretically, the symmetrical beta-carotene molecule should be cleaved into two usable molecules of vitamin A, but the actual chemistry of the conversion appears to be much less neat and efficient. The source of the provitamin influences the efficiency of conversion; root vegetables, such as carrots, are converted from provitamin A to vitamin A in the body with about half the efficiency that is demonstrated in the conversion of provitamin A from leafy vegetables. Conversion efficiency generally falls in the range from 15 to 35 percent. The recommended dietary intake of vitamin A established by the Food and Nutrition Board of the National Academy of Sciences takes cognizance of this inefficiency (Table 11.2). The recommendation of 5000 International Units of vitamin A for adult men is based on the assumption that about one half of the vitamin A will be from animal sources and one half from plant sources. As can be seen in Table 11.3, vitamin A is reasonably stable during routine food preparation.

Table 11.3 *Stability of Vitamins in Food Preparation*[a]

Vitamin	Solubility	Sensitive to				
		Acid	Alkali	Heat	Light	Oxidation
A	Fat					X[b]
D	Fat					
E[c]	Fat		X		X	
K	Fat	X	X		X	X
Thiamin	Water		X	X		X
Riboflavin	Water		X		X	
Niacin	Water					
B$_6$	Water		X		X	X
Pantothenic acid	Water	X	X	X[d]		
Biotin	Water		X			X
Folacin[e]	Water			X		X
B$_{12}$	Water		X			
Ascorbic acid	Water		X	X		X

[a] In general, vitamin retention is enhanced by short cooking times and moderate temperatures.

[b] If rancid fat is present or product is sun dried.

[c] Limited loss of vitamin E in normal food preparation.

[d] Unstable in dry heat.

[e] Long storage and long cooking times are especially detrimental.

An International Unit (I.U.) of vitamin A is equivalent to 0.344 micrograms of crystalline vitamin A acetate of 0.6 micrograms of all transforms of beta-carotene. An International Unit is the equivalent of the United States Pharmacopeia Unit (U.S.P.). In line with a previous recommendation of the 1967 FAO/WHO Expert Committee's recommendation that vitamin A values be expressed as retinol equivalents, the Food and Nutrition Board's eighth revision of the recommended Dietary Allowances for vitamin A was presented in retinol equivalents as well as in International Units. A retinol equivalent equals 3.33 International Units of retinol or 10 International Units of beta-carotene.

Deficiency conditions

The responses to a vitamin A deficiency may be somewhat varied, depending upon the severity of the condition and the duration of the problem. Symptoms of a vitamin A deficiency do not develop unless the dietary intake is inadequate, and the body stores of this vitamin are depleted. As previously mentioned, night blindness is one of the early manifestations of a vitamin A deficiency. However, occurrence of this problem cannot be used as an exclusive indicator of the vitamin deficiency since other factors can contribute to night blindness. Onset of night blindness due to insufficient vitamin A will be slow—a matter of several months—when deprivation immediately follows a regular pattern of adequate vitamin A ingestion; this is due to the storage and slow release of vitamin A from various tissues, particularly the liver.

In persons with a severe and prolonged deficiency of vitamin A, the health of the eye is endangered. The first symptoms include inflammation of the eye and Bitot's spots. Increased keratinization of the cornea and dryness of the eye are other symptoms of a serious affliction of the eye—known as xerophthalmia. Continued vitamin A deficiency causes ulceration, and ultimately leads to blindness. Xerophthalmia is a precursor of kera-

tomalacia, or softening of the eye. Collectively, these two conditions are the single greatest cause of blindness in children suffering from protein-calorie malnutrition around the world.

The changes that occur in epithelial cells in vitamin A deficiency lead to the development of hyperkeratinization of the skin. Epithelial changes in the urinary tract often result in urinary infection and the development of kidney stones. Changes in the intestinal region may play a role in the diarrheas and intestinal infections associated with this deficiency. Malformation of enamel occurs in rodents maintained on diets severely deficient in vitamin A; however, no clear evidence supports a comparable situation in man.

As described previously, growth and reproduction are impaired in vitamin A deficiency. Failure to absorb the cerebrospinal fluid surrounding the brain can increase pressure on the brain and, together with changes in bone growth, may cause paralysis of the extremities or blindness, depending upon the degree of crowding on the brain and nerves.

Although the exact mechanisms of the protective capacity of vitamin A are not known, it appears that a vitamin A deficiency may weaken the body's defense against pneumonia, tuberculosis and, possibly, other infections.

Toxicity

Excess vitamin A can create a serious health hazard, and yet any person can buy unlimited quantities of vitamin A without a physician's prescription. The only control presently in effect is the FDA measure limiting each capsule to a maximum of 10,000 I.U. and people can take as many each day as they wish. Although the level at which vitamin A becomes toxic varies from one individual to another, a daily intake of 50,000 I.U. for many months can induce toxic symptoms in adults. As little as 18,500 International Units over a period of months can produce toxicity in a young child, whose body is obviously much smaller. Symptoms of hypervitaminosis A include anorexia (or loss of appetite), blurred vision, excessive irritability, drying and cracking of the skin, hair loss, headaches, drowsiness, diarrhea, and nausea. Fortunately, recovery is accomplished in most cases when the supplement is discontinued. Certainly, these symptoms are noticeable and undesirable.

Hypervitaminosis A can easily be avoided by obtaining vitamin A only from dietary sources or low potency vitamin preparations. Resist the temptation to take high potency vitamin A capsules. With a little planning, the average diet can readily include adequate vitamin A, thus avoiding the need for vitamin A supplementation.

Some persons may consume unusually large amounts of provitamin A, but the inefficiency of the body in converting it to vitamin A virtually eliminates the possibility of developing hypervitaminosis A. In fact, when high levels of provitamin A are ingested, the body fails to convert all of the material to the vitamin form. Consequently, the pigment accumulates in the body, causing a yellowing of the skin that first appears on palms of the hands and the soles of the feet. These changes, although unattractive, do not produce a toxic effect.

Vitamin D

Although considerable research was done utilizing fish-liver oils early in the twentieth century, it was not until 1922 that McCollum noted that fish-liver oils retained their antirachitic activity after vitamin A was removed. Such an exciting observation led to closer scrutiny of this obviously nourishing, although far from palatable, food material. Eventually, 10 different forms of this antirachitic material were identified, but only two were found to be of dietary significance. Vitamin D_2 is marketed under the names of ergocalciferol, calciferol, and viosterol. The form of vitamin D that is of animal origin is termed cholecalciferol, a reflection of its cholesterol precursor.

Classification of vitamin D can become laborious if one wishes to adhere strictly to the definition of a vitamin because this substance can be formed in the body simply by exposing the skin to sunlight. However, the conditions of life often are not suitable for the production of sufficient quantities of vitamin D in the body. It then becomes necessary to include the vitamin as a dietary constituent.

Functions of vitamin D

The modus operandi of vitamin D is the subject of extensive research efforts by numerous scientists. Active vitamin D clearly performs its primary role in the absorption of calcium from the intestinal region. During recent years, exciting new studies have shown that vitamin D, as present in food, is inactive and must be hydroxylated successfully to become active metabolically. The vitamin D from food is transported via blood plasma to the liver, where it is hydroxylated and stored as 25-hydroxycholecalciferol or as 25-hydroxyergocalciferol. From storage in the liver, these compounds go to the kidney where parathyroid hormone facilitates the addition of another hydroxyl group to form 1,25-dihydroxycholecalciferol. Formation of this active form is halted when the calcium level rises to the point where calcitonin is secreted.

The absorption of calcium and phosphorus across the intestinal membrane is facilitated by active vitamin D, thus insuring that both of these minerals are available for building and maintaining bones and teeth. The precise means by which this is accomplished is not yet known.

Secondary to its role in enabling calcium absorption, adequate vitamin D enhances the levels of phosphates in the body. This is partly because of the improved absorption of phosphorus through the intestinal wall but, more importantly, because of the enhanced resorption of phosphates from the kidney tubules. Maintenance of a satisfactory phosphate level is essential to the process of bone calcification.

Various other imbalances are the result of a

vitamin D deficiency, thus indicating the regulatory functions this vitamin performs in the body. The level of amino acids excreted in the urine increases when vitamin D is inadequate, and decreases when the vitamin is administered at normal levels. The level of citrate in the blood also decreases in a vitamin D deficiency. In addition, low levels of alkaline phosphatase occur in vitamin D deficiency, thus reducing phosphate levels. Alkaline phosphatase is an enzyme playing a major role in the release of phosphate from compounds, making the mineral available for deposition as calcium phosphate. Clearly, the maintenance of alkaline phosphatase at a normal level is a significant contribution of vitamin D.

Utilization of vitamin D

Bile must be present in the intestine if fat-soluble vitamin D is to be absorbed. The factors that influence the absorption of this vitamin are the same as those for the absorption of fats. Under conditions of normal health, vitamin D is efficiently utilized by the body and limited excesses are stored in the liver, bone, adrenal glands, and the kidney. Vitamin D will ultimately be excreted in the feces.

Meeting recommended allowances

Vitamin D is unique in that it can be (1) provided entirely from the diet; (2) produced solely in the body in certain parts of the world (action of ultraviolet rays of sunlight on the skin); or (3) by a combination of the two preceding sources. Mellanby, working in England in 1919, was the first to recognize that cod-liver oil was the source of the nutrient that prevented rickets. In fact, cod-liver and other fish-liver oils were found to be some of the richest dietary sources of vitamin D. The natural occurrence of vitamin D in the diet is limited to animal foods, with eggs, cheese, and butter providing limited amounts. Fish and meats also add some vitamin D to the diet. Today milk is commonly fortified with 400 International Units

of vitamin D per quart, a practice that is highly desirable. A quart of vitamin D-fortified milk provides the amount of vitamin D recommended for one day. If vitamin D has been added, this information will be stated on the label. Unless milk is so identified, the vitamin D content will be essentially nil.

In addition to dietary sources of vitamin D, this substance is produced when sunlight irradiates 7-dehydrocholesterol, a compound present in the skin. The energy provided by ultraviolet rays causes a slight modification in the chemical structure of this sterol, thus forming active vitamin D_3. This vitamin passes from the skin into the bloodstream. Irradiation can be accomplished by direct sunlight or by the use of a sunlamp.

Anything that filters the sunlight will impede the irradiation of 7-dehydrocholesterol. One wonders why those concerned with urban ecology have not added vitamin D deficiency to their long list of complaints about smog, since the ultraviolet rays do not penetrate smog and smoke. Other obstacles of a more natural origin include clouds, fog, and latitudes far north or south of the Equator. Ordinary glass, screens, and clothing of all types also prevent irradiation of the sterol. Dark skin-tones result in less efficient formation of vitamin D in the skin than do lighter tones. Dark skin is a protection against excessive quantities of vitamin D when one frequents the beach or is in the equatorial region, but will limit vitamin D synthesis in the temperate regions of the world. However, synthesis of vitamin D in the skin is not necessary if this vitamin is ingested in food or a vitamin supplement.

As shown in Table 11.2, 400 International Units of vitamin D are recommended daily for all children, youths, and pregnant and lactating women. This level of vitamin D prevents the occurrence of rickets in young children, and is sufficiently low to avoid any possibility of a toxic dose. Although not yet proven conclusively, the suggestion has been made that a daily intake of 800 International Units may facilitate calcium absorption and thus help to main-

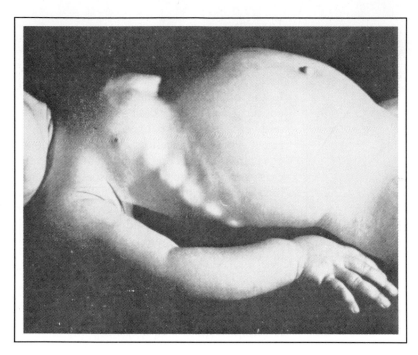

Ricketic rosary, characterized by beadlike protrusions, is a result of inadequate vitamin D intake.

tain good bone structure in aging adults. Exact recommendations for dietary vitamin D are difficult to establish because of the extreme variations that exist in the production of vitamin D in the body.

An International Unit of vitamin D is 0.025 micrograms of pure vitamin D_3. This is a considerably smaller value than the 0.3 micrograms of retinol that represent an International Unit of vitamin A.

Deficiency conditions

As with other nutritional deficiencies, it seems needless for anyone to suffer from a vitamin D deficiency today, and yet rickets and osteomalacia are still occurring. The caricature of a cowboy with legs so bowed that a horse's belly will fit easily between them may seem to be a humorous reflection of a bygone era, and yet children today are growing up with similarly

pathetic legs, simply as a result of a vitamin D deficiency early in life.

Rickets is a nutritional deficiency condition characterized by poor calcification of the bones, resulting from the insufficient calcium absorption from the intestine. Specifically, the anterior fontanel is slow to close, there is a swelling of the epiphysis of the long bones, beadlike protrusions (rachitic rosary) develop on the ribs, pigeon breast may result, and the legs will begin to bow. In some instances, knock knees result, instead of bowed legs. X rays further verify the diagnosis of rickets. Children with rickets may appear to be plump and well nourished, but they tend to be a bit retarded in the rate at which they sit, stand, and walk. (It is an ironic note that one baby contest was won by twins who were diagnosed to have rickets just two days after their triumph.) Rickets can be corrected by vitamin D therapy (3000 International Units recommended daily),

Fat-Soluble Vitamins 251

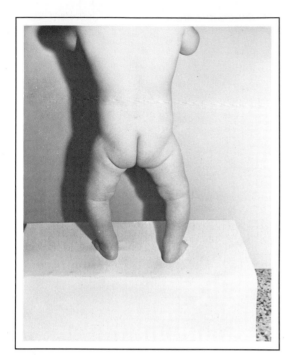

Bowed legs are the sign of rickets caused by a vitamin D deficiency during the growing years.

coupled with an adequate intake of milk. Mild bone deformities may disappear under this regimen, but serious deformities will remain throughout life.

Osteomalacia is the adult version of rickets. The usual background of the person who develops osteomalacia is a series of pregnancies and periods of lactation, combined with a low vitamin D intake and little exposure to the sun. This condition is characterized by pain in the pelvis, lower back and legs, and tenderness of the bones in these regions when pressure is placed upon them. In severe cases, bone fractures and involuntary twitching and muscle spasms occur. Extensive demineralization of the skeleton occurs. Treatment consists of administering 50,000 International Units of vitamin D daily for a period of one month (including milk at each meal) and then a daily vitamin D intake of 400 to 1000 International Units.

Toxicity

It seems ironic that a vitamin that historically has been the cause of considerable human suffering as a result of deficiency has now swung to the other extreme and has been creating concern because of possible excessive intake, and yet that is just what has happened with vitamin D in some instances. An excessive intake of vitamin D is accompanied by anorexia, excessive thirst, vomiting, weight loss, irritability, high blood calcium levels, and calcium deposition in soft tissues (including the walls of the blood vessels, kidneys, and lungs). Ultimately, continued overdosage of vitamin D can result in death.

Excessive vitamin D intake from food alone is unlikely. However, studies in England have suggested that intakes of vitamin D as low as 2500 to 4000 International Units may lead to the production of high blood-calcium levels in infants. This level of vitamin D could be reached if cod-liver oil and vitamin D-fortified infant cereals and milk were fed. These infants improved with withdrawal of vitamin D and calcium. This problem emphasizes the need for enrichment measures to be based on a consideration of the total dietary intake and not simply on a single food or narrow spectrum of the diet.

High-potency pharmaceutical preparations of vitamin D, including excessive intake of concentrated fish-liver oils, are potential sources of excessive intakes. Overdosages are far more easily reached in small children than they are in adults. Although individual sensitivity varies widely, a dosage of 10,000 International Units per day may result in toxicity in children of school age, and 10,000 International Units per day over a period of time may cause symptoms to develop in adults. Since foods in the United States have been fortified only to levels of 50 to 100 International Units per serving, and milk to 400 International Units per quart, foods in this country do not contain enough vitamin D to reach toxic levels. The difficulty with excessive dosages here is the result of self-prescribed vitamin supplements based on the theory that, if a little bit is good, still more is better.

Vitamin E

Vitamin E has caught the public's fancy under the designation of the antisterility vitamin, which presumably is fine if one is concerned about the reproductive capabilities of white rats. However, it seems safe to assume that there may be some confusion in the minds of some people who buy vitamin E in the hopes of enhancing their potency. The chemical nomenclature of the group of substances possessing vitamin E activity also reinforces the antisterility value of the vitamin for experimental animals. The group name for these substances is tocopherol, which means "to bear children." Although there are several tocopherols that occur in foods, the form with significant vitamin activity is alpha-tocopherol.

Functions

The outstanding characteristic of vitamin E is its antioxidant properties. Alpha-tocopherol is readily oxidized. As a result, other oxidizable substances such as ascorbic acid, vitamin A, and certain fats are not oxidized until all vitamin E present has been oxidized. Vitamin E, because it prevents the oxidation of both of these vitamins and unsaturated fatty acids, enables these essential nutrients to perform their specific functions in the body. Once these substances are oxidized, they can no longer react in their unique ways that are essential to the body.

In addition to the sparing action that vitamin E exerts in behalf of vitamin A, ascorbic acid, and unsaturated fatty acids, this nutrient also helps prevent hemolysis of erythrocytes. Recent research reports have indicated that smog contains various oxidants that produce peroxides that cause toxic manifestations in lung tissues and that may be lessened or prevented by vitamin E in the diet.

Dietary recommendations and sources

Vitamin E was included for the first time in the 1968 revision of the Food and Nutrition Board's recommendations for dietary allowances of essential nutrients. The 1974 recommendations, shown in Table 11.2, range from 4 International Units for the newborn to 15 International Units for adult males and pregnant and lactating women, values reduced significantly from those set originally in 1968. The International Unit for vitamin E is established as being equivalent to 1 milligram of synthetic alpha-tocopheryl acetate.

The establishment of a recommended intake of vitamin E was done on a somewhat arbitrary basis. Actually, the consumption of polyunsaturated fatty acids (PUFA), selenium, and a smoggy atmosphere may have a significant influence upon the body's need for this vitamin. The vitamin E requirement is increased by a high consumption of polyunsaturated fatty acids (and possibly smog). On the other hand, selenium, chromenols, and certain antioxidants exert a sparing action, thus decreasing the need for vitamin E.

Vitamin E is present in a wide range of foods, with particularly rich sources found in fats and polyunsaturated oils of vegetable origin. It is also found in meats, various animal products, and in green vegetables. The vitamin E value of fats and oils may be decreased by commercial processes that involve excessive heat and exposure to air (oxygen).

Deficiency

Ill health in humans specifically related to vitamin E deficiency is essentially unknown except for low-birth-weight infants, who may exhibit hemolysis of erythrocytes. This condition is corrected by feeding human milk or a commercial formula containing vitamin E.

Certain types of anemia resulting from a lack of vitamin E have been reported in the Middle East. Hemolysis of erythrocyte membranes, accompanied by decreased plasma tocopherol levels and increased urinary creatinine, have been attributed to a lack of vitamin E, but have not had an obvious impact on health.

Vitamin E deficiencies in experimental animals result in defective reproductive performance. White male rats become permanently sterile as a result of a vitamin E deficiency, while the female rarely conceives and will resorb the fetus if pregnancy is initiated. Addition of vitamin E to the diet before the fifth day of pregnancy usually remedies the problem for female rats. Similar or related effects because of a deficiency of this vitamin have never been found in man.

Various physical changes have been noted in different kinds of experimental animals when they are placed on vitamin E deficient diets. Chicks undergo changes of the central nervous system and have patchy, subcutaneous accumulations of fluids in scattered regions of the body. The muscular weakness noted in rabbits and other experimental animals suggested the possible treatment of muscular dystrophy in humans by administering vitamin E. Research on humans failed to reveal any connection between vitamin E deficiency and either muscular dystrophy or reproductive failures in humans.

Although vitamin E is a fat-soluble vitamin, it is unlike vitamins A and D in that there does not appear to be a problem with toxicity when dosages greatly in excess of the recommended level are ingested. Furthermore, this vitamin is used in the food industry as an important antioxidant additive in some foods to prolong their shelf life. Hence, addition of tocopherols to food is done for economic instead of altruistic or nutritional reasons.

Vitamin K

Vitamin K, often called the "antihemorrhagic" vitamin, has the dubious distinction of being the only fat-soluble vitamin for which no recommended allowance has been established. It was in Denmark that the role of this vitamin in blood coagulation was first noted. The name "vitamin K" signifies its role in "koagulation" (the Danish spelling).

As is true with other fat-soluble vitamins, vitamin K is actually a group of compounds, rather than a single type of structure. Vitamin K_1 is a group of phylloquinones found in plants, while the farnoquinones (vitamin K_2) are the products of microorganisms in the intestinal tract of animals. The parent compound of this group is commonly called menadione and has the impressive chemical name of 2-methyl-1, 4-naphthoquinone.

Functions

Vitamin K is intimately involved in the process of blood coagulation. One of the ways in which vitamin K functions in this important mechanism is to promote the formation of prothrombin. Prothrombin, in the presence of calcium, is converted to thrombin. Thrombin, in turn, is necessary for fibrinogen to be transformed into the clotting substance known as fibrin. Vitamin K is not a structural part of prothrombin, and yet the entire chain of reactions will not occur unless vitamin K is present to initiate prothrombin formation. Another substance required for coagulation—proconvertin —also requires the presence of vitamin K for its synthesis. Other facets of vitamin K's role in blood clotting may be discovered as the result of additional research.

Sources of vitamin K

With the tremendous strides in developing unusual food sources for human consumption, it may be of interest to point out that alfalfa is an extremely rich source of vitamin K, even though alfalfa is not (yet!) an important food for man. More conventional food sources such as dark green, leafy vegetables, liver, and egg yolks contain small amounts of vitamin K. However, there is virtually no likelihood of a deficiency occurring in any normal individual who is more than a few days old, because, as soon as the intestinal flora are established after

birth, bacteria in the intestine produce vitamin K, which is then absorbed and available. Synthesis of vitamin K by the intestinal bacteria is the main source of this vitamin, and explains why diseases characterized by chronic diarrhea or poor absorption are likely to also cause a vitamin K deficiency. This same situation may develop after prolonged use of certain types of antibiotics because they depress the intestinal flora.

Deficiency

Problems of hemorrhaging due to a vitamin K deficiency have been noted in some newborn infants and older people who have been receiving anticoagulant drugs. A vitamin K deficiency (and the potential for hemorrhaging) is a somewhat greater problem for the premature infant than for one born at full term. An injection of vitamin K during a woman's labor does enhance prothrombin formation in her offspring. Another alternative is to administer 0.5 to 1 milligram of vitamin K_1 immediately after birth. In addition, the practice of feeding infants soon after birth does begin the introduction of vitamin K. Cow's milk contains 60 micrograms of vitamin K per liter, and human milk averages approximately 15 micrograms.

Toxicity

Menadione (synthetic vitamin K_3) has been shown to be toxic to newborn infants at levels in excess of 5 milligrams. The excess of menadione apparently increases the breakdown of red-blood cells. Although placental transfer is limited, menadione is not included in vitamin preparations for pregnant women. This circumvents the possibility of building up a toxic level of vitamin K_3 in the fetus. However, vitamin K in the form of K_1 (phylloquinone) does not possess this toxic nature and, therefore, can be included in vitamin formulations.

The Water-Soluble B Vitamins

Thiamin

Thiamin is a member of the B-vitamin group and gains its distinction from the fact that it contains an atom of sulfur. The trail of research on thiamin crossed many international boundaries. Evidence of the curative powers of meat and milk, when added to the largely rice diet of the Japanese navy in the mid-nineteenth century, was clear; but the substance that accomplished the change in health was not crystallized from food until 1926. This vitamin, the first to be purified to a crystalline form, was studied intensively to determine its structure. Ten years later, in 1936, the structure was determined and the actual synthesis of the vitamin was accomplished by R. R. Williams.

Functions

As is the case with several other vitamins, thiamin is an extremely important substance in the body because of its role as a part of coenzymes essential for normal metabolism. Thiamin, as a part of the coenzyme thiamin pyrophosphate (TPP), is required in carbohydrate metabolism. Thiamin pyrophosphate is involved in decarboxylation reactions. This removal of carbon dioxide is part of the catabolic breakdown of carbohydrates. With inadequate thiamin to form the necessary thiamin pyrophosphate (TPP), intermediate metabolic compounds accumulate, causing the symptoms associated with a thiamin deficiency. For example, the decarboxylation of pyruvic acid pre-

paratory to entering the citric acid cycle (see Chapter 6) requires thiamin pyrophosphate. At yet another point in the metabolism of carbohydrates and fats, thiamin pyrophosphate is essential for the decarboxylation of alpha-ketoglutaric acid to form succinic acid.

Thiamin pyrophosphate aids in the formation of ribose (a five-carbon sugar) from glucose (six-carbon sugar) by activating the essential enzyme, transketolase. Although only a minor fraction of the body's glucose is converted into ribose, this nevertheless is a very important transformation, because ribose is a necessary constituent of DNA and RNA. Transketolase activity in the erythrocytes is directly related to the dietary adequacy of thiamin.

Beriberi

The condition that develops in humans when thiamin levels are inadequate is called beriberi. This condition, which became all too familiar in the nineteenth and early twentieth centuries, seems almost to be a product of civilization. Rice has formed a large fraction of the diet for numerous people in the world. The whole grain product, with its bran layer, was the form in which the food was commonly consumed for many generations. Gradually, the practice of eating the refined or polished rice began to be adopted by an ever-increasing number of people. Perhaps snob appeal played a significant role in stimulating this transition. Certainly, there is ample evidence that the prized polished white rice was gracing the tables of the elite long before it was generally available to the peasants. Unfortunately, the polished rice lacked something that was vital to good health. The result of the ingestion of large quantities of rice minus the bran layers was a large number of cases of beriberi.

Beriberi is characterized as causing a loss of appetite, nausea, vomiting, irritability, and depression. These symptoms appear to be the result of elevated levels of pyruvic acid as a consequence of limited thiamin pyrophosphate activity. Along with these obviously uncomfort-

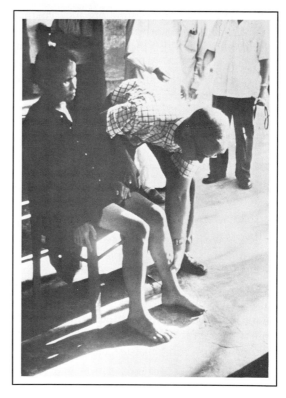

"Wet beriberi" is the result of a prolonged deficiency of thiamin. Note the indentations when the edematous legs are pressed with the finger. These depressions will swell again as the fluid collects again.

able symptoms, cramping in the legs is common; a very careful and difficult gait (much like trying to walk on marbles on a terrazzo floor) is noted; and, most important, heart functioning is impaired.

Beriberi in children up to six months of age is rapid in onset and critical in nature, because death can ensue in a very short period of time unless thiamin is administered. This problem is of greatest concern when babies are breast fed by mothers who are themselves eating diets very low in thiamin. Milk produced by thiamin-deficient mothers will be distinctly inadequate to meet the needs of the infants. In less-severe cases among older children, inadequate growth is a possible indicator of thiamin malnutrition, although other deficiencies may be contributing to the poor growth rate.

In adults, beriberi takes a more deliberate course than it does in children, but death can occur from a thiamin deficiency at any age. One form of beriberi observed in adults is termed, inelegantly, as "dry" beriberi. In dry beriberi, the patient appears emaciated and wasted. Weight loss is severe, and mental confusion and general low morale become evident. Beriberi can also take quite a different course; this second type of beriberi is referred to as "wet" beriberi. Edema or swelling of the tissues due to fluid retention is the noteworthy symptom. Ultimately, the heart muscle also becomes edematous and death results.

Utilization

Thiamin is absorbed in the small intestine in combination with various chemical compounds found in foods, such as allithiamin or thiamin hydrochloride. Although thiamin pyrophosphate is present in some foods, this molecule is not absorbed as such. The absorption of some large thiamin-complexed molecules is facilitated by the presence of hydrochloric acid in the stomach. Unfortunately, the acidity of the stomach tends to decrease in a thiamin deficiency, thus complicating the absorption of the small quantities of thiamin that may be present in the diet.

Recommended allowance

Thiamin is one of the water-soluble vitamins that has been included in the recommended allowances ever since they were first prepared by the Food and Nutrition Board. As can be seen in Table 11.4, the need for thiamin is correlated directly with the caloric intake of the individual. This comes as no surprise when one remembers the vital significance of thiamin in crucial metabolic reactions in the body. These energy-producing reactions have been clearly demonstrated to be dependent upon the availability of thiamin for the formation of the required coenzymes. For example, the highest level of thiamin recommended for males is for those in the 15 to 22 age bracket, a period in which the caloric recommendation also is at its peak. Notice, also, the increase in the thiamin recommendation for lactating women, this increase clearly paralleling the rise in caloric intake required for successful lactation. The recommendations for adults are based upon the value of 0.5 milligrams of thiamin for each 1000 kilocalories ingested. The increased allowance of 0.3 milligrams daily for the pregnant woman is based upon the modest increase in kilocalories that is recommended, although there may be a requirement for thiamin that goes beyond the need to metabolize more carbohydrates and fats during this period of stress. Older people appear to have a somewhat greater need for thiamin in proportion to the kilocalories consumed than do younger individuals, presumably because of less efficient utilization as the aging process progresses. Older persons should have a minimum intake of 1 milligram daily even if their caloric intake is less than 2000 kilocalories. Apparently more thiamin also is needed by individuals who are metabolizing a large quantity of alcohol. In contrast, a diet fairly high in fat content requires somewhat less thiamin for metabolic purposes than does a high carbohydrate diet.

Food sources

Reliable sources of thiamin include the meat group (particularly pork), the cereal group, plus additional quantities from milk and its products and the fruit and vegetable categories. Table 11.5 provides the basis for comparing some of the foods that are useful sources of thiamin, either by virtue of the content of a single serving or on the basis of the amounts ordinarily consumed as a basic part of the diet. As can be seen from this table, a wide variety of foods in the diet is useful in increasing the intake of thiamin. It is not necessary to rely on a vitamin supplement or wheat germ to procure thiamin in adequate quantities. Generally, good dietary patterns will provide this vitamin in sufficient quantities to insure satisfactory levels in the

Table 11.4 Recommended Daily Dietary Allowances for Kilocalories and the Water-Soluble Vitamins[a]

Age (years)	kcal	Thiamin (mg)	Riboflavin (mg)	Niacin (mg)[b]	B$_6$ (mg)	Folacin (μg)[c]	B$_{12}$ (μg)	Ascorbic Acid (mg)
Infants								
0.0–0.5	kg × 117	0.3	0.4	5	0.3	50	0.3	35
0.5–1.0	kg × 108	0.5	0.6	8	0.4	50	0.3	35
Children								
1–3	1300	0.7	0.8	9	0.6	100	1.0	40
4–6	1800	0.9	1.1	12	0.9	200	1.5	40
7–10	2400	1.2	1.2	16	1.2	300	2.0	40
Males								
11–14	2800	1.4	1.5	18	1.6	400	3.0	45
15–18	3000	1.5	1.8	20	2.0	400	3.0	45
19–22	3000	1.5	1.6	20	2.0	400	3.0	45
23–50	2700	1.4	1.7	18	2.0	400	3.0	45
51+	2400	1.2	1.5	16	2.0	400	3.0	45
Females								
11–14	2400	1.2	1.3	16	1.6	400	3.0	45
15–18	2100	1.1	1.4	14	2.0	400	3.0	45
19–22	2100	1.1	1.4	14	2.0	400	3.0	45
23–50	2000	1.0	1.2	13	2.0	400	3.0	45
51+	1800	1.0	1.1	12	2.0	400	3.0	45
Pregnancy	+300	+0.3	+0.3	+2	2.5	800	4.0	60
Lactation	+500	+0.3	+0.5	+4	2.5	600	4.0	80

[a] Adapted from **Recommended Daily Dietary Allowances,** revised 1974. Food and Nutrition Board, National Academy of Sciences—National Research Council.

[b] Although allowances are expressed as niacin, it is recognized that on the average 1 mg of niacin is derived from each 60 mg of dietary tryptophan.

[c] Folacin allowances refer to dietary sources as determined by **Lactobacillus casei** assay. Pure forms of folacin may be effective in doses less than one-fourth of the recommended dietary allowance.

body despite the fact that thiamin is not stored in the body.

For optimum thiamin content of foods, water losses in cooking should be held to a minimum. Where practical, the cooking water and the meat drippings can be utilized, for these often discarded liquids frequently contain appreciable amounts of the water-soluble thiamin as well as other water soluble nutrients. By avoiding the use of excessive quantities of water in food preparation, the loss of thiamin via the cooking water can be minimized. Low cooking temperatures and relatively brief duration of heating are other techniques for minimizing thiamin loss. However, palatability must also be kept in mind to enhance the likelihood that the food will be eaten. Thiamin contained in vitamin-rich foods with little eating appeal for the diner frequently is assigned to the impossible task of nourishing the plate rather than the

Table 11.5 Thiamin Content of Commonly Used Foods[a]

	Amount	Thiamin (mg)
Breads and cereals		
Bread, white enriched	1 slice	0.06
Bread, whole wheat	1 slice	0.06
Dinner roll, enriched	1 medium	0.11
Cream of wheat, cooked	1 cup	0.12
Oatmeal, cooked	1 cup	0.19
Shredded wheat	1 biscuit	0.06
Rice, cooked, enriched	1 cup	0.23
Noodles, cooked, enriched	1 cup	0.22
Spaghetti, cooked, enriched	1 cup	0.22
Macaroni, cooked, enriched	1 cup	0.20
Meat group		
Pork loin chop, lean, cooked	3 1/2 oz	1.13
center ham slice, lean, cooked	3 1/2 oz	0.58
Beef rump roast, lean, cooked	3 1/2 oz	0.07
ground, lean, cooked	3 1/2 oz	0.09
Veal loin chop, cooked	3 1/2 oz	0.07
Lamb loin chop, lean, cooked	3 1/2 oz	0.15
Chicken breast, fried	3 1/2 oz	0.05
Calf liver, fried	3 1/2 oz	0.24
Bologna	1 slice	0.08
Egg	1 medium	0.04
Peanut butter	2 tbsp	0.04
Mixed nuts	1 oz	0.17
Baked beans	1/2 cup	0.08
Split pea soup	1 cup	0.25
Vegetable—fruit group		
Asparagus spears, cooked	1/2 cup	0.11
Collard greens, cooked	1/2 cup	0.18
Peas, green, cooked	1/2 cup	0.22
Potato, baked	1 medium	0.10
Orange	1 medium	0.13
Orange juice	1/2 cup	0.11
Dairy group		
Milk, whole, 3.5% fat	1 cup	0.07
Milk, fortified low-fat	1 cup	0.10

[a] Data compiled and adapted from **Composition of Foods—Raw, Processed, Prepared.** Agriculture Handbook No. 8, U.S.D.A., 1963; **Nutritive Value of Foods,** Home and Garden Bulletin 72, U.S.D.A., 1971; and manufacturers' information.

consumer. Thiamin is more stable in an acidic than in an alkaline medium. Therefore, the use of baking soda when cooking green vegetables is not recommended, despite the fact that the green color is greatly enhanced by the soda (Table 11.3).

Riboflavin

One of the unique attributes of riboflavin is that it is a fluorescent chemical with a yellowish-green color. This fluorescent characteristic of pigments isolated from milk whey was noted in the latter part of the nineteenth century, at which time it was viewed more as an interesting phenomenon than as a nutritional discovery. In fact, the vitamin activity of this substance was not recognized until the 1930s. American and British scientists discovered independently that, although the autoclaving of yeast for a long period of time destroyed its beriberi-protective value, yet another growth factor contained in yeast remained active. This growth factor promptly received the name of vitamin G in the United States and vitamin B_2 in England. These preliminary studies were followed by the isolation of a hydrogen-carrying "yellow enzyme" by Otto Warburg of Berlin, and ultimately by the synthesis of riboflavin by Paul Karrer in Zurich, and Richard Kuhn in Heidelberg in 1935. This vitamin's name was coined by Karrer on the basis of its ribose and flavonoidlike moieties.

Functions

Riboflavin is an essential component of the coenzymes that occur in various flavoprotein enzyme systems. Riboflavin is combined with phosphoric acid to form flavin mononucleotide (FMN) or with adenine and phosphoric acid as flavin adenine dinucleotide (FAD). It is in either of these forms that riboflavin is combined with proteins to form the flavoprotein enzyme systems. These flavoprotein enzymes are essential for normal cellular respiration. Within the cell, there are numerous oxidation-reduction reactions that occur during the metabolic breakdown of carbohydrates, fats, and proteins. These reactions are dependent upon the presence of the enzyme systems that contain not only riboflavin, but also thiamin and niacin. Flavin mononucleotide and flavin adenine dinucleotide are capable of transferring a positive charge or a hydrogen atom, a process that occurs frequently when energy is being released from fatty acids, carbohydrates, and amino acids (following deamination). This vitamin functions in hydrogen transfer in protein metabolism, and specifically is needed to activate vitamin B for the conversion of the amino acid tryptophan into niacin (one of the B vitamins).

Deficiency

As a general rule, ariboflavinosis (a condition caused by a riboflavin deficiency) builds up over a period of time, instead of being sudden in its onset. Early symptoms include angular stomatitis and cheilosis. Angular stomatitis is characterized by fissures at the corners of the mouth, radiating outward to the skin and occasionally proceeding into the interior of the mouth as well. In cheilosis, there is cracking

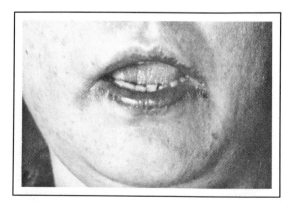

Angular fissures and cheilosis are symptoms of ariboflavinosis, a condition that is prevented by an adequate intake of riboflavin.

and soreness of both the upper and lower lips, particularly where the two lips meet. This condition may worsen, with the result that the tongue may also become involved. Glossitis develops, with its symptoms of an abnormally smooth tongue (because of papillary atrophy) and a color change to a magenta hue.

Symptoms of a riboflavin deficiency are not confined to the mouth and tongue. In children, growth failure occurs. The eyes become sensitive to light—tending to feel irritated and to water readily—and vision may be impaired. Vascularization of the cornea may cause complete opacity. The various symptoms of a riboflavin deficiency may occur in individuals with multiple nutritional deficiencies. Although this vitamin is recognized as being essential to man, a riboflavin deficiency serious enough to threaten life has not been reported. This has led to speculation that some riboflavin may be synthesized by intestinal flora and absorbed, thus somewhat minimizing the influence of a riboflavin-deficient diet.

Sources of riboflavin

As can be seen in Table 11.6, milk is the outstanding source of riboflavin. Other valuable sources of this vitamin are green vegetables, fish, eggs, and meats. Riboflavin is rather stable to heat and acid and is not readily oxidized. Unfortunately, riboflavin is very susceptible to destruction by ultraviolet light and sunlight. Consequently, the riboflavin content of milk is reduced when milk is marketed in clear glass bottles that may be exposed to direct sunlight. Despite the fact that this source of vitamin loss is well recognized, some milk still is marketed in clear glass rather than in brown-tinted glass bottles or plasticized cartons. The use of plasticized containers conserves the riboflavin content of milk, but often is criticized by consumers because of the tendency to leak. Of somewhat less significance in food preparation is the fact that riboflavin is destroyed in the presence of alkali. Since most of the foods containing riboflavin are acidic in reaction, the loss of ribo-

flavin because of the presence of alkali is largely a theoretical rather than a practical concern. Some riboflavin loss does occur when foods are cut into small pieces and cooked in water. Of course, this loss is related to the water soluble nature of riboflavin.

Recommended allowance

The 1974 recommended dietary allowances for riboflavin are based on the figure of 0.6 mg/1000 kcal consumed, a value deemed appropriate for people of all ages.

Niacin

To Joseph Goldberger, a physician with the U.S. Public Health Service, goes the credit for solving a mystery that had baffled others for more than a century. For many years, an unusual disease, known as pellagra in Italy and by various other names in other countries, had long been afflicting people with low incomes. Since this disease often developed in several members of a family, there were those who were convinced that this illness might be hereditary in origin. Others, noting that the living conditions of those afflicted with pellagra were frequently overcrowded and conducive to the spread of infectious diseases, pursued the approach of searching for a parasite or carrier that promoted the spread of pellagra. Goldberger was among those who felt that diet held the key to this condition. Through research conducted on convicts who volunteered for his project, Goldberger was able to demonstrate clearly that pellagra was indeed a dietary problem. The volunteers from the prison were placed on a diet considered to be typical of the pattern consumed by persons who had contracted pellagra. Over a period of several months, these prisoners began to develop the dermatitis, diarrhea, and dementia that are the classic symptoms of pellagra. This is considered to be the classic demonstration of the dietary causation of pellagra. Although this experiment was

Table 11.6 *Riboflavin Content of Commonly Consumed Foods*[a]

	Amount	Riboflavin (mg)
Dairy foods		
Milk, whole	1 cup	0.41
Milk, skim	1 cup	0.44
Milk, fortified low-fat	1 cup	0.51
Milk, buttermilk	1 cup	0.44
Eggnog, nonalcoholic	1 cup	0.45
"Instant" breakfast	1 cup	0.58
Yogurt, plain	1 cup	0.43
Cheese, cheddar	1 oz	0.13
Cheese, cottage	1/2 cup	0.28
Ice cream	1/2 cup	0.21
Meat group		
Beef, rump roast, lean, cooked	3 1/2 oz	0.22
Beef, sirloin steak, lean, broiled	3 1/2 oz	0.25
Veal loin chop, broiled	3 1/2 oz	0.25
Pork loin chop, lean, broiled	3 1/2 oz	0.33
center ham slice, lean	3 1/2 oz	0.23
Lamb leg roast, lean, roasted	3 1/2 oz	0.30
Chicken breast, fried	3 1/2 oz	0.22
Calf liver, fried	3 1/2 oz	4.17
Bologna	1 slice	0.07
Haddock, fried	3 1/2 oz	0.07
Tuna, oil packed	3 1/2 oz	0.12
Egg, whole	1 medium	0.12
Baked beans	1/2 cup	0.05
Peanuts, roasted	1 oz	0.07
Vegetables and fruits group		
Asparagus spears, cooked	1/2 cup	0.16
Broccoli, cooked	1/2 cup	0.15
Dandelion greens, cooked	1/2 cup	0.15
Spinach, cooked	1/2 cup	0.13
Squash, winter, cooked	1/2 cup	0.13
Sweet corn, cooked	1/2 cup	0.06
Sweet potato, cooked	1 medium	0.07
Banana	1 medium	0.07
Orange	1 medium	0.05
Watermelon	1 wedge	0.13

Table 11.6 (continued)

	Amount	Riboflavin (mg)
Breads and cereals group		
White bread, enriched	1 slice	0.05
Whole-wheat bread	1 slice	0.03
Shredded wheat	1 biscuit	0.03
Bran flakes with raisins	1 cup	0.07
Oatmeal, cooked	1 cup	0.05
Corn muffin	1 medium	0.08
Macaroni, enriched, cooked	1 cup	0.11

[a] Data compiled and adapted from **Composition of Foods—Raw, Processed, Prepared.** Agriculture Handbook No. 8, U.S.D.A., 1963; **Nutritive Value of Foods,** Home and Garden Bulletin No. 72, U.S.D.A., 1971; and manufacturers' information.

done in 1917, another 20 years of research were required before the dietary component essential to avoid pellagra was identified. In 1937, Conrad Elvehjem and some of his students, doing research at the University of Wisconsin, identified nicotinamide as the cure for "black tongue" in dogs—the analog of pellagra in man.

Functions

Niacin is a key component in two coenzymes that are vital to the release of energy from foods in the body. In the form of nicotinamide, niacin is a structural part of nicotinamide adenine dinucleotide (NAD) and nicotinamide adenine dinucleotide phosphate (NADP). These two compounds or coenzymes are identical, with one small exception. NADP contains one more phosphoric acid radical than does NAD. Both of these coenzymes are composed of ribose (a five-carbon sugar), a purine base, niacin, and phosphoric acid radicals. NAD and NADP have previously been known also as coenzymes I and II and diphosphopyridine nucleotide (DPN) and triphosphopyridine nucleotide (TPN). These coenzymes are important for the numerous reactions in tissue respiration involving the acceptance and release of hy-

drogen atoms to release energy during metabolism. Because of this capability, NAD and NADP are able to function in conjunction with the dehydrogenases (enzymes that remove hydrogen in biological reactions). NAD also serves as a coenzyme in enzyme systems that catalyze glycolysis and the reactions that are involved in fatty-acid synthesis. In metabolic reactions, niacin-containing coenzymes function in a complementary fashion with the cytochromes and flavoproteins (containing riboflavin) and other B vitamins to release energy via the electron transport system.

Recommended allowance

The recommended allowance for niacin is expressed as niacin equivalents. This terminology takes cognizance of the relationship between dietary tryptophan and niacin. Tryptophan is an essential amino acid which must be included in the human diet for normal growth and maintenance. In the presence of pyridoxine (vitamin B_6), thiamin, and riboflavin, this essential amino acid can be converted in the body to niacin. As might be anticipated, this conversion is far from being totally efficient. In fact, 60 milligrams of tryptophan are required to provide one milligram of niacin in the body. Therefore, a niacin equivalent is defined as 1 milligram of niacin or 60 milligrams of dietary tryptophan. When tryptophan is converted to niacin, it no longer is available for use in protein synthesis.

In the usual dietary patterns in the United States, approximately half of the daily intake of niacin is consumed as the vitamin itself, with the remainder being supplied by tryptophan.

As can be seen in Table 11.4, there is a gradual increase in the recommended intake of niacin equivalents throughout the growing years and again during periods of pregnancy and lactation. An infant up to 6 months of age has a recommended allowance of 5 milligrams, a recommendation which then increases to 8 milligrams. The value doubles by the time a person is 7 years old. The need for niacin reaches its peak period for males between the ages of 15 and 22, when the recommended allowance is 20 milligrams. The peak demand for niacin in females is from ages 7 to 14. These recommendations are a reflection of the body's need for this vitamin and a recognition of the relationship between the role niacin plays in energy metabolism and the total amount of food being ingested and processed by the body.

Dietary sources of niacin

Table 11.7 lists the niacin content of legumes, meats, cereals, fruits, and vegetables that are good sources of this vitamin. Niacin must be hydrolyzed in cereals to free it from the bound form in which it occurs naturally. This lack of availability of niacin may be a possible factor in the development of a niacin deficiency among individuals who rely very heavily on cereals for their sustenance. Estimates of the tryptophan contained in protein foods are based on the value of animal protein being comprised of approximately 1.4 percent tryptophan, and plant proteins being approximately 1 percent tryptophan.

The niacin content of foods is reasonably well maintained during most ordinary cooking procedures. This B vitamin is more stable to heat, light, oxidation, and variations in pH than are many of the other vitamins. Of course, there is some loss of this water-soluble vitamin when cooking procedures provide the opportunity for niacin to be leached out into the cooking water.

Deficiency

Although numerous dietary deficiencies have been considered significant problems in various parts of the world, perhaps the greatest concern historically in the United States has been the lack of niacin. A prolonged deficiency of niacin causes the disease known as pellagra. Pellagra has variously been termed the condition of the "three D's" and the "four D's." The three D's refer to the symptoms of diarrhea, dermatitis, and dementia, with the fourth D representing death. The dermatitis that develops in a niacin deficiency is somewhat unique in

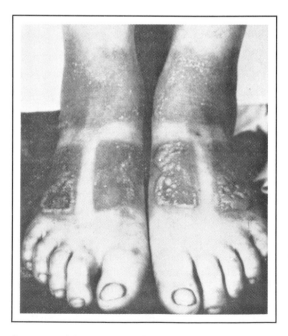

Symmetrical dermatitis of pellagra develops in a comparable manner on both sides of the body when exposed to light.

Table 11.7   Niacin Content of Commonly Used Foods[a]

	Amount	Niacin (mg)
Meat group		
Beef, sirloin steak, lean, broiled	3 1/2 oz	6.4
ground beef, lean, broiled	3 1/2 oz	6.0
Veal loin chop, lean, broiled	3 1/2 oz	5.4
Pork loin chop, lean, broiled	3 1/2 oz	6.8
center ham slice, lean, baked	3 1/2 oz	4.5
Lamb leg roast, lean, cooked	3 1/2 oz	6.2
Chicken breast, fried	3 1/2 oz	14.7
Turkey, light meat, roasted	3 1/2 oz	11.1
Calf liver, fried	3 1/2 oz	16.5
Bologna	1 slice	.8
Tuna fish, oil packed	3 1/2 oz	11.9
Swordfish, broiled	3 1/2 oz	10.9
Shrimp, cooked	3 1/2 oz	1.8
Egg	1 medium	Trace
Baked beans	1/2 cup	.7
Peanut butter	2 tbsp	4.7
Breads and cereals group		
Bread, white enriched	1 slice	.6
Bread, whole wheat	1 slice	.6
Cream of wheat	1 cup	1.0
Rice, enriched, cooked	1 cup	2.1
Noodles, enriched, cooked	1 cup	1.9
Vegetables and fruits group		
Broccoli, cooked	Medium stalk	1.4
Collard greens, cooked	1/2 cup	1.2
Peas, cooked	1/2 cup	1.8
Potato, baked	1 medium	1.7
Tomato, ripe	1 medium	1.3
Banana, ripe	1 medium	.8
Peach, ripe	1 medium	.5

[a] Data compiled and adapted from **Composition of Foods—Raw, Processed, Prepared,** Agriculture Handbook No. 8, U.S.D.A., 1963; **Nutritive Value of Foods,** Home and Garden Bulletin No. 72, U.S.D.A., 1971; and from manufacturers' information.

that it is symmetrical. Symmetrical, as used in the sense of the symmetrical dermatitis of pellagra, means that skin rashes develop in comparable positions on both sides of the body. These rashes typically are found on areas of the body that are exposed to sunlight. The skin is dry, scaly, and cracked. Caucasians with pellagra will develop discolorations similar to a sunburn, while Negroes develop hyperpigmentation. If the lower neck and upper chest are exposed to sunlight, the pellagrous individual will develop skin lesions that are referred to as Casal's neckline. The tongue may become scarlet red and smooth in appearance.

Other symptoms of pellagra are noted in the digestive tract. Abdominal pain and diarrhea may present considerable discomfort. The mental involvement may be made manifest as irritability, anxiety, poor memory, and insomnia. These disturbances sometimes become such a problem that the patient is hospitalized for mental illness, when, in fact, the cause may simply be a lack of niacin in the diet. In some instances, there may be some impairment of coordination and physical movement, but this is of limited significance. In instances where pellagra is not treated and dietary restriction is severe, the patient may die.

Satisfactory nutritional status can be restored for persons who have developed pellagra, and usually in a few days. Treatment involves niacinamide dosages of about 100 to 500 milligrams daily for a few days; regular inclusion of foods in the diet that are good sources of niacin; and a diet containing 100 grams of high-quality protein daily until all symptoms have disappeared. Of course, the diet should continue to provide the recommended allowance of niacin so that pellagra will not develop again.

The incidence of pellagra in the United States has been highest among persons eating restricted diets, generally those relying heavily on corn, molasses, and salt pork. In such diets, corn does provide protein in the diet, but zein, the predominant protein in corn, is low in tryptophan, and the small amount of niacin that is found in corn is largely unavailable. Since the use of corn is widespread in the southern part of this country, the enrichment of corn products with niacin is an effective means of helping to prevent pellagra in the southern states.

Vitamin B_6

In comparison with some of the other vitamins, vitamin B_6 is a relative newcomer. The structure and synthesis of pyridoxine were accomplished in 1939. Attention was first directed to the existence of vitamin B_6 when it was noted that pyridoxine (one form of vitamin B_6) cured a dermatitis in white rats. This vitamin has been the subject of considerable research during the past decade, as experimentalists have sought clarification of the role of vitamin B_6 in the body. Particular interest has centered on the importance of this vitamin in amino acid metabolism.

Functions

Vitamin B_6 is an inclusive term for pyridoxine, pyridoxal, and pyridoxamine. These three forms of vitamin B_6 can be phosphorylated by the enzyme phosphokinase. Pyridoxal phosphate is the primary coenzyme form of the vitamin, although pyridoxine phosphate also functions as a coenzyme in transaminases. Pyridoxal is a part of glycogen phosphorylase, and a major portion of the body stores of vitamin B_6 is found in this enzyme. Glycogen phosphorylase is needed to convert glycogen to glucose-phosphate, the first step in releasing energy from glycogen. The role of pyridoxine in fat metabolism is obscure at the present time.

It is in protein metabolism where vitamin B_6 plays a particularly significant role in the body. Pyridoxal phosphate is an important coenzyme for transaminases, deaminases, decarboxylases, and other enzymes. Transamination reactions are necessary in order that the amino group of an amino acid may be transferred to certain alpha-keto compounds to make new amino acids that may be needed by the body for protein synthesis. Deamination—the removal of an amino group from an amino acid—is a necessary step before the remainder of the amino acid radical may be metabolized for the release of energy to the body.

Decarboxylation is the removal of carbon dioxide from an amino acid. Histamine, serotonin, and norepinephrine (essential body-regulating compounds) are synthesized in the body as a result of decarboxylation. Pyridoxal phosphate also is needed for the synthesis of a precursor of porphyrin (part of the hemoglobin molecule), for the production of antibodies, and possibly for enzymes that are of importance to the normal functioning of the central nervous system.

As mentioned previously, vitamin B_6 participates in the conversion of tryptophan to niacin. Pyridoxal phosphate is needed to change 3-hydroxykynurenine (an intermediate compound formed as tryptophan is being converted to niacin) to niacin. In a vitamin B_6 deficiency, xanthurenic acid is formed from 3-hydroxykynurenine, instead of the niacin that is needed. The xanthurenic acid is excreted in the urine, where its quantitative presence can be determined. Determination of the adequacy of vitamin B_6 in the diet can be made by feeding a high level of tryptophan and then measuring the amount of xanthurenic acid in the urine. If the vitamin B_6 nutriture is inadequate, the levels of xanthurenic acid excreted will be significantly higher than for individuals who have been ingesting sufficient vitamin B_6.

Recommended allowance

The 1968 revision of the Food and Nutrition Board's recommended daily dietary allowances marked the first time that vitamin B_6 had been included. During gestation, vitamin B_6 is stored in the fetus in a quantity sufficient to enable the newborn to survive, even when his diet after birth is low in this vitamin. Because of this reservoir of vitamin B_6, the newborn is able to metabolize the relatively low quantities of protein that are found in human milk. However, the problem is intensified for utilizing the higher protein content of cow's milk formulas if the pyridoxine intake is inadequate. Proprietary formulas containing 0.015 milligrams of vitamin B_6 per gram of protein are sufficient to prevent symptoms of a vitamin B_6 deficiency. The normal growth and development (physically and mentally) of young children requires an adequate intake of vitamin B_6. The recommended intake of vitamin B_6 is high during pregnancy to insure adequate deposition of this vitamin in the fetus. The level during lactation is based on the need to provide the vitamin B_6 that will be secreted in the milk.

Sources of vitamin B_6

The food sources of pyridoxine are mainly plants; pyridoxal and pyridoxamine are found in foods of animal origin. Any of these forms of vitamin B_6 can be utilized easily in the body. Meats are particularly rich sources of vitamin B_6. Other good sources include bananas, whole-grain cereals, lima beans, cabbage, potatoes, and spinach. Although not a rich source of vitamin B_6, milk contains enough of this vitamin to be a useful source for people who drink it regularly.

Deficiency

A deficiency of vitamin B_6 is not an ordinary occurrence, but individuals with this problem have been observed. Symptoms of a deficiency include hyperirritability, convulsions, loss of weight, depression, confusion and anemia. There also is an increased tendency to excrete oxalate in the urine, which results in renal calcium oxalate stones in animals. (The fad of extremely large intakes of vitamin C for the treatment and prevention of the common cold may also cause more oxalate stones.) Hyperirritability and convulsions were observed some years ago in infants who were inadvertently fed a vitamin B_6-deficient diet, the result of a change in the processing technique that destroyed vitamin B_6 in a commercial milk formula. Adults who were intentionally depleted of vitamin B_6, with or without the use of an antagonist, developed symptoms that included loss of appetite, weight loss, general weakness, and lassitude. A hypochromic microcytic anemia and high serum-iron level also may occur.

The use of oral contraceptives by women appears to modify the body's need for this vitamin. In particular, tryptophan metabolism is impaired unless additional vitamin B_6 is administered. Up to 30 milligrams daily may be needed by some women to compensate for the effect of the estrogens.

Pantothenic acid

The ubiquitous occurrence of pantothenic acid is reflected in its name, which is derived from the Greek word meaning "everywhere". Like the other B vitamins, pantothenic acid is water soluble. It is fairly stable when food is prepared by moist heat at essentially a neutral pH. In dry heat, acid, or alkali, this vitamin is somewhat unstable. Vitamin supplements ordinarily contain the crystalline calcium pantothenate rather than the acid form.

Functions

Pantothenic acid is essential in the body because it is a component of coenzyme A (commonly referred to as CoA). This coenzyme is composed of pantothenic acid (which has been combined with a sulfur-containing substance to form pantotheine), plus a molecule of adenine and a phosphate radical. Coenzyme A is essential for accepting and transferring two carbon fragments known as acetate and for the formation of CoA derivatives of many important metabolites. Coenzyme A is required to start each cycle in the beta oxidation of fatty acids. Hence, CoA is a central substance in the numerous energy-related metabolic reactions in the body. Pantothenic acid, by virtue of its presence in CoA, is thus involved in the release of energy from carbohydrates, fats, and proteins. As shown in Chapter 6, CoA is necessary for the transfer of two-carbon acetate units for the Krebs citric acid cycle. This important coenzyme also functions in synthetic reactions. For example, coenzyme A is involved in the synthesis of porphyrin (in hemoglobin formation), some steroid hormones, and cholesterol. The synthesis of fatty acids is also dependent upon the capability of CoA to transfer acetate.

Food sources and body requirements

It is estimated that the diet of adults in the United States ordinarily provides between 10 and 15 milligrams of pantothenic acid daily. Although no recommended allowance for pantothenic acid has been proposed by the Food and Nutrition Board, it appears that an intake between 5 and 10 milligrams is sufficient for children and adults. Hence, there appears to be little likelihood of a dietary deficiency of this essential nutrient.

Food sources of pantothenic acid are very numerous. In fact, almost any food contains this vitamin. Particularly rich sources of pantothenic acid include the various organ meats. Whole-grain cereals are also excellent sources of this B vitamin. Under ordinary circumstances, it is not necessary to give special attention to the inclusion of foods rich in pantothenic acid.

Deficiency

The symptoms of a pantothenic acid deficiency are somewhat diverse from one species to another. For example, chicks develop a dermatitis around the eyes and beak, accompanied by poor feathering and impaired growth. Symptoms of a pantothenic acid deficiency were developed in man by feeding a diet relatively low in pantothenic acid and administering omega-methyl pantothenic acid, an antivitamin. Within a period of months, the experimental subjects became fatigued, slept poorly, experienced abdominal discomfort, headaches, occasional vomiting, and cramping of leg muscles, frequently accompanied by poor motor coordination. Of particular significance was the loss of ability to produce antibodies when both pantothenic acid and vitamin B_6 were lacking, and the slow production of antibodies when either of these B vitamins was deficient. A rather unusual symptom that also was noted in a pantothenic acid deficiency was a burning sensation in the feet.

Biotin

The inclusion of biotin in the B vitamins is the subject of some controversy. Certainly, biotin is required in small amounts to perform specific vital functions in the body. On that basis, there would appear to be little reason to question its classification as a vitamin. However, biotin is synthesized in the intestine and is readily absorbed. Hence, its status as a vitamin is not clear. Biotin was studied in various forms before it was finally synthesized in 1943. It is now recognized that there are at least five forms of biotin that occur in food and have activity in the body.

Functions

Biotin is needed to form aspartate from pyruvate. This vitamin functions in both carboxylation and decarboxylation reactions. In short, biotin is essential for the release of energy from carbohydrates, for the synthesis and oxidation reactions involved in fatty acid metabolism, and for the deamination of amino acids that must occur for energy to be released from proteins. Biotin may also be needed for the transformation of tryptophan to niacin and for for-

mation of pancreatic amylase, an important carbohydrase.

Recommended intake

In view of the issues regarding the inclusion of biotin as a vitamin, it is not surprising that there is no recommended allowance for this substance. The diet alone normally provides between 150 and 300 micrograms of biotin, and still more is available to the body as the result of intestinal synthesis and absorption. Therefore, a biotin deficiency cannot be viewed as a routine concern for nutritionists. Apparently, 150 micrograms of biotin is ample for the body's needs. Particularly rich sources of biotin include egg yolks, milk, and organ meats, but it is also found in cereals, legumes, and nuts.

Deficiency

Considerable ingenuity and a drastic modification in diet were required to demonstrate the effects of a biotin deficiency. Since biotin is very widespread throughout man's normal foods, the diet had to be altered to include more than 30 percent of the total caloric intake from raw egg white. In practical terms, this amounts to more than two dozen egg whites per day. The egg white contains avidin, a protein which, in its native state, forms a large complex with biotin and prevents the absorption of the biotin. One has to consider only briefly the grim prospect the experimental group faced in consuming such a diet before it becomes apparent that these men doubtless faced psychological as well as nutritional problems in adhering to the regimen. The experimental subjects showed such symptoms as loss of appetite, depression, fatigue, nausea, a scaling dermatitis, hypercholesterolemia, and changes in their electrocardiograms. It is perhaps difficult to clearly distinguish between lack of biotin and psychological responses to the diet as causes of some of these symptoms.

Experimental animals also developed dermatitis. In addition, they had some spastic paralysis of the legs and the spectacle-eye syndrome.

Folacin

One can only be grateful that scientists have chosen to use the name "folacin" rather than its chemical name "tetrahydropteroylglutamic acid" as the designation for this member of the B vitamin group. Folacin is also referred to as folic acid. Folacin is particularly appropriate nomenclature for this vitamin, which occurs abundantly in foliagelike vegetables. This B vitamin was first studied as the "Wills Factor" by Dr. Lucy Wills of India, who was searching for a cure for a megaloblastic anemia that presented a medical problem among pregnant women in India in the 1930s.

Functions

Folacin has the capability of receiving single-carbon units from one compound and transferring these units to other molecules. These single-carbon units may be in the form of methyl, formyl, or hydroxymethyl groups. The transfer mechanism is vital to the synthesis of numerous compounds in the body. Folacin, in a coenzyme form, aids in various intracellular reactions including the synthesis of (1) guanine and adenine (purines that are components of nucleic acids), (2) thymine (a pyrimidine in nucleic acids), (3) the formation of choline from ethanolamine, (4) the interconversion of various amino acids (phenylalanine to tyrosine and glycine to serine are examples), and (5) formation of the porphyrin of hemoglobin.

As a result of the vital role folacin plays in the formation of nucleic acids, it may be concluded that this vitamin is necessary for cell growth and reproduction. Folacin functions in the degradation of amino acids as well as synthesis of some nonessential amino acids.

Recommended allowance

The 1968 revision of the recommended allowances marked the first time that the Food and Nutrition Board had designated a recommendation for the intake of folacin. One of the interesting aspects of the levels recommended in both 1968 and 1974 is revealed in Table 11.4. The recommendation for pregnant women is twice that for other adult women. This reflects the rather large increase in the incidence of megaloblastic anemia during the last trimester of pregnancy, when there apparently is a stress situation placed upon the maternal supply of folacin to meet the sharply increasing demands of the fetus. In some illnesses, there is also a need for increased folacin in the diet.

The recommendations for folacin intake are the same throughout life for both men and women (with the exceptions for periods of pregnancy and lactation). This is in contrast to the larger quantities of thiamin, riboflavin, and niacin that are recommended for men in comparison with the levels recommended for women. The dietary recommendations are intended to be used as a daily value. As with the other B vitamins, storage of folacin is distinctly limited.

Food sources

Particularly important sources of folacin include spinach and other dark green, leafy vegetables, mushrooms, liver, and kidney. Various other vegetables and fruits are also generally good sources of this vitamin. Actually, the amount of folacin in a food serving may be highly variable, depending upon the preparation procedures involved. Losses may range as high as 90 percent. Storage of fresh produce for a few days and prolonged cooking periods are particularly detrimental to folacin levels in foods.

Deficiency

In healthy individuals, a folacin deficiency is not a common occurrence. However, some conditions such as sprue, pellagra, and leukemia may impair the utilization of folacin, thus causing a deficiency condition to develop. In a folacin deficiency, macrocytic anemia is noted. Along with this abnormal red-blood-cell development, lesions of the alimentary canal and diarrhea are noted. These changes in the digestive tract lead to further deficiency of folacin because of the impaired absorption of the vitamin. There is some indication that the body's ability to form antibodies is impaired as a result of a decrease in the number of white blood cells produced.

A folacin deficiency may be caused by an inadequate dietary intake of the vitamin, malabsorption of this nutrient, an unusual need for folacin, or by metabolic abnormalities. A deficiency of this vitamin is almost a routine finding among alcoholics. Infants receiving some proprietary formulas without a vitamin supplement may also develop a folacin deficiency.

The blood picture for a folacin deficiency is one factor that attracted researchers to an intensive study of this vitamin. When this nutrient's influence on the development of red blood cells was first noted, it was hoped that this might prove to be the answer to treating pernicious anemia, a condition that was eventually fatal to the patient (see next section). The ability of folacin to correct the macrocytic anemia was demonstrated conclusively, and it was first felt that pernicious anemia patients might benefit from its use. However, folacin was only effective in improving the blood picture, but not alleviating the accompanying nervous system changes. A prescription of more than 0.1 milligram of folacin daily is available only upon the written statement of a physician. This precaution is taken to avoid the possibility a high intake of folacin will mask the symptoms of the more serious problem of pernicious anemia, thus delaying treatment unnecessarily. Antifolic acid compounds have found a limited use in the treatment of leukemia by interfering with the excessive growth and proliferation of white blood cells.

Vitamin B_{12}

If one were to seek unique characteristics of vitamin B_{12}, two aspects would be noted readily. This red-colored vitamin, the most recently isolated of the vitamins, is a surprisingly large and unwieldy molecule, and it contains an atom of cobalt. Original note of this substance was made when Drs. George Minot and William Murphy of Boston found that the ingestion of large quantities of raw liver remedied pernicious anemia. It was concluded that some unknown substance in the raw liver corrected a deficiency in pernicious anemia patients. This mysterious factor was designated by Dr. William Castle, one of their co-workers, as the "extrinsic" factor, since it was obtained from an external source rather than being present naturally in the body. Researchers then clarified that normal individuals had an "intrinsic" factor as a regular component of the gastric juice/After much painstaking research, it finally became apparent that Castle's extrinsic factor was vitamin B_{12} or cobalamin, as vitamin B_{12} is frequently called.

Functions

Although vitamin B_{12} is needed by all cells, it is particularly important in the nervous system, the digestive tract, and the bone marrow. With inadequate vitamin B_{12}, erythrocytes fail to mature. Instead, the large red blood cells that are typical of pernicious anemia are produced. This appears to be the consequence of the synthesis of too little thymine to produce the necessary nucleic acid, DNA. In addition to the failure to develop a sufficient number of mature erythrocytes, nervous disorders also are observed. The problems of the central nervous system in a vitamin B_{12} deficiency appear to stem from a disruption of normal carbohydrate metabolism. This action may be the result of impaired production of enzymes that are essential to normal carbohydrate metabolism. Carbohydrates are known to be the source of energy for this system. The accumulation of pyruvic acid and lactic acid in a vitamin B_{12}-deficient individual is suggestive of the limited utilization of carbohydrates.

Cobalamin is an important key to the synthesis of numerous compounds in the body, since it is required for the formation of the single carbon radicals needed for synthesis of more complex biochemical compounds in the body. It also appears to play a role in protein and fat metabolism.

Recommended allowance

Vitamin B_{12} is another of the B vitamins that were added to the daily recommended dietary allowances in the Food and Nutrition Board's 1968 revision. The 1974 recommendations (see Table 11.4) suggest a 0.3 microgram daily for infants, with an increase to 3 micrograms for adults, and a slight increase to 4 micrograms for pregnant and lactating women. There is no variation in the recommendation for adults on the basis of either age or sex.

Sources

Animal foods are good sources of cobalamin, whereas plant foods contain none. Persons in good health normally will not need to be concerned about the adequacy of vitamin B_{12} if they are eating a normal diet that includes animal foods. This vitamin is retained reasonably well in ordinary food preparation procedures.

The problems of a deficiency condition are the result of eating a strict vegetarian diet (vegans) or of a faulty mechanism for absorbing the bulky vitamin. A deficiency due to inadequate ingestion of cobalamin can be corrected by including more animal foods, including eggs, milk, and cheese. For the individual with impaired absorption, the vitamin is administered by injection so that the absorption problem will be circumvented. In other words, a vitamin B_{12} deficiency may be either dietary or physical in origin.

Deficiency

A deficiency of vitamin B_{12} results in the condition known as pernicious anemia, a disease that formerly was always fatal. The symptoms of pernicious anemia include a general feeling of weakness and fatigue, glossitis or smoothness of the tongue, sore and cracked lips and other mucus membranes, involvement of the central nervous system, and a decrease (which may be complete) in the amount of hydrochloric acid in the stomach.

Treatment of pernicious anemia requires injections of vitamin B_{12} on a regular basis throughout life. The inability to absorb vitamin B_{12} is not corrected when the pernicious anemia itself has been relieved. The lack of availability of the intrinsic factor, which is required for absorption, is not changed. In normal individuals, the absorption of vitamin B_{12} requires intimate contact with a receptor in the intestinal wall. Calcium plays a significant role in aiding the transport of this vitamin through the intestinal wall. Other factors influencing absorption capability are age, level of thyroid activity, adequate iron, and sufficient pyridoxine.

Ascorbic acid

Frequently, the flavor of history is lost as man's heritage and happenings are transcribed onto pages that will ever after represent the era they depict. Indeed, even when such a fascinating and very human subject as nutrition is studied, the information may tend to resemble an encyclopedic presentation more closely than is desired by the student. The last of the water-soluble vitamins to be considered in this chapter, however, provides a truly colorful and fascinating opportunity to view history in the most human of terms.

Ascorbic acid, or vitamin C, long ago presented brief glimpses of today's world of nutrition to our ancestors of more than 10 generations ago. No doubt Dr. James Lind, a mid-eighteenth century physician in the British navy, would be surprised and more than a little gratified to learn that his dietary experiments, using the British sailors as subjects, are recognized as the first significant milestone in the development of the field of nutrition. Sailors had the questionable distinction of exemplifying various nutritional deficiency diseases during the period when explorers were sailing their expeditions to the many remote parts of the world formerly unknown to the Europeans.

It is easy to recognize today that the living conditions of the common seaman were ideally suited to the development of nutritional deficiencies, if not to luxurious travel. The ships sailed slowly, distances were great and generally unknown, ports of call for provisions were more a matter of chance than of predetermination, and food processing and storage were far different from the possibilities provided by food technology today. In less poetic terms, rations were distinctly a matter of expediency and space. Nutrition, as it is understood today, simply was not a part of man's knowledge. What was known was that some foods spoiled quickly and would not provide the necessary sustenance for long trips. It was also a clear and undisputed fact that many sailors would become weak or sick before the end of the journey, and indeed, that some would die. Losses of two thirds of the crew by Vasco da Gama and half by Captain Cook were simply a part of the risk of such extended exploration. The British relied heavily on their sailing forces, and such gross losses of manpower attracted the attention of Dr. Lind. He viewed the health problems of sailors with the eye of a scientist and devised a theory that various acids might be useful in preventing the scurvy he had recognized in the crew. By contemporary standards, his experimental group, each consisting of two sailors with scurvy, were distinctly small. However, he regulated the diets of each group of two. One pair was fed the ship's ration plus sulfuric acid in water, another received vinegar in addition to the normal fare, the third had a couple of cups of sea water, and the others had an added ration of oranges and a lemon daily. The scorbutic sailors on the first three supplements did not improve, but those receiving the citrus fruit recovered in about a week. The vitamin era was beginning.

Dr. Lind's findings were sufficiently dramatic to prompt interest in the value of a modified state to minimize illness on long sea voyages. However, half a century elapsed before the recommended change in diet became official. It is not clear whether the 50-year delay in the mandatory improvement of the British navy's diet stands as a tribute to the efficiency of committee action or whether this is yet another demonstration of the great difficulty that is encountered when diet modification is attempted. In any event, history loudly proclaims the fact that the British navy's diet was improved, for these proud sailors still carry the burden of the rather ignominious nickname of "limeys," a title granted in recognition of the regulation requiring that the vessels carry an adequate supply of limes (or other citrus).

All the credit for using diet to prevent scurvy should not be given to the British. Indians in Canada were credited with saving Cartier's expedition by teaching the Frenchmen to brew an infusion made from spruce bark. Spanish and French ships commonly carried large quantities of onions as routine ingredients for preparing their customary fare. Though one might speculate upon the fact that illness was reduced because of the social void that large quantities of onions might create for the crews, the practical fact is that onions, when consumed in many foods as regular fare, do provide a useful amount of ascorbic acid.

With such a rich history, it seems a bit surprising that ascorbic acid was labeled as vitamin C because vitamin A and vitamin B (as the group was first called before researchers were aware of the individual vitamins) were both studied and alphabetically designated before vitamin C came to the fore. Two different laboratories, King and Waugh's in Pittsburgh, and Szent-Gyorgi's in Szeged, Hungary, are credited with the isolation of ascorbic acid in the early 1930s.

Functions

Clarification of specific roles of ascorbic acid in the human body remains a challenge to nutrition researchers today. Despite intensive investigation, the functions this vitamin performs have not been thoroughly elucidated. One recognized role of vitamin C is in the maturation of collagen throughout all tissues of the body. Connective tissue serves to cement the cells and tissues together, and has as its principal component the unique protein, collagen. Mature collagen is unusual because it contains very high amounts of the amino acids, glycine and hydroxyproline. During the synthesis of the amino acid chains of procollagen in the cell, proline is incorporated at the appropriate points. During maturation, proline is converted to hydroxyproline by enzyme action which requires ascorbic acid.

When hydroxyproline is not present in sufficient quantities, the individual amino acid chains do not crosslink with each other adequately; collagen does not become highly insoluble and have high tensile strength. Whenever collagen does not mature, wounds do not heal properly and break down readily due to the low tensile strength of the newly forming collagen fibrils.

This function of vitamin C was rather dramatically demonstrated by a young surgeon interested in wound healing, John Crandon of Boston. He consumed a diet deficient in ascorbic acid for six months, at which time incisions were made in his skin. The wounds did not heal over a period of several weeks while he continued on the experimental diet, but healing occurred dramatically when therapeutic doses of the vitamin were administered.

It has also been observed that the protein matrix of bone and dentin form abnormally in vitamin C deficiency. In severe and prolonged deficiency, bone matrix formation ceases which, in experimental animals, leads to separation of the epiphyses from the shafts of the long bones. The odontoblasts, which are the cells in teeth required to form dentin, fail to function normally in an ascorbic acid deficiency. Again, in severe and prolonged deficiency, dentin formation ceases and the crowns of the teeth are thin and fragile due to the reduced amount of dentin in the finished product. Mineralization does not appear to be affected in vitamin C deficiency but the problem is one of insufficient matrix formation to mineralize.

Ascorbic acid also is important to maintain the elasticity and strength of normal capillary walls. With insufficient vitamin C for collagen formation, there is an accompanying increase in the fragility of blood vessels. This fragility results in minute hemorrhages subcutaneously.

As was discussed in Chapter 10, iron is more readily absorbed and utilized when it occurs as the ferrous (or reduced) iron. Since ascorbic acid is readily oxidized, it appears probable that this vitamin is effective in promoting iron utilization by simply maintaining the iron in the reduced state, thus favoring its absorption.

The conversion of folacin to the active form of the vitamin is aided by the presence of ascorbic acid. It is presumably because of this function that vitamin C is useful in preventing infants from developing a megaloblastic anemia.

Ascorbic acid also serves a function in metabolism of some amino acids. Vitamin C is important to the maintenance of normal tyrosine metabolism. An enzyme required to effect the catabolism of tyrosine so that it may be excreted is inhibited when vitamin C is lacking. The conversion of both tyrosine and phenylalanine to the hormones, thyroxine and adrenaline, may require ascorbic acid. Also, tryptophan can be converted to serotonin *in vitro* when ascorbic acid is present.

The role of ascorbic acid in preventing or overcoming infections has been fraught with controversy, and even became a topic of general conversation and heated debate as recently as 1971. Although ascorbic acid does appear to have a protective role when consumed at the recommended level, this alone is no complete guarantee that colds and other infections will never be contracted. The ingestion of the recommended quantities of ascorbic acid is to be viewed as some protection rather than complete insurance against infections. As of this writing, evidence to support the hypothesis that massive doses of ascorbic acid will prevent and cure the common cold is lacking (see Chapter 5). The lack of experimental evidence frequently tends to be obscured by the emotional fervor and conviction of persons arguing in support of this regimen. There is increasing evidence that massive doses of ascorbic acid may actually be harmful to some. The Food and Nutrition Board, in discussing the 1974 revision of recommended dietary allowances, stated that it felt that many of these claims are not sufficiently substantiated, or the effects are not of significant magnitude, and that "routine consumption of large amounts of ascorbic acid is not advisable without medical advice."[1]

Recommended allowances

The recommended allowances for ascorbic acid are presented in Table 11.4. These values are far more than minimal to prevent the development of scurvy and to provide a reasonable degree of protection against infections. Although the values that are recommended for the intake of this vitamin have varied somewhat from the initial recommendations of the Food and Nutrition Board, the trend is downward. At no time have the recommendations been anywhere near the very high levels advocated by a few individuals at the present time.

Dietary sources

Oranges and other citrus fruits and vitamin C have become virtually synonymous in the

[1] Food and Nutrition Board. *Recommended Dietary Allowances*. National Research Council–National Academy of Sciences. Washington, D.C. 8th ed. P. 64. 1974.

United States, and there is certainly no reason to question the merits of citrus in the fresh form or as processed juices. As can be seen in Table 1.5, these foods are fine sources of ascorbic acid. Other excellent sources are also included in the table. It is rather common practice among many families to include vitamin C in the diet as a supplementary nutrient rather than relying on good nutritional practices to provide this vitamin in the food consumed. The body utilizes synthetic vitamin C as effectively as it does the vitamin found in foods. When individuals are not eating sufficient vitamin C in the diet regularly, synthetic vitamin C provides an inexpensive solution to meeting the problem. However, the joy of swallowing a tablet or capsule seems a rather dreary choice in comparison with the enjoyment of getting one's ascorbic acid by eating fresh strawberries or a fresh grapefruit.

Ascorbic acid is easily oxidized and its vitamin activity lost. Food preparation procedures should be directed toward minimizing the amount of cut surfaces of foods rich in this vitamin. These foods should be served quickly after they are cut. Preparation should be done using only the water actually needed for making foods sanitary and palatable. Excess water reduces the amount of this water-soluble vitamin remaining in the food.

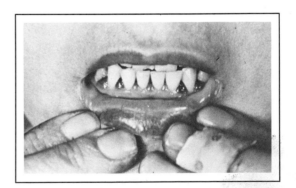

Scorbutic gums (caused by a deficiency of ascorbic acid) are swollen and inflamed.

Deficiency

Despite the fact that scurvy is recognized as a condition caused by a deficiency of ascorbic acid, there are still many cases diagnosed annually in the world. Symptoms that are noted include tenderness of the calves and muscular weakness; poor appetite; bleeding and swollen gums, sometimes accompanied by loosening of teeth; hemorrhages, including nosebleeds and subcutaneous bleeding; poor wound healing; megaloblastic anemia and shortness of breath; a typical frog-like position in infants; and sometimes sudden cardiac failure. Infantile scurvy may develop when infants are fed a formula low in ascorbic acid and no supplement is given. Either the formula should be changed or an ascorbic acid supplement should be provided to make up for the inadequacy of the formula. Symptoms can be overcome by feeding large doses of this vitamin for several days.

Summary

Vitamins are classified, according to their solubility, as water-soluble and fat-soluble. Ascorbic acid and the B vitamins, which include thiamin, riboflavin, niacin, pantothenic acid, folacin, biotin, vitamin B_6, and vitamin B_{12}, are water-soluble vitamins. Vitamins A, D, E, and K are fat-soluble (Table 11.8). Specific conditions are known to arise as a consequence of a dietary deficiency of one or more of the vitamins. A deficiency of vitamin A may lead to night blindness, xerophthalmia, or hyperkeratosis. A deficiency of vitamin D impairs absorption of calcium and causes rickets in children. Thiamin deficiency is familiar to the world because it results in beriberi. Riboflavin deficiency leads to ariboflavinosis. Pellagra, the deficiency condition resulting from too-little niacin, is all too familiar to some people in the southern United States. Low levels of folacin and vitamin B_{12} lead to the development of specific anemias characterized by large red blood cells that fail to mature normally. Scurvy results when ascorbic acid intake is too low.

A desirable and practical plan is to consume one's daily vitamin needs simply by eating well-planned and carefully prepared meals. By serving a wide variety of foods regularly, the diet will include suitable levels of all the vitamins. Fruits and vegetables that are providing useful quantities of the water-soluble vitamins should be prepared in the minimum amount of water needed to produce a palatable product. Long cooking times are to be avoided as much as possible if vitamin retention is to be maximized. By keeping food in fairly large pieces and cutting it shortly before cooking and serving, loss of ascorbic acid will be kept within practical limits. The use of added baking soda in cooking should be discouraged because the resulting alkaline reaction causes some destruction of thiamin. Milk, which is a particularly good source of riboflavin, should be marketed in tinted glass or in plasticized cartons to avoid destruction by the sunlight (Table 11.3).

Vitamins A and D are toxic in excessive amounts. This is not the

Table 11.8 *Summary of the Vitamins: Functions, Deficiency Conditions, and Food Sources*

	Vitamin	Function	Deficiency Condition	Food Sources
Fat Soluble	Vitamin A (retinal) and provitamin A (α,β,γ-carotene, cryptoxanthin)	1. Adapt to dim light 2. Promote growth 3. Prevent keratinization of skin and eye 4. Promote resistance to bacterial infection	1. Night blindness 2. Xerophthalmia 3. Hyperkeratosis 4. Poor growth	Vitamin A 　Liver 　Egg yolk 　milk, butter Provitamin A 　Sweet potatoes 　Winter squash 　Greens 　Carrots 　Cantaloupe
	Vitamin D (calciferol)	1. Facilitate absorption of calcium and phosphorus 2. Maintain alkaline phosphatase for optimum calcification	1. Rickets 2. Osteomalacia	Vitamin D-fortified milk Eggs Cheese, butter Fish
	Vitamin E (tocopherols)	1. Prevent oxidation of vitamins A and C and unsaturated fatty acids		Vegetable oils Greens
	Vitamin K (phyllo- and farnoquinone)	1. Form prothrombin and proconvertin for clotting of blood	1. Hemorrhage	Greens Liver Egg yolks
Water Soluble	Thiamin	1. Aid in releasing energy from carbohydrate and fat (as a part of coenzyme TPP) 2. Form ribose for DNA and RNA (transketolase)	1. Beriberi	Meat Whole-grain and enriched cereals Milk Legumes
	Riboflavin	1. Aid in releasing energy (as a part of FMN and FAD) 2. Activate vitamin B_6 to convert tryptophan to niacin	1. Ariboflavinosis	Milk Green vegetables Fish, meat, eggs
	Niacin	1. Aid in releasing energy (as part of NAD and NADP) 2. Promote Glycolysis 3. Aid in Fatty acid synthesis	1. Pellagra	Meat, poultry, fish Peanut butter Whole-grain and enriched cereals Greens

Table 11.8 (continued)

Vitamin	Function	Deficiency Condition	Food Sources
Vitamin B$_6$ (pyridoxine)	1. Transaminate and de-aminate amino acids 2. Aid in Porphyrin synthesis (for hemoglobin) 3. Catalyze conversion of tryptophan to niacin 4. Aid in release of energy from glycogen 5. Aid in formation of histamine, serotonin, norepinephrine		Meats Bananas Whole-grain cereals Lima beans Cabbage Potatoes Spinach
Pantothenic acid	1. Transfer 2 carbon fragments to release energy (as component of CoA 2. Synthesize porphyrin (hemoglobin formation) 3. Form cholesterol and steroids		Organ meats Whole-grain cereals
Biotin	1. Release energy from carbohydrate 2. Metabolize fatty acids 3. Deaminate protein		Egg yolks Milk Organ meats Cereals Legumes Nuts
Folacin (folic acid, pteroylglutamic acid)	1. Transfer single carbon units 2. Synthesize guanine and adenine; thymine; choline; amino acids; porphyrin (in coenzyme form)	1. Macrocytic anemia	Greens Mushrooms Liver Kidney
Vitamin B$_{12}$ (cobalamin)	1. Aid in maturing red blood cells 2. Aid in providing energy for central nervous system (from carbohydrate metabolism) 3. Form single carbon radicals 4. Convert folacin to active form	1. Pernicious anemia	Animal foods
Ascorbic acid (vitamin C)	1. Form collagen 2. Promote use of calcium in bones and teeth 3. Promote elasticity and strength of capillaries 4. Convert folacin to active form	1. Scurvy	Citrus fruits Strawberries Papayas Broccoli Cabbage Tomatoes Potatoes

usual case with any of the water-soluble vitamins, that is, any of the B vitamins or vitamin C, since they are readily excreted in the urine when taken in excessive amounts. The massive quantities of vitamin C (10 to 15 grams daily) recommended by a few scientists in 1970 as a means of prevention and treatment for the common cold are not supported by sound evidence and may, in fact, be harmful to some.

Selected References

Aly, H. E., et al. Oral contraceptives and vitamin B_6 metabolism. *Am. J. Clin. Nutr. 24:*297. 1971.

Anonymous, Vitamin E. *Consumer Reports 38,* No. 1:60. 1973.

Ariaey-Nejad, et al. Thiamin metabolism in man. *Am. J. Clin. Nutr. 23:*764. 1970.

Bailey, D. A., et al. Vitamin C supplementation related to physiological response to exercise in smoking and nonsmoking subjects. *Am. J. Clin. Nutr. 23:*905. 1970.

Cawthorne, M. A., et al. Vitamin E and heptatoxic agents. 3. Vitamin E synthetic antioxidants and carbon tetrachloride toxicity in the rat. *Brit. J. Nutr. 24:*357. 1970.

Cooper, B. A., et al. Case for folic acid supplements during pregnancy. *Am. J. Clin. Nutr. 23:*848. 1970.

Crandon, J. H., et al. Experimental human scurvy. *New Eng. J. Med. 223:*353. 1940.

DeLuca, H. F. Vitamin D: a new look at an old vitamin. *Nutrition Reviews. 29:*179. 1971.

Dowling, J. E. Night blindness. *Scientific American. 215,* No. 4:78. 1966.

Food and Nutrition Board. *Recommended Dietary Allowances.* National Research Council–National Academy of Sciences. Washington, D.C. 8th ed. 1974.

Ginter, C. E., et al. Effect of ascorbic acid on cholesterolemia in healthy subjects with seasonal deficit of vitamin C. *Nutr. and Metabolism 12,* No. 2:76. 1970.

Girdwood, R. H. Problems in the assessment of vitamin deficiency. *Proc. Nutr. Soc. 30* (May):66. 1971.

György, P. Developments leading to the metabolic role of vitamin B_6. *Am. J. Clin. Nutr. 24:*1250. 1971.

Hindson, T. C. Ascorbic acid status of Europeans resident in the tropics. *Brit. J. Nutr. 24:*801. 1970.

Hodges, R. E., et al. Experimental scurvy in man. *Amer. J. Clin. Nutr. 22:*535. 1969.

IUNS Committee. Tentative rules for generic descriptions and trivial names for vitamins and related compounds. *Nutr. Abstr. and Rev. 40*:395. 1970.

King, C. G. Present knowledge of ascorbic acid. *Nutr. Rev. 26*:33. 1968.

Kivirikko, K. I., and D. J. Prockop. Enzymatic hydroxylation of proline and lysine in protocollagen. *Proc. Nat. Acad. Sci. 57*:782. 1967.

Latham, M. C., et al. *Scope Manual on Nutrition.* Upjohn Co., Kalamazoo, Mich. 1970.

Lawson, D. E. M. Vitamin D: new findings on its metabolism and its role in calcium nutrition. *Proc. Nutr. Soc. 30 (May)*:47. 1971.

Loomis, W. F. Rickets. *Scientific American. 223,* No. 6:76. 1970.

Metz, J. Folate deficiency conditioned by lactation. *Am. J. Clin. Nutr. 23*:764. 1970.

Nammacher, M. A., et al. Vitamin K deficiency in infants beyond the neonatal period. *J. Pediatrics. 76*:549. 1970.

National Academy of Sciences. Recommended Dietary Allowances. 7th ed. Publication No. 1694. Washington, D.C. 1968.

Olson, R. E. Mode of action of vitamin K. *Nutr. Rev. 28*:171. 1970.

Osifo, B. O. A. Effect of folic acid and iron in the prevention of nutritional anaemias in pregnancy in Nigeria. *Brit. J. Nutr. 24*:689. 1970.

Pauling, L. Ascorbic acid and the common cold. *Am. J. Clin. Nutr. 24*:1294. 1971.

Phillips, D. C. Three-dimensional structure of an enzyme molecule. *Scientific American. 215,* No. 5:78. 1966.

Rivlin, R. S. Riboflavin metabolism. *New Eng. J. Med. 283*:463–472. 1970.

Rogers, W. E., Jr., et al. Vitamin A deficiency in germfree state. *Fed. Proc. 30*:1773. 1971.

Ross, R. Wound healing. *Scientific American. 220,* No. 6:40. 1969.

Schwartz, P. L. Ascorbic acid in wound healing—a review. *J. A. D. A. 56*:497. 1970.

Thomas, H. V., et al. *Science. 159*:532. 1968.

Van Reen, R., et al. Studies of bladder stone disease in Thailand. XII. Effect of methionine and pyridoxine supplements on urinary sulfate. *Am. J. Clin. Nutr. 23*:940. 1970.

NUTRITION
THROUGHOUT
LIFE

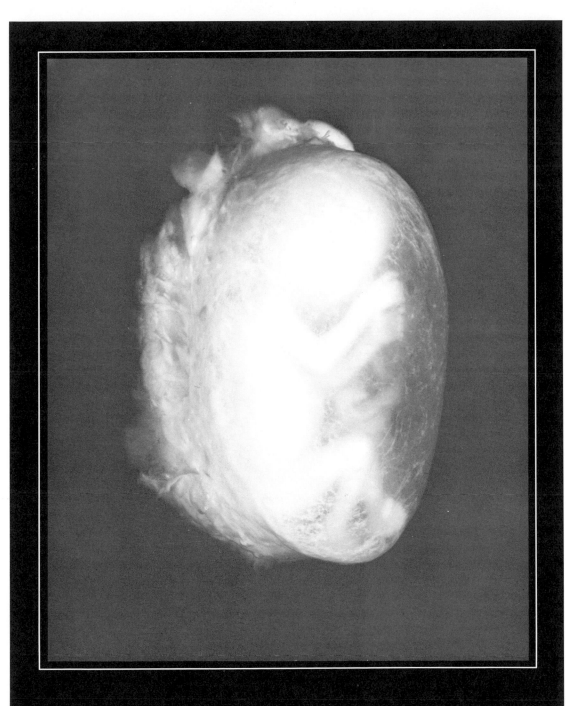

Chapter 12

Pregnancy and Lactation

The total experience of pregnancy tends to be shrouded in misconceptions and tales handed down from mother to daughter, too often with insufficient foundation in reality. From a nutritional standpoint this is an extremely important period for both the pregnant woman and the developing fetus, and there are dietary modifications that must be made to insure the optimum conditions for successful reproduction. Despite the recognized role of nutrition in reproduction, there are numerous misconceptions presently circulating regarding the dietary needs of pregnant women. Perhaps the best known and most erroneous of these is taking the old saying that "a pregnant woman is eating for two" to mean for two adults. When this often-repeated expression is misinterpreted, it lays the foundation for an unfortunate dietary pattern during this period.

The Significance of Nutrition During Pregnancy

As ever-increasing social concern is directed toward the problem of overpopulation, one natural offshoot of this concerted thought should be a growing awareness of the importance of improving the quality of both mind and body of the infants being born. Factors that may influence birth abnormalities and mental capacity already are the subjects of intensifying research efforts. The attitude that all birth defects are simply the result of a genetic defect is

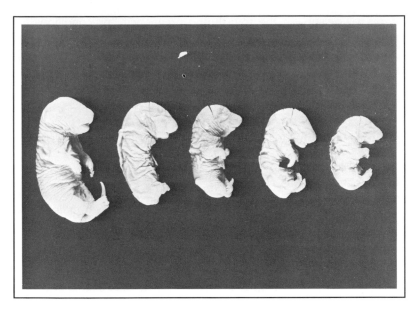

Normal, full-term rat fetus (left) and malformed fetuses from zinc-deficient rats, showing domed head, short lower jaw, fused or missing digits, clubbed feet, short or missing tail, and stunting.

giving way to one of questioning—exploring the possibility that many potential human heartbreaks can be prevented by appropriate counter-measures, often during the first 1 or 2 months of pregnancy. The specific roles of nutrients and the levels required in the diets of pregnant women are being examined as an important avenue for improving the health of the mother and the health and potential of her offspring.

Animal studies

Much of the knowledge presently available to illustrate the importance of various nutrients in pregnancy has been obtained from experiments utilizing laboratory animals. Interpretation of such animal studies and very careful examination of information collected from case studies of human pregnancies that resulted in the birth of infants with physical abnormalities form the base for the nutrition practices presently recommended for pregnant women.

Although there are serious gaps in our knowledge, a fair amount of information is being gathered that still is of immeasurable value in planning diets for the nutritional needs of pregnancy.

Since 1935, when the observation was made that some pregnant sows on a diet low in vitamin A produced broods that included pigs with cleft mouths and eye abnormalities, various physical abnormalities of offspring have been demonstrated to be the result of nutritional deficiencies in the diets of pregnant experimental animals. In 1968, Hurley reported that when female rats were kept on a zinc-deficient diet during the entire 21-day gestation period, the litters were small both in number and in physical size, the body weight being approximately half that of normal (Hurley, 1968). Congenital abnormalities were frequent and included cleft palates, cleft lips, foot and tail malformations, and brain, heart, lung, and urogenital abnormalities. Despite these dramatic problems in the offspring, the mother rats showed little change as a result of the zinc deficiency. Such results demonstrated the fallacy of the myth that the developing fetus will be supplied adequately with all the necessary nutrients at the expense of the mother's body if dietary sources alone are inadequate.

Another illustration of the impact of maternal nutrition on fetal development in animals is provided by Hurley (1968) in her work with *pallid* mice. These *pallid* mice (with the mutant gene *pallid*) characteristically have light-colored hair and are ataxic,[1] as demonstrated by their inability to swim because of the disorientation that results from abnormal vestibular (a part of the brain) reflexes. When these mice were fed a diet high in manganese throughout the period of pregnancy, the ataxia (muscular incoordination) did not develop in any of the offspring, but the hair pigmentation was still light. These offspring, seemingly normally oriented mice, were mated and fed a stock ration instead of the high-manganese diet; their offspring were ataxic.

The effect of malnutrition during pregnancy on mental development and capacity of the offspring is of considerable importance. Experimental results at the present time are not conclusive in this realm of investigation, but Barnes (1969) has found that preliminary findings in research on pigs suggest that malnutrition of

---

[1] Confused and unable to coordinate muscular movements.

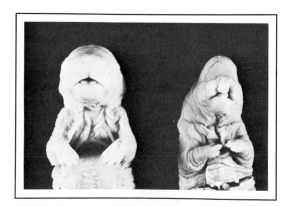

Normal (*left*) and zinc-deficient fetus showing domed skull, double cleft lip, and fused or missing digits.

the sow during pregnancy "preconditions the infant in that it has at birth a smaller weight and a smaller brain."[2] Similar findings have been noted in rats.

Malnutrition and human pregnancy

Documented evidence of congenital abnormalities in humans points suggestively to the probable relationship of various nutritional deficiencies to various conditions. In a 12-year study, the finding that many of the children born blind had a low birth weight and that their mothers had more stillbirths and gestational complications than were predictable points to the likelihood of nutritional factors being implicated in causing the blindness (McLaren, 1968). Among infants born with sight, premature infants have been found to be much more myopic than full-term infants. McLaren also reports cases where infants are born with one eye, a condition comparable to that observed in pigs born of vitamin A-deficient mothers. It is tempting to draw the analogy between species.

Other seeming relationships between nutritional impoverishment during pregnancy and physical abnormalities have been noted. A dietary relationship has been noted between inadequate iodide intake during pregnancy and the birth of a cretin. If a pregnant woman consumes a diet deficient in iodine during pregnancy, the infant often is overweight, but seemingly normal in other respects. Shortly after the middle of the first year of life, the retarded mental capacity, lethargic nature, and the stunted growth characteristic of cretinism may begin to be apparent.

The reasons for prematurity and low birth weights are diverse, but one of the common factors appears to be poor nutrition (Bagchi and Bose, 1962; Jacobson, 1972a). The duration of a state of malnutrition influences the

---

[2] R. H. Barnes. Effects of malnutrition on mental development. *J. of Home Economics.* 61:671. 1969.

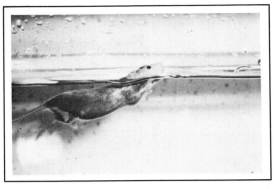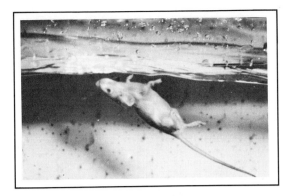

Normal and drowning mice, the result of a manganese deficiency.

reproductive capability of a woman. These workers support this conclusion by noting that there was a definite drop in the birth rate accompanied by an increased incidence of prematurity, stillbirths, miscarriages, and sterility during World War II in occupied countries where food shortages were severe for many months. These reports were in contrast to the notable lack of such difficulties in Germany, where food was very scarce for only 4 months. Although these reports cannot be supported by controlled experiments, they do add credibility to the purported importance of being well nourished both before and during pregnancy, particularly during the very early part of pregnancy.

In the United States, the persistently high incidence (Table 12.1) of fetal and neonatal deaths and physical abnormalities supports the need for the health-related professions to implement programs to overcome as many factors as possible to reduce the incidence of prematurity and its results. The infant mortality rate of 22.4 per 1000 live births in the United States in 1973 (13th among the nations of the world) is not one to be envied. The maternal mortality rate of 28.0 per 100,000 live births also carries nutritional implications and overtones. However, the nutritional status of the pregnant woman during the gestation period is only one of the factors that is important in the outcome of pregnancy.

The Psychological Impact of Pregnancy

Many adjustments, both physiological and psychological, are required during pregnancy. The preceding discussion has underlined the need for a good diet, but the actual consumption of a diet adequate in all nutrients may not become a reality unless psychological as well as physical adjustments are recognized and accomplished. The mere knowledge that a good diet is important may not provide sufficient motivation for a pregnant woman to eat a diet appropriate to her modified nutritional needs.

No pat statement can be made regarding the psychological impact of pregnancy. Seemingly, the only generalization that can be made is that a pregnant woman is psychologically different than she was before conception. For some women, the whole experience can be described as one of pleasure, a long-awaited fulfillment. For them, the doctor can give dietary recommendations and have reasonable assurance that the patients will almost religiously follow his instructions. Their nutritional man-

Table 12.1A   Fetal and Perinatal Deaths from Four Weeks Gestation to Two Years of Age (estimated and reported): United States, 1967[a,b]

Stage at Which Death Occurred	Number of Deaths
Fetal	
Between 4 and 20 weeks' gestation	1,023,880[c]
After 20 weeks' gestation	89,500[c]
After 20 weeks' gestation	54,939[d]
Perinatal	
Under 28 days	58,127[d]
28 days to 1 year	20,901[d]
1 year to 2 years	5,006[c]

[a] Reproduced by permission of the Committee on Maternal Nutrition. From **Maternal Nutrition and the Course of Pregnancy.** National Academy of Sciences—National Research Council. Washington, D.C. P. 9. 1970.

[b] Estimated number of fertilizations, 7,833,000 (derived from rates in Hertig et al. Pediatrics. 23: 202. 1959). Estimated number pregnancies at 4 weeks' gestation, 4,693,380 (based on rates in Bierman et al. **Amer. J. Obstet. Gynecol. 91:** 37. 1965). Approximate number of live births 3,521,000 (U.S. Dept. of Health, Education, and Welfare, Public Health Service. Monthly Vital Statistics Report 16, No. 13. 1968).

[c] Estimated; based on rates in Bierman et al. **Amer. J. Obstet. Gynecol. 91:** 37. 1965.

[d] Reported by U.S. Dept of Health, Education, and Welfare, Public Health Service. Monthly Vital Statistics Report 16, No. 13. 1968.

agement simply involves coordinating recognized dietary principles with their current physical condition. For many other women, the situation is vastly different; successful dietary management can only be achieved by first deriving an accurate picture of the woman's inner feelings toward the pregnancy. This is difficult to appreciate fully, but the following paragraphs will provide some insight.

For some families, a pregnancy represents a very real hardship financially. In some instances, the pregnancy means loss of income at least for a brief time, and frequently for an extended period because the woman cannot continue her job. A baby represents another financial obligation for families, a commitment that is difficult to fulfill when the family income already is too small to provide adequately for minimal needs. Under such conditions, the

pregnant woman may feel a degree of guilt and some resentment about her condition, with the result that she has little motivation to feed herself correctly during this important period.

Some women are so worn down by caring for their existing families or are so absorbed in their own activities that they genuinely deplore the prospect of the impending offspring. Still others are frightened by the experience of pregnancy and unprepared for the change this represents in their lives. These women require considerable patience, understanding, and support from those around them to help develop the confidence and interest they need if they are to be motivated to eat well during their pregnancy.

The psychological influences of pregnancy on the adolescent girl are particularly strong. Despite the fact that the number of babies born

Table 12.1B *Estimated Number of Children*
with Perinatal Handicaps Requiring Special
Care: United States, 1967[a,e]

Type of Care	Estimated Number of Children[b]
Short-term	
Low-birth-weight and preterm	
infants	125,300
Other[f]	100,240
Long-term	
Severe physical handicap[g]	68,020
Physical and mental handicap[h]	19,900
Care of mentally retarded (IQ's under 70)	46,540
Care of infants who may require special educational service (IQ's 70-79)	114,560

[e] For number of live births and number of perinatal deaths see Table 12.1A.

[f] For example, strabismus, inguinal hernia, talipes.

[g] For example, congenital heart disease, cerebral palsy.

[h] For example, multiple handicap, developmental defect (central nervous system).

to very young adolescents is increasing, there is still limited public acceptance of these girls. The social stigma that accompanies conception out of wedlock and leaving school before graduation from high school serves to only increase the apprehension and fears of the pregnant teen-ager. She may feel overwhelming disapproval from both her family and friends. She is faced with tremendous psychological adjustments as well as physiological changes. Without the assistance and understanding of those close to her, the adjustments required may be too great. These new and worrisome stresses may easily crowd nutritional concerns from the mind of the pregnant adolescent. The figures for live births to teen-agers in the United States in 1965 are a startling indicator of the magnitude of the problem: almost 8000 of the mothers were between the ages of 10 and 14, more than 29,000 were 15 or younger, more than 56,000 were 16 years old, and more than 110,000 were 17, for a total of 197,372 live births to mothers 17 years old and younger.

Cultural and religious factors can also influence a pregnant woman's attitude toward food (see Chapter 2). An illustration of these influences is provided by Matter and Wakefield (1971). These workers studied the influence of religion upon the dietary intake of Muslim, Christian, and Hindu pregnant Indian women from low-income families. The Hindu women were found to have lower intakes of protein, fat, and kilocalories than the Muslim and Christian women (the two latter groups tending to have similar dietary intakes).

In the United States, some Negro women (particularly in the South) satisfy a pica (abnormal craving) by eating clay and cornstarch. Since this is an accepted practice in certain segments of the region, starch and clay eating assumes overtones of cultural influences. Edwards et al. (1964) found that fewer babies borne by the mothers eating these substances were born in good condition than would nor-

Table 12.2 *Mean Birth Weights According to Socioeconomic Status*[a]

Place	Population	Subjects	Mean Birth Weights (g)	Source
Madras	Indian	Well-to-do "Mostly poor"	2985 2736	Achar and Yankauer[b]
South India	Indian	Wealthy Poor	3182 2810	Venkatachalam[c]
Bombay	Indian	Upper class Upper middle class Lower middle class Lower class	3247 2945 2796 2578	Udani[d]
Calcutta	Indian	Paying patients Poor class	2851 2656	Mukherjee and Biswas[e]
Congo	Bantu	"Very well nourished" "Well nourished" "Badly nourished"	3026 2965 2850	Jans[f]
	Pygmies		2635	
Ghana (Accra)	African	Prosperous General population	3188 2879	Hollingsworth[g]
Indonesia (Jogjakarta)	Javanese	Well-to-do Poor	3022 2816	Timmer[h]

[a] From World Health Organization. *Nutrition in Pregnancy and Lactation.* WHO Tech. Rep. Ser. No. 302. Geneva. 1965.

[b] S. T. Achar and A. Yankauer. Studies on the birth weight of South Indian infants. *Indian J. Child Health. 11:* 57. 1962.

[c] P. S. Venkatachalam. Effect of the nutritional status of the mother on the newborn. *Bull. WHO. 26:* 143. 1962.

[d] P. M. Udani. Physical growth of children in different socioeconomic groups in Bombay. *Indian J. Child Health. 12:* 593. 1963.

[e] S. Mukherjee and S. Biswas. Birth weight and its relationship to gestation period, sex, maternal age, parity and socioeconomic status. *J. Indian Med. Ass. 32:* 389. 1959.

[f] C. Jans. The weight increase of the Pygmy infant. *Ann. Soc. Belg. Med. Trop. 39:* 851. 1959.

[g] M. G. Hollingsworth. The birth weights of African and European babies born in Ghana. *W. Afr. Med. J. 9:* 256. 1960

[h] M. Timmer. Prosperity and birth weight of Javanese infants. *Trop. Geogr. Med. 13:* 316. 1961.

mally have been predicted. Table 12.2 provides additional information which emphasizes the relationship between socioeconomic status and mean birth weights of infants in various parts of the world.

Physiological Adjustments in Pregnancy

The stages of development during the prenatal period clearly influence the nutritional needs of the mother. During the first 2 weeks, the period known as implantation, the placenta begins to develop as the fertilized ovum is imbedded in the uterine wall. This is probably the most critical period in pregnancy, a period when nutrition is of maximal importance, and where drugs of any kind (even aspirin) should be minimal, and *unfortunately* a period when no woman can be sure she is pregnant.

The placenta is of great nutritional significance because it affords a large contact area (approximately 13 square meters) for the passage of nutrients between the maternal and fetal circulatory systems and the removal of waste products from the fetal system through the maternal system. By the end of the second month of pregnancy, the individual organs and skeletal formation are begun. This period of differentiation is deemed to be highly significant. Problems such as a cleft palate caused by a vitamin-A deficiency are postulated to develop at this time. After the gross differentiation is completed, the remainder of pregnancy is devoted to growth and refinements that will enable the newborn to flourish.

In addition to the development of the fetus,

Table 12.3 *Components of the Average Weight Gained in Normal Pregnancy*[a]

Component	Amount (g) gained at			
	10 weeks	20 weeks	30 weeks	40 weeks
A. Total gain of body weight	650	4000	8500	12,500
Fetus	5	300	1500	3300
Placenta	20	170	430	650
Liquor amnii	30	250	600	800
Increase of				
Uterus[b]	135	585	810	900
Mammary gland[c]	34	180	360	405
Maternal blood	100	600	1300	1250
B. Total (rounded)	320	2100	5000	7300
C. Weight not accounted for (A-B)	330	1900	3500	5200

[a] Committee on Maternal Nutrition. **Maternal Nutrition and the Course of Pregnancy.** Food and Nutrition Board. National Research Council. Washington, D.C. P. 64. 1970.
[b] Blood-free uterus.
[c] Blood-free mammary gland tissue.

there are also changes taking place within the tissues of the mother. Apparently in response to the ever-increasing demand upon the mother's circulatory system to supply oxygen, nourish the fetus, and remove waste (including nitrogenous wastes and carbon dioxide), there is a gradual increase in the amount of blood to more than 4 pounds (1800 milliliters) by the time of delivery. As might be anticipated, the uterus and breasts increase in mass—the uterus by as much as 2 pounds and the breasts by $1\frac{1}{2}$ to 3 pounds. Amniotic fluid, the fetus itself, increased fluid in the tissues, and some ad-

ditional fat account for the rest of the weight gain during pregnancy (Table 12.3). Jacobson (1972b) stated that the average weights of these changes associated with pregnancy, including the fetus, is 20.5 pounds.

The exact amount of weight gain considered desirable during a pregnancy is an individual matter and not a figure that can be stated for all women. There have been various ideas reflected in this topic through the years. For centuries there was little concern with the importance of weight control during pregnancy. Then the idea was embraced that too much

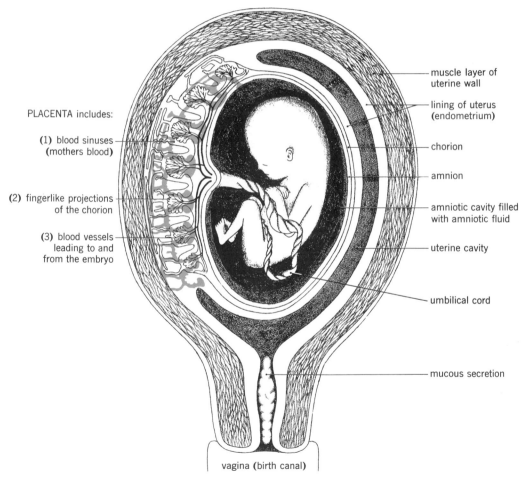

PLACENTA includes:

(1) blood sinuses (mothers blood)

(2) fingerlike projections of the chorion

(3) blood vessels leading to and from the embryo

muscle layer of uterine wall

lining of uterus (endometrium)

chorion

amnion

amniotic cavity filled with amniotic fluid

uterine cavity

umbilical cord

mucous secretion

vagina (birth canal)

Sketch of a cross-sectional view of a uterus, showing the placenta and fetus at three months.

weight gain was bad, and the trend was toward an absolute minimum gain, preferably as little as 10 pounds. Recently, data on birth weights (Table 12.3) and morbidity have been reviewed, and the recommendation for a weight gain of 22 to 27 pounds during pregnancy is emerging.

Other physiologic changes of note during pregnancy include: (1) a brief drop in basal metabolic rate to be followed by an increase to a basal metabolic rate about 13 percent higher than is normal for the nonpregnant state, (2) increase in oxygen consumption and cardiac (heart) output, (3) a reduction in the acidity of the stomach due to lowered hydrochloric acid secretion, and (4) a decrease in motility of food through the gastrointestinal tract. The modifications in oxygen consumption are important in determining caloric needs. The changes in the gastrointestinal tract may promote increased utilization of food due to the longer time the food remains in the intestine.

Nutritional Needs of Pregnancy

In view of the many changes taking place, the modifications in nutritional needs during pregnancy are not surprising. Growth of the fetal tissues and the bodily changes in the mother necessitate additional calories, protein, vitamin A, vitamin E, folic acid, niacin, riboflavin, thiamin, pyridoxine, vitamin B_{12}, ascorbic acid, iron [3], calcium, phosphorus, iodine, fluoride, zinc, and magnesium (Table 12.4). In short, all the nutrients for which daily allowances have been recommended are needed in larger quantities during pregnancy, but the amount of the increase is not uniform from one nutrient to another.

Energy

During the pregnancy of a healthy, semisedentary homemaker, the need for calories is increased by approximately 15 percent (actually only 300 kilocalories). At first impression, this seems an unreasonably small increase when one considers the fact that the woman must supply the energy required for her metabolic changes plus that needed for the growth of the fetus. Certainly, both of these factors place demands for energy upon her. However, fetal growth, in terms of actual weight gain, is relatively slow until the last trimester of pregnancy, at which time an accelerated rate of weight gain begins. Fetal weight gain in the last couple of months of pregnancy approaches $\frac{1}{2}$ pound weekly. The mother's dietary need for calories to supply energy for the rapidly growing fetus and the increased need due to an elevated energy expenditure may be counterbalanced, as pregnancy progresses, by the reduced activity of the mother. The physical inertia and slower movement, accompanied by a distinct reduction in the amount of physical activity undertaken, are typical of many women as they begin to experience the shifting of the center of gravity and the somewhat cumbersome movements characteristic of the later stages of pregnancy. However, those homemakers who also are working outside the home during pregnancy, in effect, have two jobs. There actually is very little research on the energy expenditure of pregnant women. Present knowledge indicates that pregnant women may have only a very limited need for additional calories as a consequence of pregnancy, and these can

---

[3] Although the recommendation by the Food and Nutrition Board remains constant for iron during pregnancy, many obstetricians recommend daily supplements of 30 to 60 milligrams of iron.

Table 12.4 *Comparison of Recommended Daily Dietary Allowances for Nonpregnant, Pregnant, and Lactating Women* [a]

Nutrient	Daily Recommendation for Women					
	11–14	15–18	19–22	23–50	Pregnant	Lactating
kcal	2400	2100	2100	2000	+300	+500
Protein (g)	44	48	46	46	+30	75
Vitamin A (I.U.)	4000	4000	4000	4000	5000	6000
Vitamin D (I.U.)	400	400	400	—	400	400
Vitamin E activity (I.U.)	12	12	12	12	15	15
Ascorbic acid (mg)	45	45	45	45	60	60
Folacin (μg)	400	400	400	400	800	600
Niacin (mg equiv.)	16	14	14	13	+2	+4
Riboflavin (mg)	1.3	1.4	1.4	1.2	+0.3	+0.5
Thiamin (mg)	1.2	1.1	1.1	1.0	+0.3	+0.3
Vitamin B_6 (mg)	1.6	2.0	2.0	2.0	2.5	2.5
Vitamin B_{12} (μg)	3.0	3.0	3.0	3.0	4.0	4.0
Calcium (mg)	1200	1200	800	800	1200	1200
Phosphorus (mg)	1200	1200	800	800	1200	1200
Iodine (μg)	115	115	100	100	125	150
Iron (mg)	18	18	18	18	18[b]	18
Magnesium (mg)	300	300	300	300	450	450
Zinc (mg)	15	15	15	15	20	25

[a] Adapted from Food and Nutrition Board, National Academy of Sciences—National Research Council, ***Recommended Daily Dietary Allowances,*** revised 1974. See Table 1.8 for weight and height information.
[b] Many obstetricians recommend that diets during pregnancy be supplemented with 30 to 60 mg iron per day.

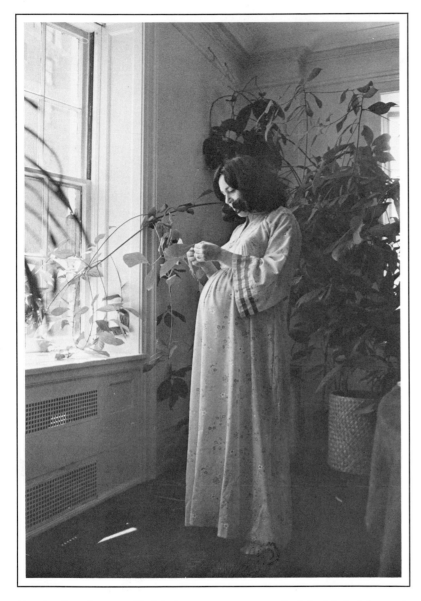

Nutritional needs are modified during pregnancy as a result of physiological changes in the mother and fetus and also as a result of modified physical activity of the mother. A total weight gain of 20—24 pounds during pregnancy is recommended.

readily be provided by increased milk consumption. Adequacy of caloric intake may be estimated by the weight gain pattern and by the total weight gain. The diet should provide sufficient calories to support a steady gain of 0.5 to 0.8 pounds per week, to a total of 22 to 27 pounds.

Protein

Perhaps the dietary modification most difficult for women to fully appreciate is that pregnant women need more protein than is required for good nutrition of adult males. The traditional pattern in the United States has

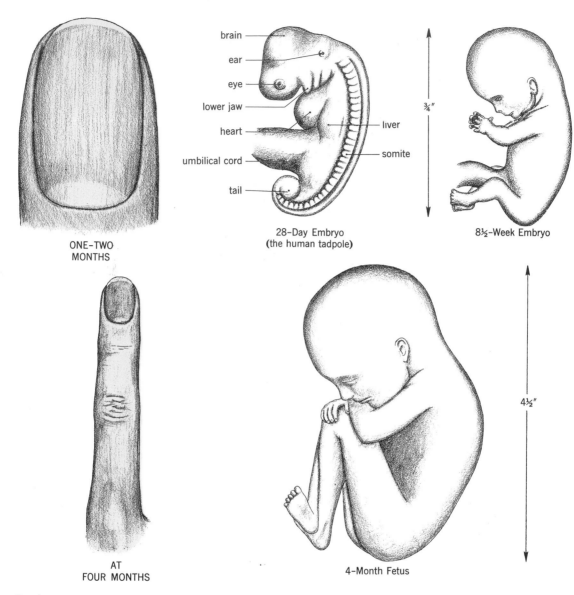

ONE–TWO
MONTHS

brain
ear
eye
lower jaw
heart
umbilical cord
tail

liver
somite

28-Day Embryo
(the human tadpole)

¾"

8½–Week Embryo

AT
FOUR MONTHS

4½"

4-Month Fetus

Development of human embryo and fetus (showing size comparisons).

been to feed the largest serving of meat to the father of the family. Although this may provide a satisfying recognition of his status as the family provider, it can present an impedance in providing a suitable diet for the pregnant woman. The recommended increase in protein intake in the healthy woman is approximately 65 percent, from the 46 grams recommended for an adult female to 76 grams during preg-

nancy. This allowance modification is based on the significant need for protein for tissue growth both in the fetus and in the maternal tissues related to reproduction. The importance of an adequate protein intake cannot be overstated. Fetal deposition of protein during the latter half of pregnancy is estimated to be approximately 1.5 grams per day. Much larger amounts of protein (1.7 grams per kilogram of body weight) may be required by pregnant adolescents and by women requiring nutritional rehabilitation.

Vitamins

The recommended intakes of the fat-soluble vitamins, A, D, and E, are increased during pregnancy for a diversity of reasons. Vitamin A probably is crucial to the development of all body cells, and as pointed out, for normally functioning eyes and a properly formed palate and skeleton in animals; such evidence strongly supports the importance of adequate vitamin A for humans, too. An increase of 25 percent, from 4000 to 5000 International Units per day, appears to be sufficient to prevent similar complications resulting from a vitamin A deficiency in humans, although as mentioned earlier, good nutrition is of most importance very early in pregnancy—a point that needs to be stressed repeatedly.

Vitamin D, important for its role in promoting the absorption of calcium and its utilization in bone formation, should be included in the diets of all pregnant women, regardless of age. The recommended level, 400 International Units per day, is simply a continuation of the recommendation for young women up to the age of 22, but is a reinstatement of the recommendation for women who become pregnant after the age of 22. A quart of milk fortified with vitamin D provides the appropriate level of vitamin D daily.

The actual role of vitamin E during pregnancy has not yet been defined. The 25 percent increase in the recommendation for vitamin E during pregnancy is based, at least in part, on the antioxidant properties of this vitamin and its consequent role in reducing the oxidation of ascorbic acid, of vitamin A, and of the polyunsaturated fatty acids in the body. Thus, vitamin E protects these important nutrients.

An important reason supporting the recommendation to increase the ascorbic acid intake from 45 milligrams to 60 milligrams daily during pregnancy is that ascorbic acid has clearly been shown to be essential for the formation of collagen. The formation of this connective tissue, although important for all individuals, assumes even greater significance in the bodies of both the mother and the developing fetus. The recommended increase of almost 35 percent during pregnancy is indicative of the significant role of ascorbic acid.

Of the B vitamins for which the National Research Council has made recommendations, the folic acid allowance is most dramatically altered by pregnancy. The recommendation for folacin is doubled (from 400 to 800 micrograms) during pregnancy to provide a sufficient amount of this vitamin to prevent the development of the macrocytic anemia that characterizes a folic acid deficiency. In animals, congenital abnormalities such as a cleft palate can result from a folic acid deficiency early in pregnancy.

Thiamin and niacin allowances are increased approximately 30 and 15 percent, respectively, to insure that they are available in adequate quantities for performing their coenzyme functions in metabolizing the small increase in total food consumed. The somewhat improved retention of thiamin during pregnancy suggests that some special requirement for this vitamin, beyond the coenzyme function, may develop in pregnancy. Riboflavin, like thiamin and niacin, is needed for metabolizing food, a role that accounts at least in part for the 25 percent increase in the recommended allowance for this vitamin.

The metabolism of amino acids is governed, in part, by pyridoxine. This B vitamin also is required by all humans for the conversion of tryptophan (an amino acid) into niacin, another one of the B vitamins. During pregnancy, there is need for an increased intake of vitamin B_6 (also called pyridoxine) if this important transformation is to take place normally. To provide sufficient pyridoxine for tryptophan conversion and also enzymatic functions involving this vitamin, the allowance for vitamin B_6 is increased by 25 percent (from 2.0 milligrams to 2.5 milligrams).

The last of the B vitamins, vitamin B_{12}, is intimately involved with the functioning of the nervous system and also with the production of normal red blood cells. This vitamin appears to be given preferentially to the fetus, at the expense of maternal supplies if necessary. The 33 percent increase in vitamin B_{12} (from 3 micrograms to 4 micrograms) recommended during pregnancy is considered sufficient to insure satisfactory levels in the mother as well as in the fetus.

Minerals

The need for calcium and phosphorus is increased despite the improved utilization of these minerals during pregnancy. The fetus will contain in the vicinity of 22 grams of calcium at birth, with almost three fourths of this amount being deposited in the last trimester. To assure an adequate supply of these important nutrients, the recommended allowance of both calcium and phosphorus is increased by 50 percent, to 1200 milligrams of each of these nutrients.

Iodide, although needed only in microgram quantities, is absolutely essential for successful reproduction because of its role as a structural component of thyroxine. When thyroxine production is very limited, conception becomes extremely unlikely, if not impossible. Also, iodide deficiency leads to the development of goiter, a result that is being noted with increasing frequency among all segments of the population and particularly among pregnant women because of their elevated need for this mineral. A severe iodide deficiency that causes goiter in the mother can lead to a goiter in the child and may result in the birth of a cretin. Adequate iodide can be obtained readily by simply using iodized salt.

The need for iron is calculated to be constant throughout a woman's reproductive lifetime. Since iron is a component of hemoglobin, any blood loss results in the loss of iron. Women have a high iron need as a consequence of regular losses during menstruation. During pregnancy, 6 to 7 milligrams of iron per day are required to meet the iron needs resulting from the increased blood volume of the mother and the fetus. An adequate intake of iron is important to insure that sufficient iron will be stored in the fetus to supply the newborn's iron needs during the first months when his iron absorption from dietary sources is poor. Since food rarely provides enough iron to permit absorption of 6 to 7 milligrams per day, diets may be supplemented with as much as 30 to 60 milligrams of iron per day when necessary.

Dietary Recommendations

Nutrition demands are great as the maternal body makes the necessary adjustments to pregnancy and as the fetus develops in preparation for birth as an independently functioning being. The modifications in nutritional recommendations have been reviewed in the preceding section, but these need to be translated into dietary terms before they assume practical meaning.

Any discussion of diet must be undertaken in relation to the usual diet of the individual. In the case of the pregnant woman, meaningful dietary recommendations can only be made after the usual dietary pattern has been determined. The assumption that women routinely eat a totally adequate diet for a period of time before beginning a pregnancy is naive. A far more realistic approach is to take into consideration the fact that dietary surveys indicate that teen-age girls are the least well-fed population group in the United States, and the group just above them in the rankings of dietary adequacy is young adult women.

From a medical viewpoint, there is value in a program that would advise and assist prospective mothers in correcting their diets *before* commencing a pregnancy. In that idealized situation, the woman could achieve her recommended weight and insure that her body is well endowed with all the dietary stores needed to optimize success in pregnancy.

One of the important items on the agenda for a woman's first visit to a doctor for obstetrical care is dietary guidance. Unfortunately this is not always given, at least not in a meaningful and useful way. If the patient has been eating an adequate diet over a period of several months and has maintained her weight within the recommended range, dietary modifications usually are not necessary during the first trimester of pregnancy unless she experiences some difficulty with nausea. In the event that nausea is preventing the utilization of her usual diet, her physician may prescribe medication that will help to control the problem. In some cases, treatment includes a nutritional supplement to supply the nutrients at a time of day when there is least likely to be rejection of the supplement. Detailed dietary instructions should be postponed until the woman is over her nausea and is more receptive to guidance.

In short, the first trimester of pregnancy, in fact, the very first month, is a time when women need to be sure they are eating a well-balanced diet to help insure that adequate nutrient stores will be available as fetal demands increase later in pregnancy. If inadequacies are noted in the diet, either because of physical problems or dietary prejudices, the use of a supplement providing the missing nutrients is advisable to complement the nutrients contained in the diet.

The dietary pattern during the second and third trimesters of pregnancy requires additional modification if all the nutrients are to be supplied in adequate amounts. The calcium re-quirement can be met by drinking 3 to 4 glasses of milk daily. If whole milk is consumed, this change from the recommended 2 glasses a day increases the kilocalorie contribution of milk from 320 to 640. Note that this change alone more than accounts for the daily recommendation of 300 additional kilocalories. There is frequently good reason for pregnant women to drink nonfat and low-fat milk. By this simple dietary modification, the 3 to 4 glasses of nonfat milk, which actually provide slightly more calcium than whole milk, total only 360 kilocalories or less of the day's intake. The diet also should include two servings of meat, chicken, or fish (*but these can be small servings*), plus one egg daily. By having one of these items plus a glass of milk at each meal and the fourth glass of milk as a snack, the protein intake is spread out over the entire day, which insures maximum utilization of this important nutrient. The remainder of the diet for the pregnant woman ideally includes four servings of breads and cereals (small servings) and at least four servings of fruits and vegetables (including citrus and dark green leafy or yellow vegetables). She usually will be more comfortable and will have less difficulty with weight control problems if she emphasizes her intake of fruits and vegetables. In general, these foods are relatively high in cellulose and water, thus helping to stimulate the intestinal tract and reduce the likelihood of constipation. Also, an extra serving of a fruit or vegetable in place of a rich dessert is a help in controlling caloric intake. The focus of the diet is on nourishing foods. The limited increase in calories during pregnancy and the large increases in the numerous nutrients needed for good health necessitate some attention to reducing the amounts of rich desserts, sauces, fats, and sweets in the diet.

With perhaps the exception of iron and folic acid, all the nutrients a woman needs for good health during pregnancy can be supplied by following the plan described above plus always drinking *fluoridated water*. An iron supplement such as ferrous sulphate can be taken to insure the adequacy of this mineral, and a folate supplement often is prescribed to provide the necessary amounts of this vitamin. In addition, care should be taken to select milk fortified with vitamin D.

For women who have persistent nausea or poor dietary patterns, the daily consumption of a supplement providing the missing nutrients in appropriate amounts may be expedient. However, care should be taken to heed the warning that both vitamins A and D are toxic in large doses. Just what the effect of continuous overdosages of these vitamins may be upon the human fetus has not yet been determined, but excessive levels of vitamin A in the pregnant rat have caused skeletal deviations in the developing fetus. In addition, actual cases have clearly demonstrated that vitamin A at levels exceeding 50,000 International Units daily and vitamin D in dosages of 100,000 International Units for several weeks will cause dangerous symptoms to develop in adults. These are levels clearly above any that can possibly be obtained from foods, even fortified foods. The excessive ingestion of the other vitamins is an unnecessary expense, but does not present a known health hazard. All nutritional supplements during pregnancy should be taken only with the advice of the physician. It is important to emphasize that vitamin supplements alone do not substitute for the need for other nutrients provided by a well-balanced diet.

Nutrition of the Pregnant Adolescent

The nutrition of pregnant teen-agers is of vital importance both to the mother and to the offspring, for the teen-ager must supply sufficient nutrients for the growth of her own body as well as that of her fetus. The earlier pregnancy occurs in the teens, the more crucial is the problem (Tables 12.5 and 12.6), but most adolescent girls achieve skeletal maturity at approximately age 17. Although much research remains to be done before the total impact of maternal nutrition on obstetric behavior of adolescents is known, some complications related to suboptimal nutrition have been noted.[4]

"The most frequently mentioned complications are premature labor and infants of low birth weight, high neonatal mortality, toxemia of pregnancy, iron-deficiency anemia, feto-pelvic disproportion, and prolonged labor. . . . Most observers cite toxemia as a special hazard of pregnancy in young girls, and some investigators note that when parity and race are held constant, the incidence rises sharply with each year of age under 20. . . . The incidence (Ed.—of iron-deficiency anemia) rises sharply in girls who have repeated pregnancies during their adolescent years, the rise suggesting cumulative deficits of iron.

"Young primigravidas present unique medical problems, and girls who experience repeated pregnancies before their 20th birthdays are at extremely high risk. Evidence suggests that nutritional reserves may be depleted. The increased incidence of iron-deficiency anemia, preeclampsia, prematurity, and neonatal mortality may well be related to this depletion. Increased efforts should be made to prevent pregnancies during the adolescent years."

When one considers the highly demanding physical needs for adequate nutrition and simultaneously reviews the psychological stresses of the pregnant teen-ager, the likelihood that she will eat a satisfactory diet for this

[4] National Academy of Sciences. *Maternal Nutrition and the Course of Pregnancy.* Washington, D.C. Pp. 148–159. 1970.

Table 12.5 *Percentage Distribution of Live Births by Birth Weight under 2500 g and by Age of Mother and Color: United States, 1965* [a]

Age of Mother (years)	Birth Weight 2500 g or Less (%)	Color White (%)	Color Nonwhite (%)
Total	8.3	7.2	13.8
Under 15	18.7	13.0	21.3
15-19	10.5	8.5	16.4
20-24	7.9	6.9	13.3
25-29	7.3	6.5	12.2
30-34	7.9	7.0	12.8
35-39	8.9	8.0	13.4
40-44	9.0	8.3	12.5
45-49	8.7	8.5	9.8

[a] Source: U.S. Department of Health, Education, and Welfare, Public Health Service (1967). *Vital Statistics of the United States, 1965: Volume 1 —Natality.* U.S. Govt. Print Office. Washington, D.C.

Table 12.6 *Mortality of White and Nonwhite Infants by Age of Mother and Age at Death: United States, 1960 Birth Cohort* [a]

Age of Mother (years)	Neonatal [b] (under 28 days) Total	White	Nonwhite	Postneonatal [b] (28 days, 11 months) Total	White	Nonwhite	Infant [b] (under 1 year) Total	White	Nonwhite
Total	18.4	16.9	26.7	6.7	5.3	14.7	25.1	22.2	41.4
Under 15	41.2	32.1	46.5	17.6	15.5	18.8	58.7	47.5	65.3
15-19	22.7	20.4	30.9	10.1	7.7	18.6	32.8	28.1	49.5
20-24	17.3	15.9	25.3	6.9	5.5	14.8	24.2	21.4	40.2
25-29	16.6	15.3	24.2	5.8	4.6	13.1	22.4	20.0	37.3
30-34	18.3	17.0	26.4	5.3	4.2	12.0	23.7	21.2	38.4
35-39	19.7	18.4	27.3	5.8	4.5	13.9	25.5	22.9	41.2
40-44	23.1	22.0	29.4	7.5	6.1	15.4	30.6	28.1	44.7
45 and over	31.3	31.8	28.9	9.8	7.1	21.6	41.1	38.9	50.5

[a] Sources: U.S. Department of Health, Education, and Welfare, Public Health Service (1967). *Vital Statistics of the United States, 1965: Volume 1— Natality.* U.S. Govt. Print. Office. Washington, D.C.
[b] Rate per 1000 live births.

stressful period is indeed slim. Her physician will need to be fully aware of her dietary pattern and work with her if she is to achieve adequate nutriture. The Committee on Maternal Nutrition (Food and Nutrition Board of the National Research Council) has emphasized the need for physicians to encourage pregnant teen-agers to consume a diet sufficiently high in caloric content (36 kilocalories per kilogram or more) so that the essential nutrients are available in adequate amounts.[5]

"A widespread practice among physicians is to place prenatal patients on restricted diets to control weight gain. Unfortunately, this practice often extends to pregnant adolescents. The effect of such restriction is illustrated by a study in Iowa. The majority of the pregnant girls' diets had been classed poor with respect to intakes of vitamin A and ascorbic acid, and borderline in calories, protein, calcium, and iron. Caloric restriction prescribed for weight-control purposes resulted in significantly lower intakes of protein and iron as well as of calories."[6]

There is valid reason to recommend routine vitamin and mineral supplements in the diet of a pregnant teen-ager to optimize her chances for good health, both for herself and for her baby. Although one can idealistically say that this is the time to improve her dietary habits, if she follows the dietary patterns of many adolescent girls, probably the additional stress of worrying about her diet is not something that will capture her interest sufficiently to guarantee that she will be well fed. Thus, a dietary supplement administered with warm understanding may be the most effective way of helping the young expectant mother. Nutrition education and some dietary change can be undertaken as she begins to adjust to her new situation. The fact that vitamin and mineral supplements do not substitute for a well-balanced diet, selected with variety from each of the Basic Four Food Groups, should be stressed, particularly with these vulnerable young girls.

Lactation

The dietary needs for the lactating woman provide some impressive statistics. Many new mothers derive considerable satisfaction from the tremendous increase in calories recommended for successful lactation. As shown in Table 12.4, there is a 500 kilocalorie increase in the recommended allowance during this important phase of the reproductive cycle.[7] This figure is calculated to be sufficient to provide the energy needed for the production of milk plus the kilocalories represented by the milk itself. To women who have been watching their diets with a constant eye to the bathroom scales during the latter phases of pregnancy, the boost in calories during lactation is a real attraction. This recommendation is based on the assumption that the new mother quickly resumes her normal range of activities plus caring for her new infant when she returns home from the hospital.

As long as she is nursing her baby, the lactating woman continues to require many nutrients at the same level recommended during pregnancy, while some other nutrients are needed in even larger quantities. The recommendations that remain the same for lactation as for pregnancy include vitamin D, vitamin E, ascorbic acid, pyridoxine, thiamin, and vitamin B_{12}. The iron allowance continues at the same

[5] National Academy of Sciences. *Maternal Nutrition and the Course of Pregnancy.* Washington, D.C. P. 152. 1970.

[6] P. A. Garcia, unpublished data.

[7] Some nutritionists deem the 1974 recommendation of 500 kilocalories to be too low and judge the 1968 value of 1000 kilocalories above the nonlactating state to be desirable.

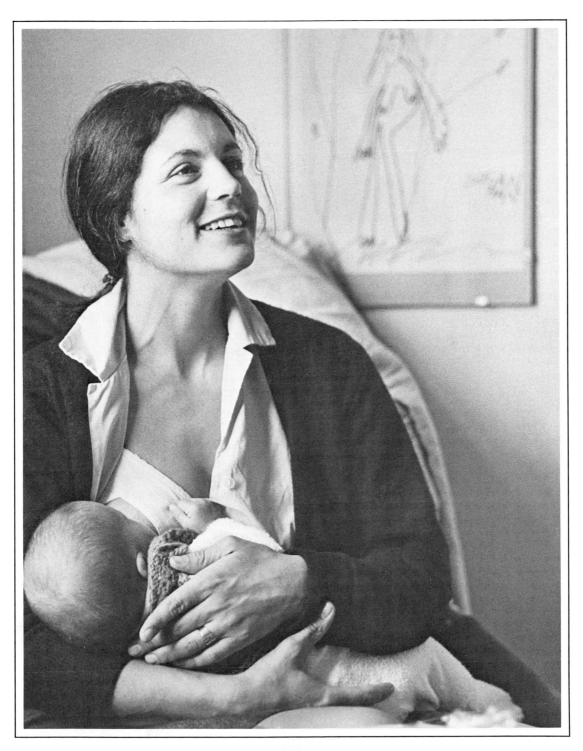

The lactating woman requires a well-planned and varied diet to meet her own need for nutrients as well as to insure that her milk will be high in nutrients. Drugs and nicotine may influence the quantity and quality of human milk.

level (18 milligrams) that is recommended for the nonpregnant adult female. The drop in the recommendation for folacin during lactation reflects the somewhat reduced need for this vitamin when the maternal blood volume begins to return to the normal amount following delivery.

Of interest is the fact that the recommended intake of 66 grams of protein daily is greater than the amount stipulated for the adult male. Protein demand during lactation is high because protein is contained in the milk being secreted, and the formation of milk is not a totally efficient process. In fact, by the time an infant is consuming 1 quart of human milk daily, the mother is estimated to need approximately 25 grams of protein simply to cover the protein requirements for lactation. Of course, she must also eat enough protein to supply the protein her body needs for normal maintenance and other functions requiring this nutrient. One excellent way of helping to provide the extra protein needed for lactation is to drink as much as 6 glasses of milk daily, preferably nonfat or low-fat milk. This dietary modification has the advantage of adding not only nutritionally complete protein, but also calcium, phosphorus, riboflavin, and vitamin D.

Since the breast-fed infant is primarily dependent on the maternal milk for practically all nutrients until additional foods are incorporated in the diet, the maternal diet should be planned to insure that the nutrient content of her milk is optimal. Calcium, protein, and phosphorus levels in milk are fairly constant regardless of the mother's diet, but the quantities of some of the other nutrients in milk are influenced by her food intake. Thiamin, ascorbic acid, iodide, and fluoride levels are definitely related to the maternal diet.

A practical daily dietary plan for the lactating woman can be outlined as follows:

Milk (preferably low fat).   Minimum of 3 to 4 glasses, frequently 5 to 6.

Meat.   Two 4-ounce servings plus 1 egg.

Vegetables and fruits.   Four ounces of orange juice or citrus; one serving of dark green leafy or yellow vegetable daily; at least 2 additional servings of fruits and/or vegetables.

Bread and cereal.   At least 4 slices of bread (or servings of cereals).

This plan still follows the same pattern that insures a varied and nourishing diet throughout life. However, the increased servings in the milk group are a highly nourishing means of helping to achieve the 500 to 1000 kilocalorie increase required for lactation. Since the lactating woman still has an allowance for vitamin D, she should be certain that the milk consumed is fortified with vitamin D. The slightly larger servings of meat and the specification of an egg are included to provide additional protein as well as good quantities of the B vitamins and iron. A good dietary source of vitamin A is recommended to insure that the fairly large increase in vitamin A is met. Although the total number of calories provided in the suggested diet plan is dependent upon the actual food selections made, there is a distinct probability that the day's energy allowance will not be met unless some additional food is eaten. The size of the servings of meat, cereals, and vegetables could be increased. Some fried foods or additional small quantities of fat in the form of salad dressings or spreads on bread can be included to meet the body's need for energy. Some desserts might be added. Attention should be given to supplying the necessary calories for lactation without establishing a permanent dietary pattern that will lead to obesity after lactation ceases.

Since the nutritional demands of lactation are even greater than those of pregnancy, the adequacy of the lactating woman's diet should be evaluated. However, with the increased requirement for calories, all the necessary nutrients will be available if good dietary patterns are followed. Unfortunately, some women simply do not eat that well nor plan that carefully. For them, a nutritional supplement may be necessary. The actual composition of the supplement needs to be based on rounding out nutritional needs instead of providing overdoses of some of the vitamins and minerals. If a woman is not drinking milk, she definitely will require a supplement containing a large fraction of the 1200 milligrams of calcium and the 1200 milligrams of phosphorus recommended daily. On the other hand, if she is drinking 4 to 5 glasses of milk regularly, her need for these minerals is supplied in her diet and supplementation is inappropriate. Particular attention should be given to the amount of iron in the diet to insure that the level is adequate to provide good protection against the development of anemia. Two additional check points in planning the diet of the lactating woman are: (1) only iodized salt should be used and (2) fluoridated water should be used for drinking water. These two minerals—iodide and fluoride—are extremely important to the infant, and they are available to the infant when the lactating woman includes these in her diet.

The actual quantity of milk produced is variable, but most women secrete close to a quart per day. Since human milk is approximately 85 percent water, this means that much water is lost from the maternal body due to the secretion of milk for her baby. To provide for this additional demand for liquid, the lactating woman usually should increase her regular fluid intake by as much as a quart if she can. This may be done by drinking extra servings of fruit or vegetable juices, tea, coffee, bouillon, or other beverages. Of course, if she is drinking 4 to 6 glasses of milk daily, she is gaining additional liquid in that manner also. This additional liquid is recommended so that the normal quantity of urine is excreted daily. If fluid intake is limited, the urine volume diminishes, and this may impair the ability of the kidneys to excrete waste materials. There is seemingly no significant relationship between the quantity of fluids ingested and the volume of milk secreted.

The ingestion of other compounds that are not ordinarily considered a part of the diet also requires consideration in a discussion of lactation. Practically all compounds that enter the mother's body will be secreted, in varying forms and quantities, in her milk. Therefore, attention should be directed to the effect of drugs, alcohol, and smoking, as well as to the dietary intake. Although considerable research still is needed to clarify the effects of drugs and medications, some answers are beginning to be available. Assessment of drug influences is made in relation to the effect upon the quantity of milk produced and the levels and forms in which the drugs are secreted in the milk. The levels need to be viewed in relation to the body weight of the infant, that is, an intake of only one twelfth of the adult dose may be expected to be comparable in effect upon the body of a very young child.

Maternal ingestion of antibiotics at usual dosage levels does not appear to present a hazard to the nursing infant. The levels of these drugs secreted in the milk are not considered to be high enough to have an effect on the infant. The same statement may be made for the use of salicylates, although very high intake apparently should be avoided during lactation.

Nicotine is secreted in milk in relation to the levels entering the lactating woman's body. Although moderate cigarette smoking perhaps is not harmful to the infant (the volume of milk may be decreased), heavy smoking is contrary to optimum lactation. The effects of smoking marijuana are deemed by Arena (1970) to be potentially far more harmful than those from cigarettes. However, extensive research data in this area are not yet available.

Yet other aspects of contemporary societal problems may be important in lactation. For example, the widespread use of oral contraceptives is a recognized fact. However, the effects of these hormones, transmitted through milk to infants, have still to be fully assessed in nursing infants. The general alarm over the use of DDT represents a different facet of societal concerns. Studies of the level of DDT in breast milk support the conclusion that present levels of DDT usage do not present a danger to nursing infants. The hazard of malaria due to reduced use of DDT, however, should be considered by those who are concerned with infant health.

The preceding suggestions provide the dietary framework needed to support successful lactation. This pattern is recommended as long as lactation continues. There is no set time for the duration of lactation, this being a largely individual matter. There is particular value in prolonging lactation for several months, even up to a year or more in areas where milk and other foods needed by infants are not readily available. Prolonged lactation requires attention to iron sources for the infant (see Chapter 13). Some mothers in the United States successfully breast feed their infants as long as 6 months, and a few continue still longer. When there is no longer sufficient milk to satisfy the infant and supplementary bottles are necessary, there usually is little value in continuing to attempt breast feeding. When practical and possible, breast feeding for at least 3 months is desirable.

Summary

Pregnancy and lactation, while normal conditions for the female, place additional nutritional demands upon the woman, and her diet needs to be adjusted to meet these requirements. The energy needs during pregnancy are increased modestly, yet the requirements for other nutrients are elevated appreciably. This necessitates careful dietary selection based on a wide variety of foods that contribute essential nutrients and modest amounts of energy. To insure optimum reproductive performance, a good diet that supplies all the necessary nutrients should be consumed prior to, early in pregnancy, and throughout the duration of pregnancy and lactation. Weight gain usually should be regulated to within the range of 22 to 27 pounds. The concern for adequate nutrition is particularly great for the pregnant adolescent because she is confronted with the need to supply her own dietary needs for growth plus those of the fetus, a taxing job at best and one that is frequently complicated both by adjustment problems and dubious dietary habits. For the pregnant woman who is experiencing difficulties in following the recommended dietary plan, or where there is uncertainty about dietary intakes, there is need to include a dietary supplement, usually of vitamins and minerals, to provide the recommended levels of nutrients not being supplied by the food she selects to eat.

Lactating women need to follow a modified diet that is an expansion of the varied diet recommended prior to pregnancy if they are to provide all their nutritional needs through food alone. This can be done by including 4 or more glasses of milk daily (preferably low fat) and by adjusting the size of the servings of the other foods eaten. A generous quantity of liquid is also recommended. The large number of calories allowed for lactation provides sufficient opportunity to obtain all the nutrients needed from the diet. However, if a review of the food intake shows that not all dietary needs are being met, a supplement may need to be provided to bring the nutritional intake to the recommended levels.

Selected References

Arena, J. M. Contamination of the ideal food. *Nutrition Today 5,* No. 4:2. 1970.

Bagchi, K., and A. K. Bose. Effect of low nutrient intake during pregnancy on obstetrical performance and offspring. *Am. J. Clin. Nutr. 11*:586–592. 1962.

Barnes, R. H. Effects of malnutrition on mental development. *J. H. Ec. 61*:671–676. 1969.

Beaton, G. H. Nutritional and physiological adaptations in pregnancy. *Fed. Proc. 20,* No. 1, Part III:196–201. 1961.

Burke, B. S. Nutrition in pregnancy. *Obstetrics,* 12th ed., by J. P. Greenhill. Saunders, Philadelphia. 1960.

Committee on Maternal Nutrition. *Maternal Nutrition and the Course of Pregnancy.* National Academy of Sciences, National Research Council. Washington, D.C. 1970.

Committee on Maternal Nutrition. *Nutritional Supplementation and Outcome of Pregnancy.* Food and Nutrition Board, NRC/NAS. Washington, D.C. 1973.

Committee on Nutrition. *Nutrition in Maternal Health Care.* American College of Obstetricians and Gynecologists. E. Wacker, Dr., Chicago. 1974.

Council on Foods and Nutrition. *Symposium 4: Nutrition in Pregnancy.* American Medical Association. Chicago. 1958.

Edwards, C. H., et al. Effect of clay and cornstarch intake on women and their infants. *J. Am. Diet. Assoc. 44*:109. 1964.

Edwards, C. H., et al. Clay- and cornstarch-eating women. *J. Am. Diet. Assoc. 35*:810. 1959.

Emerson, R. G. Obesity and its association with the complications in pregnancy. *Brit. Med. J.* Part 4:516–518. 1962.

Habicht, J. P., et al. Relation of maternal supplementary feeding during pregnancy to birth weight and other sociobiological factors. *Nutrition and Fetal Development.* Ed. by M. Winick. Wiley-Interscience. New York. P. 127. 1974.

Hurley, L. S. The consequences of fetal impoverishment. *Nutrition Today 3,* No. 4:3–10. 1968.

Josimovick, J. B., et al. *Lactogenic Hormones, Fetal Nutrition, and Lactation.* Wiley. New York. 1974.

Jacobson, H. N. Nutrition and Pregnancy. In *Maternal and Child Health Practice: Problems, Resources, and Methods of Delivery.* Ed. by H. W. Wallace et al. Charles C. Thomas. Springfield, Ill. 1973.

Jacobson, H. N. Nutrition and pregnancy. *J. Am. Diet. Assoc. 60:26.* 1972.

King, J. C., and H. N. Jacobson. Nutrition and pregnancy in adolescence. *Teenage Pregnant Girl.* Ed. by J. Zackler and W. Branstadt. Charles C. Thomas. Springfield, Ill. 1975.

Lechtig, A., et al. Maternal nutrition and fetal growth in developing countries. *Am. J. Dis. Child. 129:*553. 1975.

Matter, S. L., and L. M. Wakefield. Religious influence on dietary intake and physical condition of indigent, pregnant Indian women. *Am. J. Clin. Nutr. 24:*1097. 1971.

McGanity, W. J. Obstetric and nutritional problems. *Proceedings of the Western Hemisphere Nutrition Congress.* American Medical Association. Chicago. Pp. 199–201. 1966.

McLaren, D. S. To eat to see. *Nutrition Today 3,* No. 1:2–8. 1968.

McWilliams, M. *Nutrition for the Growing Years.* Wiley. New York. 2nd ed. 1975.

Shank, R. E. A chink in our armor. *Nutrition Today 5,* No. 2:2–11. 1970.

Simonson, M., and B. F. Chow. Maternal diet, growth and behavior. In *Nutrition and Intellectual Growth of Children.* Association for Childhood Education International. Washington, D.C. Pp. 29–32. 1969.

Stearns, G. Nutritional status of the mother prior to conception. *J. Am. Med. Assoc. 168:*1655–1659. 1958.

Subcommittee on Nutrition, Brain Development, and Behavior of Committee on International Nutrition Programs. *Relationships of Nutrition to Brain Development and Behavior.* National Academy of Sciences. National Research Council. Washington, D.C. 1973.

White, P. L. Nutrition and genetic potential. *J. School Health. 36:*337. 1966.

Winick, M., ed. *Nutrition and Development.* Wiley-Interscience. New York. 1972.

Winick, M., ed. *Nutrition and Fetal Development.* Wiley-Interscience. New York. 1974.

World Health Organization. *Nutrition in Pregnancy and Lactation.* Tech. Rept. Series No. 302. Geneva, Switzerland. 1965.

Zackler, J., and W. Branstadt. *Teenage Pregnant Girl.* Charles C. Thomas. Springfield, Ill. 1975.

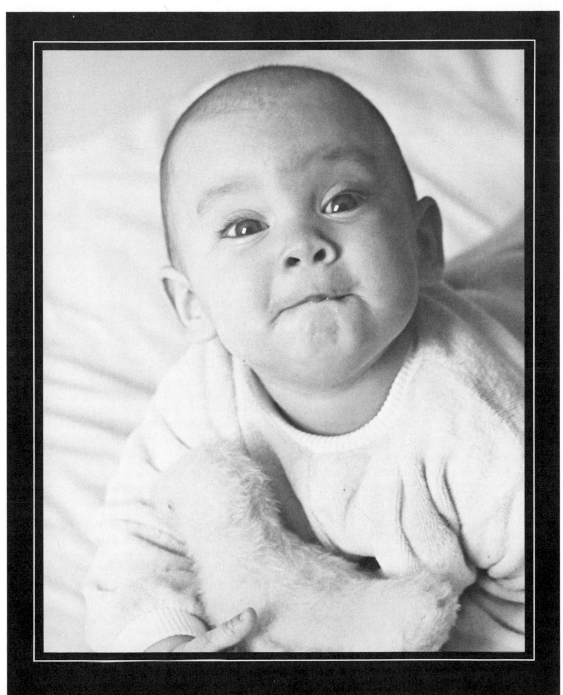

Chapter 13

Feeding the Infant

Nutrition patterns during infancy lay the foundation for the dietary habits of a lifetime. For optimal physical development, the diet must include adequate amounts of all the required nutrients. However, this is only one aspect of infant feeding. The environment in which he is fed and the attitude of those who feed him also begin to mold the infant. The person who carries the major responsibility for the care of the infant needs a good understanding of dietary requirements and hygiene, generously mixed with a blending of love and patience.

The influence of nutritional status upon mental development has been receiving increasing attention from both researchers and the public. Animal experiments, particularly with pigs and rats, have demonstrated reduced learning ability and behavioral and emotional modifications when the animals were fed inadequate diets during the early weeks of life. Malnutrition during the period of rapid cell division in pregnancy and infancy may lead to the for-mation of fewer brain cells than will be formed when the infant is well nourished. The formation of brain lipids also has been found to be reduced in young animals that are malnourished. Numerous research efforts currently in progress doubtless will contribute even more compelling findings to underline the extreme importance of adequate nutrition in the early months and years of life.

Knittle and Hirsch (1968) have drawn attention to the fact that the number of adipose tissue cells increases rapidly during early childhood. Furthermore, obesity in adults is correlated with the number of adipose cells. Such findings suggest a value in avoiding excessive weight gain during early life. Support is given to this theory by Eid's report (1970) that, among an obese group of elementary school children, a significantly greater number showed rapid weight gain during infancy (compared with those gaining at a rate of average or below during infancy).

The evidence is increasing that adequate nutrition during infancy is of permanent importance if a person is to achieve optimum development from the standpoint of both physical growth and mental capacity. Even weight control problems may have their roots in infant feeding practices. Therefore, planning of infant diets and the establishment of good dietary practices assume a significant place in discussions of human nutrition.

The Importance of Milk

The basic food in the diet of the infant, of course, is milk. This immediately leads the new mother to the question of whether the milk to be used will be human or cow's milk. For women who must return to work almost immediately, the only practical decision may well be to bottle feed. For many other women, there is need for more information on which to base their decision. A useful starting point is the comparison of the nutritive qualities of the two types of milk (Table 13.1).

For mothers electing to breast feed their infants, the first fluid to appear will be colostrum, a watery, slightly yellow liquid. The flow of colostrum begins by at least the fourth day after delivery. Colostrum is valued for the antibodies

Table 13.1 Composition of Colostrum, Human Milk, and Cow's Milk

Nutrient	Colostrum[a] (1-5 days)	Milk[b] Human	Milk[b] Cow's
	(100 g)	(100 g)	(100 g)
kcal	58	77	65
Protein (g)	2.7	1.1	3.5
Fat (g)	2.9	4.0	3.5
Carbohydrate (g)	5.3	9.5	4.9
Calcium (mg)	31	33	118
Phosphorus (mg)	14	14	93
Iron (mg)	0.09	0.1	Trace
Vitamin A (I.U.)	296	240	140
Thiamin (mg)	0.015	0.01	0.03
Riboflavin (mg)	0.029	0.04	0.17
Niacin (mg)	0.075	0.2	0.1
Ascorbic acid (mg)	4.4	5	1

[a] Data from Food and Nutrition Board, National Academy of Science. *The Composition of Milks.* National Research Council Publication No. 254. National Research Council. Washington, D.C. 1953.

[b] Data from *Composition of Foods,* Agriculture Handbook No. 8. Agricultural Research Service, U.S. Department of Agriculture. Washington, D.C. 1963.

contained in it. These antibodies are transmitted through the colostrum from mother to newborn, where they are absorbed to provide some immunity to infectious diseases (Mata and Wyatt, 1971) early in infancy. Although the caloric value is lower for colostrum than for mature human milk (defined as milk produced 10 or more days after delivery), the infant does receive a reasonable intake of most of the nutrients he needs. In addition, the sucking of the infant is important in stimulating the mammary glands to function.

Comparison of human and cow's milk

The usual assumptions are that all human milk is the same and that human milk is the ideal food for human infants since this is the natural food available. Certainly there is no question that most infants will thrive on human milk. However, many infants also grow well when fed cow's milk or formulas that are different in composition from human milk. Several distinct differences quickly become apparent when the milks are compared (Table 13.1).

1. Cow's milk contains more than three times as much protein as human milk.
2. Human milk is twice as high in carbohydrate as is cow's milk.
3. Calcium levels are approximately four times higher and the phosphorus content is six times higher in cow's milk than in human milk.
4. Cow's milk is approximately four times higher in riboflavin content than human milk.

These differences immediately raise questions regarding the efficacy of each type of milk in promoting growth. The higher content of protein, calcium, and phosphorus in cow's milk would seem to favor greater growth than would human milk, and yet infants on cow's milk

formulas grow somewhat more slowly than breast-fed infants for the first few months. By the middle of the first year, infants raised on cow's milk begin to grow more rapidly, and no observable difference is detected by the time children are 2 years old.

There are some possible explanations for this seeming paradox wherein human milk, despite its lower content of the nutrients specifically needed for growth, is able to promote growth more effectively than does cow's milk. The protein content figures tell only part of the story. The principle protein in cow's milk, casein, forms a relatively firm curd in the stomach, even when the milk has been pasteurized and homogenized. The protein in this firm curd is less easily digested by the enzymes available in the infant's digestive tract than is the curd of human milk. Dilution of cow's milk in formula preparation promotes formation of a softer protein curd and reduces renal load as a consequence of the reduced concentrations of these nutrients. Lactalbumin, the chief protein in human milk, forms a soft curd during digestion and is readily digested and absorbed by the infant.

The high level of lactose in human milk is very favorable to the increased absorption of calcium, which partially accounts for the excellent growth resulting from the consumption of human milk. Lactose is the carbohydrate in both human and cow's milk. One other compositional difference of particular interest is that the polyunsaturated, longer chain fatty acids of human milk are more readily available to the infant than are the more saturated fatty acids of cow's milk (see Chapter 7). Of course, the fatty acids in commercial formulas can be modified, a practice that is followed today in many formulas.

The decision to breast feed or bottle feed

From the foregoing discussion, it is apparent that most babies will be well nourished with either human or cow's milk as the principle source of nutrients. Hence, in the United States the selection of the source of milk enters the realm of personal preference. This is an important decision to make because reversal from bottle feeding to breast feeding is almost impossible. Success with breast feeding comes when the mother prefers this method and uses it from the beginning. In much of the world, where good cow's milk formulas are not available or economically are out of the price range of most families, breast feeding must continue to be encouraged.

Much can be said for the warm relationship breast feeding can foster between mother and infant. Many women appear to gain a real sense of fulfillment when they are able to breast feed their infants successfully. However, this is a relationship strictly between the mother and the infant, and this closeness may create feelings of insecurity and jealously in other members of the family. Some fathers feel left out when they cannot have the opportunity to feed their infants. Siblings, particularly preschoolers, may feel their mothers have lost interest in them now that the baby has arrived. When infants are bottle fed, the father and others in the family can also share in the pleasurable experience of feeding the baby. Of course, parents also should realize that the feedings in the middle of the night can only be done by the mother if she is breast feeding the infant; someone else can take over if the infant is receiving a bottle. Perhaps the practical aspects of the late-night feeding may have caused more than one father to become quite rhap-

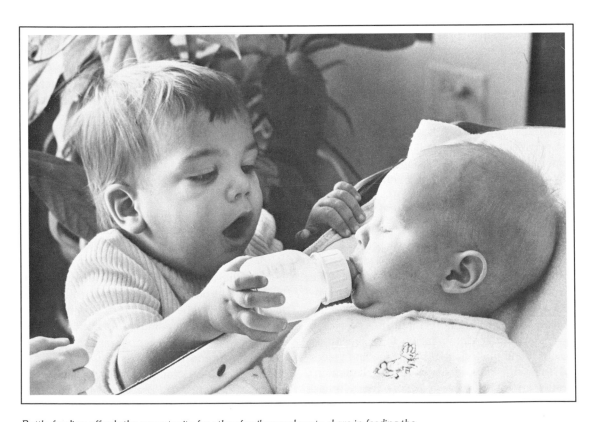

Bottle feeding affords the opportunity for other family members to share in feeding the infant. Under close supervision, this young boy has a welcome opportunity to get acquainted with his brother.

sodic about the natural beauty of the mother-child relationship that is fostered by breast feeding. In short, a warm relationship with the infant can be achieved by either breast or bottle feeding as long as the bottle is given while the baby is held rather than letting him eat alone with his bottle propped.

The safety of the milk supply is one of the important considerations in deciding whether to breast or bottle feed. In areas where a clean milk supply is readily available, sanitation is good, and cold storage facilities are adequate, many of the hazards of formula feeding are eliminated. However, in remote regions or in areas where an adequate amount of safe milk is questionable, the encouragement of breast feeding is definitely preferable for the health of the infant. Since human milk is so adequately packaged until it is consumed, the only concern is the health of the mother.

One argument for breast feeding is that there is no possibility for error in preparing the formula. Human error in formula preparation, as in many other facets of life, can cause a threat to life itself, as occurred when salt was accidentally substituted for sugar in a hospital formula some years ago. Breast feeding also eliminates the possibility of overdiluting the formula or of improperly processing it, both of which may happen when the person preparing the formula does not fully understand the procedures necessary for preparing the food.

The convenience of breast feeding is often cited by mothers who have selected this method. There is no need to budget time for preparing formula and scrubbing bottles. One is never faced with the prospect of a hungry infant and no formula when breast feeding is the choice. Other mothers feel that breast feeding places a strict confinement on their lives; they resent the limitations that breast feeding places on their activities even when supplementary bottles are given on occasion. To them, breast feeding is an inconvenience rather than a convenience.

The comparison of cost between breast and bottle feeding is difficult to make because there are so many variables involved. McKigney (1971) found that, in most cases, babies can be fed more economically by the lactating mother than when other feeding regimens are used. However, comparative costs of evaporated milk for formula preparation and food for the mother's diet may change this analysis as prices change. Despite the fact that formula ingredients must be purchased while human milk appears to be free, this is not a true picture, for the mother needs a substantial increase in her food intake to produce the milk. The cost of producing human milk is highly variable, depending upon the type of diet the woman selects to meet her nutritional needs and the degree to which she calls on her own stores in her body tissues.

Other factors that appear to influence some women's decision regarding breast feeding may also be identified. A real enticement for breast feeding is the large number of additional calories recommended during lactation. Other women will decide not to breast feed because they are fearful of permanent alterations of their figures. Newton (1971) pointed out that lactation may provide some protection against breast cancer, although other factors may reduce the effect contributed by lactation.

Another more subtle factor is that of social influences. The attitudes of relatives and friends toward breast feeding may play a large role in helping the new mother decide about breast feeding. There is prestige value attached to bottle feeding in some social classes, particularly in the lower groups. In contrast, there is increasing importance being attached to breast feeding among the upper classes, with the result that breast feeding is becoming more widely practiced in the upper classes in recent years. The trend toward less breast feeding in some of the developing countries is a reflection of the importance of "prestige value" and social attitudes in determining the extent of the practice of breast feeding. While social pressures may not be of tremendous significance in

modern countries, the serious health hazards to which the bottle-fed child is exposed in developing countries make it important to attempt to mold social acceptance back toward breast feeding.

An important factor in favor of breast feeding is the problem of allergies. Some infants are allergic to cow's milk. In such cases, the protein is absorbed intact through the intestinal wall instead of first being broken down to its component amino acids. The presence of this foreign protein in the infant can then cause rashes and other allergic manifestations. When allergies are a part of the family's history, breast feeding may help to avoid the possibility of allergy. If a child is allergic to cow's milk, other formula alternatives (such as goat's milk and formulas with a soybean or meat base) are available for feeding the infant, but the expense of most of these is substantially greater than is the cost of breast feeding. A variety of reasons should be considered in deciding whether to breast or bottle feed an infant. Since the infant can be well nourished on either regimen, the method selected should be the one that is best suited to the environmental situation and the psychological satisfactions of the family. In industrial nations, the wise choice is the method that is most likely to insure that meal time will be a joy for the infant and his family.

Meeting Nutritional Needs

The newborn

Milk, despite its many virtues, is not a totally perfect food for the infant, but it does provide most of the nutrients needed for growth and good health during infancy. A quart of vitamin D fortified milk provides 100 percent or more of the recommended daily dietary allowances for protein, riboflavin, calcium, phosphorus, and vitamin D; more than 90 percent of the recommendation for vitamin A; and approximately 65 percent of the thiamin to meet the needs of the 6-month old infant. *The notable nutritional shortcomings of milk for feeding infants are ascorbic acid and iron.* Table 13.2 lists the amounts of nutrients suggested for infants of varying ages in the 1974 revision of the Food and Nutrition Board's "Recommended Daily Dietary Allowances."

The lack of ascorbic acid is easily overcome by either feeding orange juice, a synthetic orange juice containing at least as much ascorbic acid as is found in the fresh juice, or an ascorbic acid supplement. A recommended practice is to begin adding orange juice when the baby is between 7 and 10 days old by feeding only ½ teaspoon of the juice diluted with an equal amount of water. If this is comfortably accommodated by the infant for a few days, the amount is gradually increased until an ounce (2 tablespoons) of the juice-water mixture is being given daily. Then the amount of water is gradually reduced while the juice is increased proportionally until the infant is taking an ounce of pure orange juice daily. The next step is to gradually increase the amount of pure juice given to meet the recommended allowance of 35 milligrams daily. If an infant is unable to tolerate orange juice, a vitamin supplement that includes ascorbic acid should be given until he becomes sufficiently mature for the juice.

Full-term infants born from well-nourished mothers have a supply of iron that is sufficient to last them for 3 to 6 months. Therefore, the lack of iron in milk is not an immediate concern. Dietary sources of iron are generally available to infants in the United States through their commercial baby foods in ample time to meet the body's need for this mineral.

Table 13.2 *Recommended Daily Dietary Allowance for Infants*[a]

Nutrient	Recommended Allowance for Infants	
	0–6 Months[b]	6–12 Months[c]
kcal	kg × 117	kg × 108
Protein (g)[d]	kg × 2.2	kg × 2.0
Vitamin A activity (I.U.)	1400	2000
Vitamin D (I.U.)	400	400
Vitamin E activity (I.U.)	4	5
Ascorbic acid (mg)	35	35
Folacin (μg)	50	50
Niacin (mg)	5	8
Riboflavin (mg)	0.4	0.6
Thiamin (mg)	0.3	0.5
Vitamin B_6 (mg)	0.3	0.4
Vitamin B_{12} (μg)	0.3	0.3
Calcium (mg)	360	540
Phosphorus (mg)	240	400
Iodine (μg)	35	45
Iron (mg)	10	15
Magnesium (mg)	60	70
Zinc (mg)	3	5

[a] Based on *Recommended Daily Dietary Allowances,* revised 1974. Food and Nutrition Board, National Academy of Sciences—National Research Council.
[b] Weight 6 kg (14 lb), height 60 cm (24 in.).
[c] Weight 9 kg (20 lb), height 71 cm (28 in.).
[d] Assumes protein equivalent to human milk.

Although a recommended allowance has not been established for fluoride, the content of this mineral in human milk and in formulas is still of interest because of the protection it provides against dental caries. Fluoride is a component of both cow's milk and human milk if it is present in the water regularly consumed by the milk donor. Lactating women can insure adequate fluoride for their infants if they are fortunate to live in a community that has had the good sense and courage to fluoridate their water. For infants fed by bottle, the formula can be made with fluoridated water.

The amount of vitamin D given the infant needs to be regulated. If the infant is breast fed, a supplement of approximately 400 International Units of vitamin D should be given daily to augment the limited amount of vitamin D in human milk. If the infant is fed a formula, care should be taken to select a milk source containing vitamin D. Fortification of milk products is done at the rate of 400 International Units per quart of the ready-to-drink milk. When the infant is drinking a quart of vitamin D-fortified milk daily, a vitamin D supplement is not necessary. Before the capacity of the infant reaches this point, a vitamin D supplement should be included to bring the total intake to about 400 International Units daily. This supplement should be started a few days after birth.

Feeding the infant

The nutrients in milk are not the only important contribution mealtime makes to an infant's life. Since such a large fraction of life is at first spent sleeping, mealtime represents the infant's main social contact with the world as well as his source of nutrients for physiological needs. Even this early in life a baby's attitudes toward food are beginning to be shaped by the people in his environment and by their verbal and nonverbal communications with him. When he is comfortably, but firmly and securely held and calmly fed, people look friendly and the food seems good. On the other hand, if he is held by an anxious person who holds him rigidly or insecurely or by an indifferent person who props his bottle and moves away, the infant's world is quite different. A relaxing atmosphere with perhaps some soft music and conversation can set the stage for the baby to consume the food he needs; conversely, loud, strident voices and sudden noises may frighten a baby and interrupt a satisfactory meal. However, there is some value in providing enough activity in the background to keep the baby awake until he has had enough food to sustain him comfortably for 3 to 4 hours.

Most people carry the image of the young mother carefully shaking a drop of milk on her wrist to see if she has heated the formula sufficiently to feed her baby. Certainly care must be taken to be sure that the milk is not so warm that it will burn the infant's tender mouth, but there has been considerable discussion regarding the necessity of warming the formula at all. This practice presumably was begun as an attempt to make bottle feeding as similar as possible to breast feeding. Today's rather mobile population has brought the need for warming the milk into sharp questioning. Apparently infants will thrive on formulas fed directly from the refrigerator, as they will on formulas that have been warmed. A slight warming of the milk, at least to satisfy the parents' concerns, seems appropriate for young infants when it is possible to do so, although there is no necessity for this.

Particularly for mothers who elect to breast feed their infants, it is helpful to arrange to be uninterrupted if possible during the feeding period. Breast feeding is more likely to be successful when the mother is able to relax completely, to be comfortable, and enjoy the feeding time with her infant. If she feels anxious about her life and has other small children constantly interrupting, she may find that breast feeding is a difficult choice for her. Initially, hospital personnel (Jelliffe and Jelliffe, 1971) can do much to help give a woman the confidence that she needs for successful lactation. One of the impediments to successful lactation can be fatigue, which may be alleviated with frequent rests during the day.

Timing

Most new babies will tend to vary their meal request times slightly, but in general will want to be fed approximately every 3 hours for a very small baby to every 4 hours for a large baby. By the time a baby weighs about eight pounds, he will probably be contented with six feedings each day, at approximately 4-hour intervals. As the infant becomes somewhat larger, he gradually can eliminate the middle of the night feeding.

The addition of solids

There is considerable disagreement on the age at which solid foods should be introduced into the diet (Guthrie, 1968). In fact, there seem to be more opinions than mothers, and there are certainly many more theories than pediatricians. Usually the earliest addition of solid food is no sooner than 2 weeks of age and may occur even as late as 2 months or older. In the home, the pressure to add solid food is generated more by the desire for an uninterrupted night's sleep than by a concern for improving nutrition. Many mothers are anxious to add cereal to the late-evening feeding to increase the likelihood of eliminating the middle-of-the-night feeding. For most infants, there is no harm in initiating cereal into the diet as early as 2 or 3 weeks, although there may be only limited utilization of the food. Overfeeding of infants may be a consequence of introducing relatively large quantities of cereals and other solid foods. This practice is to be avoided because of the potential for developing an excess number of adipose cells during infancy.

Cereals

Cereals especially prepared for infant feeding are nourishing and convenient to use. These products, prepared either as single-grain or mixed cereals, are processed so that the only preparation involved in the home is simply to stir in some milk. Cereals are most easily introduced to the baby if they are the consistency of a very thin gruel, just slightly more viscous than the milk itself. The first day the cereal is fed, only about ½ teaspoon of cereal is given. By gradual introduction of the new food, there is ample opportunity to observe any possible allergic response without undue discomfort to the infant.

When feeding the infant his cereal at first, parents need to realize that the young baby is unable to coordinate his tongue movements to transfer food from the tip of the tongue to the back of his mouth for swallowing. Food is as likely to come right back out as it is to move toward the back of the mouth. This is not an indication of rejection or dislike of a food when a baby spits food back out, but is simply a lack of muscular coordination. Unfortunately, parents who are apprehensive about how their babies will like a food may interpret such actions as a dislike and promptly remove the food from the baby's diet. Much of the difficulty can be avoided by diluting solid foods to a thin consistency while the infant is still very young and by placing the food toward the back of the baby's tongue rather than just spooning it onto the tip. When cereal is fed in this manner to a baby cra-

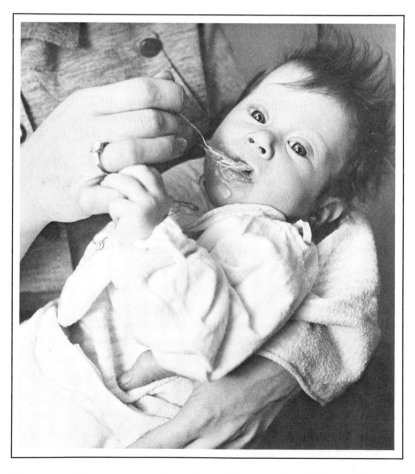

Infants are not able to move cereals and other solid foods readily to the back of the mouth for swallowing. This problem is reduced by placing the food toward the back of the tongue.

dled in the arms, the slightly thickened cereal is easily swallowed by the infant.

The age at which pediatricians currently suggest adding cereals ranges from less than 2 weeks to more than 2 months. Usually one of the single-grain cereals, such as rice, is used first because there is somewhat less likelihood of intolerance of the protein (allergy) from a single cereal than from a mixture of cereals. Most of the cereals for babies are well fortified with iron as well as the B vitamins. Although the iron appears to be virtually unavailable to the very young infant, this becomes an important source of iron and is better utilized before the infant reaches the age of 6 months. Cereals also add important new tastes and texture to help broaden the food experience of infants.

Fruits and vegetables

Usually the next food to be added will be pureed fruits, followed shortly thereafter by vegetables. Manufacturers of baby foods have made a wide array of fruits and vegetables available for feeding infants. Fruits are generally simply cooked, pureed, and canned with little modification; they are well received by almost all infants. Vegetables have undergone some flavor modification, principally in the addition of salt, seemingly to satisfy adult taste preferences. This practice of salting commercially prepared vegetables for infants has recently been questioned. Fomon et al. (1970) found that infants accepted unsalted foods as readily as the salted products. Furthermore, the use of salt increased sodium intake fourfold, and the natural levels of sodium in the foods were sufficient to meet the infant's need for this mineral nutrient. Therefore, there seems to be questionable justification for adding salt to baby food. The use of monosodium glutamate (MSG) in baby foods has also been challenged. Although evidence of possible harm was decidedly inconclusive, the major manufacturers of baby foods have voluntarily eliminated MSG and have decreased the use of salt by half or more.

Meats and eggs

The addition of strained meats, following the establishment of fruits and vegetables in the diet, provides important amounts of protein, the B vitamins, and iron. As with other new foods, a variety of strained meats should be introduced gradually to expand the baby's food experiences and nutritive intake. Meats often are added by the third month, and certainly should be a regular part of the baby's daily dietary pattern by 6 months of age. The teaspoon serving of meat used to introduce this item usually can be increased to at least 2 tablespoons by the age of 6 months.

Egg yolks, either as the canned baby food product or hard cooked in the home, are useful in providing protein, iron, and vitamin A. This food should be offered initially in ½ to 1 teaspoon quantities until it has been ascertained that the yolks do not cause an allergic response. Then the serving size can be increased to a whole yolk three or more times weekly. At approximately 10 months, most infants are ready for the white as well as the yolk. An increasing number of physicians do not recommend extensive use of the yolks because yolks are a concentrated source of cholesterol, a view with which many nutritionists agree because of future "heart health."

To an adult eye, the size of a can of baby food is small, and one might expect that a baby could readily consume the contents of the can. However, when first adding these canned solid foods to the baby's diet, only about ½ tablespoon of food is fed the first day and only slightly more is fed the second day. This means that not all the food will be eaten while the food is still reasonably fresh. Even if the remaining baby food is refrigerated as soon as the serving is removed from the can, a can of baby food should not be used more than 3 or 4 days after being opened.

One of the arguments for beginning baby foods early is to acquaint the baby with a wide variety of foods and expand his taste experiences. With that in mind, parents are wise to plan to include a broad range of foods in the diet. The addition of meats rounds out the diet so that the baby is now actually eating on the Basic Four Food Group Plan. Of course, the food may appear in a distinctly different form from that eaten by adults, but the foods are all there; and baby food manufacturers have demonstrated considerable initiative in developing a wide number of products especially for babies.

One point should be made to clarify the baby food products available on the market. There are several products that can be categorized as vegetables and meat mixtures or as casseroles. These mixtures may be quite low in meat and are not actually a replacement for the pureed meats in the diet. The so-called "high-meat dinners" actually contain somewhat less than half as much protein as the pureed meats.

As infants grow older and begin to teethe, other cereal products, such as zwieback or dry bread, are suitable additions to the diet. These provide a new experience in texture, a reasonable source of B vitamins and iron, and some comfort for teething pains. Although such foods have their place in the diet, attention should be given to avoid feeding crackers and baby cookies too close to the next meal. Poorly timed snacks can dull the appetite significantly so that milk and other nourishing foods are not consumed in adequate amounts.

Since babies have high nutritional needs (including energy requirements) and limited capacities, nourishing desserts and enriched pastas may well be included in their diets to provide the extra energy. The alternative is extra fat, most of which will be of the saturated variety (from meats and whole milk or its products), and this is not desirable. Food should supply the nutritional and energy needs of the infant without causing excessive weight gain.

Food meets psychological as well as physiological needs, even for infants and parents. The desired situation for feeding the infant is one in which a comfortable rapport is established between infant and adult, with the occasion

meeting social as well as physiological needs. In less desirable circumstances, food may assume other meanings. When food is used as a tool to salve a parent's conscience and support his ego in the raising of his child, the baby may begin to develop undesirable attitudes that may cause him to be overweight or underweight throughout his life.

The actual amounts of food required by an infant cannot be generally stated because of the variations in appetite and individual need. At first, the total nutritional needs will be provided by milk or a formula. A rough approximation of the amount of milk or formula needed daily by the newborn can be made by multiplying the baby's weight (in kilograms) times 5 ounces. Of course, this amount increases gradually as the infant grows. This intake of milk and the gradual addition of solid foods are needed to provide the increasing need for nutrients during the first year (see Table 13.2). Since milk does not, in itself, contain all the nutrients needed for good health, the amounts of the other foods served to the infant should be increased gradually so that these foods plus a maximum of a quart of milk each day satisfy the baby. Milk should not replace these other important foods in the diet.

One good way of determining that a baby is getting enough to eat is to check his weight gain. An average weight gain during the first 6 months is 6 ounces each week, with many babies doubling the birth weight around 4 months. From 6 months until a baby reaches his first birthday, the rate of gain is somewhat slower. The average baby will almost triple his birth weight by 12 months.

However, growth clearly is an individual matter. Therefore, not all well-nourished babies will gain weight at the exact rate indicated. These figures are merely a guide. Steady weight gain, even at a slower rate than indicated, is an indication of good nutrition, particularly when the baby is alert, happy, and developing some subcutaneous fat and muscles.

Feeding the older infant

As the infant's digestive tract becomes more mature and his chewing capability increases, he will be able to eat soft foods that are not pureed. To meet this transitional period to adult fare, baby food manufacturers have produced junior foods. These foods are fairly finely chopped, but provide a distinct contrast to the texture of pureed foods. Some families use the junior foods for 3 or 4 months, beginning when the baby is about 10 months old. These foods are particularly useful when the family eats on a different schedule than the baby. However, with a bit of careful planning, many young babies can make the transition from pureed

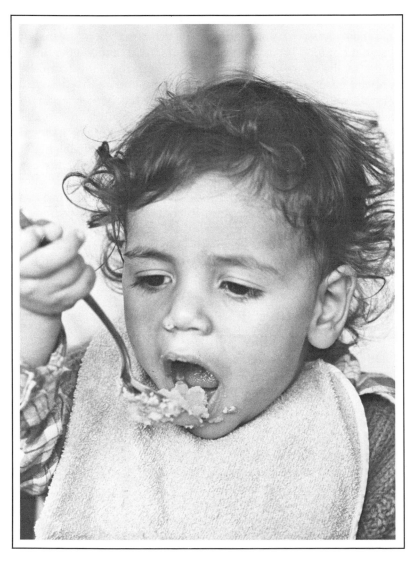

Feeding one's self is an important, although usually messy developmental task of the older infant.

foods to table foods with little or no use of junior foods. Since the cost of feeding baby foods to an infant nearing the 1-year mark is relatively high, there is some motivation to include the baby in the family's regular meals as soon as he is sufficiently mature. Extensive use of the blender is one effective way of making greater use of the family's food for feeding infants, thus reducing food costs during this period.

Babies will find that eating is an enjoyable experience if adults can avoid being over-anxious about two things: the amount of food the baby eats and the messiness of the occasion. The normal infant has a very effective hunger mechanism and will eat the amount of food he needs if he is not pressured to keep eating after he is satisfied. When a good diet is pleasantly offered in calm surroundings, the healthy infant will eat enough to be well nourished. Only when the person feeding him communicates concern and urges the baby to eat more than he needs does resistance to eating or overeating become a pattern.

As the infant grows older and begins to develop some muscular coordination, he will begin to want to feed himself sometimes. These efforts are an important developmental experience and should be encouraged. At first, the nutritional rewards of feeding oneself may be very limited, necessitating some cooperation between baby and adult. Acceptance of the learning situation involved in this period of learning to feed oneself is important. This establishes eating as a comfortable situation, a time not devoted to constant correction and complaints about what and how the baby is eating. This places food and eating in the proper context of life and lays the foundation for a lifetime of good nutrition.

In recent years there has been considerable interest as to whether poor nutrition very early in life is or is not a primary factor in mental development and learning capacity later in life. Animal studies indicate such may be the case. With humans there are so many other factors, sociologic and psychologic, that influence mental development that so far it has been impossible to separate out the purely nutritional factors. This is an active field of research at this time.

Summary

The environmental conditions and family attitudes are important considerations in the decision to breast or bottle feed the new infant. The merits of breast feeding versus bottle feeding have been reviewed in this chapter. Where possible, breast feeding is to be preferred. The newborn's diet consists of milk soon supplemented with a source of ascorbic acid and iron. The addition of solid foods is begun usually sometime between 2 and 8 weeks of age and follows the pattern of cereals first, then fruits and vegetables, and finally meats. Initial additions of food are very small, but are gradually increased as the infant's appetite grows. Milk intake is recommended to reach a maximum not exceeding 1 quart per day, with the other foods being used to round out the diet and satisfy the infant's hunger. By the time the baby is 6 months old, his daily menu can be planned around the Basic Four Food Group Plan.

Pureed foods are necessary for the young infant, but he has sufficient chewing capability by the age of 9 or 10 months to begin the transition to junior foods or selected table foods. During this important developmental period, the family can help the baby achieve a normal, interested attitude toward food without generating anxiety and undue concern about eating. The first year lays the foundation for the dietary habits of a lifetime.

Selected References

Andelman, M. B., and B. R. Sered. Utilization of dietary iron by term infants. *Am. J. Dis. Child. 113:*403. 1967.

Arroyavem, G. Biochemical characteristics of malnourished infants and children. *Proceedings of Western Hemisphere Nutrition Congress.* Chicago. Pp. 30–36. 1966.

Bakwin, H. Feeding programs for infants. *Fed. Proc. 23:*66. 1964.

Barnes, R. H. Nutrition and man's intellect and behavior. *Fed. Proc. 30:*1429. 1971.

Barnes, R. H. Effects of malnutrition on mental development. *J. Home Econ. 61:*671–676. 1969.

Beal, V. A. On the acceptance of solid foods and other food patterns of infants and children. *Pediatrics. 20:*448. 1957.

Burroughs, A. L., and R. L. Huenemann. Iron deficiency in rural infants and children. Caloric, nutrient and milk intakes. *J. Am. Diet. Assoc. 57:*122–128. 1970.

Dahl, L. K. High salt content of western infants' diets. *Nature. 198:*1204. 1963.

Darby, W. J. The rational use of vitamins in medical practice. *Med. Clin. N. Am. 48:*1203. 1964.

Dobbing, J. Nutrition and mental development. *Present Knowledge of Nutrition.* 4th ed. Nutrition Foundation. New York. 1976.

Dugdale, A. E. Effect of type of feeding on weight gain and illnesses in infants. *Br. J. Nutr. 26:*423. 1971.

Eichenwald, H. F., and P. C. Fry. Nutrition and learning. *Science 163:*644. 1969.

Fomon, S. J., et al. Acceptance of unsalted strained foods by normal infants. *J. Pediat. 76:*242–246. 1970.

Fomon, S. J., et al. Relationship between formula concentration and rate of growth of normal infants. *J. Nutr. 98:*241. 1969.

Fomon, S. J. *Infant Nutrition.* Saunders. Philadelphia. 2nd ed. 1974.

Greenwaldt, E., et al. Onset of sleeping through the night in infancy; relation to introduction of solid food in the diet, birth weight and position in the family. *Pediatrics. 26:* 667–668. 1960.

Gryboski, J. D. Swallowing mechanism of the neonate. *Pediatrics. 35:*445. 1965.

Guthrie, H. A. Nutritional intake of infants. *J. Am. Diet. Assoc. 43;* 120. 1963.

György, P. Biochemical aspects. Symposium: The uniqueness of human milk. *Am. J. Clin. Nutr. 24:*970. 1971.

Heiner, D. C., et al. Sensitivity to cow's milk. *J. Am. Med. Assoc.* 1964.

Hirsch, J. Cell number and size as a determinant of subsequent obesity. *Childhood Obesity.* Ed. by M. Winick. Wiley-Interscience. New York. 1975.

Ho, C. H., and M. L. Brown. Food intake of infants attending well-baby clinics in Honolulu. *J. Am. Diet. Assoc. 57:*17–21. 1970.

Illingsworth, R. S., and J. Lister. The critical or sensitive period, with special reference to certain feeding problems in infants and children. *J. Pediat. 65:*839. 1964.

Jackson, R. L., et al. Growth of "well-born" American infants fed human and cow's milk. *Pediatrics. 33:*642. 1964.

Jelliffe, D. B., and E. F. P. Jelliffe. Approaches to village level infant feeding. V. How breast feeding really works. *J. Trop. Pediat. and Environ. Child Health. 17* (June):62. 1971.

Jelliffe, D. B., and E. F. P. Jelliffe. The urban avalanche and child nutrition. *J. Am. Diet. Assoc. 57:*111–118. 1970.

Knittle, J. L., and J. Hirsch. Effect of early nutrition on development of rat epididymal fat pad: cellularity and metabolism. *J. Clin. Invest. 47:*2091. 1968.

Knowles, J. A. Excretion of drugs in milk—a review. *J. Pediat. 66:*1086. 1965.

Latham, M. C., and F. Cobos. Effects of malnutrition on intellectual development and learning. *Am. J. Pub. Health. 61:*1307. 1971.

Macy, I. G., et al. *Composition of milks.* Publ. 254. National Research Council of National Academy of Sciences. Washington, D.C. 1953.

Mata, L. J., and R. G. Wyatt. Host resistance to infection. Symposium: The uniqueness of human milk. *Am. J. Clin. Nutr. 24:*976. 1971.

McKigney, J. Economic aspects. Symposium: The uniqueness of human milk. *Am. J. Clin. Nutr. 24:*1005. 1971.

McLaren, D. S. To eat to see. *Nutrition Today 3,* No. 1:2–8. 1968.

McWilliams, M. *Nutrition for the Growing Years.* Wiley. New York. 2nd ed. 1975.

Meyer, H. F. *Infant Foods and Feeding Practices.* Charles C. Thomas, Springfield, Ill. 1960.

Newton, N. Mammary effects. Symposium: The uniqueness of human milk. *Am. J. Clin. Nutr. 24:*987. 1971.

Newton, N. Psychologic differences between breast and bottle feeding. Symposium: The uniqueness of human milk. *Am. J. Clin. Nutr. 24:*993. 1971.

Review. Solid foods in the nutrition of young infants. *Nutr. Rev. 25:* 233. 1967.

Seelig, M. S. Vitamin D and cardiovascular, renal, and brain damage in infancy and childhood. *Annals of the New York Acad. of Science 147:*537–582. 1969.

Shank, R. E. Is there a need to fortify infant foods? *Am. J. Pub. Health. 55:*1188. 1965.

Smith, C. A. Overuse of milk in the diets of infants and children. *J. Am. Med. Assoc. 172:*567–569. 1960.

Subcommittee of Nutrition, Brain Development, and Behavior. *Relationship of Nutrition to Brain Development and Behavior.* Food and Nutrition Board. NAS-NRC. Washington, D.C. 1973.

Tompson, M. Convenience of breast feeding. Symposium: The uniqueness of human milk. *Am. J. Clin. Nutr. 24:*991. 1971.

Weil, W. B. Infantile obesity. *Childhood Obesity.* Wiley-Interscience. New York. 1975.

Williams, H. H. Differences between cow's and human milk. *J. Am. Med. Assoc. 175:*104. 1961.

Winick, M. Nutrition and intellectual development in children. In *Nutrition and Intellectual Growth in Children.* Assoc. for Childhood Education International. Washington, D.C. 1969.

Winick, M., ed. *Childhood Obesity.* Wiley-Interscience. New York. 1975.

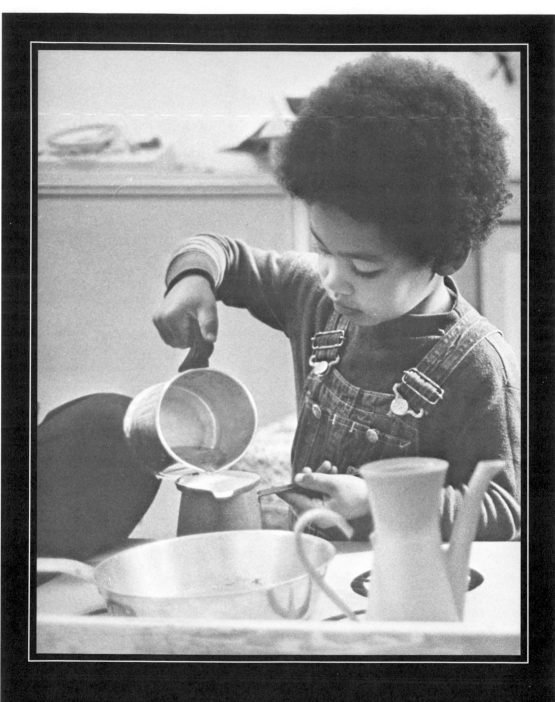

Chapter 14

The Preschool Child

During the preschool years, food begins to serve an expanded role in a child's life. The nutrients from food still are essential to him physiologically despite his slower growth rate. Also, the period between the ages of one and five is an interesting time for both parents and child as he learns about new foods. Indeed, food can be an educational medium for the preschooler. The experiences he gains as he eats with others at home and in preschool settings aid him in the complex task of becoming a social being.

Basic Characteristics of Eating Patterns

One of the most dramatic and normal changes taking place during the second year of life is the reduction in appetite. This single change may be responsible for the concern some parents begin to develop. During the first year of life, parents become accustomed to an increasingly hungry child whose appetite seemingly has amazing limits. Most infants do reduce their milk intake somewhat, beginning at about 6 months of age, as other foods begin to play a more prominent place in their diets. However, the total food intake is truly remarkable for such small bodies. Then, at approximately 1 year of age, the growth rate begins to slow, causing an accompanying decrease in appetite. During the first year, the average infant almost triples his birth weight, and he increases his length by approximately one half (Table 14.1). When one compares these impressive statistics with the gain of approximately 5.5

Table 14.1 *Average Weights and Heights of Boys and Girls from Birth to Age 5*[a]

Age	Girls		Boys	
	Weight (lb)	Height (in.)	Weight (lb)	Height (in.)
Birth	7.4	19.8	7.5	19.9
3 months	12.4	23.4	12.6	23.8
6 months	16.0	25.7	16.7	26.1
9 months	19.2	27.6	20.0	28.0
1 year	21.5	29.2	22.2	29.6
2 years	27.1	34.1	27.7	34.4
3 years	31.8	37.7	32.2	37.9
4 years	36.2	40.6	36.4	40.7
5 years	40.5	42.9	40.5	42.8

[a] Adapted from Nelson, Vaughan, and McKay. **Textbook of Pediatrics,** Ninth Edition, Saunders, Philadelphia, 1969. From data compiled originally by Harold C. Stuart, School of Public Health, Harvard University.

pounds and less than 5 inches during the entire second year, the normal reduction in appetite is not surprising.

Although subsequent pressures may cause some modifications, basic eating patterns and attitudes toward food are being established during this preschool period. Eppright et al. (1970) found that the dietary patterns of children in the North Central region of the United States gradually evolved into one of meals and snacks by age four. This stabilized for the largest percentage of children in the study into a pattern of eating four or five times daily. Such findings are totally consistent with national patterns, which have largely shifted from a strict three meals a day to at least one snack and frequently two snacks in addition to meals.

The influence both of family eating patterns and individual attitudes toward food becomes permanently etched in the preschool child's acceptance and attitudes toward food. The eating experiences of the preschool child may be limited to dining at home with his family or may include many meals away from home at children's centers or restaurants. The child whose experience is mostly in the home tends to become accustomed to the same foods as those preferred by the rest of the family. He will tend to emulate the attitudes toward food that he observes in parents and siblings. Children who frequently eat away from home may acquire more diverse food preferences and customs.

Some preschool children become highly skilled in using food intake as a means of manipulating their families to their own ends. Parents may find themselves in the position of having children dictating what will be served, or they may resort to using food as a reward. Another characteristic of this age group is the tendency to go on food jags. Among preschoolers a common phenomenon is the practice of specializing in eating certain food items for a brief period of time, and then moving on to some other favored food.

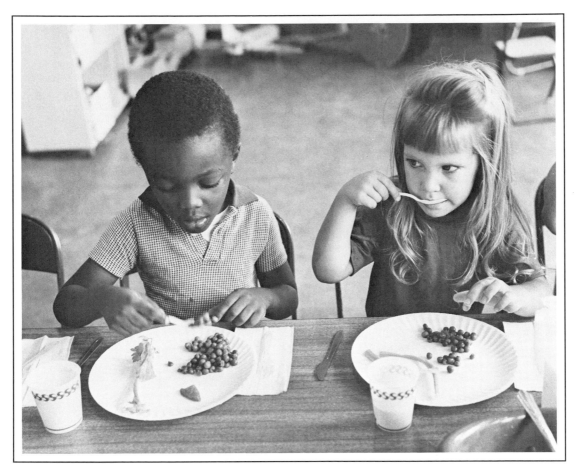

Patterns of food preferences are being formed during the preschool period. Children attending nursery school learn from watching their peers as well as from their families.

Meeting Nutritional Needs

The increasing amount of activity exhibited by the preschooler and the continuing although decelerated growth continue to dictate the need for a diet high in nutrients. Foods high in calories and low in nutrients should not be a predominant part of the diet, but they can be used in moderation to provide the needs for energy without having to rely on large amounts of fat. As seen in Table 14.2, there is a continuing need for calcium and phosphorus to provide the materials needed for continuing bone growth as well as maintenance of the existing

structure. As noted previously, the preschool child is likely to have reduced his milk intake, a change that is potentially detrimental to good nutrition if it drops below an intake of 1 to 2 glasses of milk daily. For children who are not consuming as much as a pint of milk a day, the intake of calcium and phosphorus can be increased by including cheese and ice cream in menus, by preparing items such as meat loaf with nonfat dried milk solids added to the recipe, and by generous use of cream soups and custards. An intake approaching 3 glasses of

Table 14.2 Recommended Daily Dietary Allowances for Boys and Girls Ages 1 to 6[a]

Nutrient	Age and Size	
	1–3 years 28 lb 34 in.	4–6 years 44 lb 44 in.
kcal	1300	1800
Protein (g)	23	30
Vitamin A activity (I.U.)	2000	2500
Vitamin D (I.U.)	400	400
Vitamin E activity (I.U.)	7	9
Ascorbic acid (mg)	40	40
Folacin (μg)	100	200
Niacin (mg equiv.)	9	12
Riboflavin (mg)	0.8	1.1
Thiamin (mg)	0.7	0.9
Vitamin B_6 (mg)	0.6	0.9
Vitamin B_{12} (μg)	1.0	1.5
Calcium (mg)	800	800
Phosphorus (mg)	800	800
Iodine (μg)	60	80
Iron (mg)	15	10
Magnesium (mg)	150	200
Zinc (mg)	10	10

[a] Food and Nutrition Board, National Academy of Sciences—National Research Council, 1974. Recommended Daily Dietary Allowances, revised 1974.

milk daily is helpful in insuring adequate amounts of calcium and phosphorus. If excess weight begins to be a problem, the food energy in the diet can be reduced by serving nonfat or low-fat milk (preferably fortified with vitamin D) instead of whole milk.

Some children exhibit an intolerance to lactose, the sugar in milk, following weaning. Kretchmer, et al. (1971), in studies of four major tribal groups in Nigeria, noted that the malabsorption of lactose ranged from 20 per-

cent in one group to 99 percent in another. Young children with lactose intolerance can be given smaller amounts of milk at each feeding to avoid symptoms, or lactose-free milk can be fed, thus avoiding the diarrhea caused by the presence of excessive amounts of lactose. This problem is far more common among blacks than Caucasians.

The meat category provides a particular challenge in feeding the 1-year-old child adequately. Many of the meats served to older members of the family are too tough for the toddler's chewing capability and interest. If the child is eating with the rest of the family, an important step is to be sure to cook less tender cuts such as pot roasts until they are thoroughly tender so that chewing problems are minimized. However, the stringiness of cuts such as flank steak make these meats difficult for some preschoolers to chew. Some so-called "tender cuts" actually are extremely difficult for youngsters to chew. When such meats are being served, some other product from the meat category should be served to the child until he develops to the point where he can chew steaks

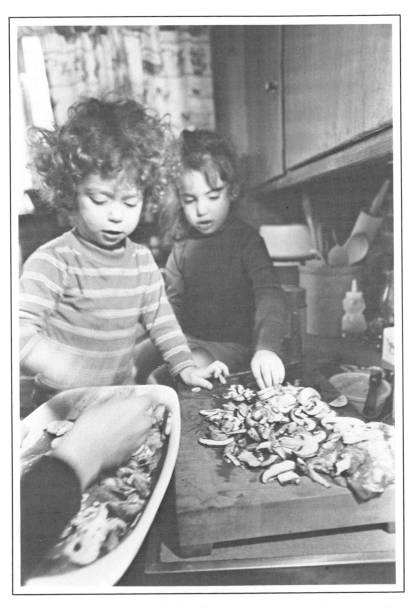

Children may enjoy some vegetables raw. These are particularly tempting and nourishing for snacks.

and similar cuts. In the meantime, suitable substitutes might be a small hamburger patty, cheese, carefully boned fish, or an egg. A satisfactory serving size for preschoolers may be as small as only 1 tablespoon of meat for each year of age. Certainly there is no objection to using somewhat larger servings if they are desired. The recommendation is at least two servings in the meat category daily. From the standpoint of economy as well as good nutrition, serving beans or other legumes for one of these servings is very practical. Also, poultry, fish, eggs, and cheese offer other opportunities for reducing costs in this food category.

Fruits and vegetables are recommended for this age group, as for all other ages. Eppright, et al. (1970) have noted that particular attention is warranted in educating parents to the need for including a citrus fruit daily and a good source of vitamin A at least every other day. Other fruit juices fortified with vitamin C or tomato juice also are useful. The total of four *small* servings of fruits and vegetables daily can readily be consumed if they are prepared attractively and enjoyed by the entire family. Many parents express considerable concern about their children's resistance to eating vegetables, although fruits usually are well accepted. The underlying resistance frequently appears to be the result of poor acceptance of vegetables by other members of the family, a problem that often originates from indifferent preparation, which leads to cooked vegetables with little appeal in texture, color, flavor, or aroma. Dutiful, but unenthusiastic and unimaginative presentation of vegetables usually results in total rejection of numerous vegetables from the diet or a dedicated consumption of vegetables simply because "they are good for you." Quite a different attitude toward vegetables can be developed when they are prepared and cooked with attention and interest or appropriate ones are served raw. One simple way of encouraging the acceptance of cooked vegetables is to serve them when they just lose their crispness and become tender, rather than cooking them until they become mushy and

faded. Acceptance of fruits is usually high, perhaps because they are often incorporated in sweet desserts, or when they are ripe and served raw, the flavor is naturally sweet.

The four servings of the bread and cereal group are met and even exceeded in the preschool period by many youngsters, partly because these items are easily chewed and are readily enjoyed by children and partly because mothers often give crackers and cookies as pacifiers to boost hungry children along toward the family mealtime. For these foods, one should select whole-grain products or those made with enriched flour so that important B vitamins and iron will be consumed along with the calories and protein of these items. Although bread and cereals are nutritionally valuable foods, they should be limited to four servings (each equivalent to approximately one half slice of bread) per day during the preschool period to insure that sufficient space is left in the small stomach for the other foods that also are required for optimum nutrition.

The total dietary intake for the preschool child usually consists of three meals plus a small midmorning and midafternoon snack. Average serving sizes for preschoolers are suggested as being approximately 1 level tablespoon for each year of age. The meals and snacks need to be spaced suitably to promote a good appetite at mealtime without generating undue hunger and fatigue. A suggested schedule is to serve breakfast at 7:30 A.M., midmorning snack at 10 A.M., lunch at noon, midafternoon snack at 3:45 P.M., and supper at 6 P.M.

A suggested menu for a summer day in the life of a 3-year-old child might be:

Breakfast. Orange juice; toast; cereal with milk.

Snack. Milk.

Lunch. Tuna salad sandwich; sliced tomato; fresh apricot; milk.

Snack. Slice of cheese; cracker.

Dinner. Meat loaf; baked potato; green beans; fruit gelatin; milk.

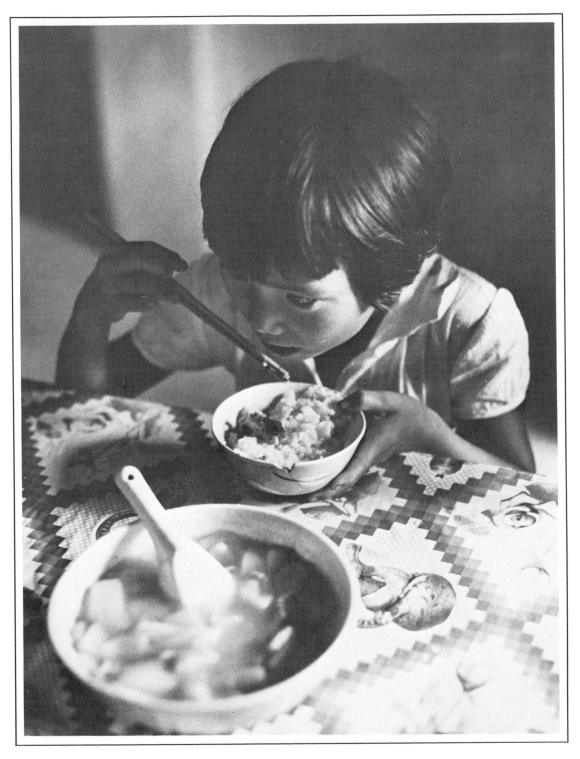

Cultural patterns will influence selections in the diet. Enriched and brown rice are excellent choices in the bread and cereal group.

In addition to the preceding recommendations for the preschooler's diet, two minerals—iodide and fluoride—are very important for growing children. To provide the iodide needed by the preschool child, iodized salt should be used for all food preparation and at the table. Fluoride has been demonstrated to be a mineral nutrient that is effective in reducing the incidence of dental caries. Maximum benefit for children is derived by always using fluoridated water for drinking and in food preparation. This nutrient is most easily provided by adjusting the level of fluoride in the community water supply to a level of 1 part fluoride per million parts of water (1 part per million), a process known as fluoridation. In the event that a city's water is not fluoridated, parents of preschoolers should consult their physician or dentist for a fluoride preparation, although this is not as effective as fluoridated water (see Chapter 10).

Limiting the intake of candy and other sugar-containing foods is of importance during the preschool period, just as it is throughout life. These foods are appealing to many children but excessive use tends to replace more nourishing foods in the diet when they are regularly available to the young child. In addition, caramels, taffy, and lollipops are pertinent examples of ''sticky'' sugar-containing foods that remain in the mouth for a relatively long period of time. The presence of sugar in the mouth between meals provides an environment that favors activity of caries-inducing bac-

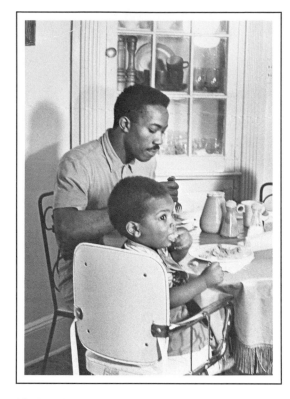

Meals at the table are more pleasant for preschooler and parent when the young child has a chair that is the right height for him to reach the table. The foot rest also is important.

teria. Sugar in moderation at meals can be a part of good nutrition. Excessive use of sugar such that other foods providing protein, minerals, and vitamins are crowded out of the diet is to be discouraged.

Developing Good Dietary Patterns

The meal setting

The goal of establishing good dietary patterns is a reasonable one for the preschool years if parents work constructively toward this end. The first step is to provide a good physical arrangement for the toddler when he begins to eat with the family. This means that a comfortable chair and appropriate tableware are essential. The chair must have a footrest the child can reach easily so he can avoid the problem of dangling feet. It should fit conveniently to the table or provide its own table so that the young diner can reach all of his food easily. His glass will spill less frequently if it is small enough to be held easily with small hands, and if the bottom is weighted to minimize tipping hazards. Silverware designed to meet the specifications of junior-sized hands and mouths is helpful when the youngster is striving to improve his mastery of eating. Easily laundered or plastic mats also help to ease the concerns of the adults when young children join the family at the table.

Usually young children find the dinner table a very stimulating place where there are many new things to learn. The actual consumption of food is only a part of what they are experiencing. This total social experience is important to the development of children, but the ingestion of an adequate diet is essential to building healthy bodies. The attitudes children

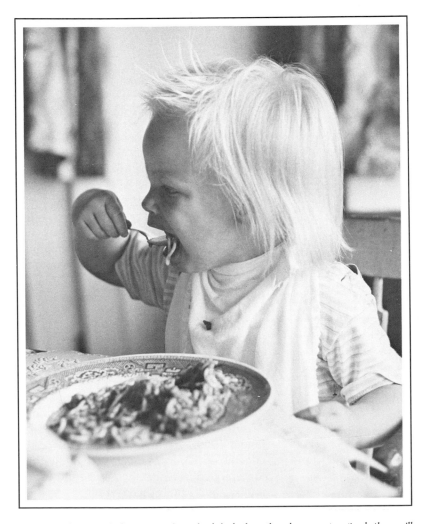

When children are fed on a regular schedule before they become too tired, they will be better able to form good dietary patterns. Note the ease with which this eager diner manages the small spoon.

develop toward eating at the family table are influenced by the general atmosphere. By creating a congenial atmosphere and conversation at the table, all family members, including young children, will find that mealtime is a pleasant and sociable occasion.

A child is encouraged to eat well: (1) if meals are served on a regular schedule at times when the child is hungry and yet not overtired, (2) if the food is already served on his plate when he comes to the table so that he can start to eat without waiting a long time for the food to be served, (3) if adults accept the variations in his appetite from day to day and resist the temptation to coax him to eat, and (4) if table manners are quietly developed over a period of several years. Comments that characterize a child's eating habits, whether they are complimentary or derogatory, are best avoided. A child's dietary patterns may be influenced by adults. Praise for being a "good eater" may encourage a child to eat more than he needs; negative reminders about a "fussy eater" may discourage food intake.

Parental influences

The task of being a parent is a responsibility with many facets. When a youngster begins eating with his parents, the father and mother suddenly are placed in the position of setting the example that influences their child's dietary pattern. Whether or not parents wish this role, it nevertheless is theirs, because children observe and often try to imitate those around them. Ideally, parents will set a fine example by eating a varied diet that provides optimum nutrition while maintaining a desirable weight. Of course, the ideal often is not possible, but some parents may be able to make some improvements in their own diet patterns. Such changes as increasing the variety of foods, drinking milk at some meals, and eating modest amounts of food that lead toward achieving and maintaining a desirable weight may be possible to achieve.

Both the father and mother have a responsibility when the child is eating with the family, but the mother's role often goes beyond the example she sets as she eats. In most families the mother is responsible for planning and preparing the meals and for supervising the schedule of the child. Thus, it becomes her role to gradually introduce a wide variety of well-prepared foods to the young child. She can help to maintain sufficient organization in the family so that the meal schedule is generally the same from day to day and meals are served at times compatible with the young child's need for food and rest, yet not stifling to the needs of other family members.

Preparing food for preschoolers

There are some guidelines that can be used when preparing food for young children. Although not all children will agree with these suggestions, they serve as a convenient starting point in planning food for preschoolers.

1. Generally mild flavors and aromas are preferred. Children have a very sensitive sense of taste because of the large number of functioning taste buds. In addition, mild food aromas generally are preferred because children normally have a keen sense of smell. Strong odors drifting the short distance from the food to the small child may be so intense that there is little motivation to taste the food.

2. Finger foods are tempting to many children who find it frustrating and tiring to persevere with silverware throughout the meal. Finger foods, including strips of uncooked vegetables, slivers of meat, and sandwiches, are enjoyed because they invite the use of fingers rather than silverware.

3. Extreme temperatures in foods are not likely to be well received. The mouth of a child is very sensitive to heat and will be

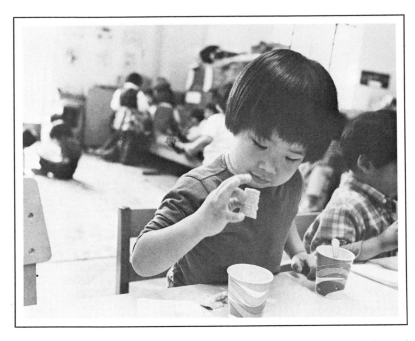

Finger foods provide an invitation to young children to try them even when the food is a new one.

burned at temperatures that adults may find pleasing. At the other end of the continuum, some children object to ice cream straight from the freezer because it is too cold. The problem of temperature extremes can easily be handled by serving the child's plate a brief time before the others are served.

4. Simple and familiar foods are favored by most children. Children, like adults, seem to gain some security by eating foods they recognize. Therefore children often prefer foods served alone instead of as a small part of a casserole or elaborate dish.

5. As preschoolers develop and more teeth come in, they can chew foods that were difficult to manage at the age of one or two. Celery sticks and other foods high in cellulose that present a chewing problem and choking hazard to a very young child can be added when children are about 3 years old.

6. Encourage children to participate in plan-

ning and preparing meals. Children feel more a part of the family group when their favorites are included in the menu occasionally. When they see others respecting their food preferences, they are likely to be willing to try the favorites of others in the family. Even young children can do simple food preparation tasks. Such achievements as pulling the strings from fresh green beans or shucking corn give them a feeling of helping to create the food, thus increasing acceptance of the food at mealtime.

7. Provide opportunities for children to help at the table. For example, when a child has a small pitcher from which he can pour milk into his own glass, he is subtly encouraged to drink the milk he needs.

8. Serve children with the approximate amount of food they usually will eat at a meal. It is generally better to put too little rather than too much food on the plate at

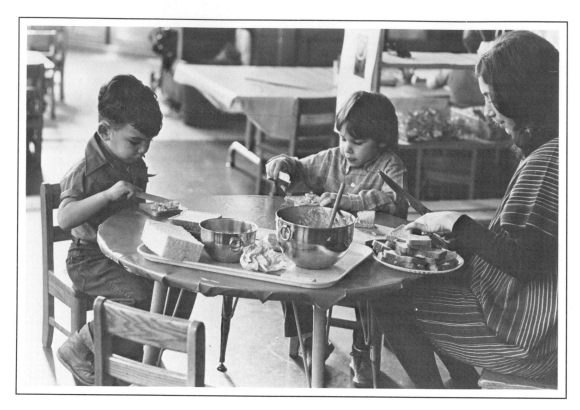

When children help with food preparation, they are likely to become eager consumers.

first. Some children may feel defeated when they have more food than they can eat on their plates and have difficulty mounting any sort of an offensive to eat these imposing quantities. A more successful approach in such cases is to give them only a little food at first and then to offer seconds. Some highly active children will eat better if they are given approximately the amount of food that they will eat, because they simply are too busy to bother to get more food on their plates to satisfy their hunger.

9. Aid children to keep their activity level relatively high so the need for energy in the diet will be correspondingly high. This helps to insure adequate intake of various nutrients. Limited use of television and encourage-

ment in games and sports are of merit in this regard. Adult participation also helps.

The preceding suggestions may be applied at home and also in a nursery school setting. When a preschooler obtains part of his food at home and part away from home, parents and the other adults involved with the child's welfare should work together to achieve good nutrition for him. This can best be accomplished by frequent conferences and by posting menus if the child is fed in an organized group situation where menus are available. The influences outside the home are becoming increasingly significant in achieving good nutrition as more mothers enter the work force and enroll their preschoolers in either a day care or nursery school situation.

Summary

The year-old child has need for a well-balanced diet, but will begin to show less appetite than the infant because his growth rate is reduced. Also at the age of about 1 year, most children will begin to eat with the family. At this time, parental and sibling influences are important factors in molding the nutrition pattern of the toddler.

The 1- and 2-year old's usual dietary pattern of three meals and two snacks a day can be based on the Basic Four Food Group Plan, with particular attention being given to providing meats and vegetables that can be chewed satisfactorily. As the child grows somewhat older, fewer modifications in the family's fare will need to be made. Although preschoolers will sometimes go on food jags for a limited time, they will gradually expand their food preferences to a very wide range by age 5 if the home environment encourages this attitude.

Since the preschooler has proportionately high nutritional needs in relation to his volume of food intake, the foods selected need to be good sources of nutrients. Rich desserts and candy should not be the predominant part of the total food intake, but occasionally they may help provide the large amounts of energy needed by active children in this age group. The nutritional status of the preschooler is significantly enhanced by using water that is fluoridated, salt that is iodized, milk fortified with vitamin D, and enriched or whole-grain breads and cereals.

The goals of achieving normal weight control and good nutritional status can be accomplished while helping the preschooler establish sound nutritional habits that will provide a workable foundation for a lifetime of good eating. Success can be gained by the cooperative efforts of parents who practice good nutrition and are well informed about nutrition and the coordination of nutrition programs if the child regularly eats part of his meals away from home.

Selected References

Beal, V. A. Dietary intake of individuals followed through infancy and childhood. *Am. J. Pub. Health. 51:*1107–1117. 1961.

Brown, A. M., and A. P. Matheny, Jr. Feeding problems and preschool intelligence scores: a study using the co-twin method. *Am. J. Clin. Nutr. 24:*1207. 1971.

Brown, M. L., et al. Diet and nutriture of preschool children in Honolulu. *J. Am. Diet. Assoc. 57,* No. 6:22–28. 1970.

Council on Foods and Nutrition. Symposium 8. *Nutrition in Tooth Formation and Dental Caries.* American Med. Assoc. Chicago. 1960.

Eppright, E. S., et al. North Central regional study of diets of preschool children. 1. Family environment. *J. Home Econ. 62:*241–245. 1970.

Eppright, E. S., et al. North Central regional study of diets of preschool children. 2. Nutrition knowledge and attitudes of mothers. *J. Home Econ. 62:*327–332. 1970.

Eppright, F. S., et al. North Central regional study of diets of preschool children. 3. Frequency of eating. *J. Home Econ. 62:*407–410. 1970.

Food and Nutrition Board. *Pre-school Child Malnutrition.* National Research Council of the National Academy of Sciences. Washington, D.C. 1964.

Garn, S. M., et al. Growth, body composition, and development of obese and lean children. *Childhood Obesity.* Ed. by M. Winick. Wiley-Interscience. New York. 1975.

Hathaway, M. L., and D. W. Sargent. Overweight in children. *J. Am. Diet. Assoc. 40:*511. 1962.

Hendel, C. M., et al. Socioeconomic factors influence children's diets. *J. Home Econ. 57:*205. 1965.

Holt, L. E., Jr., and S. E. Snyderman. Protein and amino acid requirements of infants and children. *Nutr. Abst. Rev. 35:*1. 1965.

Latham, M. C., and F. Cobos. Effects of malnutrition on intellectual development and learning. *Am. J. Publ. Health. 61:*1307. 1971.

Kretchmer, N. Intestinal absorption of lactose in Nigerian ethnic groups. *Lancet. 7721:*392. 1971.

Mayer, J. Obesity during childhood. *Childhood Obesity.* Ed. by M. Winick. Wiley-Interscience. New York. 1975.

McWilliams, M. *Nutrition for the Growing Years.* Wiley. New York. 2nd ed. 1975.

Milner, R. D. G. Protein-calorie malnutrition. In *Present Knowledge of Nutrition.* 4th ed. Nutrition Foundation. New York. 1976.

Scrimshaw, N. S. Malnutrition and health of children. *J. Am. Diet. Assoc. 43:*203–208. 1963.

Seelig, M. S. Vitamin D and cardiovascular, renal, and brain damage in infancy and childhood. *Annals of N.Y. Acad. Sciences. 147:*537—582. 1969.

Smith, C. A. Overuse of milk in the diets of infants and children. *J. Am. Med. Assoc. 172:*567–569. 1960.

Schaefer, A. E. *Statement before Senate Select Committee on Nutrition and Related Human Needs.* Washington, D.C. Jan. 22, 1969.

Teply, L. J. Nutritional needs of the preschool child. *Nutr. Rev. 22:*65. 1964.

Winick, M., ed. *Childhood Obesity.* Wiley-Interscience. New York. 1975.

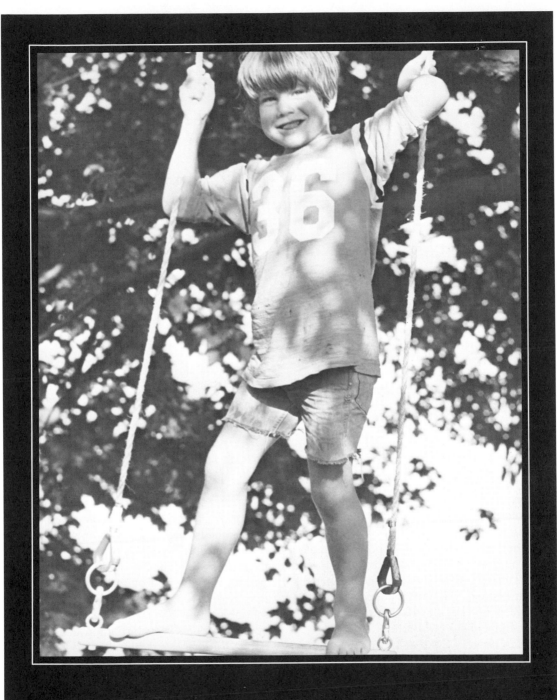

Chapter 15

Nutrition in the School Years

Elementary School Years

Nutrition patterns in the elementary school years generally follow the familial dietary habits established during the preschool period. This preadolescent period may be characterized as a time when children are likely to be well nourished. They are usually at home for meals, with the frequent exception of lunch, and parents still supervise and watch what their children are eating. The independence of adolescence has not begun; this is a period when parental influences are strong.

As described in Chapter 14, one might conclude that all elementary-age schoolchildren are well nourished. Obviously, however, this is not the case. Some children enter school with poor nutrition habits stemming from a variety of familial situations that existed during the preschool period. In families with limited incomes, adequate food simply is not always available to provide the variety and quantity of food that may be deemed desirable for developing good nutrition habits during the preschool years. Parents may have food prejudices that mold their children's dietary habits even before children enter school. For still other children, food has become a weapon or means of negotiation during the early developmental period. In these and other instances, nutrition may not be optimum during the elementary school years. However, educators can help young students develop improved nutrition habits through good nutrition education and school lunch programs in the elementary grades.

In a 1965 survey of dietary intake in the United States (conducted by the Agricultural Research Service), children through the age of eight generally were found to have adequate diets, with the exception of iron intake. Older children were found to be less adequately fed than this younger group, and boys were eating a more adequate diet than girls. As a group, boys between the ages of 9 and 11 were well fed, except for the slightly low calcium intakes that reflected the small decrease in consumption of milk. Girls in this same age bracket were already exhibiting some of the dietary patterns typical of many teen-age girls, resulting in inadequate intakes of calcium, iron, and thiamin.

Nutritional requirements

As can be seen in Table 15.1, there is a gradual increase in energy requirements throughout the elementary school period to cover the energy needs of growth and considerable physical activity. The recommended allowances for the other nutrients are also increased, with the exception of vitamin D, ascorbic acid, calcium, phosphorus, zinc, and iron, which remain constant throughout this age span. The increases in niacin, riboflavin, and thiamin are a reflection of the need for these vitamins to assist in releasing energy from food. The sharp increase in the recommendation for iodide anticipates the metabolic changes of puberty and the need for thyroxine. During this period, often described as the period of latency, the dietary needs are basically for a well-balanced diet with attention being given to maintenance of a sufficient intake of protein foods, milk, fruits, and vegetables, and a minimum of candy and soft drinks.

Dietary influences

The dietary pattern is modified for some children when they begin school. Breakfast may begin to be a more hurried affair or may even be skipped in the rush to get to school. The midmorning snack that is so frequently a part of the routine for preschoolers will become only a memory unless the school has a so-called "nutrition break." Lunch for some children continues to be a meal at home, but for many others this meal is eaten at school, either as a

Table 15.1 Recommended Daily Dietary Allowances for Children Ages 7 to 10[a]

Nutrient	Age and Size
	7–10 years 61 lb 54 in.
kcal	2400
Protein (g)	36
Vitamin A activity (I.U.)	3300
Vitamin D (I.U.)	400
Vitamin E activity (I.U.)	10
Ascorbic acid (mg)	40
Folacin (μg)	300
Niacin (mg equiv.)	16
Riboflavin (mg)	1.2
Thiamin (mg)	1.2
Vitamin B$_6$ (mg)	1.2
Vitamin B$_{12}$ (μg)	2.0
Calcium (mg)	800
Phosphorus (mg)	800
Iodine (μg)	110
Iron (mg)	10
Magnesium (mg)	250
Zinc (mg)	10

[a] Food and Nutrition Board, National Academy of Sciences—National Research Council, *Recommended Daily Dietary Allowances,* revised 1974.

sack lunch or as a part of the school lunch program. A brief examination of each of these influences will give a clearer picture of the nutrition pattern of many elementary school children.

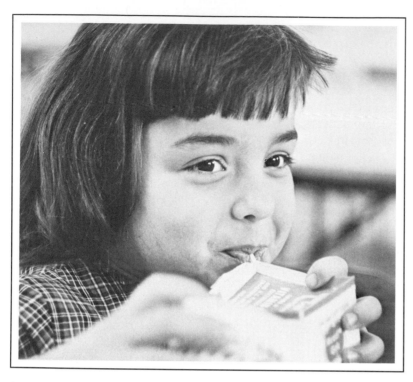

School breakfast programs provide an important foundation for learning for many children who do not have breakfast at home.

Breakfast pattern

The importance of breakfast has been researched and summarized by the Cereal Institute (1962). In tests on schoolboys, their maximum work rate and maximum work output were greater when they ate a basic breakfast[1] than when they skipped breakfast. Their teacher reported better attitudes and greater scholastic achievement when the boys were eating the basic breakfast than when breakfast was omitted. Efficiency in the late morning hours was particularly altered. The study also determined that a midmorning break was not significant in increasing work output if breakfast had been eaten, but did increase work output

[1] Basic breakfast consisted of either: (1) fruit or juice, cereal, two slices of toast with butter, and milk, or (2) fruit or juice, soft-cooked egg, bacon, two slices of toast with butter and jelly, and milk.

for almost half of the people who had not had breakfast. Results indicated that breakfast is of more value than a midmorning break.

The reasons for a child missing breakfast may be varied, but the net result is usually inadequate nutrition. As a means of attempting to insure better nutrition for school-age children, the federal government initiated the Child Nutrition Act of 1966, which included the potential for schools to provide breakfast as well as lunch for pupils. The pattern for school breakfasts includes, as a minimum, any kind of milk, fruit or vegetable juice or fruit, bread or biscuits or muffins, and cereal. The U.S. Department of Agriculture, the agency responsible for the School Breakfast Program, also urges the inclusion of such protein-rich foods as eggs, meat, fish, poultry, cheese, and peanut butter when possible. This program was extended to various other institutions, such as day care centers for young children, in 1968. Although the breakfast program has been of limited scope, indications are strong that there will be a considerable increase in the number of participating schools as federal funding is increased. Schools given top priority to participate in this program are those serving children from families with limited incomes or students who travel very long distances between home and school. The cost to students for breakfast generally ranged between 10 and 15 cents in this nonprofit service in 1973. For children unable to pay the full price, breakfast is to be served free or at a reduced price.

The problem of an adequate breakfast could be overcome in many homes if families would develop a greater appreciation for the merits of breakfast for all family members. Whether a family elects to sleep longer or to get up in time to eat breakfast is partially a matter of values. The preparation and supervision of breakfast in the home usually is principally a management problem for mothers, even when they are employed outside the home. When parents provide the example and motivation to eat a good breakfast, their elementary-age schoolchildren will almost certainly eat breakfast, too.

Lunch at home or school

Lunch is always an important meal, but it becomes particularly significant for the elementary school child who is adjusting to a structured routine away from the comfortable home environment. No longer is it possible for him to get a snack before mealtime if he is hungry. Some children will be able to have lunch at home. In this situation, parents can easily maintain a fairly accurate check of what a child eats each day. However, with the increasing numbers of working mothers and the necessity of bussing some elementary schoolchildren, lunch at home often simply is not possible. In many schools, children now have a choice between participating in the school lunch program or bringing their own lunches from home; in other schools lacking food facilities, a bag lunch is presently the only solution. However, with the modern equipment and delivery systems now available, even schools without facilities should be able to offer a school lunch program to all children.

Considerable imagination and effort are required to regularly pack a bag lunch that is adequate nutritionally, safely kept for several hours without refrigeration, and tempting to eat when lunchtime finally arrives. Ideally, the bag lunch will include a good source of protein, either a fruit or a vegetable, and bread or a cereal product. Milk to round out the meal can be carried from home or purchased at school. The nutritional merits of this type of lunch are considerably greater than the jelly sandwich and candy bar comprising the lunches of some children.

The Special Milk Program is one of the components of the federal government's child nutrition programs. Its specific purpose is to encourage children to drink more milk. Partial reimbursement for the cost of the milk is made

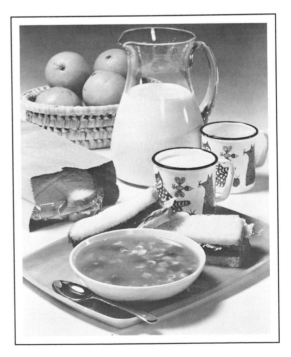

A lunch of soup, a hearty meat sandwich, fruit, and milk can be eaten at home or carried to school.

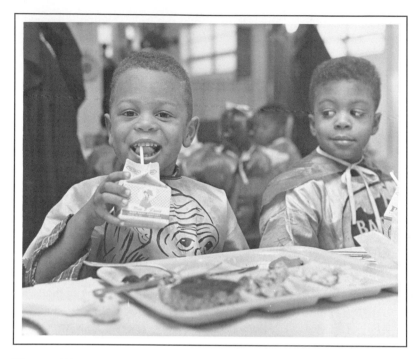

The typical Type A school lunch is a pattern familiar to the nation's school children. This program is under the direction of the U.S. Department of Agriculture.

to schools so that children may buy their milk at a reduced price—a food bargain designed to increase participation in this program. In fact, some schools in low-income areas are able to qualify for total reimbursement, which enables these schools to provide milk free to the children. Although the Special Milk Program is useful in all schools and child-care institutions that participate, the contribution is especially significant where lunch or breakfast programs are not available to the children.

The school lunch menus are planned to meet the guidelines established for a Type A lunch under the National School Lunch Program. The Type A lunch menu served must meet the following requirements:

1. Eight ounces ($\frac{1}{2}$ pint) of fluid whole milk.[2]

2. Meat or meat alternate: 2 ounces of cooked or canned lean meat, fish, or poultry; or 2 ounces of cheese; or one egg; or $\frac{1}{2}$ cup cooked dry beans or peas; or 4 tablespoons of peanut butter; or an equivalent combination of these foods.

3. Vegetables and fruits: two or more to equal $\frac{3}{4}$ cup total. Undiluted juice can be used as the equivalent of $\frac{1}{4}$ cup of the total. The daily inclusion of foods rich in vitamin A, ascorbic acid, and iron helps to meet recognized shortages in the diets of some of the children.

4. Bread or a bread substitute, either whole grain or made with enriched flour or meal: one slice or its equivalent.

5. Butter or fortified margarine: 1 teaspoon used as a spread or in preparation of other foods.

Actual planning and preparation of school lunches are the responsibilities of the local school districts, although the Food and Nutri-

[2] Alternatives include low fat, skimmed, buttermilk, or flavored milks made from these types of milks which meet state and local standards.

tion Service of the United States Department of Agriculture does provide ongoing leadership in the federal program. Some states, through the Department of Education, also provide valuable leadership and service in nutrition programs. The physical facilities for preparing and serving the food, the available budget, and the food preferences of the children all must be incorporated in the planning if a school lunch program is to be successful.

When menus are structured carefully along the guidelines for Type A lunches, the lunch served each child should provide approximately one third of the daily Recommended

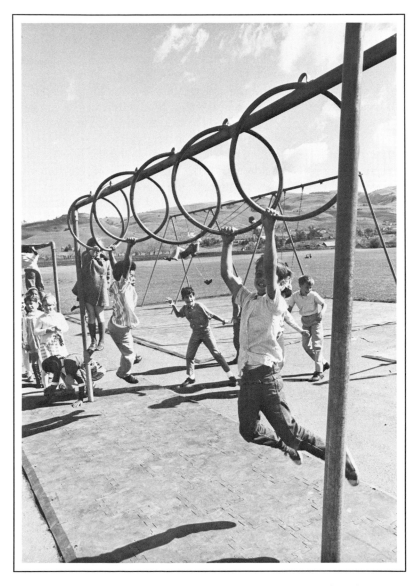

For optimum health, elementary school children require plenty of physical activity as well as adequate nutrition.

Dietary Allowances. A nationwide survey conducted by the Agricultural Research Service (1964–65) revealed that the 300 schools surveyed were serving lunches adequate in protein, niacin, and riboflavin. The levels of thiamin and calcium were close to the recommended amounts, and they also probably contained sufficient ascorbic acid. However, the following inadequacies were found: two thirds of the school menus were low in iron, one third of the lunches were short in vitamin A, the percentage of kilocalories from fat tended to be too high, and kilocalorie levels tended to be too low, particularly for older students. Simply by increasing the size of the servings or by allowing second servings for older children, most of the shortcomings of the school lunch menus can be corrected.

The successful operation of a nationwide school lunch program is a very complex program that requires skilled and dedicated personnel at all levels. Local planning and purchasing are necessary to achieve nutritious, yet economical meals suited to the food preferences of the students. About 80 percent of the foods used in school lunches are purchased at local markets. The remainder is donated food, distributed by the U.S. Department of Agriculture under the Food Distribution Program. Some foods donated to schools have been purchased by the U.S.D.A. specifically for utilization in the National School Lunch Program. Additional commodities are purchased by the government to remove surplus foods that would tend to drive market prices lower than government economists calculate to be healthy for the farm economy. Still other foods are purchased because of farm subsidy commitments made to farmers by the government. The use of foods obtained through the Food Distribution Program is a boon to keeping food costs for lunches at a price the public can afford.

Good nutrition at lunch extends beyond the provision of an adequate bag lunch or hot lunch. There may be a wide breech between the availability of a nutritionally adequate lunch and its consumption. In some schools, lunchtime is very brief, hectic, and noisy. Particularly for some of the younger elementary schoolchildren, such an atmosphere is not conducive to eating. There may also be the possibility of an active bartering economy existing in the school lunchroom. Some children are truly expert in their trading abilities where food is involved. Children with limited food acceptance may refuse to eat or only nibble at many of the foods served at school.

Inadequate money prevents some children from buying the school lunch. Federal regulations require lunches to be sold at a reduced price or given free to children whose families cannot afford to buy them. Despite careful attempts to avoid letting children know who is getting assistance in obtaining the lunches, the children usually find out. Some children are very sensitive to the reaction of their peers and may elect to stay out of the program simply to avoid the stigma of being identified as poor. Despite the problems of providing free or reduced-cost lunches, participation increased from 2,800,000 needy children in 1967 to 8,900,000 in 1973. Increased support from the federal government since the 1969 White House Conference on Food, Nutrition, and Health has been instrumental in achieving this growth.

Some children may have forgotten or lost their money for lunch. Or they may have elected to spend their lunch money at a store on their way to school. Unfortunately, a common sight is schoolchildren of all ages clustered around the candy counter or soft-drink dispenser in a drug or grocery store before school starts in the morning. This phenomenon can be encountered whenever children walk past such stores on their way to school. Soft drinks and candy can be a part of the total daily food intake, but by themselves they do not provide a good breakfast or any other good meal.

A 1969 nutrition survey of 80,000 public

schoolchildren in Massachusetts[3] revealed that participation in the Type A school lunch was the safest way to assure an adequate noon meal. Almost three fourths of the children buying the Type A lunch on the survey day had an adequate meal. In contrast, nearly two thirds of the children going home for lunch, bringing lunch from home, buying a la carte items in school, or eating in a neighborhood store ate an inadequate noon meal that day.

In view of the fiscal limitations in school budgets, schools may not, realistically, be expected to serve both a good breakfast and a good lunch. The answer may be to serve the good Type A lunch at about 10 A.M. so it may serve as a breakfast for those who have had none or only a skimpy one, and yet serve the purpose of a lunch as well. A few studies along the line of this suggestion (one good school meal in midmorning) should be done.

Rounding out the diet

The nutritional pattern for most elementary schoolchildren is rounded out by a snack after school and a family dinner. Recommended snack items are foods such as juice, milk, fresh fruits, strips of raw vegetables, or a small sandwich. Although candy, potato chips, and so-called "empty calorie" foods are convenient snacks for children to fix for themselves, regular snacking on these items is to be discouraged. Such foods add significantly to caloric intake and may lead to the gradual onset of obesity while contributing little to the body's need for nutrients. Foods high in calories and low in nutrients can be a part of meals and snacks, but they should not completely replace those foods that provide the key nutrients—proteins, vitamins, and minerals. Smart food selection in snacking is becoming increasingly important as many families shift to more snacking and less formal meals. This also places an increased

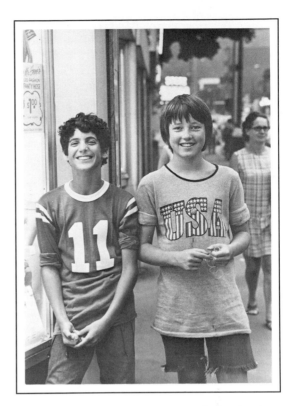

Teen-age boys have high nutritional needs, but their large appetites ordinarily will be sufficient to motivate them to eat enough food to provide most of the nutrients. Even so, it still is important for them to learn how to meet those needs.

responsibility on the food industry to provide more nutritious, yet tasty snacks.

When an elementary schoolchild has a consistent dietary pattern of breakfast, lunch, possibly a snack, and dinner that meets the recommendations of the Basic Four Food Group Plan, plus providing sufficient calories to achieve and maintain a desirable weight for his height, he should be well nourished. However, families should be certain that (1) the milk served is fortified with vitamin D, (2) iodized salt is used, (3) whole-grain or enriched cereal products are selected, and (4) fluoridated water is available through fluoridation of the city water supply.

[3] Unpublished data. Department of Education, School Food Service, Commonwealth of Massachusetts, Boston.

Recommended dietary allowances

In the teen-age period, nutritional requirements for the body are at a maximum. The growth spurt preceding sexual maturation generally occurs in girls between the ages of 11 and 13 and in boys from 13 to 15. As is to be predicted, the nutritional requirements are increased significantly above those of younger individuals to accommodate the nutritional demands of a rapidly growing body. The highest daily Recommended Dietary Allowances for girls, exclusive of pregnancy and lactation, are

Table 15.2   *Recommended Daily Dietary Allowances for Teen-agers*[a]

Nutrient	Age and Body Size			
	Boys		Girls	
	11–14 years 97 lb 63 in.	15–18 years 134 lb 69 in.	11–14 years 97 lb 62 in.	15–18 years 119 lb 65 in.
kcal	2800	3000	2400	2100
Protein (g)	44	54	44	48
Vitamin A activity (I.U.)	5000	5000	4000	4000
Vitamin D (I.U.)	400	400	400	400
Vitamin E activity (I.U.)	15	15	12	12
Ascorbic acid (mg)	45	45	45	45
Folacin (μg)	400	400	400	400
Niacin (mg equiv.)	18	20	16	14
Riboflavin (mg)	1.5	1.8	1.3	1.4
Thiamin (mg)	1.4	1.5	1.2	1.1
Vitamin B_6 (mg)	1.6	2.0	1.6	2.0
Vitamin B_{12} (μg)	3.0	3.0	3.0	3.0
Calcium (mg)	1200	1200	1200	1200
Phosphorus (mg)	1200	1200	1200	1200
Iodine (μg)	130	150	115	115
Iron (mg)	18	18	18	18
Magnesium (mg)	350	400	300	300
Zinc (mg)	15	15	15	15

[a] Adapted from the ***Recommended Daily Dietary Allowances,*** revised 1974. Food and Nutrition Board, National Academy of Sciences—National Research Council.

in the 11 to 18-year-old bracket; for boys, the peak is from 15 to 18. For many of the nutrients, the recommendation for girls is not as high as for boys. These recommended values take into consideration the somewhat more rapid growth rate, greater ultimate body size, and generally greater physical activity of boys in comparison with girls during this period of life. The Recommended Dietary Allowances for ages 11 through 18 are given in Table 15.2.

If good nutrition were simply a matter of making appropriate dietary recommendations to individuals, one could safely say that teen-agers would very likely be adequately nourished. They have a rather large number of kilocalories recommended, so they can eat a relatively large amount of food to obtain the nutrients required for good health. Teen-age boys have greater caloric latitude available to them than do the girls, but teen-age girls can easily get all the nutrients they need without excessive caloric intake if they select foods sensibly. Therefore, the fact that teen-agers may not always be well nourished may seem surprising. In fact, teen-age girls are cited as having the poorest diets of any age group in the United States. This paradox exists as the result of some sociopsychological influences.

Impact of socio-psychological influences

One of the very important developmental tasks of adolescence is the achievement of self-identity. The path toward this goal leads to the need for establishing independence from parents, acceptance by friends, and the acquisition of a self-satisfying personal image. All three of these factors are significant influences in determining the dietary patterns of each teen-ager.

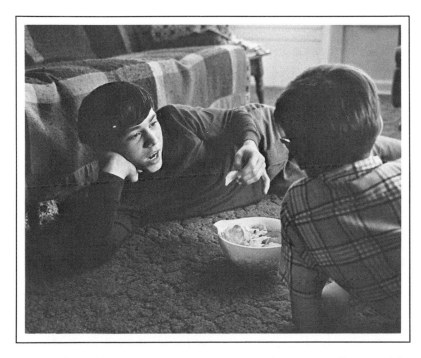

Simple-to-prepare snacks often are a part of the teens' diet pattern. Because of the prominent role of snacks at this age, the nutritional value of these snack foods is a question of importance.

Desire for independence

If nutrition habits have been a matter of controversy and debate between parent and child prior to the teen-age period, there is little reason to be surprised when the teen-ager may choose to defy parental dictates regarding food habits. This is one tangible means of establishing independence in action and image. Another aspect of achieving independence is the pursuit of the numerous activities in which many teen-agers are involved. These activities place scheduling and time demands on participants and may make it difficult for teen-agers to mesh their meal schedules with the rest of the family. Thus, the increasing independence and mobility of teen-agers lead to some modification in dietary patterns. The influences of parents and familiar family food patterns no longer completely dominate and determine food consumption.

Acceptance by peer group

During adolescence there is typically a strong need to be accepted by the peer group. Even when the interests of the group center upon activities far removed from eating, there is almost always some snacking included as part of the sociability. This social aspect of food may range from attention-getting diversions, such as the goldfish-swallowing fad or the gulping of raw liver at fraternity initiations of some years ago to simply sharing a pizza or to the macrobiotic diets of more recent times. When the group adopts certain foods or eating practices, individuals are strongly compelled to eat with the group regardless of their own personal preferences or appetite. The food consumed as snacks by teenagers in groups is often a significant part of the day's intake. Of course, the nutrient content of the snack foods is important as a part of the day's diet, but the influence of the snack may extend beyond the value of the snack itself. The timing and the quantity of food in the snack are also important because of the influence snacking may have on the appetite at mealtime.

Achieving a desirable self-image

Nutrition is closely linked to the self-image a teen-ager develops. The adolescent usually is aware that the actual image he presents to the world is greatly influenced by his nutrition pattern over a period of time. A well-nourished and healthy adolescent will have a well-developed body with straight bones, appropriate fatty deposits, good musculature, shiny hair, healthy skin, and strong teeth quite free of decay. These attributes are important to anyone's self-image and are definitely enhanced by good nutrition.

Although many teen-agers recognize the contribution of a proper diet, the difficult problem for many of them is to translate this recognition into a meaningful and realistic dietary regimen to be lived each day. Part of the problem is due to limited knowledge of basic nutrition, but the difficulties of learning to be one's own master may contribute still more to the impedance in eating a nourishing diet.

Societal pressures

Today's social pressures have added to adolescent nutrition problems, also. The gross malnutrition exhibited by some of the "flower children," "hippies," and others in subcultures, some of whom have so enthusiastically substituted drugs for a large part of their sustenance, is an exaggerated illustration of how sociological and psychological adjustments can influence the nutritional status of individuals.

Some teen-agers (and adults, too) have become so engulfed in the tide of concern over the basic nature of man and the environmental problems developing in our technological society that they have modified their diets significantly. The desire to return to the simple, agrarian life of ages past has led some adolescents to eat rather restricted vegetarian diets. In some instances, the diet has been selected from such a narrow range of plant foods that the total nutritional needs of the body were not supplied (see Chapter 5).

The tremendous preoccupation of the teen

with the importance of achieving a slim body is a reflection of the population's emphasis on sexual attractiveness. As teen-agers strive to achieve an image pleasing to themselves, they are also attempting to be as attractive as possible to their peers, for physical attractiveness is important for entry into a peer group, one of the compelling goals of the teens. The adolescent's preferred figure for today is one bordering on underweight, particularly for girls.

Huenemann et al. (1966) surveyed nearly 1000 students from Berkeley when they were high school freshmen and again when they were juniors. They found that over half of the girls were worried about being overweight, although actually only one fourth were found to be overweight. Boys revealed just the opposite concern. Over half of the boys were concerned about being underweight. The boys generally felt that exercise was the best solution to their problem; the girls preferred dieting instead of increased exercise.

Some adolescents do, indeed, have a weight problem that can be helped through more exercise and proper nutrition. However, as indicated in the Berkeley study, there is considerable unwarranted concern about body weight. This rather pervading preoccupation with weight among teen-age girls appears to influence the dietary patterns of some of the girls. One indication of this is the alacrity with which some teen-age girls omit breakfast. However, the concern with weight often appears to be less strong than the need to conform to the peer group. Even girls who are in need of weight reduction will have difficulty in eliminating snacks or selecting a food low in calories when others in the group are having pie a la mode or some other delectable treat.

Emotional stresses

The teen-age period is frequently depicted as a time of strong emotions and stressful interaction with adults, as contrasted to the latency of the preceding developmental period. Although many teen-agers make the transition from child to adult in a generally routine, non-stressful manner, many others do experience emotional stress. Such stress may not only influence appetite, but also may result in poor utilization of the nutrients that are consumed. Even for the relatively quiescent adolescent, some stresses are hard to ignore. For example, the stress of taking examinations is difficult to minimize when the grades earned in high school have so much influence on admission to colleges. Unhappy social relationships can create considerable stress in adolescence (as well as later in life). Discussions between teen-agers and their parents may develop into arguments full of emotional stress. Disagreements between teen-agers also may be laden with intense emotions. Perhaps the greatest stresses are generated by premarital pregnancies that are becoming increasingly frequent prior to graduation from high school. Good nutrition in times of emotional crisis is very difficult, but not impossible to achieve.

Nutritional status

In the United States, the dietary patterns of adolescents have been the subject of several research studies. One general conclusion has been that young men are better nourished than young women. This is influenced by the fact that the greater total amount of calories recommended for males provides more opportunity for variety and choice within the diet. Also, the observation by Huenemann et al. (1966) that boys frequently imagined themselves as underweight suggests that boys are not as likely to skimp on food as are the many girls who are concerned about their weight. Blewett and Schuck (1950) found that young men consumed more milk, cereal, and meat than women, while the young women ate more fruit. Although these data were obtained for a different generation, current information regarding dietary intake of people in the United States suggests that these patterns may still be valid.

Teen-agers' diets have occasionally been found to be low in calcium, ascorbic acid, and vitamin A. However, one of the nutrients most likely to be inadequate in adolescent diets, particularly girls' diets, is iron. This deficiency results in low hemoglobin levels in the blood, which in turn leads to a constant feeling of being tired. This continual fatigue is scarcely compatible with encouraging greater activity among adolescents who are overweight. In fact, a self-defeating cycle, one in which iron intake is seriously limited by a poorly planned reducing diet, may evolve gradually. Too little iron in the diet results in anemia. The anemia leads to decreased physical activity and caloric expenditure. The decreased need for energy from food requires an even greater decrease in food intake. This reduction means less iron is consumed. And so the cycle goes round and round.

Particular attention should be given in the adolescent period to insuring that calcium and phosphorus intake are adequate and that protein is available in the plentiful quantities needed for growth. By including 3 to 4 glasses of milk in the diet each day, calcium and phosphorus will be adequate, and the protein intake will be enhanced greatly. If overweight is a problem, the milk consumed should be low-fat or nonfat. Iodized salt is important in helping to prevent the development of goiter, which is a problem among teen-agers when iodine intake is inadequate. To meet the possible problem of providing sufficient ascorbic acid and vitamin A, families are wise to maintain an environment that encourages the consumption of a breakfast providing the recommended amount of ascorbic acid daily. Other meals served at home should feature well-prepared fruits and vegetables, with attention being given to serving a good source of vitamin A at least every other day. Prominent displays of attractive fruits and ready-to-eat raw vegetables in the refrigerator are open invitations to nourishing snacks.

The incidence of tuberculosis among adolescents, particularly among those who are underweight, may be a reflection of the reduced resistance to infection that is an outgrowth of inadequate nutrition. The inadequate intake of essential nutrients over a period of time in the teens may result in increased susceptibility to various contagious diseases. This can lead to frequent absences from school or the job and result in increased anxiety about personal adequacy and the reality of failure.

The health hazard of malnutrition during teen-age pregnancies is of great significance and is one that cannot be overcome in a few days, even if the expectant teen-ager could be persuaded to begin to suddenly eat an adequate diet. If the period of malnutrition has extended over several months or even years, a number of months may be required to replenish the calcium stores that are so important to both mother and fetus. Everson (1960) cited the poor reproductive records of pregnant girls from the lowest two social classes in Scotland, who were small and in poor physical condition.

Dental health can be influenced in an important way by teen-age dietary practices. The practice of frequent snacking on high-carbohydrate foods, so common in adolescence, creates an environment in the mouth that is favorable to the development of dental caries, particularly if the carbohydrate is in a sticky form that adheres to the teeth for periods of several minutes. The cariogenic effect of snacks can be greatly reduced by being sure that the mouth is at least rinsed well with water as soon as the snack is eaten. But, most important in reducing tooth decay is the continued use of fluoridated water from birth throughout life.

Recent research strongly suggests that nutritional status of teen-agers can be improved in the direction of avoiding the substantial rise in blood cholesterol that usually occurs in adolescence. This undoubtedly is important in slowing down the development of coronary heart disease later in life. To accomplish this, the dietary changes are similar to those given in Chapter 16: less saturated fat (meaning less meat and whole milk products, these being replaced by more chicken and fish, low-fat or skim milks, and ice creams), a polyunsaturated margarine, and fewer eggs and more cereals.

Nutrition and athletics

Many coaches and athletes attach considerable importance to the idea that athletes need a diet significantly different from the average individual. The ideas espoused in the locker room range from the very essential nature of a high-protein diet to the critical need for wheat germ oil and other so-called "health foods." Stringent rules for diet are forcefully announced and faithfully followed. Some schools require that all the members of the team eat at the training table so that the diet will follow the exact dictates of the coach. This dictatorial and somewhat emotional approach to the problem of feeding athletes an adequate diet may serve psychological purposes in raising team morale to an appropriate level for good competitive sports, but research studies have not substantiated the merits of such nutrition measures.

Not less than three meals a day are recommended for good nutrition of athletes. For athletes participating in cross-country track, tennis, and other events of rather long duration, the pattern of five lighter meals daily may be preferable. These meals generally should follow the same food patterns that are suggested for the average person, with the exception that the

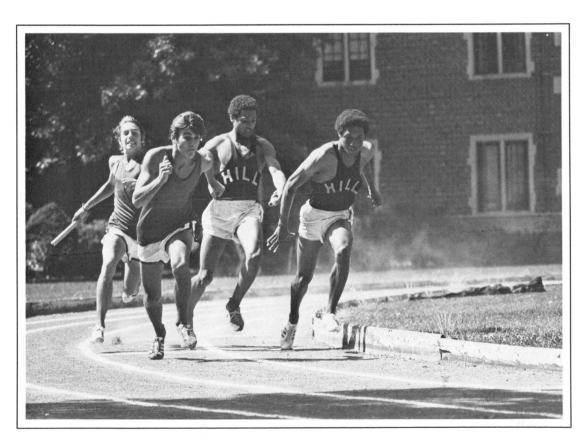

Sound nutrition practices are valuable during training as well as at the actual events.

total amount of food consumed will need to be increased. The increased quantity, of course, is needed to provide the energy required for participation in practices and sporting events. If any adjustment is to be made in the percentage of calories derived from protein, carbohydrate, and fat, the shift suggested is toward more carbohydrate and less fat. Several researchers (Mayer and Bullen, 1959) have shown that a high-carbohydrate diet allowed a person to maintain strenuous activity for sustained periods of time, a fact of interest to athletes participating in events that are long. The value of the high-carbohydrate diet for short-term exercise is not conclusive. A high-fat diet, when maintained more than 3 days, decreased performance in both short- and long-term activities. Thus, athletes may improve their performance a little by increasing carbohydrate intake instead of obtaining the usually large fraction of calories from fats.

Contrary to popular beliefs stemming from the times of the Greeks, athletes do not require a higher percentage of protein from the diet than other people do. Serving sizes of meat and other protein foods will be increased slightly, just as is true for servings of other foods, to increase the total caloric intake required by high energy expenditure.

Some coaches have recommended vitamin supplements for their players in the belief that this will give the athletes more vitality and endurance. Keys and Henschel (1942), Vytchikova (1958), and others did not find any improvement in physical performance when levels of vitamin intake were increased. Of course, the increased amounts of carbohydrate, protein, and fat that must be metabolized in the body require somewhat higher levels of the B vitamins. However, these vitamins are included in the additional food that is eaten. The use of vitamin E and wheat germ oil in experimental studies has not been shown to be of value in improving athletic performance (Sharman et al., 1971).

Some coaches do not allow the use of alcoholic beverages, tea, or coffee for their athletes because of possible harmful effects. There appears to be no difficulty in permitting these beverages in small amounts, although they may impair performance if consumed within 4 hours of the contest.

Salt consumption of athletes should be geared to the replacement of salt lost through perspiration, just as is true for workers in hot climates. Except in unusually hot weather, the salt needed to season the food will be sufficient.

Recommendations for nutrition just prior to an athletic event include (Mayer and Bullen, 1959):

1. Drink bouillon at least 3 hours before the event. This provides salt, yet allows time for thirst to develop and for water to be consumed and excreted before activity is begun.

2. The last meal should be eaten at least 3 hours before the activity. The menu for this meal should be high in carbohydrate content. Protein intake should be minimal. Foods such as lettuce or celery, which are high in cellulose, are best excluded from the diet for the 48 hours preceding the event.

3. During long athletic events, sugar may be used to provide additional energy.

Fait (1961) refutes the idea of many athletes that milk is detrimental to athletic performances. He even states that milk may be included in the pre-game meal. The "cotton mouth" sometimes attributed to drinking milk seems not to be changed when milk is deleted from the diet. Unquestionably, athletes need the minerals, vitamins, and protein of milk just as much as do nonathletes.

Summary

Nutritional needs are likely to be met by the diets of elementary school-children, but the increasing independence of adolescence may lead to inadequate nutrition. Elementary schoolchildren usually eat breakfast, lunch, an after-school snack, and dinner. Teen-agers, particularly girls, exhibit some tendency to omit breakfast and substitute with snacks. Optimum health, better achievement in school, a feeling of vitality, and an attractive, strong body are the rewards of good nutritional practices. These are within the reach of most elementary and high school students if they take advantage of the nutrition education and school lunch programs available to them.

Many rumors and misunderstandings surround the problem of providing good nutrition for athletes. Rather than feeding athletes an exotic array of "health foods" and vitamin supplements, they should be fed the same diet (only in slightly larger quantities) that non-athletes eat.

Selected References

Agricultural Research Service. A better school lunch for your child. In *Toward the New*. Agriculture Information Bulletin. *341*:49–54. Washington, D.C. 1970.

Agricultural Research Service. *Food Intake and Nutritive Value of Diets of Men, Women, and Children in the United States.* Spring 1965. A Preliminary Report, ARS 62–18. U.S. Department of Agriculture. Washington, D.C. 1969.

American Association for Health, Physical Education, and Recreation. *Nutrition for Athletes, a Handbook for Coaches.* Washington, D.C. 1971.

Blewett, G. W., and C. Schuck. Comparison of food consumption of men and women college students. *J. Am. Diet. Assoc. 26*:525–528. 1950.

Bullen, B., et al. Athletics and nutrition. *Am. J. Surg. 98*:343. 1959.

Cereal Institute, Inc. *Complete Survey of the Iowa Breakfast Studies.* Chicago. 1962.

Dwyer, J. T., et al. New vegetarians. *J. Am. Diet. Assoc. 64*:376. 1974.

Everson, G. J. Bases for concern about teen-agers' diets. *J. Am. Diet. Assoc. 36*:17–21. 1960.

Fait, H. F. *What Research Shows about the Effects of Milk in the Athletes' Diet.* University of Conn. Physical Efficiency Research Lab. 1961.

Ford, C. H., et al. An Institutional Approach to the Dietary Regulation of Blood Cholesterol in Adolescent Males. *Preventive Medicine. 1*:426–445. 1972.

Friedman, G. M. Atherosclerosis and the pediatrician. *Childhood Obesity.* Ed. by M. Winick. Wiley-Interscience. New York. 1975.

Heald, F. P. Juvenile obesity. *Childhood Obesity*. Ed. by M. Winick. Wiley-Interscience. New York. 1975.

Huenemann, R. L., et al. A longitudinal study of gross body composition and body conformation and their association with food and activity in a teen-age population. View of teen-age subjects on body conformation, food and activity. *Am. J. Clin. Nutr. 18*:325. 1966.

Keys, A., and A. F. Henschel. Vitamin supplementation of U.S. Army rations in relation to fatigue and the ability to do muscular work. *J. Nutrition. 23*:259. 1942.

Law, H. M., et al. Sophomore high school students' attitudes toward school lunch. *J. Am. Diet. Assoc. 60*:38. 1972.

Mayer, J., and B. Bullen. Nutrition and athletic performance. *Postgraduate Medicine. 26,* No. 6:848. 1959.

Mitchell, H. S. Protein limitations and human growth. *J. Am. Diet. Assoc. 44*:165–172. 1964.

Morgan, A. F. Nutritional Status U.S.A. *Calif. Ag. Expt. Sta. Bull. 769*. Berkeley, Calif. 1959.

Ohlson, M. A., and B. P. Hart. Influence of breakfast on total day's food intake. *J. Am. Diet. Assoc. 47*:282–286. 1965.

Sharman, I. M., et al. Effects of vitamin E and training on physiological function and athletic performance in adolescent swimmers. *British J. Nutr. 26*:265. 1971.

Vanneman, S. C. School lunch to food stamp: America cares for its hungry. In *Food for Us All*. The Yearbook of Agriculture, 1969. Washington, D.C. P. 69–74. 1969.

Vytchkova, M. A. Increasing the vitamin B_1 content in the ration of athletes. *Chem Abstr. 52*:14787. 1958.

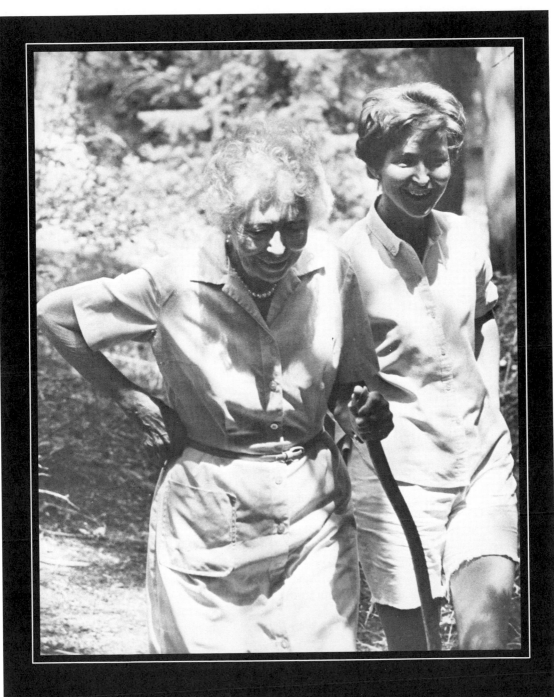

Chapter 16

Nutrition for Adults

The Twenties to The Sixties

An individual, upon reaching maturity, bears the imprint of his nutrition during infancy, childhood, and adolescence. Adulthood should be a time of achievement. A person's health, vigor, work capacity, happiness, and contentment reflect, in part, the kind of nutrition that has marked his previous life. The level of cellular nutrition determines in part, at least, the age at which he displays the physical, mental, and emotional changes one associates with the aging process.

Thus, some people reach adulthood with vigorous, normally functioning bodies and minds. Others permanently carry many nutritional scars as a result of tissue injury. The scars may not be immediately detectable, but animal experiments have shown that faulty nutrition in early life—acting like a time bomb—may induce physical breaks in later life. The nutritional needs of the adult must, therefore, be considered both from the standpoint of those who have been well nourished as children and those whose diets were inadequate in the early years or teens.

Sociopsychological Influences on Diet

One might be tempted to assume that a person who is well nourished when he reaches adulthood has established the dietary patterns needed for a lifetime of good nutrition. Certainly this would be helpful if it were true, but many physiological, psychological, and sociological changes occur that influence dietary patterns during the remaining stages of the life cycle. When people marry, there is usually at least a small change in dietary patterns as two people blend their tastes into a single menu, and if the new mate is from a distant part of the world, the dietary alterations may be significant. The increasing rate of divorce and remarriage means that this adjustment may be made more than once.

The occupation of an adult may be responsible for other dietary shifts a person makes after he matures. Corporation men in the sales division and other professional people are confronted with the prospect of many a round of cocktails and elaborate meals away from home when they entertain business clients. Heavy schedule pressures may interfere so that other professional people may not have time to eat lunch at all. Still others may have jobs with heavy responsibilities and considerable tension, which culminate in physical problems such as ulcers, thus necessitating dietary changes not necessarily of the patient's choosing. Some women who have been calorically indiscreet during pregnancy may also join the ranks of those who are modifying their diets. Home-makers continually are confronted with ready access to food and the problems of excess weight if they yield to the urge to snack frequently. Food provides a strong temptation for women who have a propensity to sample frequently while cooking. Those who find homemaking a lonely or frustrating occupation may use food as a means of escape.

During the last three decades, many dietary modifications have occurred among the adult population, partially as a result of sociological factors and partly because of technological changes. The work week has been shortened for many workers and is showing a continuing trend toward a 4-day week. Particularly for the hourly worker, this is creating more free time, and eating is a favorite use of leisure. The urbanization movement is further modifying living patterns and promoting a more sedentary society. Distances in the city to work and school frequently are too great for people to walk or ride a bicycle. The job itself often provides less opportunity for exercise than was available in the past. Machines in the home, factory, and office are continually being developed to reduce human labor.

Food science has done much to modify dining fare. At the grocery store, the food products prominently displayed today are quite different from many that were featured only a few years ago. The TV dinners, frozen lobster tails, dehydrated soups, instant mashed potatoes, and puddings in pull-open cans are only a few of the items now available as a result of technological advances. These are only some of the numerous illustrations of the significant point that many factors are influencing and changing the dietary patterns of adults.

While external influences are contributing to change, there are also internal changes that modify the dietary allowances recommended for adults. The young adult needs to make the dietary transition to a somewhat reduced intake to compensate for the fact that he is no longer growing. High school and college athletes usually become much less active after their days of interscholastic competition have faded to a display of trophies or a box of carefully preserved school letters in the closet. This rather definite change in physical activity requires a modification in dietary habits if the former athlete is to retain his figure. The somewhat slower basal metabolism of adults further contributes to the need to reduce caloric intake by dietary adjustments.

Problems stemming from malnutrition prior to adulthood

During the two decades leading to adulthood, many people experience malnutrition of varying intensity and duration. The nutrients lacking in the diet also differ from one adult to another. Examples, therefore, are diverse.

Some people entering adulthood bring with them the problem of prolonged overnutrition. The added physical strain, such as the extra burden obesity places on the heart and blood vessels, has long been contributing to their physical condition. Overweight originating in childhood often is accompanied by less physical activity, which also is detrimental to optimum health. The prognosis for changing from being overweight to achieving and maintaining normal weight is poor, although the condition can be corrected.

Undernutrition is a general term for any condition in which dietary intake is inadequate in one or more nutrients. Sometimes the calcium intake is low for extended periods of time, which can cause poor calcification of bones and teeth. The results of this problem that can be observed in adults include such possibilities as a short body, a small rib cage, relatively high incidence of decayed or missing teeth, or osteoporosis. Inadequate intake of iodide during childhood can cause the gradual growth of the thyroid gland, known as goiter. Iron deficiency results in anemia, which impairs performance in school and physical activities. No doubt the most common malnutrition problem prior to adulthood is lack of the mineral nutrient fluoride—a lack that results in the high incidence of tooth decay and may contribute to osteoporosis in aging.

Although not a common problem in the United States, protein deficiency in early childhood can cause permanent stunting of growth. Mental development may be slowed, and the consequences become a lifelong concern.

Eating for optimum health

The problems of atherosclerosis and obesity are two common concerns of the American adult population—both those who reached adulthood in a well-nourished state and those who were overweight in childhood. Improper diet is certainly not likely to be the single causative culprit, but it can play a prominent role in the development of physical problems.

Atherosclerosis and coronary heart disease

Atherosclerosis is a condition in which the blood vessels become narrowed by deposits (atheroma) that thicken the walls in certain areas. This condition presents a potential hazard to many adults because blood clots may become lodged in the narrowed vessels and slow down or completely block the flow of blood to a part of the heart. The result is a heart attack or "coronary." Approximately 200,000 Americans under age 65 died from heart attacks in 1965 and almost three times that many suffered nonfatal heart attacks of varying

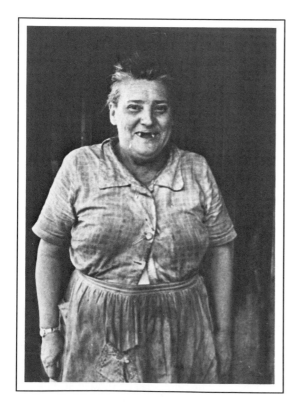

Overweight and missing teeth are possible problems in adulthood which may be the result of poor nutrition in childhood. Impaired chewing ability probably contributes to poor nutrition by limiting the choice and variety of foods.

intensity. Such statistics have provided the impetus for extensive research into the causative agents of these attacks. While results to date have helped to increase understanding of this important health problem, considerably more research is needed because of the numerous variables involved and also because of the diversity of suspected factors being studied.

The remarks that can be made relative to the relationship of diet and heart disease represent a partial summation of dietary studies relating to this health hazard. Subsequent research may modify these views. However, today's widespread concern with this problem dictates the inclusion of present knowledge of the influence of diet on the development of atherosclerosis.

As research has progressed on heart disease, diverse risk factors have been noted. Foremost is probably genetic predisposition. Next would be high blood pressure and an elevated level of serum (blood) cholesterol, and sometimes other blood fats (triglycerides). Smoking, lethargy, obesity, diabetes, and possibly stress (Rosenman and Friedman, 1971), are other "risk" factors. The greater the number of these "risk" factors present in one individual, the greater his likelihood of having a heart attack.

Since serum cholesterol is one of the risk factors that is related to diet, nutrition research in the realm of heart disease has centered around exploration of this relationship. Cholesterol is an organic, waxy compound (technically a higher alcohol), which is only found in foods of animal origin. This compound normally is synthesized by the human body. Diets in the United States (Table 16.1) ordinarily contain between $\frac{1}{2}$ and 1 gram of cholesterol daily (largely from egg yolks and a little from meats, whole milk, and other dairy products). Although opinions vary, experts who work in this field of research believe that levels of more than 210 to 220 milligrams of cholesterol per 100 milliliters of serum are a factor in predisposing an individual to heart disease.

In addition to the possible influence of dietary cholesterol, some interesting observations regarding dietary fat and heart disease have been noted. Diets low in total fat have been typical of the Japanese. Interestingly, the Japanese have a far lower incidence of heart disease than people in the United States do. The average percentage of calories from fat is approximately 20 percent or less in Japanese diets and 35 percent or more in American diets.

The type of fat consumed also influences serum cholesterol values. When the fats consumed are high in saturated fats—meats, dairy products, and coconut oil—serum cholesterol levels are higher than when saturated fats are low and monounsaturated and polyunsaturated fats are high. Certain vegetable oils, particularly soya, cottonseed, corn, and safflower are relatively high in polyunsaturated fatty acids (PUFA) and low in the saturated fatty acids. Olive oil is low in saturated fat and high in monounsaturated fat. In comparison, the fats of animal origin are relatively high in saturated fatty acids and low in polyunsaturated fatty acids. Exceptions are coconut oil, palm kernel oil, and cocoa fat which are mostly saturated despite the fact that they are of plant origin.

Elevated serum triglyceride levels are another factor predisposing some few individuals to heart disease. In a very few individuals, the blood's serum triglyceride level is increased when a diet high in sucrose (sugar) is consumed—that is, a diet significantly higher in sugar than is eaten by the general population. However, sugar is not an important factor in influencing serum cholesterol in most people. High alcohol consumption, including liquors, wine, and beer, may lead to elevated serum triglycerides. Hypertriglyceridemia (high serum triglyceride level) is more prevalent in the obese than in patients of normal weight. This condition in the obese is partially alleviated when weight reduction is accomplished.

General dietary modifications for individuals who are potential candidates for heart attacks, because of having a number of the "risk" factors mentioned earlier, include:

1. Limitation in total caloric intake to achieve

Table 16.1 *Cholesterol Value of Selected Foods* [a]

Food	Cholesterol (mg)
Milk	
Whole, 3.5% fat (1 cup)	34
Nonfat (skim) (1 cup)	5
Low-fat (1 cup)	22
Cheese	
Blue or Roquefort type (1 cu in.)	15
Camembert (1 wedge)	35
Cheddar (1 cu in.)	17
Cottage cheese, creamed (1 pkg)	65
Cottage cheese, uncreamed (1 pkg)	24
Cream cheese (1 pkg, 3 oz)	94
Parmesan (1 tbsp)	5
Swiss cheese (1 cu in.)	15
Processed cheese (1 cu in.)	16
American pasteurized process cheese food (1 tbsp)	10
American process cheese spread (1 oz)	18
Cream	
Half-and-half (1 tbsp)	6
Light, coffee or table (1 tbsp)	10
Sour (1 tbsp)	8
Whipped topping (1 cup), pressurized	51
Milk Beverages	
Cocoa, homemade (1 cup)	35
Chocolate-flavored drink (skim milk) (1 cup)	20
Milk Desserts	
Custard, baked (1 cup)	278
Ice cream, regular (1 cup)	53
Ice milk, hardened (1 cup)	26
Ice milk, soft serve (1 cup)	36
Yogurt (made from partially skimmed milk) (1 cup)	17
Yogurt (made from whole milk) (1 cup)	30
Yogurt (sweetened with fruit added) (1 cup)	15
Eggs	
Whole, (large size)	252
White of egg	0
Yolk of egg	252
Meat, Poultry, Fish, Shellfish, Related Products	
Bacon (2 slices)	16
Beef (lean only) (2.5 oz)	66
Hamburger, broiled, lean (3 oz)	77
Rib roast, oven cooked, lean and fat (3 oz)	80
Rib roast, oven cooked, lean only (1.8 oz)	46
Steak, broiled, lean and fat (6 oz)	160

[a] Cholesterol values calculated from R. M. Feeley, et al. Cholesterol content of foods. *J. Am Diet. Assoc. 61*:134. 1972.

Table 16.1   (continued)

Food	Cholesterol (mg)
Steak, broiled, lean only (6 oz)	153
Corned beef (3 oz)	85
Chicken, flesh only, broiled (3 oz)	74
Chicken, breast, fried (with bone), (3 oz)	75
Chicken, breast, fried (flesh and skin only) (2.7 oz)	68
Chili con carne, canned, with beans (1 cup)	77
Chili con carne, canned, without beans (1 cup)	153
Lamb chop, broiled with bone (1 chop) (4.8 oz)	74
Roast leg of lamb, lean and fat (3 oz)	83
Roast lamb shoulder, lean and fat (3 oz)	83
Beef liver, fried (2 oz)	250
Roast ham, lean and fat (3 oz)	76
Boiled ham, sliced (2 oz)	51
Canned, spiced or unspiced ham (2 oz)	51
Pork chop, thick with bone (1 chop) (3.5 oz)	59
Pork chop, lean only (1 chop) (1.7 oz)	42
Bologna (2 slices)	26
Braunschweiger (2 slices)	20
Frankfurter, heated (1 frank)	56
Pork links, cooked (2 links)	26
Salami, dry type (1 oz)	28
Vienna sausage, canned (1 sausage)	16
Veal cutlet (3 oz)	86
Veal roast (3 oz)	86
Bluefish, baked (3 oz)	60
Clams, raw (3 oz)	43
Clams, canned (3 oz)	86
Crabmeat, canned (3 oz)	86
Fishsticks, frozen (2 sticks)	46
Haddock, fried (3 oz)	51
Ocean perch, fried (3 oz)	51
Oysters, raw (1 cup)	120
Salmon, pink, canned (3 oz)	30
Sardines, Atlantic (3 oz)	119
Shrimp, canned (3 oz)	128
Tuna, canned in oil (3 oz)	55
Grain Products	
Angel-food cake (whole cake) (1 cake)	0
Devil's-food cake with chocolate icing (1 cake)	531
Cupcake (1)	17
Gingerbread (1 cake)	6
White layer cake with chocolate icing (1 cake)	23
Boston cream pie (1 piece)	33
Fruitcake, dark (1 slice)	7
Pound cake (1 slice)	30

Table 16.1 (continued)

Food	Cholesterol (mg)
Sponge cake (1 piece)	162
Yellow cake without icing (1 piece)	26
Yellow cake (1 piece)	36
Brownies with nuts (1 brownie)	17
Doughnuts, cake type (1)	27
Macaroni and cheese, baked (1 cup)	42
Muffins (1)	21
Egg noodles (1 cup)	50
Pancakes (1 cake)	20
Apple pie (1 piece)	0
Custard pie (1 piece)	137
Lemon meringue pie (1 piece)	112
Mince pie (1 piece)	16
Pecan pie (1 piece)	57
Pumpkin pie (1 piece)	79
Spaghetti with meat balls and tomato sauce (1 cup)	75
Spaghetti with meat balls and tomato sauce, canned (1 cup)	39
Waffles (1)	45
Fats and Oils	
Butter (1 tbsp)	35
Butter (1 pat)	13
Whipped butter (1 tbsp)	22
Whipped butter (1 pat)	10
Lard (1 tbsp)	12
Mayonnaise, regular (1 tbsp)	8
Sugars and Sweets	
Chocolate candy, milk, plain (1 oz)	21
Miscellaneous Items	
Chocolate pudding (1 cup)	30
Vanilla pudding (1 cup)	35
Tapicoa cream pudding (1 cup)	159

and maintain a weight appropriate to one's height.

2. A decrease by half or more in the consumption of saturated fat. This means less meat because of the generous amounts of saturated fat in meat, less butter and cream, and less lard used in cooking. Meat chosen should be lean. The consumption of poultry and fish should be increased except for shellfish (lobster and shrimp), as the latter contain about twice the amount of cholesterol as meat or ordinary fish, but far less than egg yolks.

3. Restriction of egg yolks to no more than two or three per week.

4. An increase in the amount of polyunsaturated oils in the form of polyunsaturated margarines, salad oils, and oils used for

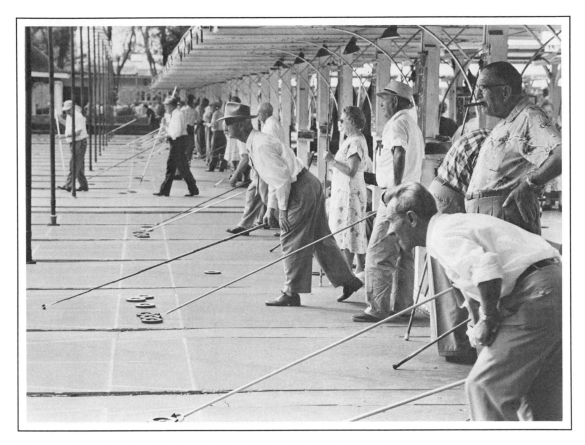

Decreasing physical activity and a slower basal metabolic rate in adulthood necessitate a reduction in food intake if weight control is to be achieved.

cooking. Thus the total amount of fat can be about as usual, though a modest reduction in the total calories coming from fat to between 30 and 35[1] percent may be helpful in obtaining or maintaining a desirable weight.

In addition, moderate physical activity is strongly recommended both for its contribution toward maintaining a desirable weight (thus helping to reduce serum cholesterol levels) and also for other health benefits such as improved blood circulation and muscle tone.

Obesity

Gradual onset of obesity plagues many adults in the United States, where overnutrition is frequently a greater problem than undernutrition. Probably the gradual nature of the onset of this problem is one reason that obesity is so common and so difficult to treat. If a person suddenly put on 5 or 10 pounds, he would be sure to notice the change and likely would do something about it. However, when the weight creeps on over a period of several months or years, one adjusts to the change in appearance

[1.] For those interested in "numbers," typical American diets provide an average of 18 percent of the calories from saturated fats, 18 percent from monounsaturates, and 4 percent from polyunsaturates, for a total of 40 percent. The preceding recommendation should be followed so that saturates provide 8 to 9 percent, monounsaturates 16 to 17 percent, and polyunsaturates 10 to 12 percent, for a total of 35 percent of calories from fat.

and the slow change in clothing sizes without giving it too much thought. The problem of obesity during the adult years is caused mostly by the reduction in activity and an increased consumption of alcoholic beverages (alcohol provides 7 kilocalories per gram). The slow reduction of basal metabolic rate throughout adulthood may also be a factor. These factors dictate a reduction in the total number of calories ingested daily. However, dietary patterns are rather firmly established even in early adulthood, and adults often continue to eat approximately the same number of calories as in younger years, despite their decreasing need for them. The reader is referred to Chapter 4 for a more thorough discussion of the causes and treatment of obesity.

Diet recommendations

Dietary needs of adults are the same in quality as those of children. However, these nutrients need to be provided by gradually smaller quantities of food. This means that the calorie content of the diet should be decreased as energy needs decrease, but that the intake of the other nutrients should remain high (Table 16.2). As declining activity and basal metabolic rate effect this reduction in energy needs, the selection of foods becomes more critical if one is to provide all the nutrients the body needs for optimum health. An adequate diet for adults can be provided by following the Basic Four Food Group Plan, just as has been recommended for the younger ages. While the numbers of recommended servings of the Basic Four remain the same, the serving size should be smaller. There is a continuing need for calcium and phosphorus for maintenance purposes although growth has ceased. One or two glasses of milk daily are sufficient, particularly if the water consumed has adequate amounts of fluoride (fluoridated water). One of the more recent discoveries in nutrition is that the mineral nutrient fluoride helps the body keep calcium in the hard tissues of the

body—teeth and bones—and prevents it from being deposited in the soft tissues.

The difficulty in maintaining a desired weight in adulthood is reflected in Swanson's (1956) report of the mean body weights of 1072 adult women in Iowa. Her figures showed a steady gain in mean weight through the age range 50 to 59; mean weight for women at ages 30 to 39 was approximately 141 pounds; ages 40 to 49, 148 pounds; 50 to 59, 153 pounds. In later life, a distinct decline was noted; ages 60 to 69 had an approximate mean weight of 147 pounds, and past the age of 70, 138 pounds.

The dietary allowances recommended for adults are rather simple to meet if an adult is careful to eat three meals a day and take into consideration the calories in snacks and cocktails. One of the greatest impediments to good nutrition in adults is the attitude that nutrition is not important once growth has ceased. This simply is not so. Every person reflects physically what he eats over a period of time, and adults are the result of dietary patterns over a long period. As in the teen-age period, females are less likely to be well nourished than males during the adult years. Adults need to be aware of shifts in food intake that result from physical alterations such as poor digestion or impaired absorption. If specific foods are eliminated from the diet, other foods containing the needed nutrients or a nutritional supplement will be needed to maintain good nutritional status.

Persons who are malnourished when they reach adulthood can instrument changes to fortify their diets and improve their nutritional status. Overweight individuals can achieve and maintain normal weight. Undernourished adults are encouraged to follow these recommendations:

1. Generous amounts of protein and fats, including unsaturated fats.

2. Regular use of whole or skim milk or their products.

3. Recommended, but not excessive use of green, leafy, and yellow vegetables and cit-

Table 16.2 *Recommended Daily Dietary Allowances for Men and Women*[a]

Nutrient	Men[b]			Women[c]		
	19–22	23–50	51+	19–22	23–50	51+
kcal	3000	2700	2400	2100	2000	1800
Protein (g)	54	56	56	46	46	46
Vitamin A activity (I.U.)	5000	5000	5000	4000	4000	4000
Vitamin D (I.U.)	400	—	—	400	—	—
Vitamin E activity (I.U.)	15	15	15	12	12	12
Ascorbic acid (mg)	45	45	45	45	45	45
Folacin (μg)	400	400	400	400	400	400
Niacin (mg equiv.)	20	18	16	14	13	12
Riboflavin (mg)	1.8	1.6	1.5	1.4	1.2	1.1
Thiamin (mg)	1.5	1.4	1.2	1.1	1.0	1.0
Vitamin B_6 (mg)	2.0	2.0	2.0	2.0	2.0	2.0
Vitamin B_{12} (μg)	3.0	3.0	3.0	3.0	3.0	3.0
Calcium (mg)	800	800	800	800	800	800
Phosphorus (mg)	800	800	800	800	800	800
Iodine (μg)	140	130	110	100	100	80
Iron (mg)	10	10	10	18	18	10
Magnesium (mg)	350	350	350	300	300	300
Zinc (mg)	15	15	15	15	15	15

[a] Food and Nutrition Board, National Academy of Sciences—National Research Council, *Recommended Daily Dietary Allowances,* revised 1974.

[b] Weight for men ages 19–22 is based on 67 kg, and for ages 23 and older on 70 kg; height for ages 19 and older is based on 69 in.

[c] Weight for women ages 19 and older is based on 58 kg; height is based on 65 in.

rus fruits (to leave space for higher calorie foods).

4. When desired weight is achieved, control of caloric intake to avoid becoming heavier.

Improvement of the diet of previously malnourished people is needed to at least partially improve health in adulthood. For example, improving calcium and iron intake to achieve normal body stores of minerals is an important step in preparing for pregnancy and lactation. Building calcium stores is an aid in preventing the onset of osteoporosis.

Influences of adult diets on children

The discussion to this point has focused on the importance of diet for the adult himself. Many adults, however, need to consider their dietary habits from the viewpoint of their role as parents. The impact of the pregnant woman's diet on her offspring has been discussed in Chapter 12.

From the period of infancy and throughout childhood, parents are vital influences in establishing dietary patterns and molding the food preferences of their children. Children quickly notice their parents' attitude toward various foods. If the father does not like vegetables, it is likely that his children may be unenthusiastic about them also. Foods that are disliked by the mother are usually on the rejected list for children both because of the mother's attitude toward the food and because of the probable infrequency with which the item is served. Perhaps the most subtle influence is the example parents set toward milk. If parents do not drink milk regularly, children may drink milk a bit reluctantly when young and then eliminate it from their diets when they reach adulthood.

Adults, particularly mothers, can assist in the development of good dietary patterns in their children (while helping themselves) if they form the habit of eating a good breakfast with their children. Setting a good example is far more effective than lecturing children about the merits of breakfast while neglecting to practice one's own advice. This becomes particularly important in maintaining good dietary patterns for teen-agers. The subtlety of example does not create the resistance and hostility that may develop when parent and teen-ager loudly discuss why adolescents need breakfast.

When parents have a wholesome attitude toward food instead of using it as a panacea for their own troubles, they are able to help their children also develop a healthy perspective toward food. Parents of normal weight, who appreciate food for its social, psychological,

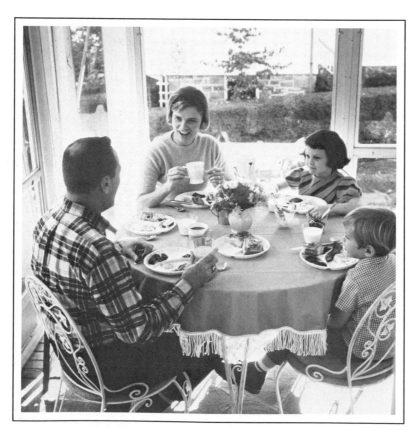

Parents who regularly drink milk provide the example needed to encourage children to continue to drink milk when they reach adulthood.

and physiological contributions without letting it become the dominating force in their lives, naturally guide their children into similar attitudes toward food. Healthful weight control presents little difficulty for such people throughout their lives.

Nutrition After 65

Nutrition for people in the retirement years is a subject of growing interest in the United States, for this segment of the population is growing disproportionately to the population as a whole. In 1970 there were more than 20 million people age 65 or more, or approximately 10 percent of the total population in the United States. A century ago only 2.5 percent of the nation's people were 65 or older. The increasing numbers of older people are the result of (1) many discoveries and advances in the medical and nutritional fields, (2) improved living conditions, and (3) greater availability of health services.

As this segment of the population becomes larger, there is an increasing awareness of the unique problems faced by people after age 65. These problems are intertwined and frequently complex, but with the growing social consciousness of many citizens, it is realistic to predict that some of the difficulties of the elderly will come into sharper focus and begin to be alleviated. Adequate nutrition for this age group is an achievable goal if environmental, social, and psychological influences do not interfere with the nutritional process. These influences, therefore, need to be understood clearly and taken into account.

Sociopsychological aspects

Although there is variation among individuals, there are problems that are common to a large fraction of the elderly. In the United States, with its youth-oriented culture, there is an emphasis on the relationship of social status to job status. A person who occupies a position of authority in the business world is treated with dignity and respect. However, when he retires, he may find that he no longer has the social status that was inherently attached to his position. He then may join the ranks of the elderly who have the task of searching once again for the tangible and satisfactory identity that will give status in the eyes of the world. The dignity accorded the elderly in cultures that embrace the aged within the family circle is denied a distressing fraction of people in the United States following their retirement.

Despite the fact that a person's ability to work is not magically ended on his 65th birthday, most employees automatically receive their accolades and termination papers without consideration for their actual physical and mental capabilities. The self-employed are more fortunate, because they are in the position of being able to continue to work if they wish. Some retired people find new recognition and status through volunteer work. Others may tend to brood over their totally different way of life, finding little reason for existing, and simply wait for death.

Many older citizens have made virtually no preparation for the ever-lengthening years of retirement. People who have worked long hours for many years may not have developed hobbies that are of value when the pressures of work have been left behind. Their lives may become filled only with ennui and boredom. Golden Age Clubs and Senior Citizen Centers have sprung up in many cities and towns to combat the empty hours. There are even whole towns dedicated to the retired citizen. These retirement villages specialize in providing the practical and human needs that are difficult to manage in the workaday world. Recreation facilities are geared toward the capabilities of the older citizen, and the emphasis is on compatible companionship. For the person in good health who chooses to gravitate toward these clubs and communities, the empty hours of the day become very full.

The void created by lack of employment during the retirement years is but one of the adjustments frequently required. The loss of one's mate requires considerable adaptation on the part of the bereaved at any point in life, but in the later years, there is less activity to direct the mind away from the immediate problems one faces. Adjustments during the time of bereavment may mean giving up the home that has been the family gathering place for many years; feelings of depression may be very intense and life may seem overwhelmingly empty. For a woman, widowhood may impose financial responsibilities she has never had to understand and handle before. For a widower, the problems of managing one's home and meals become immediately pressing. Previously shared responsibilities become the sole burden of the survivor, and the golden years may abruptly lose their burnish.

Some people have sufficient funds to make these remaining years comfortable and free of financial worry, but the large majority of the elderly are tightly caught in the press created by the inflationary spiral of the economy and the very limited income available under most retirement plans. The picture is complicated still farther by the prolonged period of retirement that must be financed. About 5 million people over age 65 have to live on fixed incomes that are too little to enable them to live in the manner that they did when they were still working. This obvious deterioration in the standard of living is degrading to anyone, and is no more acceptable to the aged than to younger people. In some instances, this shortage of funds freezes older people into life in a portion of town where the life is changing. The more affluent residents may have moved away, to be replaced by people who cannot or do not maintain the area. There is less pleasure to be drawn from the immediate environment, and the rate of crimes in the area may rise. Cramped budgets of the elderly require skillful management if they are to cover the bare necessities. A move to a more pleasant area is not a financial possibility for them.

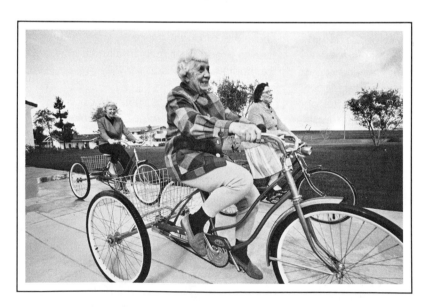

A retirement village has numerous recreation facilities geared to the interests of older people.

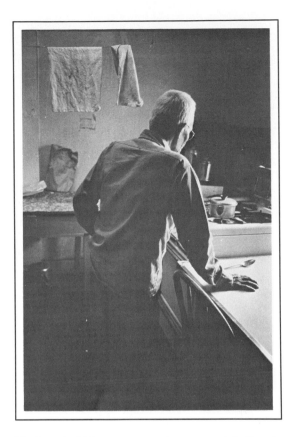

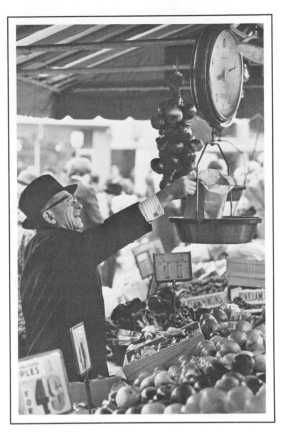

The loss of a lifelong mate may plunge a man into the role of total responsibility for preparing all of his food, but with no help in learning how to do this task.

High food costs and the fixed incomes of retired persons present serious impediments to achieving good nutrition.

As if these problems were not sufficient, general health will deteriorate eventually. Concern with health is very real to the aged. Some of the problems can be treated very well; others are costly and threatening to life itself; others are merely imagined. In the desire to avoid possible ailments or to improve ailments resulting from hypochondriacal musing, older people are easy prey for the hawker of patent medicines and "health foods." Today's older generation grew up when the general pattern was to see a doctor only when virtually on one's deathbed. To them it may seem less ominous (and less costly) to try the wares of the "health-peddling" entrepreneur in preference to visiting the physician, a choice that may be injurious to the health of the individual.

This overview of the realities of being a part of this somewhat isolated generation, of course, is not complete in all aspects, nor is it all true for any one individual. However, this provides the background needed to view the nutritional needs and problems of the elderly in the perspective of today's world. This population group, perhaps more than any other, can only be aided nutritionally when those who work with them see the total picture in which they live.

Physiological factors

Aging is a process that continues throughout the duration of one's lifetime, but by the time a

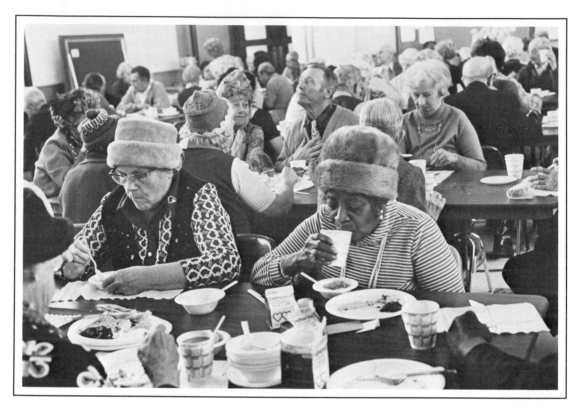

Older women have been found to have deficient intakes of several nutrients. For women living alone, meals providing social contact with others are a pleasant way of promoting better nutrition practices.

person has lived 65 years, there are significant differences between his body and that of a person of 20. These changes alter the amounts of nutrients needed and the utilization of the nutrients ingested.

With advancing years, the heart may be less able to pump the volume of blood that was circulated earlier in life, and waste products are removed less efficiently from the blood by filtration in the kidneys. Blood vessels may have become somewhat clogged with atherosclerotic deposits and the walls may thicken, calcify, and become less elastic, thus reducing blood flow.

The flow of saliva may decrease, the result of some degeneration of the saliva glands. This change may make food less palatable because of greater difficulty in swallowing without the lubricating effect of adequate saliva. The re-

duced sensitivity of taste buds and the olfactory receptor cells also decreases the flavor sensations of food for older people, making food less appealing than it was earlier in life.

Digestion becomes slightly impaired as a result of several physical alterations in the body. There is poorer digestion of fats when the amount of bile secreted is reduced. In the aging process, there is a gradual reduction in the quantity of digestive enzymes being secreted.

There is a slowing of the body processes with an accompanying decrease in basal metabolic rate. Although the overall pattern for basal metabolism shows a general decline throughout life, there is a more pronounced decrease during the later years of life than there is at any other time. This reduction in basal metabolic rate reflects the decline in muscle tonus that results from the reduced activity that is the typical pattern during the later years.

Osteoporosis (reduced bone mass) is a disease associated with aging. This progressive disease commonly occurs in women in their mid-50s, and in men in their mid-60s. The causes of the gradually decreasing bone mass are not clearly understood. In osteoporosis there is greater likelihood of breaking bones. There also may be severe pain in the back as a result of the collapse of vertebrae.

Diets that are inadequate in calcium, phosphorus, and vitamin D, as are the diets of the elderly who do not drink milk, may favor the development of osteoporosis. This condition is a particular problem for older women and appears to be aggravated by poor nutritional practices over the years.

The relationship of fluoride intake to osteoporotic changes was suggested by Leone, et al. in 1955. These workers observed that fluoride, when consumed at the level of 8 parts per million over the period of a lifetime, had some benefit in counteracting the tendency toward osteoporosis in the aged. Gron, et al. (1966) reported that fluoride is incorporated into the crystalline structure of bones in a manner similar to its deposition in teeth. They reported that high fluoride intake (10 to 66 milligrams of fluoride daily) for at least a year by adults produced changes in bone, making them similar to the structure found in the bones of adults who had been drinking water containing between four and eight parts of fluoride throughout their lives. Bernstein and Cohen (1967) treated 200 adults over 50 years of age with levels of fluoride ranging from 10 to 66 milligrams for several months to 1 or 2 years. In several patients treated in this manner for more than 18 months, recalcification was initiated. A shift in the calcium balance was achieved in 90 percent of the subjects receiving fluoride. The observations by Bernstein, et al. (1966) in North Dakota further support the suggestion that fluoride throughout life is an important mineral in the diet as protection not only against dental caries and resulting potential loss of teeth, but also against the rarefaction of bones in the later years.

Loss of teeth presents a significant obstacle to the achievement of an adequate dietary intake for a large number of senior citizens. Yurkstas (1954) reported a loss of 33 percent efficiency in chewing when persons lost the first permanent molar; with loss of the second, a drop in efficiency of 44 percent; and with that of the third molar, 66 percent. Manly and Vinton (1951) found that denture wearers had to chew their food approximately four times as much as the average person to reach the same end point in mastication. With such differences, many people with dentures tend to restrict their diets to foods that are easily chewed. Such a change is likely to mean a reduction in the amount of protein foods and fruits and vegetables included in the diet. By using a blender or chopping foods that are difficult to chew, one can readily maintain the full spectrum of the menu for denture wearers. Of course, such sobering thoughts underscore the importance of proper diet and fluoridated water throughout life so that the teeth remain sound throughout the person's lifetime. These data also demonstrate that even perfectly designed and fitted dentures used in these studies were poor substitutes for good natural teeth.

Dietary recommendations

The National Academy of Sciences—National Research Council's daily dietary recommendations (1974 revision) for women 51 and older show a decrease in calories, niacin, riboflavin, iodine, and iron in comparison with the recommendations for young adult women. The 10 percent reduction in calories is particularly significant because this figure means that the older woman needs to reduce her total intake of food significantly while still consuming the same amounts of protein, vitamin A, vitamin E, ascorbic acid, folacin, thiamin, vitamin B_6, vitamin B_{12}, calcium, phosphorus, zinc, and magnesium that she required as a young woman.

To maintain a state of good nutriture without gradually acquiring excess poundage, the diet will have to be modified so that a higher percentage of the diet contains protein. The decreased amount of iron recommended is explained on the basis of the cessation of menstruation; iodine at the somewhat reduced level recommended is still sufficient to prevent development of goiter in older people. Increased amounts of fluoride are desirable to maintain the strength of their bones.

The recommended daily dietary allowances for men show a calorie decrease of just over 11 percent for men 51 and over, in comparison with the recommendation for young adult males; the decreases in thiamin, riboflavin, and niacin recommendations are associated with the 300-kilocalorie reduction during this age span.

Of interest is the fact that the recommended level of calcium and phosphorus for both men and women in the age bracket 51 and older remains constant. This recommendation is based on the continuing need for these minerals to maintain the integrity of bones.

Results presented in the 1969 preliminary report of the dietary survey conducted in Spring 1965 by the Agricultural Research Service clearly highlighted the need to improve dietary intakes of the elderly in the United States. As was true from the teen-age years onward, elderly males were found to be better fed than were their female counterparts. However, the trend for both men and women is toward a poorer diet late in life. Men between the ages of 55 and 74 were found, as a group, to be deficient in calcium intake; after age 75, the deficiency of calcium was more of a problem than previously, and in addition, vitamin A values, riboflavin, and ascorbic acid were also low. Women aged 55 to 64 were low in their consumption of calcium, thiamin, and riboflavin; at age 65 and over, the inadequacies included not only calcium, thiamin, and riboflavin, but also iron and vitamin A, with the problem growing in severity among women age 75 or older. Since the dietary survey included assessment of the adequacy of only protein, calcium, iron, vitamin A, thiamin, riboflavin, and ascorbic acid, there is some likelihood that other vitamins and minerals are also inadequate in the diets of older people.

One may assume, however, that people who have successfully lived to old age and are enjoying reasonably good health must have been eating a diet that was generally supportive of their physical condition throughout their lives. However, changes in their living patterns that result from the social, economic, and physical events that alter their lives during the later years are likely to cause some modifications in their traditional dietary patterns. These adaptations take place despite the fact that the basic dietary habits are strongly ingrained by the time the age of retirement is reached.

The Basic Four Food Group Plan is a suitable pattern for the diets of the elderly. This is to be expected since the dietary allowances are not greatly modified (with the exception of calories) during this period. There are some apparent but small changes that will facilitate the consumption of an adequate diet. The inclusion of 2 glasses of milk daily presents no problem for the individual who has regularly consumed milk throughout his life. However, some older people view milk strictly as food only for children and therefore have not formed the habit of drinking milk as adults. Even in the later years, there is value in reinstituting the practice of drinking milk daily. This could be done by drinking a large glass of milk twice daily or by having three or four smaller glasses. If this proves to be difficult to achieve, milk-containing soups, puddings, cottage cheese, and other foods made with milk or consumed with milk, such as cereals, can occupy a prominent position in the diet. There is considerable merit in using nonfat or low-fat rather than whole milk for at least two reasons: (1) this substitution is one simple and palatable way of reducing caloric intake during this period of relatively low caloric need, and (2) the reduced intake of saturated fat will be beneficial to persons with cardiovascular problems.

The amount of protein in the diet needs to be maintained during the later years at about the same level as was consumed earlier. This can be accomplished by continuing to eat a minimum of two servings daily from the meat group. Loss of teeth and poorly fitting dentures present particular problems for the elderly when they are trying to provide for their needs in this category. Ground meats, fish, cheese, and less tender cuts of meat cooked until tender or with the use of a tenderizer then become particularly important in the planning of menus. That the intake of protein foods is likely to be more limited in the later years has been documented by Swanson (1964). She found that women over 70 years of age ingested only about half as many calories from meat, fish, and poultry as did women between the ages of 30 and 39. In addition, she found a small decrease in the calories available from milk, eggs, cheese, and legumes in the diet. The summation clearly indicated a reduction in the amount of protein in the diet, despite the fact that the body still has a need for protein for tissue maintenance that is not diminished by the aging process. Steinkamp, et al. (1965) did not report a deficit of protein in the diets of the California population they studied, but they did note a

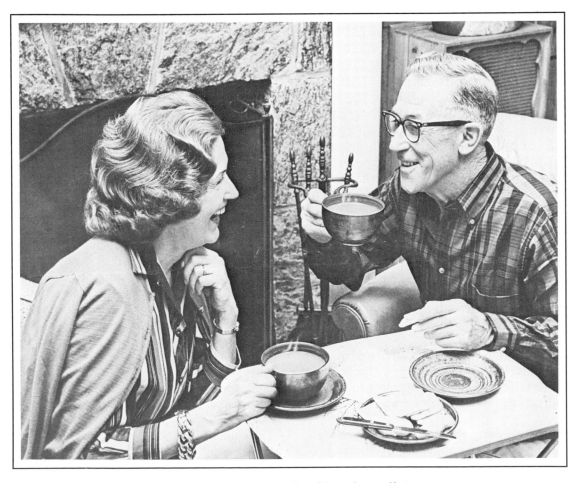

Frequent small meals may suit the life-style of older people well, and the inclusion of hot soups is a good means of increasing liquid intake.

significant decrease in the adequacy of diets after people reached the age of 75.

The recommendations for four or more servings of fruits and vegetables, with at least one serving of a citrus fruit daily and a good source of vitamin A every other day, may not be met by senior citizens, as indicated by the 1965 ARS dietary survey which reported inadequacies of both vitamin A and ascorbic acid for older men and vitamin A deficiencies among older women. When planning menus for this age group, one must consider the chewing capabilities and the digestive prowess of the individual so that the fruits and vegetables are tempting and easily consumed. Denture wearers may experience considerable difficulty eating corn on the cob, while others may experience some discomfort when fed beans, raw onions, or various other vegetables or fruits. With the wide range of foods available in this category, the preparation of fruits and vegetables so that they are highly palatable as well as nourishing becomes a relatively simple matter.

The four servings in the bread and cereal group are likely to be consumed by people in this age bracket. The reasons for this are related to the ease with which these foods can be eaten and their relatively low cost. For example, Swanson (1964) noted a drop of only 5 kilocalories contributed by breads and cereals to the diets of women over 70 in comparison with the intake of women ages 30 to 39.

Liquid and fiber or roughage are important in the diet of the elderly if constipation is to be avoided. At least 6 or 8 glasses of liquid are recommended daily. If desired, the liquid may be hot bouillon, coffee, tea, and fruit and vegetable juices. These add interest as well as liquid to the diet. Fiber comes from whole grain breads and cereals, and roughage from the skins of fruits.

The preceding recommendations point out the importance of maintaining a wide range of foods in the diets of the elderly so that the nutrients, water, and necessary roughage are provided on a daily basis. To protect against the consumption of too many calories, smaller servings are important. Most elderly people will need to minimize the amount of sweets they eat and reduce the total amount of fat, while substituting polyunsaturated vegetable oil products for much of the fat from animal sources. Frequent small meals, perhaps as many as five daily, are better suited to the desires of some elderly people rather than the usual three meals. The frequent service of hot beverages or soups may be a source of comfort as well as a useful addition to the liquid intake for the day.

Improving nutrition of the aged

Of course, adequate diet is not simply a matter of planning menus. The food must be purchased, prepared, and then served in an attractive manner in pleasant surroundings if older people are truly to enjoy eating. For the fortunate elderly with excellent income, a comfortable place to live, good health, and companionship, good nutritional status is a relatively simple matter except for caloric intake. Only minor modifications from the previous dietary pattern are required.

However, for a large number of the elderly, one or more factors will greatly impede an individual's efforts to be well fed. A tightly limited budget may require more marketing skill than he has acquired by previous experience if the money is to cover even the bare necessities. It may be that transportation for shopping is not readily available, so that he must impose on someone else for grocery shopping or make numerous trips to the market if there is one within a reasonable walking distance. Economical shopping is not enhanced under transportation handicaps.

Still other older people have poor facilities for preparing food. It is difficult for anyone to become very inspired about cooking when refrigerator facilities are absent and hot foods can only be prepared on a hot plate in the same room where one eats and sleeps. Older men, who have not had to do food preparation earlier in life, may get totally discouraged when they suddenly become responsible for all their own cooking. The prospect that they will prepare tempting and nutritionally adequate meals for themselves is remote. Even older women, who have had considerable experience in food preparation, may fail to eat well when they have only themselves to cook for.

Problems are magnified when the individual living alone is not in good health. To the preceding picture, one certainly must add that a rather substantial amount of advertising regarding so-called "health foods" is directed toward older people. When the elderly have very limited understanding of the sciences of medicine and nutrition and a painful familiarity with the various physical problems they have acquired as they aged, there is little reason to be surprised that they are courted into parting with some of their limited dollars to buy products that are touted to cure existing problems or to prevent the development of others yet unknown.

While not all of these problems will confront any one person, the general picture for the elderly is that care must be given to planning and eating an adequate diet. With some attention, many older people can handle this phase of their lives very adequately for several years. For numerous others, some form of assistance is needed if good nutrition is to be achieved.

One interesting approach to the problems of the elderly in the inner city of Los Angeles has been to provide a highly nourishing, hot meal free of charge and served in a congenial setting one noon a week to all interested persons over 64 who live in this low-income area. The meals are served at various points in the city with the aid of volunteers from the churches where the meals are served. Leftover foods that do not require refrigeration are given to guests who wish to take them home, thus adding to the nutritional benefit of the program. To date, the program has been very well received by the numerous elderly who participate regularly in this sociable and nourishing weekly event. Obviously, such a service can alleviate loneliness, provide at least some good food each week, and teach a little about shopping and preparation of nourishing food the remainder of the

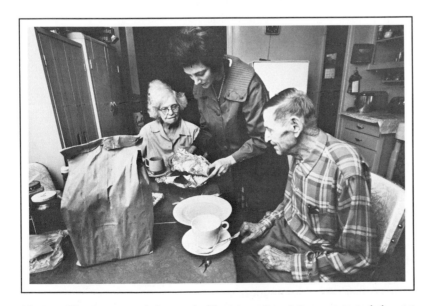

Meals-on-Wheels are provided as a valuable community nutrition program to help meet the needs of homebound older people in many places.

week. This program is a very useful aid for the aged, but unfortunately cannot provide a guarantee that its participants will be well fed all week. Community support, in the form of money, facilities, and volunteer labor, is needed for this type of program.

Meals-on-Wheels programs have been available as an assistance to the elderly who are living in their own homes, but who may have difficulty in preparing adequate meals for themselves. The mechanics of the programs vary from city to city, but the underlying goal of the Meals-on-Wheels is to provide a hot meal in the home each day at a low cost. The meals usually are prepared in a central kitchen and then delivered by truck to the participants in the program. The success of this approach to good nutrition for the elderly is largely dependent upon the local situation. When supervision, planning, and administration are good, the food is of high quality and reasonable in price. In short, the program is highly successful. Where quality control and other facets of administration have been weak, the program has failed. Certainly, the basic concepts of this type of program are sound. Meals-on-Wheels has the potential for enabling many elderly people to maintain their independence longer than they could if they did not have this nutritional assistance available to them.

Of growing importance in the feeding of the elderly have been nursing and convalescent homes. As the numbers of older citizens have been increasing, institutional care for the elderly has grown significantly. The quality of the meals in these various institutions is highly variable, again reflecting the general competence and skills of the person supervising this aspect of the unit. Theoretically, trained personnel can provide optimum nutrition and very broad acceptance of the food in these institutions for the elderly. Meals need not be eaten alone, meal preparation and planning are done by persons skilled in the art and science of feeding people, and the total physical environment is centered around the needs and interests of this age group. In practice, this idealized circumstance is achieved in some nursing and convalescent homes, but undoubtedly some owners and managers are motivated more by profits and practical concerns than they are by the desire to care for the elderly to the very best of their ability. Nursing homes can brighten the lives of their patients if the staff recognizes the role of good food as being a link with the past. Mealtime may be the only pleasurable activity for some of the patients. Good food is a real morale builder.

Summary

Dietary needs throughout adulthood can be met by following the Basic Four Food Group Plan. In early adulthood, attention should be given to eating three meals a day, planned so that all the necessary nutrients are consumed in sufficient quantities. The importance of maintaining a desirable weight throughout adulthood must be appreciated and practiced. Parents have the responsibility of not only feeding themselves appropriately, but also of setting a good example for their children. Adult women, because of both the documented likelihood of dietary indiscretions and because of their probable pregnancy and lactation periods, need to be particularly careful to maintain an appropriate dietary regimen.

The elderly in our society are required to make many social and psychological adjustments in addition to the physiological changes that accompany the aging process. Modifications in the life-style of the individual and in the functioning of the body result in modified dietary patterns during this phase of life. In particular, the elderly well need to reduce caloric intake while maintaining a highly nourishing diet. Modifications may include a shift toward eating more frequent, smaller meals, a diet generous in fiber and roughage to avoid constipation, and the ingestion of more liquid. As a result of growing community awareness of the problems of the elderly, some programs have been implemented to assist its senior residents in overcoming the problems that may cause them to be poorly nourished.

Selected References

Agricultural Research Service. *Food Intake and Nutritive Value of Diets of Men, Women, and Children in the United States.* Spring 1965. ARS 62-18. U.S. Department of Agriculture. 1969.

Beeuwkes, A. M. Studying the food habits of the elderly. *J. Am. Diet. Assoc.* 37:215. 1960.

Bernstein, D. S., and P. Cohen. Use of sodium fluoride in the treatment of osteoporosis. *J. Clin. Endr. Metab.* 27:197. 1967.

Bernstein, D. S., et al. Prevalence of osteoporosis in high- and low-fluoride areas in North Dakota. *J. Am. Med. Assoc.* 198:499. 1966.

Bierman, E. L., and R. Nelson. Carbohydrates, diabetes, and blood lipids. *World Rev. Nutr. Diet* 22:280. 1975.

Brine, R. The old in the country of the young. *Time.* August 3, 1970. P. 49–54.

Brown, A. T. Oral biology. *Present Knowledge of Nutrition.* 4th ed. Nutrition Foundation. New York. 1976.

Brusis, O. A., and R. B. McGandy. Nutrition and man's heart and blood vessels. *Fed. Proc.* 30:1417. 1971.

Darby, W. J. Nutrition and noma. *Present Knowledge of Nutrition.* 4th ed. Nutrition Foundation. New York. 1976.

Friedman, M., et al. Coronary-prone individuals. *J. Am. Med. Assoc.* 217:929. 1971.

Fry, P. C., H. M. Fox, and H. Linkswiler. Nutrient intakes of healthy older women. *J. Am. Diet. Assoc.* 42:218–222. 1963.

Graude, F. Sugar and cardiovascular disease. *World Rev. Nutr. Diet* 22:248. 1975.

Gron, P., et al. Effect of fluoride on human osteoporotic bone mineral: a chemical and crystallographic study. *J. Bone Joint Surg. (Amer.).* 48:892. 1966.

Halsted,C. Nutritional implications of alcohol. *Present Knowledge of Nutrition.* 4th ed. Nutrition Foundation. New York. 1976.

Hathcock, J. Nutrition, toxicology and pharmacology. *Present Knowledge of Nutrition.* 4th ed. Nutrition Foundation. New York. 1976.

LeBovit, C. The food of older persons living at home. *J. Am. Diet. Assoc. 46:285–289.* 1965.

Leone, N. C., et al. A roentgenologic study of a human population exposed to high-fluoride domestic water. *Amer. J. Roentgen Rad. Ther. Nuc. Med. 74:874.* 1955.

Lutwak, L. Osteoporosis—a mineral deficiency disease. *J. Am. Diet. Assoc. 44:173.* 1964.

Manly, R. S., and P. Vinton. A survey of the chewing ability of denture wearers. *J. Den. Res. 30:314–321.* 1951.

Mayer, J. Nutrition in the aged. *Postgrad. Med. 32:394.* 1962.

Mayer, J. Aging and nutrition. *Geriatrics 29:57.* 1974.

McGill, H. C., Jr. Coronary artery disease. *Present Knowledge of Nutrition.* 4th ed. Nutrition Foundation. New York. 1976.

Mitra, M. L. Confusional states in relation to vitamin deficiencies in the elderly. *J. Am. Geriatrics Soc. 19:536.* 1971.

National Academy of Sciences. *Dietary Fat and Human Health.* Publication No. 1147. National Research Council. Washington, D.C. 1966.

Qureshi, R. U., et al. Effect of an "atherogenic" diet containing starch or sucrose upon carcass composition and plasma lipids in the rat. *Nutr. and Metab. 12,* No. 6:341. 1970.

Review. Fluoride, bony structure and aortic calcification. *Nutrition Rev. 25:100.* 1967.

Rosenman, R. H., and M. Friedman. Observations on the pathogenesis of coronary heart disease. *Nutrition News. 34,* No. 3:9. 1971.

Shock, N. W. Physiological aspects of aging. *J. Am. Diet. Assoc. 56:491–496.* 1970.

Stare, F. J. Nondental use of fluoride. *Dental Abstracts. 13:202.* April, 1968.

Steinkamp, R. C., N. L. Cohen, and H. E. Walsh. Resurvey of an aging population—fourteen year follow-up. *J. Am. Diet. Assoc. 46:103–110.* 1965.

Swanson, P. Adequacy in old age. Part I. Role of Nutrition. *J. Home Econ. 56:651–658.* 1964.

Swanson, P. Adequacy in old age. Part II. Nutrition education programs for the aging. *J. Home Econ. 56:728—734.* 1964.

Swanson, P. From the standpoint of a nutritionist. In *Potentialities of Women in the Middle Years.* I. H. Gross, ed. Michigan State U. Press. East Lansing. P. 59–86. 1956.

Vanamee, P. Intravenous alimentation. *Present Knowledge of Nutrition.* 4th ed. Nutrition Foundation. New York. 1976.

Watkin, D. M. New findings in the nutrition of older people. *Am. J. Pub. Health. 55:548–553.* 1965.

Weinberg, J. Psychologic implications of nutritional needs of elderly. *J. Am. Diet. Assoc. 60:293.* 1972.

Wolgamot, I. H. Helping older persons meet their nutritional needs. *Nutrition Program News*. U.S. Department of Agriculture, Washington. January–February 1970.

Young, C. Nutrition counseling for better health. *Geriatrics 29:*83. 1974.

Yurkstas, A. A. The effect of missing teeth on masticatory performance and efficiency. *J. Pros. Dent. 4:*120–123.

APPLYING NUTRITION

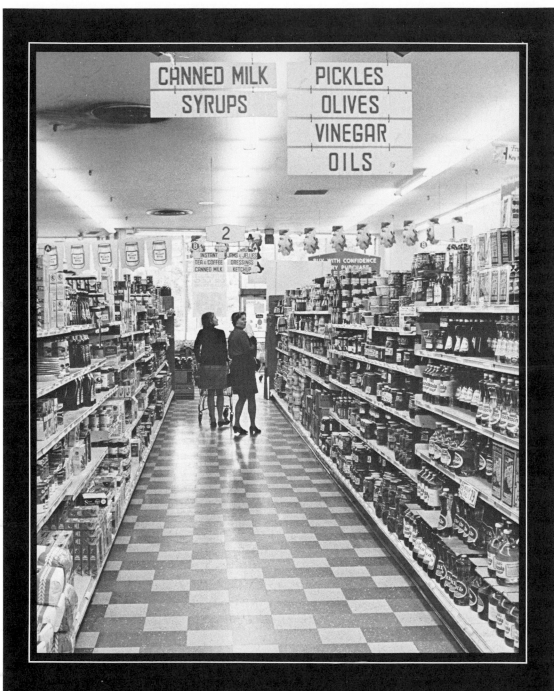

CANNED MILK
SYRUPS

PICKLES
OLIVES
VINEGAR
OILS

Chapter 17

Shopping for Good Nutrition

Nutrition is more than a subject to learn about from a book and from lectures. For this fascinating field to be seen in total perspective, the wealth of knowledge about nutrition must be translated from a passive to an active role. Only by actually practicing the recommendations for good dietary patterns regularly can an individual gain the greatest possible benefits from the science of nutrition. This is a subject which has potential benefits for all of its students throughout life and is not limited simply to the campus or to a selected career. Every person practices nutrition throughout life, but whether the patterns followed prove to be a benefit or a hindrance to good health is very much an individual matter.

Accurate knowledge of nutritional needs and food sources of these nutrients is a valuable tool for achieving good nutritional status; unfortunately, knowledge alone is not enough. A nourishing array of foods consumed in the right quantities is essential on a reasonably reg-

ular basis if good nutritional status is to be achieved and maintained. There is no single set of menus which must be followed to be well nourished. The actual foods, the ways in which they are prepared, and the quantities eaten are all very individual matters. There are many ways of achieving the same end. The routes used can be chosen to add interest and pleasure to life while meeting physiological and psychological needs.

Food certainly is one of the true pleasures of life, and eating for good nutrition can be done while enhancing this enjoyment. Good nutrition does not need to be synonymous with self-denial and menus featuring foods that are *good* for you but which may have little psychological satisfaction. Anytime is a good time to begin eating for enjoyment and optimum health; the sooner the better. The pleasures are many, and the cost in time and money need be no more, and well may be less, than the resources presently being used to be fed. The key is to translate nutritional needs and food preferences into appealing foods which are served and eaten in desirable quantities. This can be achieved through intelligent shopping, appropriate storage, and careful preparation and service of food.

The Consumer in the Market

One of the most important decision points in achieving a good diet is the grocery store. The choices made there greatly influence dietary practices. A kitchen supplied primarily with carbonated beverages, potato chips, and sour cream stimulates a family toward snacking as a pattern. A tempting bowl of fresh fruits ready to eat may also stimulate snacking, but the nutrient intake of the two types of snacks will be quite different. When one shops with the idea of the role of the pantry and its contents in shaping dietary patterns, the choices can be made to help encourage family members to select impulse snacks that make a nutritional contribution while also adding pleasure to the day.

In many instances nutritional choices are made at the store, decisions which modify the nutritive value of the diet while having very little influence upon the psychological value of the food. For example, the nutritional value of meats varies widely from one source or cut to another depending largely on the amount and kind of fat. The choice of milks will have dietary implications. Salad dressings represent still other types of products where the shopper is faced with choices having nutritional implications. Throughout the store similar choices which influence nutritional status need to be made. The shopper today is faced with numerous decisions regarding the purchase of the ingredients for good nutrition. The nutritional choices are not made in an isolated fashion, but actually have to be made in the context of price considerations, quality, and family food preferences. Decisions in the market are becoming increasingly complex, and television and advertising have not made the choices simpler.

An examination of some of the products presently available, which have nutritional implications, provides interesting ideas and questions for individual consumers. The actual best choice of a product will vary in individual cases, but the points to consider can be identified. Examples of foods causing questions among consumers include margarines, eggs, cereals, and fruit juices. Also raising questions among consumers is the nutrition labeling which is now available as an aid in providing answers to many questions about products. Considerable information is available. The need is to be able to utilize this information to make the best individual choice.

Nutrition labeling

Many food products available in the grocery store carry nutrition-labeling information for consumers. This information must be provided if nutritional claims are made for the product, and the information is required by law to be listed in a prescribed format. Each nutrition label must have the following information:

1. Serving size for which the nutrition information is given. The serving size must be clearly stated, but is not necessarily the exact amount that a person actually eats.
2. The number of servings of the stated size which are provided in the container. This figure is particularly useful when a comparison in cost per serving between similar products is desired.
3. Number of kilocalories per serving size indicated. When a serving provides up to 20

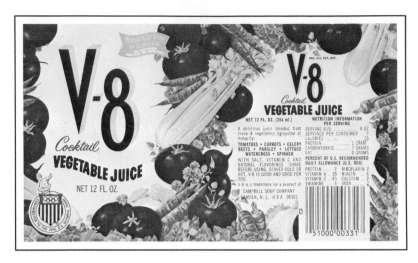

The statement "naturally low in calories" whether appearing in advertising or as shown on the label, is a sufficient nutritional claim to trigger the requirement for nutritional labeling.

kilocalories (small), the value is shown to the nearest 2 kilocalories, to the nearest 5 up to 50, and to the nearest 10 above 50.

4. Grams of protein per serving size indicated.

5. Grams of carbohydrate per serving size indicated. The label provides information only on total carbohydrate and gives no breakdown regarding the type of carbohydrate and the relative amounts of starch, sugar, and fiber.

6. Grams of fat per serving indicated. Some food products will also carry information about the amounts of polyunsaturated and saturated fats in them. This information is provided at the option of the manufacturer.

7. The percentage of the U.S. Recommended Daily Allowance (U.S. RDA) for protein, vitamin A, vitamin C, thiamin, riboflavin, niacin, calcium, and iron provided by the serving indicated also are stated on the label. The U.S. RDA's (Table 17.1) are derived from the RDA's (Table 1.8) and, for adults and children, are usually the highest RDA of all sex-age categories; commercial baby and junior foods are labeled

with special U.S. RDA's for infants and young children.

The U.S. RDA's are based on the needs of healthy people and, with the exception of kilocalories, represent an excess of 30 to 50 percent above actual needs to allow for individual variations with a margin of safety. Many adults may need only between two-thirds and three-fourths of the U.S. RDA, while half the value may be enough for many children. Thus, it is possible to be well nourished without always consuming 100 percent of the U.S. RDA. A comparison of the U.S. RDA and RDA is presented in Table 17.2.

8. Nutrient information does not have to be restricted to the listing of the eight nutrients which are mandated to be listed. Twelve additional vitamins and minerals have established U.S. RDA values, and the nutritional contribution of a food toward these values also may be provided if a manufacturer wishes to do so. These optional nutrient listings include vitamin D, vitamin E, vitamin B_6, folic acid, vitamin B_{12}, phosphorus, io-

Table 17.1 *U.S. Recommended Daily Allowances (U.S. RDA)*

Nutrient	Amount		
	Adults and Children 4 Years or Older	Under 4 Years	Pregnant or Lactating Women
Required Listings on Labels			
Protein	45 or 65 g[a]		
Vitamin A	5,000 I.U.	2,500 I.U.	8,000 I.U.
Vitamin C (ascorbic acid)	60 mg	40 mg	60 mg
Thiamin (vitamin B_1)	1.5 mg	0.7 mg	1.7 mg
Riboflavin (vitamin B_2)	1.7 mg	0.8 mg	2.0 mg
Niacin	20 mg	9.0 mg	20 mg
Calcium	1.0 g	0.8 g	1.3 g
Iron	18 mg	10 mg	18 mg
Optional Listings on Labels			
Vitamin D	400 I.U.	400 I.U.	400 I.U.
Vitamin E	30 I.U.	10 I.U.	30 I.U.
Vitamin B_6	2.0 mg	0.7 mg	2.5 mg
Folic acid (folacin)	0.4 mg	0.2 mg	0.8 mg
Vitamin B_{12}	6.0 mcg	3.0 mcg	8.0 mcg
Phosphorus	1.0 g	0.8 g	1.3 g
Iodine	150 mcg	70 mcg	150 mcg
Magnesium	400 mg	200 mg	450 mg
Zinc	15 mg	8 mg	15 mg
Copper	2 mg	1 mg	2 mg
Biotin	0.3 mg	0.15 mg	0.3 mg
Pantothenic acid	10 mg	5 mg	10 mg

[a] Forty-five grams if protein quality is equal to or greater than milk protein, 65 grams if protein quality is less than milk protein.

dide, magnesium, zinc, copper, biotin, and pantothenic acid.

9. As an aid to some individuals on special diets, a few products also will be labeled with the level of cholesterol contained in a serving. For persons on salt-restricted diets, the sodium content is of interest. This information also may be included on the label.

10. Since some foods traditionally are eaten with another food added rather than being eaten alone, a second column of nutrition information may be presented to show the total contribution of the food combination as it is eaten. Such a listing, for example, usually is provided for breakfast cereals plus milk.

By taking the time to read nutrition labels on food products, it is possible to gain a good picture of one's diet. However, it is necessary to consider the total food intake for the day and not merely to rely on labeled foods for information. Fresh fruits and vegetables, for example,

Table 17.2 *Percentage of the U.S. RDA needed to meet the Recommended Dietary Allowances for children, men, and women of different ages*

Age Years	Protein[a]	Vitamin A	Vitamin C	Thiamin	Ribo-flavin	Niacin[b]	Calcium	Iron
	Percent of U.S. Recommended Daily Allowance							
Child:								
1–3	35	40	70	50	50	30	80	85
4–6	50	50	70	60	65	35	80	60
7–10	55	70	70	80	75	50	80	60
Male:								
11–14	70	100	75	95	90	55	120	100
15–18	85	100	75	100	110	55	120	100
19–22	85	100	75	100	110	60	80	60
23–50	90	100	75	95	95	45	80	60
51+	90	100	75	80	90	35	80	60
Female:								
11–14	70	80	75	80	80	45	120	100
15–18	75	80	75	75	85	30	120	100
19–22	75	80	75	75	85	35	80	100
23–50	75	80	75	70	75	30	80	100
51+	75	80	75	70	65	25	80	60
Pregnant	+50[c]	100	100	+20[c]	+20[c]	35	120	100+
Nursing	+35[c]	120	135	+20[c]	+30[c]	35	120	100

[a] U.S. RDA of 65 grams is used for this table. In labeling, a U.S. RDA of 45 grams is used for foods providing high-quality protein, such as milk, meat, and eggs.

[b] The percentage of the U.S. RDA shown for niacin will provide the RDA for niacin if the RDA for protein is met. Some niacin is derived in the body from tryptophan, an amino acid present in protein.

[c] To be added to the percentage for the girl or woman of the appropriate age.

Source: U.S. Recommended Daily Allowance. "Food Labeling." *Federal Register.* Vol. 38, No. 49. Part II. March 14, 1973. Recommended Dietary Allowances. 8th ed. 1974. National Academy of Sciences—National Research Council.

are excellent sources of nutrients, but their contributions are not identified in the clear-cut manner available for processed foods. This seeming discrepancy in information is the result of the variability that occurs in fresh produce as a result of nutrient losses during the harvesting and marketing processes. This variability makes meaningful legislation regarding nutritional information for fresh fruits and vegetables very difficult to write, and, at the time of this revision, no laws have been passed to provide this information to consumers. The most practical approach to obtaining this information is from tables of food composition, such as those contained in the Appendix. These values approximate the expected levels of nutrients in fresh produce, and thus are of merit in calculating dietary adequacy.

Responsibility for the enforcement of the provisions regarding nutrition labeling lies with the Food and Drug Administration of the Department of Health, Education and Welfare and with the Animal and Plant Health Inspection Service of the Department of Agriculture. Food manufacturers have the option of providing nutrition labeling on any food they package, but they are required by law to provide nutrition labeling only if they make claims regarding the nutritional merits of the product. If they do provide nutrition labeling, they must provide information on all the eight nutrients listed in the legislation, not just on one or two.

Other consumer information

The Universal Product Code (UPC) is a prominent marking on a number of food products in the market. This code represents a nationally coordinated system of product identification which has a goal of facilitating checkout lines at grocery stores by permitting use of an electronic scanner for calculating the total cost of a grocery order. The system has the potential for printing the cost and name of each item purchased to be presented as a receipt to the

Universal product code is the combination of lines of varying width and numbers contained in lower right-hand corner of the package.

consumer while also maintaining a current inventory of all grocery items for the store. The Universal Product Code is based on a linear bar system and a 10-digit number. The first five numbers identify the manufacturer; the last 5 digits identify the individual product made by the manufacturer. The line pattern is read by a scanner, and this information is fed to a computer coupled to a cash register. Although this system has some clear advantages, there is considerable consumer resistance to the use of the system because of the lack of readable prices. As a result, many stores using the system are also continuing stamping the prices on individual packages.

Open dating is another piece of information often available to today's consumer. The dating is intended to give assurance of having purchased a reasonably fresh product. Dating is strictly optional at this time, with no legal or practical guidelines having yet been established. This lack of guidelines has caused some problems because some manufacturers will indicate the date of manufacture, some may indicate the date when the product should be removed from the shelves if it has not been sold, and still others may indicate the date after which the food is not considered to be safe. To help remove such ambiguity, a few manufacturers now are beginning to indicate on the package just what the meaning of the date is.

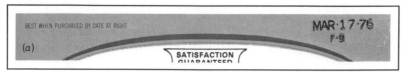

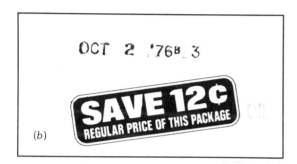

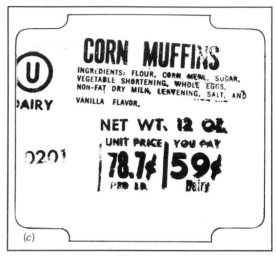

Examples of code dating. The most useful type of coding (a) explains the meaning of the date in understandable language; (b) a clear, but unexplained date is of little value to consumers (this date appeared on a box of margarine purchased on December 17, 1975); and (c) a well-disguised and unexplained date, such as this (0201 indicating February 1) that appeared on a package purchased on January 30, 1976, is likely to go unnoticed.

Food buying

Numerous choices need to be made in the grocery store. Some of these doubtless will be based on cost considerations, while nutrition and personal preferences will dictate others. It is possible to use the nutrition-labeling information to good advantage when making these selections. Application of this information in making shopping decisions can be made in a number of different food products. Some examples are discussed in the following sections.

Salad dressings

Salad dressings afford an excellent opportunity for reviewing the value of nutrition labeling. They also can serve as a useful introduction to the other consumer information

available on labels. In addition to nutritive value, labels carry a listing of the ingredients contained in a product. The contents must be listed in sequence, beginning with the ingredient present in the largest amount and ending with the ingredient used in the smallest amount. On most salad dressing labels, a list of ingredients will be found, but this may not be true in the case of mayonnaise, for this is an example of a food product for which a *standard of identity* has been established. The simple act of labeling the product as mayonnaise is sufficient from a legal standpoint because the formulation for mayonnaise is established and thus need not be restated on the label. Standards of identity and ingredient labeling are under the jurisdiction of the Food and Drug Administration.

Salad dressings other than mayonnaise will

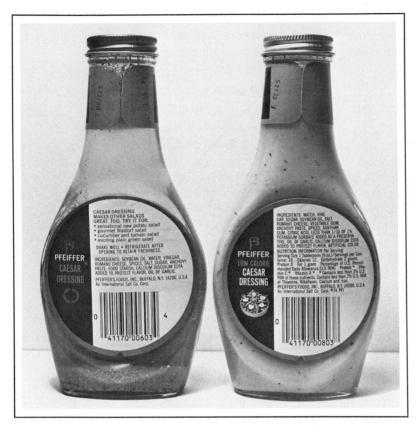

The order of ingredients listed on these labels indicates clearly that the oil content is also lower in the "low-calorie" version than in the regular dressing.

carry a listing of ingredients. Most salad dressings will have vegetable oil listed as the first ingredient, followed by water and vinegar plus other flavoring ingredients. The usual practice is to market these dressings without nutrition labeling. However, some salad dressings may be billed as low-calorie dressings, a designation which now requires that they carry all of the prescribed nutrition information. Of course, the promotional point for these dressings is their lower calorie content, and the label states clearly the actual caloric content per tablespoon (the serving size indicated). The usual value for these dressings is approximately 30 kilocalories per tablespoon. Although this information is of interest to the consumer when purchasing salad dressings, he usually will not have comparative information available because the labels on the regular dressings do not carry the information that they contain 100 kilocalories per tablespoon.

A reading of regular salad dressing ingredients compared with the listing of the low-calorie dressings helps to pinpoint the reason for the difference in caloric content. Low calorie dressings will have water listed as the first ingredient, followed by vinegar. The principal source of calories will be from the oil in the dressing, and that is the third ingredient. This is in contrast to the regular dressings, which list oil as the most abundant ingredient. From a nutritional viewpoint, either type of salad dressing is acceptable. The actual choice revolves around the individual's need for calories and upon the amount of salad dressing ordinarily consumed.

Mayonnaise is a popular type of salad

dressing, yet it is quite expensive in price as well as being a relatively concentrated source of calories. An imitation mayonnaise now is available at a substantially lower price both in money and in calories. This imitation product has water as its first ingredient, a fact which explains why the calorie content is only half that of regular mayonnaise. The soybean oil used in formulating the imitation mayonnaise is partially hardened, making this product somewhat less useful as a source of polyunsaturated vegetable oils than is mayonnaise. Despite this small disadvantage, the imitation mayonnaise is a perfectly suitable choice for price- and weight-conscious consumers.

Still other choices might be of interest when selecting salad dressings. Some people are concerned about the types of vegetable oils they consume. It is possible in some instances to tell from the label what type of oil is used in the dressing. Safflower oil is an example of a vegetable oil which may be identified on a label; when this is specified, the product usually will be higher in price because the oil is more costly. Some persons with a strong interest in weight control may choose a dressing which is marketed in individual packages. The use of these controlled portions may be of particular value to people who are trying to limit their food intake, but who find it difficult to control portion size.

When the complete list of ingredients in salad dressings or most other manufactured foods is reviewed, it is apparent that a number of specialized ingredients are used to improve the marketability and shelf life. For example, a label for a Thousand Island dressing lists vegetable oil, vinegar, water, pickle relish, sugar, tomato paste, salt, egg yolk solids, spice, algin derivative, xanthan gum, hydroxypropyl methylcellulose and polysorbate 60 for consistency, dehydrated onion, dehydrated bell peppers, natural flavors, and calcium disodium EDTA. Although these substances are perfectly safe in the diet, consumers are able to read labels and make the choice of purchasing the commercial product or of buying the plain salad oil, vin-

egar, and flavoring ingredients to make their own dressing without the additives needed for commercial marketing.

Margarines

Choices between margarines as well as between margarine and butter also need to be made at the market. In the past there was a significant price difference between margarines and butter, a difference which tended to give butter a prestigious appeal for some consumers—"the expensive spread." This difference has tended to disappear, and the decision now often revolves around the nutritional merits of the various products.

Butter is not subject to manufacturing changes other than the option of whipping it to make whipped butter. This operation introduces air, thus increasing the volume so that a tablespoon of whipped butter contributes only 65 kilocalories rather than the 100 kilocalories persent in butter. Butter does not carry nutrition labeling; for comparison with margarine information it would be necessary for the consumer to know that butter has very little polyunsaturated fatty acids (3 percent or less) and a large amount of saturated fatty acids (approximately 30 percent).

Margarines are manufactured from a variety of different vegetable oils. Choices include the type of oil used, soft or regular margarines, and whipped products. Label reading will reveal a considerable amount of information about the various products in the case. The caloric content of the margarines is identical to that of butter; the ratio of polyunsaturated fatty acids to saturated fatty acids is distinctly different. The ratio will vary with the specific margarine being studied, but the ratio will usually be either 3:2 or 4:2. When diets are planned for persons to lessen the possibility of heart disease, the ratios in margarines are considered to be distinctly advantageous compared with the reverse ratios found in butter and butterfat. The ratio of polyunsaturates to saturates in the soft margarines ordinarily is higher than is found in the regular margarines. Although this listing is optional on labels, the ratio often is included. Another means of evaluating margarines is to note the first ingredient listed. When an oil is listed as the first ingredient, the content of polyunsaturates ordinarily is higher than when a partially hardened or hydrogenated fat or oil is listed first.

Eggs

Eggs in the shell present choices between grades, sizes, and, in some instances, between the polyunsaturated fat content of the yolk. The highest eating quality in eggs at the time of grading is indicated by the Grade AA designation. However, the nutritive value of Grade A or even Grade B is just as high. The size designations range from jumbo to peewee, with the extremes often not being available. Recipes can be made very satisfactorily with either medium or large eggs. It is not necessary to buy extra large eggs.

Eggs from chickens fed special diets often are available at a premium price in the market. It is possible to modify slightly the polyunsaturate content of the fat (but not the cholesterol content) in the yolk by altering the chicken's diet, but this small change is insignificant when choosing eggs. If a person is on a strictly controlled diet for managing heart disease, it is far more important to reduce the number of egg yolks eaten than to use these special "polyunsaturated" eggs.

The chicken has received considerable assistance from food technologists in the form of products which could be characterized as *imitation* eggs. These modified egg products can be purchased either as a liquid in the refrigerator section of the market or in a frozen form. In either event, the food is fabricated to produce a product with virtually no cholesterol in it. On the negative side, these products have a higher sodium content and a more limited storage life than shell eggs. Perhaps the greatest concern is the sharp difference in price between man's and the chicken's efforts. It is important to note that eggs are sold by the dozen while the artificial products are marketed in packages which usually are equivalent to less than a dozen eggs. The egg substitutes are usually appreciably more costly per egg than fresh eggs.

Milks

Milk may be purchased as whole milk, low-fat, or nonfat. In addition, there may be a choice of imitation or filled milks. For persons of normal weight and with no apparent predisposition toward developing heart disease, homogenized and pasteurized whole milk probably will be the milk of preference. The use of low-fat or nonfat milk provides minerals and protein in amounts slightly in excess of the quantities found in whole milk. The vitamin A level is reduced when milk fat is removed. However, skim or low-fat milk with added vitamin A and vitamin D usually can be purchased. The lower fat and calorie content of low-fat and nonfat milks are important for people who are attempting to lose weight and yet maintain a good intake of nutrients.

A very suitable and economical choice of milk is instant nonfat dry milk. The dry product has excellent shelf life, is comparable to fluid nonfat milk in nutritive value when reconstituted, and is easy to use. The powdered milk can be used in meat loaf, soups, casseroles, and a variety of other recipes to increase nutritive value. This is particularly useful when preparing food for people who drink little milk. Some people like to prepare a combination of fresh homogenized whole milk and reconstituted nonfat dry milk. This aids the budget yet provides the richness of flavor that many people prefer.

Filled milks actually are not as remote from their bovine origin as the name might suggest. The only significant change is the removal of butter fat and the replacement with a vegetable oil, usually coconut oil. This change is not as beneficial as might be thought because coconut oil, despite its plant origin, actually is rich in saturated fatty acids, in fact, more so than butter

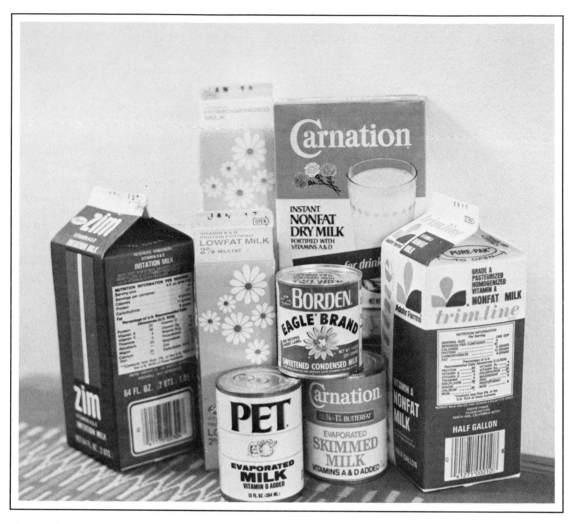

Shoppers have a choice of a wide variety of milk products: (left to right) imitation milk, low-fat milk, homogenized milk, evaporated milk, evaporated skimmed milk, sweetened condensed milk, instant nonfat dry milk, and nonfat milk. Some markets also carry low-fat and whole dry milk solids, as well as goat's milk and soy milks.

fat. An economic advantage of filled milks is that they cost less.

In some parts of the country imitation milks are available. These bear little nutritive resemblance to bovine milk. They usually contain a soy protein, corn syrup, coconut oil, and various added vitamins and minerals. To our knowledge they have not yet been made the equivalent of cow's milk. For individuals who

cannot properly digest milk sugar (lactose) they may be useful.

Canned milks also are available. Evaporated milk is a relatively inexpensive form of milk with an excellent shelf life. When reconstituted with an equal volume of water, its nutritive value is comparable to the original milk. Another type of canned milk which can be purchased is sweetened condensed milk. This milk also has an excellent shelf life, but its price is substantially higher than evaporated milk because this product has a high level of sugar (44 percent concentration) added to it. This high sugar level makes this type of milk much higher in calories than other milks. Although sweetened condensed milk is useful in preparing some desserts, it is not well suited for regular use as a beverage in the diet.

Cereals

There may have been more controversy and public clamor over cereals than over any other class of products in the grocery store. Nutrition labeling is particularly good news in making informed cereal selections for it is simply impossible for anyone to memorize the composition of the innumerable cereals available for consideration by shoppers. Comparison at the point of purchase is the easiest approach to the problem.

Since nutrition labeling does not break down carbohydrate into starch and sugar as separate categories, it is helpful to read the ingredient label on cereal boxes as well as the nutrition label. It may come as a real shock to discover that some cereals list sugar as the first ingredient, meaning that there is a greater weight of sugar than cereal present in the product as it is marketed. There are many other cereal products where sugar is listed after the grain. When making a selection, be sure to note the number of servings per package and the size of the serving as well as the nutritional contribution per serving. There is a particularly wide range of cost comparisons to be found in the cereal section. There also is a broad range of nutritive value in various products.

In many cereal products, the food has been fortified with added nutrients to provide significant levels of minerals and vitamins. In other cereals these nutrient levels may be low. The mere fact that a cereal has undergone extensive processing does not tell the entire story. An interesting comparison can be seen in Table 17.3 in which corn flakes and a granola-type cereal are listed. Note the greater breadth and value of nutrients in the corn flakes. At the time of this survey, the granola cereal cost approximately eight times more than the corn flakes per serving. Consider also the psychological value to a dieter of having a large bowl (1⅓ cups) of corn flakes compared with the small (¼ cup) serving of granola. A quarter cup serving of a granola cereal looks rather lonesome in a cereal bowl and the natural tendency is to use more—and there go more calories! Another observation in the market was that only one of the granolas provided nutrition labeling despite the fact that there is considerable lip service given to the nutritional significance of such foods by some persons.

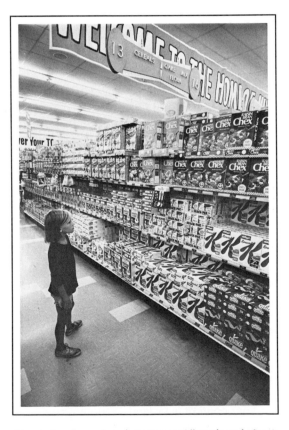

The choice of cereal products is unusually wide and often is as influenced by television advertising as by nutritive and economic considerations.

Nutrient/Serving[b]	Corn Flakes	Granola
Kilocalories	110	125
Protein	2 g	3.7 g
Fat	0 g	4.1 g
Carbohydrate	24 g	18.5 g
Vitamin A	25%	—
Vitamin C	25%	—
Thiamin	25%	9.4%
Riboflavin	25%	—
Niacin	25%	—
Calcium	—	9.4%
Iron	10%	7.5%
Vitamin D	10%	—
Vitamin B_6	25%	—
Folacin	25%	—

[a] Values are listed as percentage of U.S. RDA's for minerals and vitamins.
[b] Serving of corn flakes is 1⅓ cups; of granola it is ¼ cup.

Hot cereals are also available in the market. Again the nutritional value will vary from one product to another. In general, the price per serving for hot cereals is less than for many of the cold cereals. Unique among cereals is the very high iron level (45 percent of the U.S. RDA) available in a serving of hot farina. The caloric content of hot cereals per serving is approximately that of ready-to-eat cereals, with the exception of granolas.

In a sense, the instant breakfast products also represent a choice related to cereals because these products are used by some people to replace cereals or other breakfast items. An envelope of an instant breakfast is comparable to granolas in calories (130 kilocalories) and contains more calories than many of the ready-to-eat or hot cereals. The protein, fat, and carbohydrate content of these formulated products also is higher than cereals. Of course, the bulk or fiber content is lacking. A more recent alternative for breakfast is bars or squares of formulated materials. These are being questioned by nutritionists because of their high sugar content (46 grams of carbohydrate in a recommended serving of one commercial product) and also the high amount of fat (15 grams of fat in the recommended serving of two squares of the same commercial product). The intent of this formulation is to provide a fourth of the U.S. RDA's in a recommended serving. The actual consumer acceptance of products such as these is not apparent yet at the time of this revision.

Juices of various types also confront the shopper. Choices range from the fresh fruit, to the frozen juice concentrates, to freshly bottled juices, to the canned product, and even dehydrated powders. One consideration, of course, is storage space. The powdered product might be valued if emergency rations were being considered or if a camping trip is being planned. Others with limited refrigerator space and a large family might select the canned product. Often the best buy from a nutritional and price standpoint will be the frozen concentrate. Fresh fruit may be the most expensive, depending on the season.

Of particular interest from the viewpoint of

Table 17.4 *Selected Fruit Drinks and Their Ascorbic Acid Content*

Fruit Beverage	Fortification	Mg Vitamin C/100 ml
Fruit juices		
Apple juice (canned)	No	1
Cranberry juice (canned)	Yes	33
Grapefruit juice (fresh)	No	36–40
Grapefruit juice (canned)	No	34
Grapefruit juice (frozen conc., reconstituted)	No	39
Grapefruit juice (dehydrated, reconstituted)	No	37
Orange juice (fresh)	No	54
Orange juice (frozen conc., reconstituted)	No	45
Vegetable juice cocktail	Yes	15
Grape juice drink	Yes	11
Powdered breakfast drinks	Yes	50
Powdered fruit flavored drinks	Yes	4

nutrition is the ascorbic acid content. Many juice products are fortified with this vitamin now. Selected samples are presented in Table 17.4.

From the wide range of ascorbic acid values shown in this table, it is clear that it is necessary to check carefully to see just what the level of fortification is. The simple act of emblazoning the message "Vitamin C Added" in large letters does not insure the consumer of adequate intake of this vitamin.

Some examples of food products and nutrition choices have been cited above. There are many other illustrations available to all consumers in the market. In the final analysis it is necessary to weigh nutritional content with cost, eating quality, and consumer acceptance of each item being considered. This is a time-consuming task, yet is an extremely important step in selecting a good diet, for this is the point at which the decision is made as to whether or not a food will be available to family members at home. Shopping choices will influence the consumption patterns for protein food sources of all types and fruits and vegetables as well as for carbonated beverages and candy.

Preparing the Food

Preferences for the ways food is prepared are as personal as the foods selected in individual diets. However, preparation choices and practices also play important roles in achieving good nutrition. The amount of salt contained in a person's diet often is influenced by practices in the kitchen. In a similar way the fat content of a diet can be modified markedly by the way food is prepared. Acceptance of foods also can be determined in large measure by the standards of quality maintained in preparation of foods. The amount of additives contained in foods as served also is influenced by the preparation practices in a home. Total food consumption also stems from the philosophy practiced in the kitchen.

A concern of some individuals is the need to decrease the intake of salt, or more specifically, sodium. This intake can be modified by using very little or no salt in preparing foods. The actual amount to use will need to be adjusted to the individual practices of salting food at the table.

One of the concerns about the "typical" American diet is the high intake of fat, particularly the saturated type. This intake can be modified significantly in the kitchen. Meats can be cooked without added fat, and the fat they contain can be removed from the meat as it cooks out and collects in the frying pan. More use of broiled meats can be included rather than doing so much frying. Broiling, when done properly, keeps the meat completely out of the fat collecting in the pan. Fat also can be drained completely from meats that are to be incorporated in casseroles. Ground meats can be extended with the use of soy protein as yet another means of reducing the total amount of fat available through meat choices. Another significant decrease in the amount of fat can be accomplished by actually serving smaller servings of meat. The recommended serving size is only 3 ounces, a serving far smaller than is commonly provided in many homes. Other ways of reducing fat intake include avoiding French fries and other fried foods, less use of sour cream and butter on baked potatoes or in dips, and encouraging smaller amounts of spreads on breads and dressings on salads.

Emphasis is being given today on the importance of fruits and vegetables in the diet. Fruits are often served raw, thus presenting minimal preparation problems. Vegetables are used raw in salads many times, but still many vegetables need to be cooked before they reach the table. It is the preparation of cooked vegetables which demands interest and skill in the kitchen. Color of cooked vegetables is important. The best color for green vegetables is achieved by placing the vegetables in boiling water and cooking them without a cover just until the vegetables are tender enough to cut, but are not mushy. Longer cooking will cause the green to change to a less-appealing olive-green color. The flavor of cabbage and related vegetables will be best when cooked without a cover and

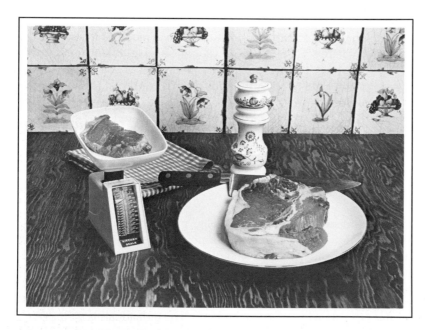

A 3-ounce serving of meat, the recommended serving size, is significantly smaller than the size of the serving of steak often selected. The smaller size provides sufficient protein without contributing excessively to the fat and caloric intake.

cooking time is kept to a minimum; longer cooking develops stronger odors and flavors, both of which often deter acceptance.

People who are concerned about the additives used in commercially prepared foods may prefer to prepare many of their foods at home (see Chapter 5). Bread can be baked at home without adding the preservatives considered to be necessary for regular marketing channels. Salad dressings, casseroles, and all types of baked products can be made at home. Such a choice involves more time in food preparation, but it affords the option of fewer additives and improved palatability if the preparation is well done. The relative cost of home prepared versus commercially prepared foods varies with the type of product and with the recipe used at home. Such comparisons would need to be done by the individual if they are to be meaningful.

A very significant factor in achieving optimal nutrition for a family is the philosophy of the person preparing the food. Intimately related is the concern for planning and preparing pleasing meals. The needs of individual family members can best be met when meals are prepared at times convenient to the family and the food is available in appropriate quantities. The preparation of even small excesses of food can lead to overeating and weight problems over a period of time. Since weight control is a common concern in this country, preparation of appropriate amounts of food rather than an overabundance is an important philosophical and practical consideration.

A person who is genuinely concerned with the adequacy of a family's diet will evaluate menu planning and food preparation practices regularly and make appropriate modifications as needed. When certain nutrients are found to be present in less than recommended quantities, some ideas for including foods that are particularly good sources of the nutrient will be helpful. Suggestions for sources of vitamin A, vitamin C, thiamin, riboflavin, niacin, calcium, and iron are provided in Appendix C.

Summary

Considerable information is available in the market and in the literature to aid consumers in selecting and consuming adequate diets. By taking advantage of aids such as nutrition labeling, studying food choices carefully, and preparing foods tastefully in appropriate quantities, it is very possible for families to be well nourished today. The achievement of good nutrition is a personal matter with significant health benefits to individuals and families.

Selected References

Kramer, M., and M. Spader. *Contemporary Meal Management.* Wiley. New York. 1972.

McWilliams, M. *Food Fundamentals.* Wiley. New York. 2nd ed. 1974.

Peterkin, B., et al. *Nutrition Labeling—Tools for Its Use.* U.S. Dept. of Agriculture Information Bulletin No. 382. Washington, D.C. 1975.

Whelan, E. M., and F. J. Stare. *Panic in The Pantry.* Atheneum. New York. 1975.

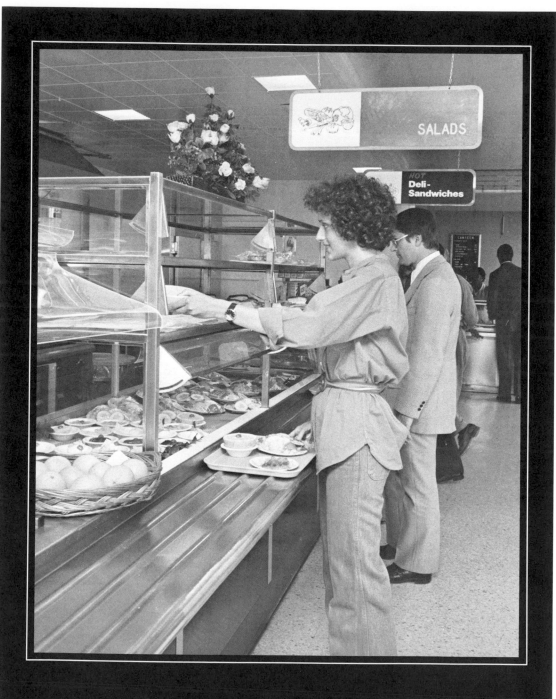

Chapter 18

Nutrition in Practice

The achievement of good nutritional status is very much an individual option for most people. Although purchasing power, life-styles, and food preferences vary widely, most people in the United States have the opportunity to be well nourished. Whether the goal actually is achieved is a matter of choice and knowledge. For almost all people, eating is a very pleasant part of life, a satisfying and contenting experience. To change eating from this pleasurable context to a spartan dedication to good nutrition is neither wise nor necessary. The secret of achieving good nutrition for a lifetime is to translate the knowledge of nutrients needed for good health into a food pattern that satisfies an individual's taste preferences on a continuing basis. There are innumerable combinations of foods and patterns of eating which can provide adequate nutrition and psychological satisfaction. In fact, variety is the cornerstone of good nutrition.

The Individual

A realistic starting point for achieving good nutrition is to stand back and take a hard look at oneself. This look is needed to see the present nutritional status, consumption patterns, and food preferences. To be effective and useful, this assessment should be very objective and accurate.

Since the figure represents, in part, the nutritional status achieved by present dietary and exercise practices, a good look at the physical shape is a reasonable place to start considering adequacy. Consideration of weight in relation to height is discussed in Chapter 4. With the use of a scale and height-weight tables it is a simple matter to determine whether the caloric intake in the present diet is appropriate to maintain body weight within the recommended range.

If a person's weight is outside the recommended range, either too high or too low, the question arises as to whether or not the diet and exercise could or should be modified to adjust and maintain body weight within the recommended range. This answer must lie with the individual because actual food consumption and exercise decisions and practices are the province of oneself. Others may offer advice and opinions, but what actually is eaten is determined by the individual eating the food. Therefore any commitment to modify physical weight must be an internal commitment and goal of an individual.

Weight change will require a modification in dietary and exercise habits that are already firmly established. Unless a change in weight is identified as a high priority, it is not realistic to expect to improve this aspect of nutritional status by assessing dietary and exercise patterns and suggesting changes. It is important to be really honest with oneself and to decide whether any dissatisfaction with weight is sufficient to motivate permanent changes in eating and exercise patterns. If weight control is determined to be really important to an individual, appropriate dietary and exercise changes can be made to achieve and maintain the desired weight.

A review of consumption patterns is a good way of seeing how adequate the diet actually is and identifying potential problem areas that may interfere with the achievement of good nutritional status. A practical approach to reviewing consumption patterns is to keep a daily log of all foods eaten, the approximate amounts consumed, and the time of day. This log can be reviewed at the end of a week. When each day's total intake is compared with the Basic Four, any obvious weaknesses in dietary intake will be quite apparent and suitable modifications can be made.

This dietary log is important as a means of seeing just what eating patterns are preferred

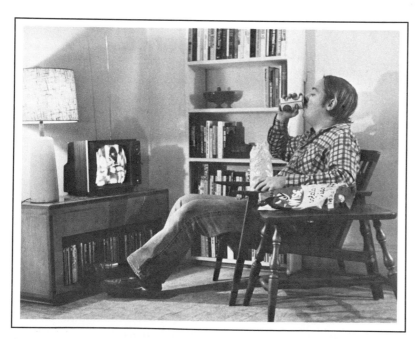

Television viewing, combined with snacks and lack of exercise, leads to overweight, a common problem in the United States.

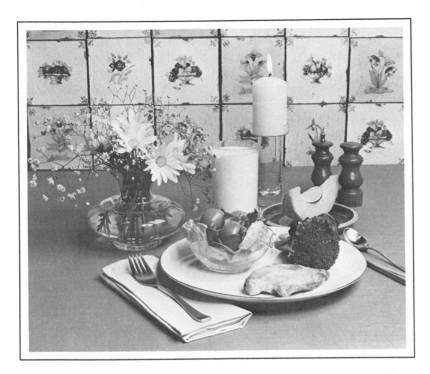

The use of a smaller plate and appropriately smaller servings to fit the plate is a useful, yet easily accomplished change which can be effective in helping to reduce total food intake and thus aid in weight control.

by an individual. Look particularly for the timing of snacks and the frequency with which breakfast is eaten. Note whether snacks are a regular part of the pattern. Observe also the number of meals that ordinarily are eaten. From a summary of the comparison of the intake with the Basic Four and an analysis of the meal and snacking pattern, personal habits and preferences will begin to be clear. Any personal plan for improving one's nutritional status will be easier to follow if it is adapted to the snack schedule and meal patterns already established.

The matter of personal food preferences also needs to be considered. When dietary plans are made to overcome weight difficulties and other possible nutritional problems, they usually will be followed only to the extent that they provide psychological satisfaction and fulfill personal desires for specific foods. An inventory of foods an individual wishes to eat frequently serves as a practical basis for dietary planning to achieve an adequate state of nutrition.

Any shortcomings that have been identified in the study of a week's intake can be corrected, but merely to recommend to a person that specific changes be made is not enough to insure that nutritional status will be changed. Recommendations need to be put into practice, and to change the dietary patterns established over a lifetime is a difficult task. However, subtle minor changes can be made when they are based on preferences and present practices. Small changes can be accomplished when a person is interested in improving the diet; large changes may prove to be too hard to make.

The success of making very minor changes reinforces the sense of accomplishment and encourages a person to continue with the improved diet. If the changes are so large that they cannot be followed fairly easily, there is likely to be a feeling of frustration and failure. This feeling does not reinforce the commitment to improved nutrition, but rather tends to give a person the negative feeling that there is no way for him to modify his diet successfully. The satisfactions of eating what is familiar and desired will often outweigh the perceived value of consuming a nutritionally adequate diet. This reinforces the comfort and satisfaction provided by the usual diet and reduces the motivation and interest in making any modifications.

For long range, continuing success in achieving good nutrition, it is wise to be content with making changes in very small steps. When one small change becomes habit and an accepted part of the pattern, then another small step can be tried. After all, eating is a lifetime proposition and can well be done to provide a great deal of pleasure along with necessary nutrients. Everything does not need to be accomplished in a matter of a day or two. The important thing is to develop a rational and workable individual plan for being well nourished and to continue to review the adequacy of one's diet throughout life. An awareness of the importance of good nutrition and the application of nutrition knowledge are of value throughout life.

Planning the Day's Intake

Since eating is such an individual matter, there are many approaches to meeting the body's total dietary needs each day. A good breakfast generally is recommended. Studies have demonstrated the importance of a good meal in the morning to break the fast and provide the energy needed for good work performance during the morning.

The recommendation is to provide approximately one-fourth the nutritional needs for the day at the morning's meal. A quick, practical, and enjoyable way of meeting this recommendation is by a meal of orange juice, milk, and cereal, with some toast, too, if desired. A totally different approach, such as a hamburger sandwich, milkshake, and a bowl of strawberries might be preferred by a hungry teen-age boy. Still other ideas for a tempting breakfast might include a hot dog, perhaps a taco, or even a casserole or stew left over from the previous day. The important point is to consume a meal which is tempting and satisfying, one which motivates a person to eat when his day begins. This helps to promote successful performance in the morning and sets the stage for a day of good nutrition.

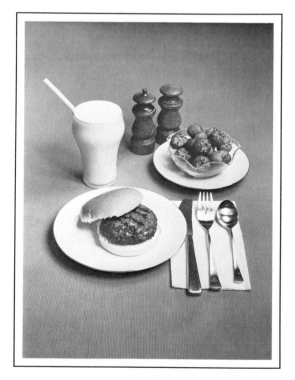

Although this may not meet the expected picture of a nourishing breakfast, this menu is an appropriate way of providing a nutritionally adequate breakfast for a teen-age boy.

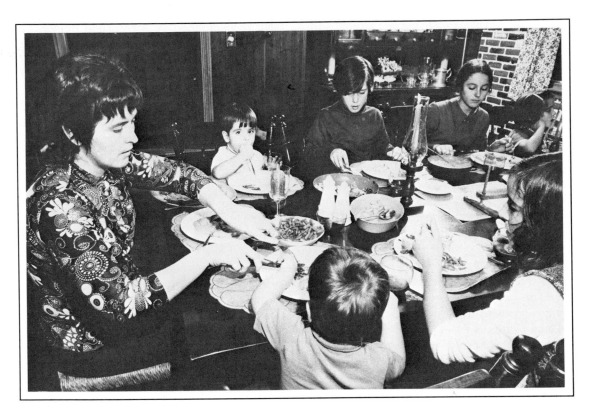

Family dinners are important for sociability as well as for good nutrition.

Although there is only limited physiological need for a mid-morning snack, social pressure or habit may prompt people to eat something at break time. If this is a preferred way of living, then the snack should be viewed as being a part of the total day's intake. Rather than eating quite so much at breakfast or lunch, these meals can be cut back slightly and part of the food that would have been eaten at mealtime can be used for the snack, what we call a "scientific snack" rather than an "extra." This helps to avoid having snacks amount to becoming extra calories that help to cause weight gain. These snack foods can be valuable in helping to meet the body's nutritional needs if they are selected with an eye to nutritive value as well as pleasure. A bag of peanuts or a glass of milk are examples of foods that often are available at snack time.

A wide range of food choices usually can be found to satisfy lunch-time appetites. Soup, a sandwich with meat or other protein-containing filling, fruit, and milk make a nutritionally adequate and satisfying lunch that can be carried to work or to school. Other possibilities open up when a hot lunch is available. A pattern of a protein-containing main dish, vegetable, salad, bread, and beverage is a reasonable guide to follow in selecting lunch. This meal may be somewhat smaller if the preferred pattern of eating is to include "scientific" morning and afternoon snacks.

Afternoon snacks are popular with many people. The choice of snack foods varies widely, ranging from non-nourishing calorie-containing beverages to foods such as fruits and whole grain breads that are useful in meeting the day's nutrient needs. The key is to pick snacks that add pleasure to the day without adding too many calories to the day's input and without impairing appetite for dinner.

The point to keep in mind is that snacks do contribute to the day's total intake and need to be selected in relation to the entire day's food pattern. Ice cream or even potato chips or candy may be selected as snack foods without causing feelings of guilt if planned as part of a balanced diet for the total day. The key is to keep such selections in perspective and to acknowledge their caloric contribution. A nourishing, yet low calorie dinner, perhaps with fish as the entree, could be eaten the same evening to help avoid too high an intake of calories. Infrequent snacks of this nature will not create a nutrition problem. The difficulty arises when these are consumed frequently and nourishing foods are crowded from the menu.

Dinner often is the largest meal of the day. This practice is born of tradition and is not one representing physiological need only. Actually, most persons have the largest amount of physical activity earlier in the day and require less energy for activity during the evening hours. However, dinner still remains a pleasant social event for a number of families, and the socia-bility is heightened by a complete dinner. Of course, a broad menu for dinner helps to insure a broad range of nutrients, but it may also contribute to an excess intake for the day. This potential problem can be avoided by preparing just the amount of food that is needed for serving each individual in the family. Very large servings and second helpings are usually not necessary in relatively sedentary families.

The usual plan for dinner includes a serving of meat or a meat substitute such as poultry or fish, a vegetable, potato or a cereal product such as rice, a fruit or vegetable salad, bread, and a beverage (preferably low-fat or skim milk). Within this general framework for a dinner menu, numerous variations are possible to incorporate the food preferences of family members. The preparation of foods popular with individuals in the group helps to make the dinner more sociable and pleasing to all. By varying the menus at dinner a wide range of foods with significant nutritional contributions can be included in the diet. This variety is an aid in assuring that adequate amounts of the many essential nutrients are available in the daily diet.

Planning for Family Needs

Although living patterns and family management styles vary, menu planning usually is part of the daily or weekly tasks handled by a family member. In families where all adults are working, a single weekly grocery shopping expedition often is a part of the plan. Time and money can be saved by shopping once a week if the menus have been planned for the week and the shopping list has been prepared carefully. Over a long period of time, much of this responsibility may become so familiar that it can be handled easily and without a detailed list.

As an aid to shoppers facing this weekly shopping event, the U.S. Department of Agri-culture has developed food plans for families with different income levels. These plans outline the quantities of food to buy for families with members of various ages. On a monthly basis the cost of buying representative foods under each of the plans is determined and published. These figures are available in *Family Economic Review,* which is published by the Consumer and Food Economics Institute, Agricultural Research Service, U.S. Department of Agriculture. The suggested amounts of food to buy under the three food plans are presented in Table 18.1. These values are for a hypothetical family of four which includes a couple between the ages of 20 and 54 and a child

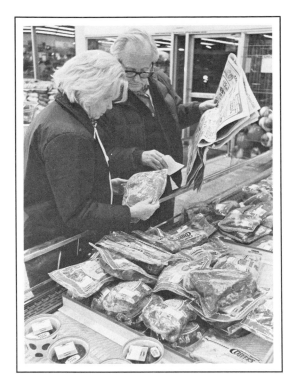

Weekly shopping for groceries, aided by a prepared shopping list and information on grocery store specials, is a good way of buying the foods needed for adequate nutrition while keeping food costs under control.

between the ages of 6 and 8 and a second child between 9 and 11 years old. Of course, many families do not fit this model. Specific recommendations for individual family members are available from the same source. By using these more specific recommendations, any family group plan can be calculated.

The figures on the following page are those recommended if a family is to provide optimal nutrition for all family members. Note that the recommended purchases on the low-cost plan call for smaller amounts of most foods; in particular, somewhat smaller quantities of milk, meats and related foods, and fruits and vegetables other than potatoes are suggested while more cereal products are recommended. The lower-cost items within each of the categories also need to be selected as a means of helping to keep cost down. With some care and knowledge, it is possible to be well nourished on a realtively limited budget. However, wise shopping, knowledge of nutrition and alternative sources of nutrients, plus excellent food preparation skills are very useful tools when food costs need to be kept at very low levels. The responsibility for providing tempting and nourishing meals is simplified by having a more generous budget.

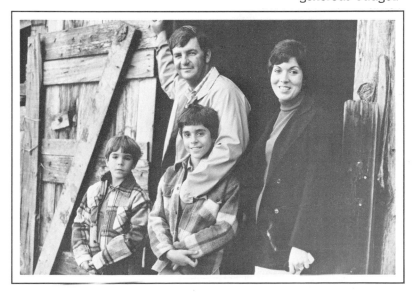

A family typical of the hypothetical family on which the U.S.D.A. food plans are based.

Table 18.1   *Weekly Family Food Plans of Varying Cost for a Family of Four*[a]

Food Group	Unit	Low Cost	Plan Moderate Cost	Liberal
Milk, cheese, ice cream	Quart	16.0	19.2	20.7
Meat, poultry, fish	Pound	12.4	15.8	18.9
Eggs	Dozen	1.2	1.3	1.3
Dry beans and peas, nuts	Pound	1.4	1.2	1.3
Vegetables, fruit	Pound	33.3	39.2	45.3
Grain products	Pound	17.1	16.4	16.9
Cost in Jan., 1976 (estimated)		$50.20	$63.00	$75.90

[a] From Family Economics Review, Winter, 1975. USDA, Agricultural Research Service. Washington, D.C.

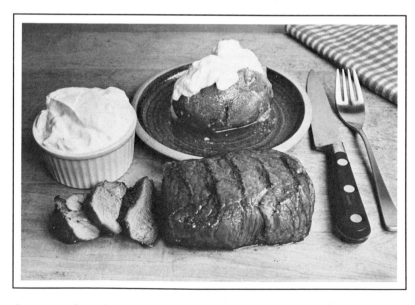

A restaurant dinner featuring a steak well-marbled with fat and baked potato generously piled with sour cream and/or butter is a meal preferred by many diners, but is one providing a very high intake of fat and a restricted content of some essential minerals and vitamins.

Meals Away From Home

Several factors have contributed to the trend for family members to eat away from home at least part of the time each week. The impact of restaurant meals on nutrition needs to be considered when dietary adequacy is being assessed. Obviously, there are many different kinds of restaurants and innumerable selections can be made. In a cafeteria there usually will be a sufficient range of foods offered to enable the diner to select a broader menu than would be available at home. The potential for eating a nutritionally adequate meal exists, but it is up to the individual to make the selections that will provide a balanced meal. A relatively small proportion of restaurants with table service will serve vegetables as a part of the dinner menu. However, in a far larger proportion of restaurants the emphasis is given to meat, potatoes in the form of French fries or baked (usually served with generous portions of butter or sour cream), rolls, and salad. Vegetables and fruits often are not included. Milk is available at additional cost. Restaurateurs report that vegetables have been deleted from their menus because so many of their customers were not eating them. The preparation of fresh vegetables also is somewhat time-consuming, and their quality suffers as a result of being held on a steam table until they are served.

A particularly popular segment of the restau-

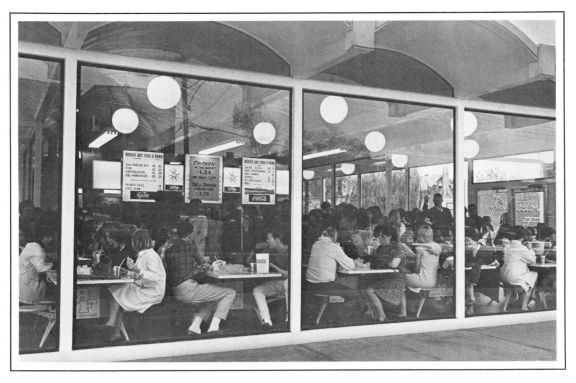

Fast food operations are an increasingly significant part of the American dietary pattern. The choices made from their menus can contribute significant amounts of nutrients as well as calories, but less wise choices may contribute to a high caloric intake with little nutritive value. The most serious limitation is the lack of vegetables or fruits available here.

rant business is the fast-food chains. Like their more formal restaurant cohorts, fast-food operators have opted to eliminate essentially all vegetables except potatoes in the form of French fries, cabbage in cole slaw, and tomato slices in some hamburgers. With the increasing frequency with which the public is dining at this type of facility, there is reason to explore rather carefully the nutritive value of the types of meals that are purchased in a fast-food operation. Despite the fact that these establishments are extremely limited in their utilization of fruits and vegetables, they actually are making more of a contribution to nutrition than some of their sharper critics suggest. The nutritional assessments of selected menu items and meal combinations are presented in Tables 18.2 and 18.3, respectively.

Another problem of dining away from home is cited by persons who either need to do significant amounts of entertaining in line with their professional commitments or who are required to attend a number of banquets and other gatherings where an abundance of food is available. It is not unusual to hear persons with such occupational hazards bemoaning their weight problems and rationalizing them with the statement that their work requires them to attend too many social functions and banquets. For politicians and other people who must live this kind of life, it still is possible to be well nourished and not gain weight. The usual banquet or big dinner is a good source of a wide range of nutrients. Perhaps the greatest criticism of banquets is that usually simply too much food is served. However, it is not re-

Table 18.2 Nutritional Evaluation of Selected Food Items Commonly Available at a Fast-Food Operation[a]

Nutrient	Egg McMuffin Actual	%[b]	Hamburger Actual	%	Cheeseburger Actual	%	¼ lb Hamburger Actual	%	¼ lb Cheeseburger Actual	%	Big Mac Actual	%
Calories	310	[c]	250	[c]	310	[c]	415	[c]	520	[c]	560	[c]
Protein (g)	18	27	13	20	16	25	27	41	41	48	26	40
Fat (g)	11	[c]	10	[c]	14	[c]	19	[c]	28	[c]	32	[c]
Carbohydrate (g)	35	[c]	28	[c]	30	[c]	33	[c]	36	[c]	41	[c]
Vitamin A (I.U.)	460	9	165	3	315	6	260	5	395	8	210	4
Vitamin D (I.U.)	80	20	17	4	25	6	45	11	50	13	33	8
Vitamin E (mg)	0.7	2	0.3	1	0.2	1	0.3	1	0.5	2	1.3	4
Vitamin C (mg)	4	6	4	6	4	6	3	5	5	9	5	8
Folic acid (mg)	0.02	5	0.02	5	0.02	6	0.02	7	0.03	8	0.03	8
Niacin (mg)	3.1	16	3.7	19	3.9	20	6.5	32	7.1	36	6.3	32
Riboflavin (mg)	0.5	27	0.4	21	0.5	30	0.6	37	0.7	42	0.6	38
Thiamin (mg)	0.4	25	0.2	12	0.2	13	0.2	15	0.3	17	0.3	18
Vitamin B_6 (mg)	0.14	7	0.14	7	0.15	7	0.30	15	0.31	16	0.24	12
Vitamin B_{12} (μg)	0.9	15	0.8	13	1.0	17	1.9	31	2.3	39	1.5	26
Calcium (g)	0.17	17	0.05	5	0.14	14	0.07	7	0.23	23	0.16	16
Phosphorus (g)	0.38	38	0.12	12	0.19	19	0.23	23	0.37	37	0.29	29
Iodide (μg)	27	18	47	31	47	31	66	44	84	56	77	51
Iron (mg)	2.5	14	2.6	14	2.3	13	3.8	21	3.9	22	3.8	21
Magnesium (g)	0.02	4	0.02	4	0.02	4	0.03	7	0.03	8	0.03	8
Sodium (g)	1.3	[c]	0.5	[c]	0.8	[c]	0.7	[c]	1.2	[c]	1.1	[c]

[a] Adapted from **Nutritional Analysis of Food Served at McDonald's Restaurants.** Warf Institute, Inc. P.O. Box 2599, Madison, Wis. 53701.
[b] Percent of U.S. RDA's.
[c] No U.S. RDA established.

Table 18.3 *Nutritional Evaluation of Various Menus Available at a Fast-Food Operation*[a]

Nutrient	Percent of U.S. RDA Provided by Menu Consisting of French Fries, Chocolate Shake, and:						
	2 Hamburgers	½ lb Cheeseburger	½ lb Hamburger	Big Mac	Filet of fish	Cheeseburger	Hamburger
Kilocalories	1030[b]	1055[b]	950[b]	1090[b]	940[b]	840[b]	780[b]
Protein	62	70	63	62	45	47	42
Vitamin A	7	8	5	4	2	6	3
Vitamin D	17	22	20	17	18	15	13
Vitamin E	2	2	1	5	4	1	1
Vitamin C	28	24	20	23	17	21	21
Folic acid	16	14	12	13	11	12	11
Niacin	51	50	47	46	29	34	33
Riboflavin	78	78	73	73	57	66	57
Thiamin	32	30	28	30	28	26	24
Vitamin B_6	27	29	28	26	19	21	20
Vitamin B_{12}	52	65	57	52	39	43	39
Phosphorus	65	78	64	60	65	60	53
Iodide	156	149	137	145	169	125	125
Iron	35	29	28	28	16	20	21
Magnesium	22	23	22	23	20	19	19
Calcium	52	65	48	58	51	55	47

[a] Adapted from *Nutritional Analysis of Food Served at McDonald's Restaurants.* Warf Institute, Inc. P.O. Box 2599. Madison, Wis. 53701.

[b] There are no U.S. RDA's for kilocalories. Figures represent actual kilocalories available, rounded off to the nearest 5.

quired that every scrap of food be consumed from one's plate. Rich sauces and gravies on the main course and generous servings of dressings on salads can be left quietly on the plate. Even the very simple act of skipping dessert can be accomplished with grace and effectiveness. The most important single act for most people on the banquet circuit is just to eat less food than is served, but to be sure to concentrate on eating a balanced diet in reasonable quantities. Emphasize consumption of the fruits and vegetables and minimize desserts and alcoholic beverages.

Summary

Living a life keyed to good nutrition and regular activity has benefits for anyone. This book has been written to help you achieve a better understanding of nutrition, its principles, and applications for daily living. The pleasures of eating are an important part of life. Good nutrition combines the psychological and the physiological satisfactions available from food.

Appendix A
Nutritive Values of the Edible Part of Foods[a]

[a] From *Home and Garden Bulletin No. 72*. USDA. Washington, D.C. Revised 1971.

Table 1   Nutritive Values of the Edible Part of Foods

	Food, Approximate Measure, and Weight (in Grams)		Weight (g)	Water (%)	Food Energy (kcal)	Protein (g)	Fat (g)	Fatty Acids Saturated (total) (g)	Unsaturated Oleic (g)	Linoleic (g)	Carbohydrate (g)	Calcium (mg)	Iron (mg)	Vitamin A value (I.U.)	Thiamin (mg)	Riboflavin (mg)	Niacin (mg)	Ascorbic acid (mg)
	MILK, CHEESE, CREAM, IMITATION CREAM; RELATED PRODUCTS																	
	Milk:																	
	Fluid:																	
1	Whole, 3.5% fat	1 cup	244	87	160	9	9	5	3	Trace	12	288	0.1	350	0.07	0.41	0.2	2
2	Nonfat (skim)	1 cup	245	90	90	9	Trace	—	—	—	12	296	.1	10	.09	.44	.2	2
3	Partly skimmed, 2% nonfat milk solids added	1 cup	246	87	145	10	5	3	2	Trace	15	352	.1	200	.10	.52	.2	2
	Canned, concentrated, undiluted:																	
4	Evaporated, unsweetened	1 cup	252	74	345	18	20	11	7	1	24	635	.3	810	.10	.86	.5	3
5	Condensed, sweetened	1 cup	306	27	980	25	27	15	9	1	166	802	.3	1100	.24	1.16	.6	3
	Dry, nonfat instant:																	
6	Low-density (1 1/3 cups needed for reconstitution to 1 qt)	1 cup	68	4	245	24	Trace	—	—	—	35	879	.4	20[a]	.24	1.21	.6	5
7	High-density (7/8 cup needed for reconstitution to 1 qt)	1 cup	104	4	375	37	1	—	—	—	54	1345	.6	30[a]	.36	1.85	.9	7
	Buttermilk:																	
8	Fluid, cultured, made from skim milk	1 cup	245	90	90	9	Trace	—	—	—	12	296	.1	10	.10	.44	.2	2
9	Dried, packaged	1 cup	120	3	465	41	6	3	2	Trace	60	1498	.7	260	.31	2.06	1.1	—
	Cheese:																	
	Natural:																	
	Blue or Roquefort type:																	
10	Ounce	1 oz	28	40	105	6	9	5	3	Trace	1	89	.1	350	.01	.17	.3	0
11	Cubic inch	1 cu in.	17	40	65	4	5	3	2	Trace	Trace	54	.1	210	.01	.11	.2	0
12	Camembert, packaged in 4-oz pkg. with 3 wedges per pkg.	1 wedge	38	52	115	7	9	5	3	Trace	1	40	.2	380	.02	.29	.3	0

a Value applies to unfortified product; value for fortified low-density product would be 1500 I.U. and the fortified high-density product would be 2290 I.U.

Table 1 (continued)

MILK, CHEESE, CREAM, IMITATION CREAM; RELATED PRODUCTS—Con.

	Food, Approximate Measure, and Weight (in Grams)		Weight (g)	Water (%)	Food Energy (kcal)	Protein (g)	Fat (g)	Fatty Acids Saturated (total) (g)	Unsaturated Oleic (g)	Unsaturated Linoleic (g)	Carbohydrate (g)	Calcium (mg)	Iron (mg)	Vitamin A value (I.U.)	Thiamin (mg)	Riboflavin (mg)	Niacin (mg)	Ascorbic acid (mg)
	Cheese—Continued																	
	Cheddar:																	
13	Ounce	1 oz	28	37	115	7	9	5	3	Trace	1	213	0.3	370	0.01	0.13	Trace	0
14	Cubic inch	1 cu in.	17	37	70	4	6	3	2	Trace	Trace	129	.2	230	.01	.08	Trace	0
	Cottage, large or small curd:																	
	Creamed:																	
15	Package of 12-oz net wt	1 pkg	340	78	360	46	14	8	5	Trace	10	320	1.0	580	.10	.85	0.3	0
16	Cup, curd pressed down	1 cup	245	78	260	33	10	6	3	Trace	7	230	.7	420	.07	.61	.2	0
	Uncreamed:																	
17	Package of 12-oz net wt	1 pkg	340	79	290	58	1	1	Trace	Trace	9	306	1.4	30	.10	.95	.3	0
18	Cup, curd pressed down	1 cup	200	79	170	34	1	Trace	Trace	Trace	5	180	.8	20	.06	.56	.2	0
	Cream:																	
19	Package of 8-oz, net wt	1 pkg	227	51	850	18	86	48	28	3	5	141	.5	3500	.05	.54	.2	0
20	Package of 3-oz, net wt	1 pkg	85	51	320	7	32	18	11	1	2	53	.2	1310	.02	.20	.1	0
21	Cubic inch	1 cu in.	16	51	60	1	6	3	2	Trace	Trace	10	Trace	250	Trace	.04	Trace	0
	Parmesan, grated:																	
22	Cup, pressed down	1 cup	140	17	655	60	43	24	14	1	5	1893	.7	1760	.05	1.22	.3	0
23	Tablespoon	1 tbsp	5	17	25	2	2	1	Trace	Trace	Trace	68	Trace	60	Trace	.04	Trace	0
24	Ounce	1 oz	28	17	130	12	9	5	3	Trace	1	383	.1	360	.01	.25	.1	0
	Swiss:																	
25	Ounce	1 oz	28	39	105	8	8	4	3	Trace	1	262	.3	320	Trace	.11	Trace	0
26	Cubic inch	1 cu in.	15	39	55	4	4	2	1	Trace	Trace	139	.1	170	Trace	.06	Trace	0
	Pasteurized processed cheese:																	
	American:																	
27	Ounce	1 oz	28	40	105	7	9	5	3	Trace	1	198	.3	350	.01	.12	Trace	0
28	Cubic inch	1 cu in.	18	40	65	4	5	3	2	Trace	Trace	122	.2	210	Trace	.07	Trace	0

#	Food	Measure	Grams																
	Swiss:																		
29	Ounce	1 oz	28	40	100	8	8	4	3	Trace	1	251	.3	310	Trace	.11	Trace	0
30	Cubic inch	1 cu in.	18	40	65	5	5	3	2	Trace	Trace	159	.2	200	Trace	.07	Trace	0
	Pasteurized process cheese food,																	
	American:																	
31	Tablespoon	1 tbsp	14	43	45	3	3	2	1	Trace	1	80	.1	140	Trace	.08	Trace	0
32	Cubic inch	1 cu in.	18	43	60	4	4	2	1	Trace	1	100	.1	170	Trace	.10	Trace	0
33	Pasteurized process cheese spread, American	1 oz	28	49	80	5	6	3	2	Trace	2	160	.2	250	Trace	.15	Trace	0
	Cream:																	
34	Half-and-half (cream and milk)	1 cup	242	80	325	8	28	15	9	1	11	261	.1	1160	.07	.39	.1	2
35		1 tbsp	15	80	20	1	2	1	1	Trace	1	16	Trace	70	Trace	.02	Trace	Trace
36	Light, coffee or table	1 cup	240	72	505	7	49	27	16	1	10	245	.1	2020	.07	.36	.1	2
37		1 tbsp	15	72	30	1	3	2	1	Trace	1	15	Trace	130	Trace	.02	Trace	Trace
38	Sour	1 cup	230	72	485	7	47	26	16	1	10	235	.1	1930	.07	.35	.1	2
39		1 tbsp	12	72	25	Trace	2	1	1	Trace	1	12	Trace	100	Trace	.02	Trace	Trace
40	Whipped topping (pressurized)	1 cup	60	62	155	2	14	8	5	Trace	6	67	–	570	–	.04	–	–
41		1 tbsp	3	62	10	Trace	1	Trace	Trace	Trace	Trace	3	–	30	–	Trace	–	–
	Whipping, unwhipped (volume about double when whipped):																	
42	Light	1 cup	239	62	715	6	75	41	25	2	9	203	.1	3060	.05	.29	.1	2
43		1 tbsp	15	62	45	Trace	5	3	2	Trace	1	13	Trace	190	Trace	.02	Trace	Trace
44	Heavy	1 cup	238	57	840	5	90	50	30	3	7	179	.1	3670	.05	.26	.1	2
45		1 tbsp	15	57	55	Trace	6	3	2	Trace	1	11	Trace	230	Trace	.02	Trace	Trace
	Imitation cream products (made with vegetable fat):																	
	Creamers:																	
46	Powdered	1 cup	94	2	505	4	33	31	1	0	52	21	.6	200[b]	–	–	Trace	–
47		1 tsp	2	2	10	Trace	1	Trace	Trace	0	1	1	Trace	Trace[b]	–	–	–	–
48	Liquid (frozen)	1 cup	245	77	345	3	27	25	1	0	25	29	–	100[b]	0	0	–	–
49		1 tbsp	15	77	20	Trace	2	1	Trace	0	2	2	–	10[b]	0	0	–	–
50	Sour dressing (imitation sour cream) made with nonfat dry milk	1 cup	235	72	440	9	38	35	1	Trace	17	277	.1	10	.07	.38	.2	1
51		1 tbsp	12	72	20	Trace	2	2	Trace	Trace	1	14	Trace	Trace	Trace	Trace	Trace	Trace

[b] Contributed largely from beta-carotene used for coloring.

Table 1 (continued)

MILK, CHEESE, CREAM, IMITATION CREAM; RELATED PRODUCTS—Con.

#	Food, Approximate Measure, and Weight (in Grams)		Weight (g)	Water (%)	Food Energy (kcal)	Protein (g)	Fat (g)	Fatty Acids			Carbo-hydrate (g)	Calcium (mg)	Iron (mg)	Vitamin A value (I.U.)	Thiamin (mg)	Riboflavin (mg)	Niacin (mg)	Ascorbic acid (mg)
								Saturated (total) (g)	Unsaturated Oleic (g)	Linoleic (g)								
	Imitation cream products (made with vegetable fat):—Con. Whipped topping:																	
52	Pressurized	1 cup	70	61	190	1	17	15	1	0	9	5	—	340[b]	—	0	—	—
53		1 tbsp	4	61	10	Trace	1	1	Trace	0	Trace	Trace	—	20[b]	—	0	—	—
54	Frozen	1 cup	75	52	230	1	20	18	Trace	0	15	5	—	560[b]	—	0	—	—
55		1 tbsp	4	52	10	Trace	1	1	Trace	0	1	Trace	—	30[b]	—	0	—	—
56	Powdered, made with whole milk	1 cup	75	58	175	3	12	10	1	Trace	15	62	Trace	330[b]	.02	.08	.1	Trace
57		1 tbsp	4	58	10	Trace	1	1	Trace	Trace	1	3	Trace	20	Trace	Trace	Trace	Trace
	Milk beverages:																	
58	Cocoa, homemade	1 cup	250	79	245	10	12	7	4	Trace	27	295	1.0	400	.10	.45	.5	3
59	Chocolate-flavored drink made with skim milk and 2% added butterfat.	1 cup	250	83	190	8	6	3	2	Trace	27	270	.5	210	.10	.40	.3	3
	Malted milk:																	
60	Dry powder, approx. 3 heaping teaspoons per ounce	1 oz	28	3	115	4	2	—	—	—	20	82	.6	290	.09	.15	.1	0
61	Beverage	1 cup	235	78	245	11	10	—	—	—	28	317	.7	590	.14	.49	.2	2
	Milk desserts:																	
62	Custard, baked	1 cup	265	77	305	14	15	7	5	1	29	297	1.1	930	.11	.50	.3	1
	Ice cream:																	
63	Regular (approx. 10% fat)	½ gal	1064	63	2055	48	113	62	37	3	221	1553	.5	4680	.43	2.23	1.1	11
64		1 cup	133	63	255	6	14	8	5	Trace	28	194	.1	590	.05	.28	.1	1
65		3 fl oz cup	50	63	95	2	5	3	2	Trace	10	73	Trace	220	.02	.11	.1	1
66	Rich (approx. 16% fat)	½ gal	1188	63	2635	31	191	105	63	6	214	927	.2	7840	.24	1.31	1.2	12
67		1 cup	148	63	330	4	24	13	8	1	27	115	Trace	980	.03	.16	.1	1

No.	Food	Measure	Grams															
	Ice milk:																	
68	Hardened	½ gal	1048	67	1595	50	53	29	17	2	235	1635	1.0	2200	.52	2.31	1.0	10
69		1 cup	131	67	200	6	7	4	2	Trace	29	204	.1	280	.07	.29	.1	1
70	Soft-serve	1 cup	175	67	265	8	9	5	3	Trace	39	273	.2	370	.09	.39	.2	2
	Yogurt																	
71	Made from partially skimmed milk	1 cup	245	89	125	8	4	2	1	Trace	13	294	.1	170	.10	.44	.2	2
72	Made from whole milk	1 cup	245	88	150	7	8	5	3	Trace	12	272	.1	340	.07	.39	.2	2
	EGGS																	
	Eggs, large, 24 ounces per dozen:																	
	Raw or cooked in shell or with nothing added:																	
73	Whole, without shell	1 egg	50	74	80	6	6	2	3	Trace	Trace	27	1.1	590	.05	.15	Trace	0
74	White of egg	1 white	33	88	15	4	Trace	—	—	—	Trace	3	Trace	0	Trace	.09	Trace	0
75	Yolk of egg	1 yolk	17	51	60	3	5	2	2	Trace	Trace	24	.9	580	.04	.07	Trace	0
76	Scrambled with milk and fat	1 egg	64	72	110	7	8	3	3	Trace	1	51	1.1	690	.05	.18	Trace	0
	MEAT, POULTRY, FISH, SHELLFISH; RELATED PRODUCTS																	
77	Bacon, (20 slices per lb raw), broiled or fried, crisp	2 slices	15	8	90	5	8	3	4	1	1	2	.5	0	.08	.05	.8	—
	Beef,[c] cooked:																	
	Cuts braised, simmered, or pot roasted:																	
78	Lean and fat	3 oz	85	53	245	23	16	8	7	Trace	0	10	2.9	30	.04	.18	3.5	—
79	Lean only	2.5 oz	72	62	140	22	5	2	2	Trace	0	10	2.7	10	.04	.16	3.3	—
	Hamburger (ground beef), broiled:																	
80	Lean	3 oz	85	60	185	23	10	5	4	Trace	0	10	3.0	20	.08	.20	5.1	—
81	Regular	3 oz	85	54	245	21	17	8	8	Trace	0	9	2.7	30	.07	.18	4.6	—
	Roast, overcooked, no liquid added:																	
	Relatively fat, such as rib:																	
82	Lean and fat	3 oz	85	40	375	17	34	16	15	1	0	8	2.2	70	.05	.13	3.1	—
83	Lean only	1.8 oz	51	57	125	14	7	3	3	Trace	0	6	1.8	10	.04	.11	2.6	—
	Relatively lean, such as heel of round:																	
84	Lean and fat	3 oz	85	62	165	25	7	3	3	Trace	0	11	3.2	10	.06	.19	4.5	—
85	Lean only	2.7 oz	78	65	125	24	3	1	1	Trace	0	10	3.0	Trace	.06	.18	4.3	—

[b] Contributed largely from beta-carotene used for coloring.

[c] Outer layer of fat on the cut was removed to within approximately ½-in. of the lean. Deposits of fat within the cut were not removed.

Table 1 (continued)

		Water (%)	Food Energy (kcal)	Protein (g)	Fat (g)	Fatty Acids Saturated (total) (g)	Unsaturated Oleic (g)	Unsaturated Linoleic (g)	Carbohydrate (g)	Calcium (mg)	Iron (mg)	Vitamin A value (I.U.)	Thiamin (mg)	Riboflavin (mg)	Niacin (mg)	Ascorbic acid (mg)
	MEAT, POULTRY, FISH, SHELLFISH; RELATED PRODUCTS—Con.															
	Steak, broiled:															
	Relatively fat, such as sirloin:															
86	Lean and fat 3 oz 85	44	330	20	27	13	12	1	0	9	2.5	50	.05	.16	4.0	—
87	Lean only 2.0 oz 56	59	115	18	4	2	2	Trace	0	7	2.2	10	.05	.14	3.6	—
	Relatively lean, such as round:															
88	Lean and fat 3 oz 85	55	220	24	13	6	6	Trace	0	10	3.0	20	.07	.19	4.8	—
89	Lean only 2.4 oz 68	61	130	21	4	2	2	Trace	0	9	2.5	10	.06	.16	4.1	—
	Beef, canned:															
90	Corned beef 3 oz 85	59	185	22	10	5	4	Trace	0	17	3.7	20	.01	.20	2.9	—
91	Corned beef hash 3 oz 85	67	155	7	10	5	4	Trace	9	11	1.7	—	.01	.08	1.8	—
92	Beef, dried or chipped 2 oz 57	48	115	19	4	2	2	Trace	0	11	2.9	—	.04	.18	2.2	—
93	Beef and vegetable stew 1 cup 235	82	210	15	10	5	4	Trace	15	28	2.8	2310	.13	.17	4.4	15
94	Beef pot pie, baked 4¼-in. diam., weight before baking about 8 oz 1 pie 227	55	560	23	33	9	20	2	43	32	4.1	1860	.25	.27	4.5	7
	Chicken, cooked:															
95	Flesh only, broiled 3 oz 85	71	115	20	3	1	1	1	0	8	1.4	80	.05	.16	7.4	—
	Breast, fried, ½ breast:															
96	With bone 3.3 oz 94	58	155	25	5	1	2	1	1	9	1.3	70	.04	.17	11.2	—
97	Flesh and skin only 2.7 oz 76	58	155	25	5	1	2	1	1	9	1.3	70	.04	.17	11.2	—
	Drumstick, fried:															
98	With bone 2.1 oz 59	55	90	12	4	1	2	1	Trace	6	.9	50	.03	.15	2.7	—
99	Flesh and skin only 1.3 oz 38	55	90	12	4	1	2	1	Trace	6	.9	50	.03	.15	2.7	—
100	Chicken, canned, boneless 3 oz 85	65	170	18	10	3	4	2	0	18	1.3	200	.03	.11	3.7	3
101	Chicken pot pie, baked 4¼-in. diam., weight before baking about 8 oz 1 pie 227	57	535	23	31	10	15	3	42	68	3.0	3020	.25	.26	4.1	5

	Food	Measure	Grams	Water (%)	Food energy (cal)	Protein (g)	Fat (g)	Saturated fatty acids (g)	Unsaturated Oleic (g)	Unsaturated Linoleic (g)	Carbohydrate (g)	Calcium (mg)	Iron (mg)	Vitamin A (IU)	Thiamine (mg)	Riboflavin (mg)	Niacin (mg)	Ascorbic acid (mg)
	Chili con carne, canned:																	
102	With beans	1 cup	250	72	335	19	15	7	7	Trace	30	80	4.2	150	.08	.18	3.2	—
103	Without beans	1 cup	255	67	510	26	38	18	17	1	15	97	3.6	380	.05	.31	5.6	—
104	Heart, beef, lean, braised	3 oz	85	61	160	27	5	—	—	—	1	5	5.0	20	.21	1.04	6.5	1
	Lamb,ᶜ cooked:																	
105	Chop, thick, with bone, 1 chop, broiled	4.8 oz	137	47	400	25	33	18	12	1	0	10	1.5	—	.14	.25	5.6	—
106	Lean and fat	4.0 oz	112	47	400	25	33	18	12	1	0	10	1.5	—	.14	.25	5.6	—
107	Lean only	2.6 oz	74	62	140	21	6	3	2	Trace	0	9	1.5	—	.11	.20	4.5	—
	Leg roasted:																	
108	Lean and fat	3 oz	85	54	235	22	16	9	6	Trace	0	9	1.4	—	.13	.23	4.7	—
109	Lean only	2.5 oz	71	62	130	20	5	3	2	Trace	0	9	1.4	—	.12	.21	4.4	—
	Shoulder, roasted:																	
110	Lean and fat	3 oz	85	50	285	18	23	13	8	1	0	9	1.0	—	.11	.20	4.0	—
111	Lean only	2.3 oz	64	61	130	17	6	3	2	Trace	0	8	1.0	—	.10	.18	3.7	—
112	Liver, beef, fried	2 oz	57	57	130	15	6	—	—	—	3	6	5.0	30,280	.15	2.37	9.4	15
	Pork, cured, cooked:																	
113	Ham, light cure, lean and fat, roasted	3 oz	85	54	245	18	19	7	8	2	0	8	2.2	0	.40	.16	3.1	—
	Luncheon meat:																	
114	Boiled ham, sliced	2 oz	57	59	135	11	10	4	4	1	0	6	1.6	0	.25	.09	1.5	—
115	Canned, spiced or unspiced	2 oz	57	55	165	8	14	5	6	1	1	5	1.2	0	.18	.12	1.6	—
	Pork, fresh,ᶜ cooked:																	
116	Chop, thick, with bone 1 chop	3.5 oz	98	42	260	16	21	8	9	2	0	8	2.2	0	.63	.18	3.8	—
117	Lean and fat	2.3 oz	66	42	260	16	21	8	9	2	0	8	2.2	0	.63	.18	3.8	—
118	Lean only	1.7 oz	48	53	130	15	7	2	3	1	0	7	1.9	0	.54	.16	3.3	—
	Roast, oven-cooked, no liquid added:																	
119	Lean and fat	3 oz	85	46	310	21	24	9	10	2	0	9	2.7	0	.78	.22	4.7	—
120	Lean only	2.4 oz	68	55	175	20	10	3	4	1	0	9	2.6	0	.73	.21	4.4	—
	Cuts, simmered:																	
121	Lean and fat	3 oz	85	46	320	20	26	9	11	2	0	8	2.5	0	.46	.21	4.1	—
122	Lean only	2.2 oz	63	60	135	18	6	2	3	1	0	8	2.3	0	.42	.19	3.7	—
	Sausage:																	
123	Bologna, slice, 3-in. diam. by 1/8 in.	2 slices	26	56	80	3	7	—	—	—	Trace	2	.5	—	.04	.06	.7	—

ᶜ Outer layer of fat on the cut was removed to within approximately ½-in. of the lean. Deposits of fat within the cut were not removed.

Table 1 (continued)

	Food, Approximate Measure, and Weight (in Grams)		Water (%)	Food Energy (kcal)	Protein (g)	Fat (g)	Fatty Acids Saturated (total) (g)	Unsaturated Oleic (g)	Unsaturated Linoleic (g)	Carbohydrate (g)	Calcium (mg)	Iron (mg)	Vitamin A value (I.U.)	Thiamin (mg)	Riboflavin (mg)	Niacin (mg)	Ascorbic acid (mg)
	MEAT, POULTRY, FISH, SHELLFISH; RELATED PRODUCTS—Con.																
	Sausage:—con.																
124	Braunschweiger, slice 2-in. diam. by ¼ in.	2 slices 20	53	65	3	5	—	—	—	Trace	2	1.2	1310	.03	.29	1.6	—
125	Deviled ham, canned	1 tbsp 13	51	45	2	4	2	2	Trace	0	1	.3	—	.02	.01	.2	—
126	Frankfurter, heated (8 per lb. purchased pkg)	1 frank 56	57	170	7	15	—	—	—	1	3	.8	—	.08	.11	1.4	—
127	Pork links, cooked (16 links per lb raw)	2 links 26	35	125	5	11	4	5	1	Trace	2	.6	0	.21	.09	1.0	—
128	Salami, dry type	1 oz 28	30	130	7	11	—	—	—	Trace	4	1.0	—	.10	.07	1.5	—
129	Salami, cooked	1 oz 28	51	90	5	7	—	—	—	Trace	3	.7	—	.07	.07	1.2	—
130	Vienna, canned (7 sausages per 5-oz can)	1 sausage 16	63	40	2	3	—	—	—	Trace	1	.3	—	.01	.02	.4	—
	Veal, medium fat, cooked, bone removed:																
131	Cutlet	3 oz 85	60	185	23	9	5	4	Trace	—	9	2.7	—	.06	.21	4.6	—
132	Roast	3 oz 85	55	230	23	14	7	6	Trace	0	10	2.9	—	.11	.26	6.6	—
	Fish and shellfish:																
133	Bluefish, baked with table fat	3 oz 85	68	135	22	4	—	—	—	0	25	.6	40	.09	.08	1.6	—
	Clams:																
134	Raw, meat only	3 oz 85	82	65	11	1	—	—	—	2	59	5.2	90	.08	.15	1.1	8
135	Canned, solids and liquid	3 oz 85	86	45	7	1	—	—	—	2	47	3.5	—	.01	.09	.9	—
136	Crabmeat, canned	3 oz 85	77	85	15	2	—	—	—	1	38	.7	—	.07	.07	1.6	—
137	Fish sticks, breaded, cooked frozen; stick 3¾ by 1 by ½ in.	10 sticks or 8 oz pkg 227	66	400	38	20	5	4	10	15	25	0.9	—	.09	.16	3.6	—
138	Haddock, breaded, fried	3 oz 85	66	140	17	5	1	3	Trace	5	34	1.0	—	.03	.06	2.7	—
139	Ocean perch, breaded, fried	3 oz 85	59	195	16	11	1	—	—	6	28	1.1	—	.08	.09	1.5	2
140	Oysters, raw, meat only (13-19 med. selects)	1 cup 240	85	160	20	4	—	—	—	8	226	13.2	740	.33	.43	6.0	—
141	Salmon, pink, canned	3 oz 85	71	120	17	5	1	1	Trace	0	167[d]	.7	60	.03	.16	6.8	—
142	Sardines, Atlantic, canned in oil, drained solids	3 oz 85	62	175	20	9	—	—	—	0	372	2.5	190	.02	.17	4.6	—

143	Shad, baked with table fat and bacon[a]	3 oz	85	64	170	20	10	—	—	—	0	20	.5	20	.11	.22	7.3	—
144	Shrimp, canned, meat	3 oz	85	70	100	21	1	—	—	—	1	98	2.6	50	.01	.03	1.5	—
145	Swordfish, broiled with butter or margarine	3 oz	85	65	150	24	5	—	—	—	0	23	1.1	1750	.03	.04	9.3	—
146	Tuna, canned in oil, drained solids	3 oz	85	61	170	24	7	2	1	1	0	7	1.6	70	.04	.10	10.1	—
	MATURE DRY BEANS AND PEAS, NUTS, PEANUTS; RELATED PRODUCTS																	
147	Almonds, shelled, whole kernels	1 cup	142	5	850	26	77	6	52	15	28	332	6.7	0	.34	1.31	5.0	Trace
	Beans, dry:																	
	Common varieties as Great Northern, navy, and others:																	
	Cooked, drained:																	
148	Great Northern	1 cup	180	69	210	14	1	—	—	—	38	90	4.9	0	.25	.13	1.3	0
149	Navy (pea)	1 cup	190	69	225	15	1	—	—	—	40	95	5.1	0	.27	.13	1.3	0
	Canned, solids and liquid:																	
	White with —																	
150	Frankfurters (sliced)	1 cup	255	71	365	19	18	—	—	—	32	94	4.8	330	.18	.15	3.3	Trace
151	Pork and tomato sauce	1 cup	255	71	310	16	7	2	3	1	49	138	4.6	330	.20	.08	1.5	5
152	Pork and sweet sauce	1 cup	255	66	385	16	12	4	5	1	54	161	5.9	—	.15	.10	1.3	—
153	Red kidney	1 cup	255	76	230	15	1	—	—	—	42	74	4.6	10	.13	.10	1.5	—
154	Lima, cooked, drained	1 cup	190	64	260	16	1	—	—	—	49	55	5.9	—	.25	.11	1.3	—
155	Cashew nuts, roasted	1 cup	140	5	785	24	64	11	45	4	41	53	5.3	140	.60	.35	2.5	—
	Coconut, fresh, meat only:																	
156	Pieces, approx. 2 by 2 by ½ in.	1 piece	45	51	155	2	16	14	1	Trace	4	6	.8	0	.02	.01	.2	1
157	Shredded or grated, firmly packed	1 cup	130	51	450	5	46	39	3	Trace	12	17	2.2	0	.07	.03	.7	4
158	Cowpeas or blackeye peas, dry, cooked	1 cup	248	80	190	13	1	—	—	—	34	42	3.2	20	.41	.11	1.1	Trace
159	Peanuts, roasted, salted, halves	1 cup	144	2	840	37	72	16	31	21	27	107	3.0	—	.46	.19	24.7	0

[a] If bones are discarded, value will be greatly reduced.

Table 1 (continued)

MATURE DRY BEANS AND PEAS, NUTS, PEANUTS; RELATED PRODUCTS—Con.

	Food, Approximate Measure, and Weight (in Grams)	Water (%)	Food Energy (kcal)	Protein (g)	Fat (g)	Saturated (total) (g)	Oleic (g)	Linoleic (g)	Carbohydrate (g)	Calcium (mg)	Iron (mg)	Vitamin A value (I.U.)	Thiamin (mg)	Riboflavin (mg)	Niacin (mg)	Ascorbic acid (mg)
160	Peanut butter, 1 tbsp, 16	2	95	4	8	2	4	2	3	9	.3	–	.02	.02	2.4	0
161	Peas, split, dry, cooked, 1 cup, 250	70	290	20	1	–	–	–	52	28	4.2	100	.37	.22	2.2	–
162	Pecans, halves, 1 cup, 108	3	740	10	77	5	48	15	16	79	2.6	140	.93	.14	1.0	2
163	Walnuts, black or native, chopped, 1 cup, 126	3	790	26	75	4	26	36	19	Trace	7.6	380	.28	.14	.9	–
	VEGETABLES AND VEGETABLE PRODUCTS															
	Asparagus, green: Cooked, drained:															
164	Spears, ½-in. diam. at base, 4 spears, 60	94	10	1	Trace	–	–	–	2	13	.4	540	.10	.11	.8	16
165	Pieces, 1½ to 2-in. lengths, 1 cup, 145	94	30	3	Trace	–	–	–	5	30	.9	1310	.23	.26	2.0	38
166	Canned, solids and liquid, 1 cup, 244	94	45	5	1	–	–	–	7	44	4.1	1240	.15	.22	2.0	37
	Beans:															
167	Lima, immature seeds, cooked, drained, 1 cup, 170	71	190	13	1	–	–	–	34	80	4.3	480	.31	.17	2.2	29
	Snap: Green:															
168	Cooked, drained, 1 cup, 125	92	30	2	Trace	–	–	–	7	63	.8	680	.09	.11	.6	15
169	Canned, solids and liquid, 1 cup, 239	94	45	2	Trace	–	–	–	10	81	2.9	690	.07	.10	.7	10
	Yellow or wax:															
170	Cooked, drained, 1 cup, 125	93	30	2	Trace	–	–	–	6	63	0.8	290	.09	.11	.6	16
171	Canned, solids and liquid, 1 cup, 239	94	45	2	1	–	–	–	10	81	2.9	140	.07	.10	.7	12
172	Sprouted mung beans, cooked, drained, 1 cup, 125	91	35	4	Trace	–	–	–	7	21	1.1	30	.11	.13	.9	8

No.	Food, approximate measure, and weight (in grams)	Measure	Grams	Water (%)	Food energy	Protein	Fat	Saturated	Unsaturated Oleic	Unsaturated Linoleic	Carbohydrate	Calcium	Iron	Vitamin A	Thiamin	Riboflavin	Niacin	Ascorbic acid
	Beets																	
	Cooked, drained, peeled:																	
173	Whole beets, 2-in. diam.	2 beets	100	91	30	1	Trace	—	—	—	7	14	.5	20	.03	.04	.3	6
174	Diced or sliced	1 cup	170	91	55	2	Trace	—	—	—	12	24	.9	30	.05	.07	.5	10
175	Canned, solids and liquid	1 cup	246	90	85	2	Trace	—	—	—	19	34	1.5	20	.02	.05	.2	7
176	Beet greens, leaves and stems, cooked, drained	1 cup	145	94	25	3	Trace	—	—	—	5	144	2.8	7,400	.10	.22	.4	22
	Blackeye peas. See Cowpeas.																	
	Broccoli, cooked, drained:																	
177	Whole stalks, medium size	1 stalk	180	91	45	6	1	—	—	—	8	158	1.4	4,500	.16	.36	1.4	162
178	Stalks cut into ½-in. pieces	1 cup	155	91	40	5	1	—	—	—	7	136	1.2	3,880	.14	.31	1.2	140
179	Chopped, yield from 10-oz frozen pkg	1 3/8 cups	250	92	65	7	1	—	—	—	12	135	1.8	6,500	.15	.30	1.3	143
180	Brussels sprouts, 7-8 sprouts (1¼ to 1½ in. diam.) per cup, cooked	1 cup	155	88	55	7	1	—	—	—	10	50	1.7	810	.12	.22	1.2	135
	Cabbage:																	
	Common varieties:																	
	Raw:																	
181	Coarsely shredded or sliced	1 cup	70	92	15	1	Trace	—	—	—	4	34	.3	90	.04	.04	.2	33
182	Finely shredded or chopped	1 cup	90	92	20	1	Trace	—	—	—	5	44	.4	120	.05	.05	.3	42
183	Cooked	1 cup	145	94	30	2	Trace	—	—	—	6	64	.4	190	.06	.06	.4	48
184	Red, raw, coarsely shredded	1 cup	70	90	20	1	Trace	—	—	—	5	29	.6	30	.06	.04	.3	43
185	Savoy, raw, coarsely shredded	1 cup	70	92	15	2	Trace	—	—	—	3	47	.6	140	.04	.06	.2	39
186	Cabbage, celery or Chinese, raw, cut in 1-in. pieces	1 cup	75	95	10	1	Trace	—	—	—	2	32	.5	110	.04	.03	.5	19
187	Cabbage, spoon (or pakchoy), cooked	1 cup	170	95	25	2	Trace	—	—	—	4	252	1.0	5,270	.07	.14	1.2	26
	Carrots:																	
	Raw:																	
188	Whole, 5½ by 1 in. (25 thin strips)	1 carrot	50	88	20	1	Trace	—	—	—	5	18	.4	5,500	.03	.03	.3	4
189	Grated	1 cup	110	88	45	1	Trace	—	—	—	11	41	.8	12,100	.06	.06	.7	9

Table 1 (continued)

VEGETABLES AND VEGETABLE PRODUCTS—Continued

	Food, Approximate Measure, and Weight (in Grams)		Water (%)	Food Energy (kcal)	Protein (g)	Fat (g)	Fatty Acids Saturated (total) (g)	Unsaturated Oleic (g)	Linoleic (g)	Carbohydrate (g)	Calcium (mg)	Iron (mg)	Vitamin A value (I.U.)	Thiamin (mg)	Riboflavin (mg)	Niacin (mg)	Ascorbic acid (mg)
190	Cooked, diced	1 cup	145	91	45	1	Trace	—	—	—	10	48	.9	15,220	.08	.07	.7	9
191	Canned, strained or chopped (baby food)	1 oz	28	92	10	Trace	Trace	—	—	—	2	7	.1	3,690	.01	.01	.1	1
192	Cauliflower, cooked, flowerbuds	1 cup	120	93	25	3	Trace	—	—	—	5	25	.8	70	.11	.10	.7	66
193	Celery, raw: Stalk, large outer, 8 by about 1½ in., at root end	1 stalk	40	94	5	Trace	Trace	—	—	—	2	16	.1	100	.01	.01	.1	4
194	Pieces, diced	1 cup	100	94	15	1	Trace	—	—	—	4	39	.3	240	.03	.03	.3	9
195	Collards, cooked	1 cup	190	91	55	5	1	—	—	—	9	289	1.1	10,260	.27	.37	2.4	87
196	Corn, sweet: Cooked, ear 5 by 1¾ in.e	1 ear	140	74	70	3	1	—	—	—	16	2	.5	310f	.09	.08	1.0	7
197	Canned, solids and liquid	1 cup	256	81	170	5	2	—	—	—	40	10	1.0	690f	.07	.12	2.3	13
198	Cowpeas, cooked, immature seeds	1 cup	160	72	175	13	1	—	—	—	29	38	3.4	560	.49	.18	2.3	28
199	Cucumbers, 10 oz; 7½ by about 2 in.: Raw, pared	1 cucumber	207	96	30	1	Trace	—	—	—	7	35	.6	Trace	.07	.09	.4	23
200	Raw, pared, center slice 1/8-in. thick	6 slices	50	96	5	Trace	Trace	—	—	—	2	8	.2	Trace	.02	.02	.1	6
201	Dandelion greens, cooked	1 cup	180	90	60	4	1	—	—	—	12	252	3.2	21,060	.24	.29	—	32
202	Endive, curly (including escarole)	2 oz	57	93	10	1	Trace	—	—	—	2	46	1.0	1,870	.04	.08	.3	6
203	Kale, leaves including stems, cooked	1 cup	110	91	30	4	1	—	—	—	4	147	1.3	8,140	—	—	—	68

No.	Food	Measure	Weight (g)	Water (%)	Food energy	Protein	Fat	Saturated	Oleic	Linoleic	Carbo-hydrate	Calcium	Iron	Vitamin A	Thiamin	Ribo-flavin	Niacin	Ascorbic acid
204	Lettuce, raw: Butterhead, as Boston types; head, 4-in. diameter	1 head	220	95	30	3	Trace	—	—	—	6	77	4.4	2,130	.14	.13	.6	18
205	Crisphead, as Iceberg; head, 4¾-in. diameter	1 head	454	96	60	4	Trace	—	—	—	13	91	2.3	1,500	.29	.27	1.3	29
206	Looseleaf, or bunching varieties, leaves	2 large	50	94	10	1	Trace	—	—	—	2	34	.7	950	.03	.04	.2	9
207	Mushrooms, canned, solids and liquid	1 cup	244	93	40	5	Trace	—	—	—	6	15	1.2	Trace	.04	.60	4.8	4
208	Mustard greens, cooked	1 cup	140	93	35	3	1	—	—	—	6	193	2.5	8,120	.11	.19	.9	68
209	Okra, cooked, pod 3 by 5/8 in.	8 pods	85	91	25	2	Trace	—	—	—	5	78	.4	420	.11	.15	.8	17
	Onions: Mature:																	
210	Raw, onion 2½-in. diameter	1 onion	110	89	40	2	Trace	—	—	—	10	30	.6	40	.04	.04	.2	11
211	Cooked	1 cup	210	92	60	3	Trace	—	—	—	14	50	.8	80	.06	.06	.4	14
212	Young green, small, without tops	6 onions	50	88	20	1	Trace	—	—	—	5	20	.3	Trace	.02	.02	.2	12
213	Parsley, raw, chopped	1 tbsp.	4	85	Trace	Trace	Trace	—	—	—	Trace	8	.2	340	Trace	.01	Trace	7
214	Parsnips, cooked	1 cup	155	82	100	2	1	—	—	—	23	70	.9	50	.11	.12	.2	16
	Peas, green:																	
215	Cooked	1 cup	160	82	115	9	1	—	—	—	19	37	2.9	860	.44	.17	3.7	33
216	Canned, solids and liquid	1 cup	249	83	165	9	1	—	—	—	31	50	4.2	1,120	.23	.13	2.2	22
217	Canned, strained (baby food)	1 oz.	28	86	15	1	Trace	—	—	—	3	3	.4	140	.02	.02	.4	3
218	Peppers, hot, red, without seeds, dried (ground chili powder, added seasonings)	1 tbsp.	15	8	50	2	2	—	—	—	8	40	2.3	9,750	.03	.17	1.3	2
	Peppers, sweet: Raw, about 5 per pound:																	
219	Green pod without stem and seeds	1 pod	74	93	15	1	Trace	—	—	—	4	7	.5	310	.06	.06	.4	94

e Measure and weight apply to entire vegetable or fruit including parts not usually eaten.

f Based on yellow varieties; white varieties contain only a trace of cryptoxanthin and carotenes, the pigments in corn that have biological activity.

Table 1 (continued)

	Food, Approximate Measure, and Weight (in Grams)		Water (%)	Food Energy (kcal)	Protein (g)	Fat (g)	Fatty Acids Saturated (total) (g)	Unsaturated Oleic (g)	Linoleic (g)	Carbohydrate (g)	Calcium (mg)	Iron (mg)	Vitamin A value (I.U.)	Thiamin (mg)	Riboflavin (mg)	Niacin (mg)	Ascorbic acid (mg)
	VEGETABLES AND VEGETABLE PRODUCTS—Continued																
220	Cooked, boiled, drained	1 pod	73	95	15	1	Trace	—	—	—	3	7	.4	310	.05	.05	.4	70
221	Potatoes, medium (about 3 per pound raw): Baked, peeled after baking	1 potato	99	75	90	3	Trace	—	—	—	21	9	.7	Trace	.10	.04	1.7	20
	Boiled:																	
222	Peeled after boiling	1 potato	136	80	105	3	Trace	—	—	—	23	10	.8	Trace	.13	.05	2.0	22
223	Peeled before boiling	1 potato	122	83	80	2	Trace	—	—	—	18	7	.6	Trace	.11	.04	1.4	20
	French-fried, piece 2 by ½ by ½ in.:																	
224	Cooked in deep fat	10 pieces	57	45	155	2	7	2	2	4	20	9	.7	Trace	.07	.04	1.8	12
225	Frozen, heated	10 pieces	57	53	125	2	5	1	1	2	19	5	1.0	Trace	.08	.01	1.5	12
	Mashed:																	
226	Milk added	1 cup	195	83	125	4	1	—	—	—	25	47	.8	50	.16	.10	2.0	19
227	Milk and butter added	1 cup	195	80	185	4	8	4	3	Trace	24	47	.8	330	.16	.10	1.9	18
228	Potato chips, medium, 2-in. diameter	10 chips	20	2	115	1	8	2	2	4	10	8	.4	Trace	.04	.01	1.0	3
229	Pumpkin, canned	1 cup	228	90	75	2	1	—	—	—	18	57	.9	14,590	.07	.12	1.3	12
230	Radishes, raw, small, without tops	4 radishes	40	94	5	Trace	Trace	—	—	—	1	12	.4	Trace	.01	.01	.1	10
231	Sauerkraut, canned, solids and liquid	1 cup	235	93	45	2	Trace	—	—	—	9	85	1.2	120	.07	.09	.4	33
	Spinach:																	
232	Cooked	1 cup	180	92	40	5	1	—	—	—	6	167	4.0	14,580	.13	.25	1.0	50
233	Canned, drained solids	1 cup	180	91	45	5	1	—	—	—	6	212	4.7	14,400	.03	.21	.6	24
	Squash: Cooked:																	
234	Summer, diced	1 cup	210	96	30	2	Trace	—	—	—	7	52	.8	820	.10	.16	1.6	21
235	Winter, baked, mashed	1 cup	205	81	130	4	1	—	—	—	32	57	1.6	8,610	.10	.27	1.4	27

No.	Food, approximate measure, and weight		grams	Water (%)	Food energy	Protein	Fat	Saturated	Oleic	Linoleic	Carbohydrate	Calcium	Iron	Vitamin A	Thiamine	Riboflavin	Niacin	Ascorbic acid
	Sweetpotatoes: Cooked, medium, 5 by 2 inches, weight raw about 6 ounces:																	
236	Baked, peeled after baking.	1 sweetpotato	110	64	155	2	1	—	—	—	36	44	1.0	8,910	.10	.07	.7	24
237	Boiled, peeled after boiling.	1 sweetpotato	147	71	170	2	1	—	—	—	39	47	1.0	11,610	.13	.09	.9	25
238	Candied, 3½ by 2¼ inches.	1 sweetpotato	175	60	295	2	6	2	3	1	60	65	1.6	11,030	.10	.08	.8	17
239	Canned, vacuum or solid pack.	1 cup	218	72	235	4	Trace	—	—	—	54	54	1.7	17,000	.10	.10	1.4	30
	Tomatoes:																	
240	Raw, approx. 3-in. diam. 2 1/8 in. high; wt., 7 oz.	1 tomato	200	90	40	2	Trace	—	—	—	9	24	.9	1,640	.11	.07	1.3	42[g]
241	Canned, solids and liquid.	1 cup	241	94	50	2	1	—	—	—	10	14	1.2	2,170	.12	.07	1.7	41
	Tomato catsup:																	
242	Cup	1 cup	273	69	290	6	1	—	—	—	69	60	2.2	3,820	.25	.19	4.4	41
243	Tablespoon	1 tbsp.	15	69	15	Trace	Trace	—	—	—	4	3	.1	210	.01	.01	.2	2
	Tomato juice, canned:																	
244	Cup	1 cup	243	94	45	2	Trace	—	—	—	10	17	2.2	1,940	.12	.07	1.9	39
245	Glass (6 fl. oz.)	1 glass	182	94	35	2	Trace	—	—	—	8	13	1.6	1,460	.09	.05	1.5	29
246	Turnips, cooked, diced	1 cup	155	94	35	1	Trace	—	—	—	8	54	.6	Trace	.06	.08	.5	34
247	Turnip greens, cooked	1 cup	145	94	30	3	Trace	—	—	—	5	252	1.5	8,270	.15	.33	.7	68
	FRUITS AND FRUIT PRODUCTS																	
248	Apples, raw (about 3 per lb.).[e]	1 apple	150	85	70	Trace	Trace	—	—	—	18	8	.4	50	.04	.02	.1	3
249	Apple juice, bottled or canned.	1 cup	248	88	120	Trace	Trace	—	—	—	30	15	1.5	—	.02	.05	.2	2
	Applesauce, canned:																	
250	Sweetened	1 cup	255	76	230	1	Trace	—	—	—	61	10	1.3	100	.05	.03	.1	3[h]
251	Unsweetened or artificially sweetened.	1 cup	244	88	100	1	Trace	—	—	—	26	10	1.2	100	.05	.02	.1	2[h]

[e] Measure and weight apply to entire vegetable or fruit including parts not usually eaten.

[g] Year-round average. Samples marketed from November through May, average 20 milligrams per 200-gram tomato; from June through October, around 52 milligrams.

[h] This is the amount from the fruit. Additional ascorbic acid may be added by the manufacturer. Refer to the label for this information.

Table 1 (continued)

| | Food, Approximate Measure, and Weight (in Grams) | | Water (%) | Food Energy (kcal) | Protein (g) | Fat (g) | Fatty Acids | | | Carbohydrate (g) | Calcium (mg) | Iron (mg) | Vitamin A value (I.U.) | Thiamin (mg) | Riboflavin (mg) | Niacin (mg) | Ascorbic acid (mg) |
							Saturated (total) (g)	Unsaturated Oleic (g)	Unsaturated Linoleic (g)								
	FRUITS AND FRUIT PRODUCTS—Con.																
	Apricots:																
252	Raw (about 12 per lb)[e]	3 apricots 114	85	55	1	Trace	—	—	—	14	18	.5	2,890	.03	.04	.7	10
253	Canned in heavy sirup	1 cup 259	77	220	2	Trace	—	—	—	57	28	.8	4,510	.05	.06	.9	10
254	Dried, uncooked (40 halves per cup)	1 cup 150	25	390	8	1	—	—	—	100	100	8.2	16,350	.02	.23	4.9	19
255	Cooked, unsweetened, fruit and liquid	1 cup 285	76	240	5	1	—	—	—	62	63	5.1	8,550	.01	.13	2.8	8
256	Apricot nectar, canned	1 cup 251	85	140	1	Trace	—	—	—	37	23	.5	2,380	.03	.03	.5	8[h]
	Avocados, whole fruit, raw:[e]																
257	California (mid- and late-winter; diam. 3 1/8 in.)	1 avocado 284	74	370	5	37	7	17	5	13	22	1.3	630	.24	.43	3.5	30
258	Florida (late summer, fall diam. 3 5/8 in.)	1 avocado 454	78	390	4	33	7	15	4	27	30	1.8	880	.33	.61	4.9	43
259	Bananas, raw, medium size[e]	1 banana 175	76	100	1	Trace	—	—	—	26	10	.8	230	.06	.07	.8	12
260	Banana flakes	1 cup 100	3	340	4	1	—	—	—	89	32	2.8	760	.18	.24	2.8	7
261	Blackberries, raw	1 cup 144	84	85	2	1	—	—	—	19	46	1.3	290	.05	.06	.5	30
262	Blueberries, raw	1 cup 140	83	85	1	1	—	—	—	21	21	1.4	140	.04	.08	.6	20
263	Cantaloupes, raw; medium, 5-inch diameter about 1 2/3 pounds[e]	½ melon 385	91	60	1	Trace	—	—	—	14	27	.8	6,540[i]	.08	.06	1.2	63
264	Cherries, canned, red, sour, pitted, water pack	1 cup 244	88	105	2	Trace	—	—	—	26	37	.7	1,660	.07	.05	.5	12
265	Cranberry juice cocktail, canned	1 cup 250	83	165	Trace	Trace	—	—	—	42	13	.8	Trace	.03	.03	.1	40[j]
266	Cranberry sauce, sweetened, canned, strained	1 cup 277	62	405	Trace	1	—	—	—	104	17	.6	60	.03	.03	.1	6
267	Dates, pitted, cut	1 cup 178	22	490	4	1	—	—	—	130	105	5.3	90	.16	.17	3.9	0
268	Figs, dried, large, 2 by 1 in.	1 fig 21	23	60	1	Trace	—	—	—	15	26	.6	20	.02	.02	.1	0

No.	Food	Measure	Weight (g)	Water (%)	Food energy (cal)	Protein (g)	Fat (g)	Saturated fatty acids (g)	Unsaturated oleic (g)	Unsaturated linoleic (g)	Carbohydrate (g)	Calcium (mg)	Iron (mg)	Vitamin A (I.U.)	Thiamin (mg)	Riboflavin (mg)	Niacin (mg)	Ascorbic acid (mg)
269	Fruit cocktail, canned, in heavy sirup	1 cup	256	80	195	1	Trace	—	—	—	50	23	1.0	360	.05	.03	1.3	5
	Grapefruit:																	
270	Raw, medium, 3¾-in. diam.[e] White	½ grapefruit	241	89	45	1	Trace	—	—	—	12	19	.5	10	.05	.02	.2	44
271	Pink or red	½ grapefruit	241	89	50	1	Trace	—	—	—	13	20	.5	540	.05	.02	.2	44
272	Canned, sirup pack	1 cup	254	81	180	2	Trace	—	—	—	45	33	.8	30	.08	.05	.5	76
273	Grapefruit juice: Fresh	1 cup	246	90	95	1	Trace	—	—	—	23	22	.5	k	.09	.04	.4	92
	Canned, white:																	
274	Unsweetened	1 cup	247	89	100	1	Trace	—	—	—	24	20	1.0	20	.07	.04	.4	84
275	Sweetened	1 cup	250	86	130	1	Trace	—	—	—	32	20	1.0	20	.07	.04	.4	78
	Frozen, concentrate, unsweetened:																	
276	Undiluted, can, 6 fl oz	1 can	207	62	300	4	1	—	—	—	72	70	.8	60	.29	.12	1.4	286
277	Diluted with 3 parts water, by volume	1 cup	247	89	100	1	Trace	—	—	—	24	25	.2	20	.10	.04	.5	96
278	Dehydrated crystals	4 oz	113	1	410	6	1	—	—	—	102	100	1.2	80	.40	.20	2.0	396
279	Prepared with water (1 pound yields about 1 gal)	1 cup	247	90	100	1	Trace	—	—	—	24	22	.2	20	.10	.05	.5	91
	Grapes, raw:[e]																	
280	American type (slip skin)	1 cup	153	82	65	1	1	—	—	—	15	15	.4	100	.05	.03	.2	3
281	European type (adherent skin)	1 cup	160	81	95	1	Trace	—	—	—	25	17	.6	140	.07	.04	.4	6
	Grapejuice:																	
282	Canned or bottled	1 cup	253	83	165	1	Trace	—	—	—	42	28	.8	—	.10	.05	.5	Trace
	Frozen concentrate, sweetened:																	
283	Undiluted, can, 6 fl oz	1 can	216	53	395	1	Trace	—	—	—	100	22	.9	40	.13	.22	1.5	12

e Measure and weight apply to entire vegetable or fruit including parts not usually eaten.

h This is the amount from the fruit. Additional ascorbic acid may be added by the manufacturer. Refer to the label for this information.

i Value for varieties with orange-colored flesh; value for varieties with green flesh would be about 540 I.U.

j Value listed is based on products with label stating 30 milligrams per 6 fl. oz. serving.

k For white-fleshed varieties value is about 20 I.U. per cup; for red-fleshed varieties, 1,080 I.U. per cup.

l Present only if added by the manufacturer. Refer to the label for this information.

Table 1 (continued)

FRUITS AND FRUIT PRODUCTS—Con.

	Food, Approximate Measure, and Weight (in Grams)		Water (%)	Food Energy (kcal)	Protein (g)	Fat (g)	Saturated (total) (g)	Unsaturated Oleic (g)	Unsaturated Linoleic (g)	Carbohydrate (g)	Calcium (mg)	Iron (mg)	Vitamin A value (I.U.)	Thiamin (mg)	Riboflavin (mg)	Niacin (mg)	Ascorbic acid (mg)
	Grapejuice:--Con.																
284	Diluted with 3 parts water, by volume	1 cup	250	86	135	1	Trace	—	—	—	33	8	.3	10	.05	.08	.5	—
285	Grapejuice drink, canned	1 cup	250	86	135	Trace	Trace	—	—	—	35	8	.3	—	.03	.03	.3	—
286	Lemons, raw, 2 1/8-in. diam., size 165.[e] Used for juice	1 lemon	110	90	20	1	Trace	—	—	—	6	19	.4	10	.03	.01	.1	39
287	Lemon juice, raw	1 cup	244	91	60	1	Trace	—	—	—	20	17	.5	50	.07	.02	.2	112
	Lemonade concentrate:																
288	Frozen, 6 fl oz per can	1 can	219	48	430	Trace	Trace	—	—	—	112	9	.4	40	.04	.07	.7	66
289	Diluted with 4 1/3 parts water, by volume	1 cup	248	88	110	Trace	Trace	—	—	—	28	2	Trace	Trace	Trace	.02	.2	17
	Lime juice:																
290	Fresh	1 cup	246	90	65	1	Trace	—	—	—	22	22	.5	20	.05	.02	.2	79
291	Canned, unsweetened	1 cup	246	90	65	1	Trace	—	—	—	22	22	.5	20	.05	.02	.2	52
	Limeade concentrate, frozen:																
292	Undiluted, can, 6 fl oz	1 can	218	50	410	Trace	Trace	—	—	—	108	11	.2	Trace	.02	.02	.2	26
293	Diluted with 4 1/3 parts water by volume	1 cup	247	90	100	Trace	Trace	—	—	—	27	2	Trace	Trace	Trace	Trace	Trace	5
294	Oranges, raw 2 5/8-in. diam., all commercial, varieties[e]	1 orange	180	86	65	1	Trace	—	—	—	16	54	.5	260	.13	.05	.5	66
295	Orange juice, fresh, all varieties	1 cup	248	88	110	2	1	—	—	—	26	27	.5	500	.22	.07	1.0	124
296	Canned, unsweetened	1 cup	249	87	120	2	Trace	—	—	—	28	25	1.0	500	.17	.05	.7	100
	Frozen concentrate:																
297	Undiluted, can, 6 fl oz	1 can	213	55	360	5	Trace	—	—	—	87	75	.9	1620	.63	.11	2.8	360
298	Diluted with 3 parts water by volume	1 cup	249	87	120	2	Trace	—	—	—	29	25	.2	550	.22	.02	1.0	120
299	Dehydrated crystals	4 oz	113	1	430	6	2	—	—	—	100	95	1.9	1900	.76	.24	3.3	408
300	Prepared with water (1 pound yields about 1 gal)	1 cup	248	88	115	2	1	—	—	—	27	25	.5	500	.20	.07	1.0	109

Item No.	Food, approximate measure, and weight		Water (%)	Food energy (cal)	Protein (g)	Fat (g)	Fatty acids, Saturated (total) (g)	Unsaturated Oleic (g)	Unsaturated Linoleic (g)	Carbohydrate (g)	Calcium (mg)	Iron (mg)	Vitamin A (I.U.)	Thiamin (mg)	Riboflavin (mg)	Niacin (mg)	Ascorbic acid (mg)
301	Orange-apricot juice drink	1 cup 249	87	125	1	Trace	—	—	—	32	12	.2	1440	.05	.02	.5	40[j]
	Orange and grapefruit juice: Frozen concentrate:																
302	Undiluted, can, 6 fl oz	1 can 210	59	330	4	1	—	—	—	78	61	.8	800	.48	.06	2.3	302
303	Diluted with 3 parts water by volume	1 cup 248	88	110	1	Trace	—	—	—	26	20	.2	270	.16	.02	.8	102
304	Papayas, raw, ½-in. cubes	1 cup 182	89	70	1	Trace	—	—	—	18	36	.5	3190	.07	.08	.5	102
	Peaches: Raw:																
305	Whole, medium, 2-in. diameter, about 4 per pound.[e]	1 peach 114	89	35	1	Trace	—	—	—	10	9	.5	1320[m]	.02	.05	1.0	7
306	Sliced	1 cup 168	89	65	1	Trace	—	—	—	16	15	.8	2230[m]	.03	.08	1.6	12
	Canned, yellow-fleshed, solids and liquid: Sirup pack, heavy:																
307	Halves or slices	1 cup 257	79	200	1	Trace	—	—	—	52	10	.8	1100	.02	.06	1.4	7
308	Water pack	1 cup 245	91	75	1	Trace	—	—	—	20	10	.7	1100	.02	.06	1.4	7
309	Dried, uncooked	1 cup 160	25	420	5	1	—	—	—	109	77	9.6	6240	.02	.31	8.5	28
310	Cooked, unsweetened, 10-12 halves and juice	1 cup 270	77	220	3	1	—	—	—	58	41	5.1	3290	.01	.15	4.2	6
	Frozen:																
311	Carton, 12 oz, not thawed	1 carton 340	76	300	1	Trace	—	—	—	77	14	1.7	2210	.03	.14	2.4	135[n]
	Pears:																
312	Raw, 3 by 2½-in. diam.[e]	1 pear 182	83	100	1	1	—	—	—	25	13	.5	30	.04	.07	.2	7
	Canned, solids and liquid: Sirup pack, heavy:																
313	Halves or slices	1 cup 255	80	195	1	1	—	—	—	50	13	.5	Trace	.03	.05	.3	4
	Pineapple:																
314	Raw, diced	1 cup 140	85	75	1	Trace	—	—	—	19	24	.7	100	.12	.04	.3	24
	Canned, heavy sirup pack, solids and liquid:																
315	Crushed	1 cup 260	80	195	1	Trace	—	—	—	50	29	.8	120	.20	.06	.5	17
316	Sliced, slices and juice	2 small or 1 large 122	80	90	Trace	Trace	—	—	—	24	13	.4	50	.09	.03	.2	8

[e] Measure and weight apply to entire vegetable or fruit including parts not usually eaten.

[j] Value listed is based on product with label stating 30 milligrams per 6 fl oz serving.

[l] Present only if added by the manufacturer. Refer to the label for this information.

[m] Based on yellow-fleshed varieties; for white-fleshed varieties value is about 50 I.U. per 114-gram peach and 80 I.U. per cup of sliced peaches.

[n] This value includes ascorbic acid added by manufacturer.

Table 1 (continued)

FRUITS AND FRUIT PRODUCTS—Con.

	Food, Approximate Measure, and Weight (in Grams)			Water (%)	Food Energy (kcal)	Protein (g)	Fat (g)	Fatty Acids Saturated (total) (g)	Unsaturated Oleic (g)	Linoleic (g)	Carbohydrate (g)	Calcium (mg)	Iron (mg)	Vitamin A value (I.U.)	Thiamin (mg)	Riboflavin (mg)	Niacin (mg)	Ascorbic acid (mg)
317	Pineapple juice, canned	1 cup	249	86	135	1	Trace	–	–	–	34	37	.7	120	.12	.04	.5	22[h]
318	Plums, all except prunes: Raw, 2-in. diameter, about 2 oz[e]	1 plum	60	87	25	Trace	Trace	–	–	–	7	7	.3	140	.02	.02	.3	3
319	Canned, sirup pack (Italian prunes): Plums (with pits) and juice[e]	1 cup	256	77	205	1	Trace	–	–	–	53	22	2.2	2970	.05	.05	.9	4
320	Prunes, dried, "softenized", medium: Uncooked[e]	4 prunes	32	28	70	1	Trace	–	–	–	18	14	1.1	440	.02	.04	.4	1
321	Cooked, unsweetened, 17-18 prunes and 1/3 cup liquid[e]	1 cup	270	66	295	2	1	–	–	–	78	60	4.5	1860	.08	.18	1.7	2
322	Prune juice, canned or bottled	1 cup	256	80	200	1	Trace	–	–	–	49	36	10.5	–	.03	.03	1.0	5[h]
323	Raisins, seedless: Packaged, ½ oz or 1½ tbsp per pkg	1 pkg	14	18	40	Trace	Trace	–	–	–	11	9	.5	Trace	.02	.01	.1	Trace
324	Cup, pressed down	1 cup	165	18	480	4	Trace	–	–	–	128	102	5.8	30	.18	.13	.8	2
325	Raspberries, red: Raw	1 cup	123	84	70	1	1	–	–	–	17	27	1.1	160	.04	.11	1.1	31
326	Frozen, 10-oz carton, not thawed	1 carton	284	74	275	2	1	–	–	–	70	37	1.7	200	.06	.17	1.7	59
327	Rhubarb, cooked, sugar added	1 cup	272	63	385	1	Trace	–	–	–	98	212	1.6	220	.06	.15	.7	17
328	Strawberries: Raw, capped	1 cup	149	90	55	1	1	–	–	–	13	31	1.5	90	.04	.10	1.0	88
329	Frozen, 10-oz carton, not thawed	1 carton	284	71	310	1	1	–	–	–	79	40	2.0	90	.06	.17	1.5	150
330	Tangerines, raw, medium, 2 3/8-in. diam., size 176[e]	1 tangerine	116	87	40	1	Trace	–	–	–	10	34	.3	360	.05	.02	.1	27

No.	Food	Measure	Grams	Water (%)	Food energy (cal)	Protein (g)	Fat (g)	Saturated fatty acids (g)	Unsaturated Oleic (g)	Unsaturated Linoleic (g)	Carbohydrate (g)	Calcium (mg)	Iron (mg)	Vitamin A (IU)	Thiamin (mg)	Riboflavin (mg)	Niacin (mg)	Ascorbic acid (mg)
331	Tangerine juice, canned, sweetened.	1 cup	249	87	125	1	Trace	—	—	—	30	45	.5	1050	.15	.05	.2	55
332	Watermelon, raw, wedge, 4 by 8 in. (1/16 of 10 by 16-inch melon, about 2 pounds with rind)[e]	1 wedge	925	93	115	2	1	—	—	—	27	30	2.1	2510	.13	.13	.7	30
	GRAIN PRODUCTS																	
333	Bagel, 3-in. diam.: Egg	1 bagel	55	32	165	6	2	—	—	—	28	9	1.2	30	.14	.10	1.2	0
334	Water	1 bagel	55	29	165	6	2	—	—	—	30	8	1.2	0	.15	.11	1.4	0
335	Barley, pearled, light, uncooked	1 cup	200	11	700	16	2	Trace	—	—	158	32	4.0	0	.24	.10	6.2	0
336	Biscuits, baking powder from home recipe with enriched flour, 2-in. diam.	1 biscuit	28	27	105	2	5	1	2	1	13	34	.4	Trace	.06	.06	.1	Trace
337	Biscuits, baking powder from mix, 2-in. diam.	1 biscuit	28	28	90	2	3	1	1	1	15	19	.6	Trace	.08	.07	.6	Trace
338	Bran flakes (40% bran), added thiamin and iron	1 cup	35	3	105	4	1	—	—	—	28	25	12.3	0	.14	.06	2.2	0
339	Bran flakes with raisins, added thiamin and iron	1 cup	50	7	145	4	1	—	—	—	40	28	13.5	Trace	.16	.07	2.7	0
340	Breads: Boston brown bread, slice 3 by ¾ in.	1 slice	48	45	100	3	1	—	—	—	22	43	.9	0	.05	.03	.6	0
341	Cracked-wheat bread: Loaf, 1 lb	1 loaf	454	35	1190	40	10	2	5	2	236	399	5.0	Trace	.53	.41	5.9	Trace
342	Slice, 18 slices per loaf	1 slice	25	35	65	2	1	—	—	—	13	22	.3	Trace	.03	.02	.3	Trace
343	French or Vienna bread: Enriched, 1 lb loaf	1 loaf	454	31	1315	41	14	3	8	2	251	195	10.0	Trace	1.27	1.00	11.3	Trace
344	Unenriched, 1 lb loaf	1 loaf	454	31	1315	41	14	3	8	2	251	195	3.2	Trace	.36	.36	3.6	Trace
345	Italian bread: Enriched, 1 lb loaf	1 loaf	454	32	1250	41	4	Trace	1	2	256	77	10.0	0	1.32	.91	11.8	0
346	Unenriched, 1 lb loaf	1 loaf	454	32	1250	41	4	Trace	1	2	256	77	3.2	0	.41	.27	3.6	0

[e] Measure and weight apply to entire vegetable or fruit including parts not usually eaten.

[h] This is the amount from the fruit. Additional ascorbic acid may be added by the manufacturer. Refer to the label for this information.

Table 1 (continued)

GRAIN PRODUCTS—Continued

	Food, Approximate Measure, and Weight (in Grams)		Weight (g)	Water (%)	Food Energy (kcal)	Protein (g)	Fat (g)	Fatty Acids Saturated (total) (g)	Unsaturated Oleic (g)	Linoleic (g)	Carbohydrate (g)	Calcium (mg)	Iron (mg)	Vitamin A value (I.U.)	Thiamin (mg)	Riboflavin (mg)	Niacin (mg)	Ascorbic acid (mg)
	Raisin bread:																	
347	Loaf, 1 lb	454		35	1190	30	13	3	8	2	243	322	5.9	Trace	.23	.41	3.2	Trace
348	Slice, 18 slices per loaf	25		35	65	2	1	—	—	—	13	18	.3	Trace	.01	.02	.2	Trace
	Rye bread:																	
	American, light (1/3 rye, 2/3 wheat):																	
349	Loaf, 1 lb	454		36	1100	41	5	—	—	—	236	340	7.3	0	.82	.32	6.4	0
350	Slice, 18 slices per loaf	25		36	60	2	Trace	—	—	—	13	19	.4	0	.05	.02	.4	0
351	Pumpernickel, loaf, 1 lb	454		34	1115	41	5	—	—	—	241	381	10.9	0	1.04	.64	5.4	0
	White bread, enriched:[o]																	
	Soft-crumb type:																	
352	Loaf, 1 lb	454		36	1225	39	15	3	8	2	229	381	11.3	Trace	1.13	.95	10.9	Trace
353	Slice, 18 slices per loaf	25		36	70	2	1	—	—	—	13	21	.6	Trace	.06	.05	.6	Trace
354	Slice, toasted	22		25	70	2	1	—	—	—	13	21	.6	Trace	.06	.05	.6	Trace
355	Slice, 22 slices per loaf	20		36	55	2	1	—	—	—	10	17	.5	Trace	.05	.04	.5	Trace
356	Slice, toasted	17		25	55	2	1	—	—	—	10	17	.5	Trace	.05	.04	.5	Trace
357	Loaf, 1½ lb	680		36	1835	59	22	5	12	3	343	571	17.0	Trace	1.70	1.43	16.3	Trace
358	Slice, 24 slices per loaf	28		36	75	2	1	—	—	—	14	24	.7	Trace	.07	.06	.7	Trace
359	Slice, toasted	24		25	75	2	1	—	—	—	14	24	.7	Trace	.07	.06	.7	Trace
360	Slice, 28 slices per loaf	24		36	65	2	1	—	—	—	12	20	.6	Trace	.06	.05	.6	Trace
361	Slice, toasted	21		25	65	2	1	—	—	—	12	20	.6	Trace	.06	.05	.6	Trace
	Firm-crumb type:																	
362	Loaf, 1 lb	454		35	1245	41	17	4	10	2	228	435	11.3	Trace	1.22	.91	10.9	Trace
363	Slice, 20 slices per loaf	23		35	65	2	1	—	—	—	12	22	.6	Trace	.06	.05	.6	Trace
364	Slice, toasted	20		24	65	2	1	—	—	—	12	22	.6	Trace	.06	.05	.6	Trace
365	Loaf, 2 lb	907		35	2495	82	34	8	20	4	455	871	22.7	Trace	2.45	1.81	21.8	Trace
366	Slice, 34 slices per loaf	27		35	75	2	1	—	—	—	14	26	.7	Trace	.07	.05	.6	Trace
367	Slice, toasted	23		35	75	2	1	—	—	—	14	26	.7	Trace	.07	.05	.6	Trace
	Whole-wheat bread, soft-crumb type:																	
368	Loaf, 1 lb	454		36	1095	41	12	2	6	2	224	381	13.6	Trace	1.36	.45	12.7	Trace
369	Slice, 16 slices per loaf	28		36	65	3	1	—	—	—	14	24	.8	Trace	.09	.03	.8	Trace
370	Slice, toasted	24		24	65	3	1	—	—	—	14	24	.8	Trace	.09	.03	.8	Trace
	Whole-wheat bread, firm-crumb type:																	
371	Loaf, 1 lb	454		36	1100	48	14	3	6	3	216	449	13.6	Trace	1.18	.54	12.7	Trace

No.	Food	Measure	Grams	Water (%)	Food energy (cal)	Protein (g)	Fat (g)	Saturated (g)	Oleic (g)	Linoleic (g)	Carbohydrate (g)	Calcium (mg)	Iron (mg)	Vitamin A (IU)	Thiamin (mg)	Riboflavin (mg)	Niacin (mg)	Ascorbic acid (mg)
372	Slice, 18 slices per loaf	1 slice	25	36	60	3	1	—	—	—	12	25	.8	Trace	.06	.03	.7	Trace
373	Slice, toasted	1 slice	21	24	60	3	1	—	—	—	12	25	.8	Trace	.06	.03	.7	Trace
374	Breadcrumbs, dry, grated	1 cup	100	6	390	13	5	1	2	1	73	122	3.6	Trace	.22	.30	3.5	Trace
375	Buckwheat flour, light, sifted	1 cup	98	12	340	6	1	—	—	—	78	11	1.0	0	.08	.04	.4	0
376	Bulgur, canned, seasoned	1 cup	135	56	245	8	4	—	—	—	44	27	1.9	0	.08	.05	4.1	0
	Cakes made from cake mixes:																	
	Angelfood:																	
377	Whole cake	1 cake	635	34	1645	36	1	—	—	—	377	603	1.9	0	.03	.70	.6	0
378	Piece, 1/12 of 10-in. diam. cake	1 piece	53	34	135	3	Trace	—	—	—	32	50	.2	0	Trace	.06	.1	0
	Cupcakes, small, 2½ in. diam.:																	
379	Without icing	1 cupcake	25	26	90	1	3	1	1	1	14	40	.1	40	.01	.03	.1	Trace
380	With chocolate icing	1 cupcake	36	22	130	2	5	2	2	1	21	47	.3	60	.01	.04	.1	Trace
	Devil's food, 2-layer, with chocolate icing:																	
381	Whole cake	1 cake	1107	24	3755	49	136	54	58	16	645	653	8.9	1660	.33	.89	3.3	1
382	Piece, 1/16 of 9-in. diam. cake	1 piece	69	24	235	3	9	3	4	1	40	41	.6	100	.02	.06	.2	Trace
383	Cupcake, small, 2½ in. diam.	1 cupcake	35	24	120	2	4	1	2	Trace	20	21	.3	50	.01	.03	.1	Trace
	Gingerbread:																	
384	Whole cake	1 cake	570	37	1575	18	39	10	19	9	291	513	9.1	Trace	.17	.51	4.6	2
385	Piece, 1/9 of 8-in. square cake	1 piece	63	37	175	2	4	1	2	1	32	57	1.0	Trace	.02	.06	.5	Trace
	White, 2-layer, with chocolate icing:																	
386	Whole cake	1 cake	1140	21	4000	45	122	45	54	17	716	1129	5.7	680	.23	.91	2.3	2
387	Piece, 1/16 of 9-in. diam. cake	1 piece	71	21	250	3	8	3	3	1	45	70	.4	40	.01	.06	.1	Trace
	Cakes made from home recipes:[p]																	
388	Boston cream pie; piece 1/12 of 8-in. diam.	1 piece	69	35	210	4	6	2	3	1	34	46	.3	140	.02	.08	.1	Trace
	Fruitcake, dark, made with enriched flour::																	
389	Loaf, 1-lb	1 loaf	454	18	1720	22	69	15	37	13	271	327	11.8	540	.59	.64	3.6	2
390	Slice, 1/30 of 8-in. loaf	1 slice	15	18	55	1	2	Trace	1	Trace	9	11	.4	20	.02	.02	.1	Trace

° Values for iron, thiamin, riboflavin, and niacin per pound of unenriched white bread would be as follows:

	Iron (mg)	Thiamin (mg)	Riboflavin (mg)	Niacin (mg)
Soft crumb	3.2	.31	.39	5.0
Firm crumb	3.2	.32	.59	4.1

[p] Unenriched cake flour used unless otherwise specified.

Table 1 (continued)

	Food, Approximate Measure, and Weight (in Grams)		Water (%)	Food Energy (kcal)	Protein (g)	Fat (g)	Saturated (total) (g)	Unsaturated Oleic (g)	Unsaturated Linoleic (g)	Carbohydrate (g)	Calcium (mg)	Iron (mg)	Vitamin A value (I.U.)	Thiamin (mg)	Riboflavin (mg)	Niacin (mg)	Ascorbic acid (mg)
	GRAIN PRODUCTS—Continued																
	Plain sheet cake:																
	Without icing:																
391	Whole cake	1 cake 777	25	2830	35	108	30	52	21	434	497	3.1	1320	.16	.70	1.6	2
392	Piece, 1/9 of 9-in. square cake	1 piece 86	25	315	4	12	3	6	2	48	55	.3	150	.02	.08	.2	Trace
393	With boiled white icing, piece, 1/9 of 9-in. square cake	1 piece 114	23	400	4	12	3	6	2	71	56	.3	150	.02	.08	.2	Trace
	Pound:																
394	Loaf, 8½ by 3½ by 3 in.	1 loaf 514	17	2430	29	152	34	68	17	242	108	4.1	1440	.15	.46	1.0	0
395	Slice, ½-in. thick	1 slice 30	17	140	2	9	2	4	1	14	6	.2	80	.01	.03	.1	0
	Sponge:																
396	Whole cake	1 cake 790	32	2345	60	45	14	20	4	427	237	9.5	3560	.40	1.11	1.6	Trace
397	Piece, 1/12 of 10-in. diam. cake	1 piece 66	32	195	5	4	1	2	Trace	36	20	.8	300	.03	.09	.1	Trace
	Yellow, 2-layer, without icing:																
398	Whole cake	1 cake 870	24	3160	39	111	31	53	22	506	618	3.5	1310	.17	.70	1.7	2
399	Piece, 1/16 of 9-in. diam. cake	1 piece 54	24	200	2	7	2	3	1	32	39	.2	80	.01	.04	.1	Trace
	Yellow, 2-layer, with chocolate icing:																
400	Whole cake	1 cake 1203	21	4390	51	156	55	69	23	727	818	7.2	1920	.24	.96	2.4	Trace
401	Piece, 1/16 of 9-in. diam. cake	1 piece 75	21	275	3	10	3	4	1	45	51	.5	120	.02	.06	.2	Trace
	Cake icings. See Sugars, Sweets,																
	Cookies:																
	Brownies with nuts:																
402	Made from home recipe with enriched flour	1 brownie 20	10	95	1	6	1	3	1	10	8	.4	40	.04	.02	.1	Trace
403	Made from mix	1 brownie 20	11	85	1	4	1	2	1	13	9	.4	20	.03	.02	.1	Trace
	Chocolate chip:																
404	Made from home recipe with enriched flour	1 cookie 10	3	50	1	3	1	1	1	6	4	.2	10	.01	.01	.1	Trace
405	Commercial	1 cookie 10	3	50	1	2	1	1	Trace	7	4	.2	10	Trace	Trace	Trace	Trace

No.	Food	Measure																
406	Fig bars, commercial	1 cookie	14	14	50	1	1	—	—	—	11	11	.2	20	Trace	.01	.1	Trace
407	Sandwich, chocolate or vanilla, commercial	1 cookie	10	2	50	1	2	1	1	Trace	7	2	.1	0	Trace	Trace	.1	0
	Corn flakes, added nutrients:																	
408	Plain	1 cup	25	4	100	2	Trace	—	—	—	21	4	.4	0	.11	.02	.5	0
409	Sugar-covered	1 cup	40	2	155	2	Trace	—	—	—	36	5	.4	0	.16	.02	.8	0
	Corn (hominy) grits, degermed, cooked:																	
410	Enriched	1 cup	245	87	125	3	Trace	—	—	—	27	2	.7	150[q]	.10	.07	1.0	0
411	Unenriched	1 cup	245	87	125	3	Trace	—	—	—	27	2	.2	150[q]	.05	.02	.5	0
	Cornmeal:																	
412	Whole-ground, unbolted, dry	1 cup	122	12	435	11	5	1	1	2	90	24	2.9	620[q]	.46	.13	2.4	0
413	Bolted (nearly whole-grain) dry	1 cup	122	12	440	11	4	Trace	1	2	91	21	2.2	590[q]	.37	.10	2.3	0
	Degermed, enriched:																	
414	Dry form	1 cup	138	12	550	11	2	—	—	—	108	8	4.0	610[q]	.61	.36	4.8	0
415	Cooked	1 cup	240	88	120	3	1	—	—	—	26	2	1.0	140[q]	.14	.10	1.2	0
	Degermed, unenriched:																	
416	Dry form	1 cup	138	12	500	11	2	—	—	—	108	8	1.5	610[q]	.19	.07	1.4	0
417	Cooked	1 cup	240	88	120	3	1	—	—	—	26	2	.5	140[q]	.05	.02	.2	0
418	Corn muffins, made with enriched degermed cornmeal and enriched flour; muffin 2 3/8-in. diam.	1 muffin	40	33	125	3	4	2	2	Trace	19	42	.7	120[q]	.08	.09	.6	Trace
419	Corn muffins, made with mix, egg, and milk; muffin 2 3/8-in. diam.	1 muffin	40	30	130	3	4	1	2	1	20	96	.6	100	.07	.08	.6	Trace
420	Corn, puffed, presweetened, added nutrients	1 cup	30	2	115	1	Trace	—	—	—	27	3	.5	0	.13	.05	.6	0
421	Corn, shredded, added nutrients	1 cup	25	3	100	2	Trace	—	—	—	22	1	.6	0	.11	.05	.5	0
	Crackers:																	
422	Graham, 2½-in. square	4 crackers	28	6	110	2	3	1	1	—	21	11	.4	0	.01	.06	.4	0
423	Saltines	4 crackers	11	4	50	1	1	—	—	—	8	2	.1	0	Trace	Trace	.1	0
424	Danish pastry, plain (without fruit or nuts): Packaged ring, 12 oz	1 ring	340	22	1435	25	80	24	37	15	155	170	3.1	1050	.24	.51	2.7	Trace

[q] This value is based on product made from yellow varieties of corn; white varieties contain only a trace.

Table 1 (continued)

	Food, Approximate Measure, and Weight (in Grams)		Weight (g)	Water (%)	Food Energy (kcal)	Protein (g)	Fat (g)	Fatty Acids			Carbohydrate (g)	Calcium (mg)	Iron (mg)	Vitamin A value (I.U.)	Thiamin (mg)	Riboflavin (mg)	Niacin (mg)	Ascorbic acid (mg)
								Saturated (total) (g)	Unsaturated Oleic (g)	Unsaturated Linoleic (g)								
	GRAIN PRODUCTS—Continued																	
425	Round piece, approx. 4¼-in. diam. by 1 in.	1 pastry	65	22	275	5	15	5	7	3	30	33	.6	200	.05	.10	.5	Trace
426	Ounce	1 oz	28	22	120	2	7	2	3	1	13	14	.3	90	.02	.04	.2	Trace
427	Doughnuts, cake type	1 doughnut	32	24	125	1	6	1	4	Trace	16	13	.4[r]	30	.05[r]	.05[r]	.4[r]	Trace
428	Farina, quick-cooking, enriched, cooked	1 cup	245	89	105	3	Trace	—	—	—	22	147	.7[s]	0	.12[s]	.07[s]	1.0[s]	0
	Macaroni, cooked: Enriched:																	
429	Cooked, firm stage (undergoes additional cooking in a food mixture)	1 cup	130	64	190	6	1	—	—	—	39	14	1.4[s]	0	.23[s]	.14[s]	1.8[s]	0
430	Cooked until tender	1 cup	140	72	155	5	1	—	—	—	32	8	1.3[s]	0	.20[s]	.11[s]	1.5[s]	0
	Unenriched:																	
431	Cooked, firm stage (undergoes additional cooking in a food mixture)	1 cup	130	64	190	6	1	—	—	—	39	14	.7	0	.03	.03	.5	0
432	Cooked until tender	1 cup	140	72	155	5	1	—	—	—	32	11	.6	0	.01	.01	.4	0
433	Macaroni (enriched) and cheese, baked	1 cup	200	58	430	17	22	10	9	2	40	362	1.8	860	.20	.40	1.8	Trace
434	Canned	1 cup	240	80	230	9	10	4	3	1	26	199	1.0	260	.12	.24	1.0	Trace
435	Muffins, with enriched white flour; muffin, 3-in. diam.	1 muffin	40	38	120	3	4	1	2	1	17	42	.6	40	.07	.09	.6	Trace
	Noodles (egg noodles), cooked:																	
436	Enriched	1 cup	160	70	200	7	2	1	1	Trace	37	16	1.4[s]	110	.22[s]	.13[s]	1.9[s]	0
437	Unenriched	1 cup	160	70	200	7	2	1	1	Trace	37	16	1.0	110	.05	.03	.6	0
438	Oats (with or without corn) puffed, added nutrients	1 cup	25	3	100	3	1	—	—	—	19	44	1.2	0	.24	.04	.5	0
439	Oatmeal or rolled oats, cooked	1 cup	240	87	130	5	2	—	—	1	23	22	1.4	0	.19	.05	.2	0

No.	Food	Measure																
	Pancakes, 4-inch diam.:																	
440	Wheat, enriched flour (home recipe)	1 cake	27	50	60	2	2	Trace	1	Trace	9	27	.4	30	.05	.06	.4	Trace
441	Buckwheat (made from mix with egg and milk)	1 cake	27	58	55	2	2	1	1	Trace	6	59	.4	60	.03	.04	.2	Trace
442	Plain or buttermilk (made from mix with egg and milk)	1 cake	27	51	60	2	2	1	1	Trace	9	58	.3	70	.04	.06	.2	Trace
	Pie (piecrust made with unenriched flour): Sector, 4-in., 1/7 of 9-in. diam. pie:																	
443	Apple (2-crust)	1 sector	135	48	350	3	15	4	7	3	51	11	.4	40	.03	.03	.5	1
444	Butterscotch (1-crust)	1 sector	130	45	350	6	14	5	6	2	50	98	1.2	340	.04	.13	.3	Trace
445	Cherry (2-crust)	1 sector	135	47	350	4	15	4	7	3	52	19	.4	590	.03	.03	.7	Trace
446	Custard (1-crust)	1 sector	130	58	285	8	14	5	6	2	30	125	.8	300	.07	.21	.4	0
447	Lemon meringue (1-crust)	1 sector	120	47	305	4	12	4	6	2	45	17	.6	200	.04	.10	.2	4
448	Mince (2-crust)	1 sector	135	43	365	3	16	4	8	3	56	38	1.4	Trace	.09	.05	.5	1
449	Pecan (1-crust)	1 sector	118	20	490	6	27	4	16	5	60	55	3.3	190	.19	.08	.4	Trace
450	Pineapple chiffon (1-crust)	1 sector	93	41	265	6	11	3	5	2	36	22	.8	320	.04	.08	.4	1
451	Pumpkin (1-crust)	1 sector	130	59	275	5	15	5	6	2	32	66	.7	3210	.04	.13	.7	Trace
	Piecrust, baked shell for pie made with:																	
452	Enriched flour	1 shell	180	15	900	11	60	16	28	12	79	25	3.1	0	.36	.25	3.2	0
453	Unenriched flour	1 shell	180	15	900	11	60	16	28	12	79	25	.9	0	.05	.05	.9	0
	Piecrust mix including stick form:																	
454	Package, 10-oz, for double crust	1 pkg	284	9	1480	20	93	23	46	21	141	131	1.4	0	.11	.11	2.0	0
455	Pizza (cheese) 5½-in. sector; 1/8 of 14-in. diam. pie	1 sector	75	45	185	7	6	2	3	Trace	27	107	.7	290	.04	.12	.7	4
	Popcorn, popped:																	
456	Plain, large kernel	1 cup	6	4	25	1	Trace	—	—	—	5	1	.2	—	—	.01	.1	0
457	With oil and salt	1 cup	9	3	40	1	2	1	Trace	Trace	5	1	.2	—	—	.01	.2	0
458	Sugar coated	1 cup	35	4	135	2	1	—	—	—	30	2	.5	—	—	.02	.4	0

r Based on product made with enriched flour. With unenriched flour, approximate values per doughnut are: Iron, 0.2 milligram; thiamin, 0.01 milligram; riboflavin, 0.03 milligram; niacin, 0.2 milligram.

s Iron, thiamin, riboflavin, and niacin are based on the minimum levels of enrichment specified in standards of identity promulgated under the Federal Food, Drug, and Cosmetic Act.

Table 1 (continued)

#	Food, Approximate Measure, and Weight (in Grams)		Water (%)	Food Energy (kcal)	Protein (g)	Fat (g)	Fatty Acids Saturated (total) (g)	Fatty Acids Unsaturated Oleic (g)	Fatty Acids Unsaturated Linoleic (g)	Carbohydrate (g)	Calcium (mg)	Iron (mg)	Vitamin A value (I.U.)	Thiamin (mg)	Riboflavin (mg)	Niacin (mg)	Ascorbic acid (mg)
	GRAIN PRODUCTS—Continued																
	Pretzels:																
459	Dutch, twisted	1 pretzel	16	5	60	2	1	—	—	—	12	4	.2	0	Trace	Trace	.1	0
460	Thin, twisted	1 pretzel	6	5	25	1	Trace	—	—	—	5	1	.1	0	Trace	Trace	Trace	0
461	Stick, small, 2¼ in.	10 sticks	3	5	10	Trace	Trace	—	—	—	2	1	Trace	0	Trace	Trace	Trace	0
462	Stick, regular, 3 1/8 inches	5 sticks	3	5	10	Trace	Trace	—	—	—	2	1	Trace	0	Trace	Trace	Trace	0
	Rice, white:																	
	Enriched:																	
463	Raw	1 cup	185	12	670	12	1	—	—	—	149	44	5.4t	0	.81t	.06t	6.5t	0
464	Cooked	1 cup	205	73	225	4	Trace	—	—	—	50	21	1.8t	0	.23t	.02t	2.1t	0
465	Instant, ready-to-serve	1 cup	165	73	180	4	Trace	—	—	—	40	5	1.3t	0	.21t	–t	1.7t	0
466	Unenriched, cooked	1 cup	205	73	225	4	Trace	—	—	—	50	21	.4	0	.04	.02	.8	0
467	Parboiled, cooked	1 cup	175	73	185	4	Trace	—	—	—	41	33	1.4t	0	.19t	–t	2.1t	0
468	Rice, puffed, added nutrients	1 cup	15	4	60	1	Trace	—	—	—	13	3	.3	0	.07	.01	.7	0
	Rolls, enriched:																	
	Cloverleaf or pan:																	
469	Home recipe	1 roll	35	26	120	3	3	1	1	1	20	16	.7	30	.09	.09	.8	Trace
470	Commercial	1 roll	28	31	85	2	2	Trace	1	Trace	15	21	.5	Trace	.08	.05	.6	Trace
471	Frankfurter or hamburger	1 roll	40	31	120	3	2	1	1	1	21	30	.8	Trace	.11	.07	.9	Trace
472	Hard, round or rectangular	1 roll	50	25	155	5	2	Trace	1	Trace	30	24	1.2	Trace	.13	.12	1.4	Trace
473	Rye wafers, whole-grain, 1 7/8 by 3 1/2 in.	2 wafers	13	6	45	2	Trace	—	—	—	10	7	.5	0	.04	.03	.2	0
474	Spaghetti, cooked, tender stage, enriched	1 cup	140	72	155	5	1	—	—	—	32	11	1.3s	0	.20t	.11s	1.5s	0
	Spaghetti with meat balls, and tomato sauce:																	
475	Home recipe	1 cup	248	70	330	19	12	4	6	1	39	124	3.7	1590	.25	.30	4.0	22
476	Canned	1 cup	250	78	260	12	10	2	3	4	28	53	3.3	1000	.15	.18	2.3	5
	Spaghetti in tomato sauce with cheese:																	
477	Home recipe	1 cup	250	77	260	9	9	2	5	1	37	80	2.3	1080	.25	.18	2.3	13
478	Canned	1 cup	250	80	190	6	2	1	1	1	38	40	2.8	930	.35	.28	4.5	10
479	Waffles, with enriched flour, 7-in. diam.	1 waffle	75	41	210	7	7	2	4	1	28	85	1.3	250	.13	.19	1.0	Trace

No.	Food, approximate measure, and weight (in grams)	Measure	Grams	Water (%)	Food energy (cal)	Protein (g)	Fat (g)	Saturated (g)	Oleic (g)	Linoleic (g)	Carbohydrate (g)	Calcium (mg)	Iron (mg)	Vitamin A (I.U.)	Thiamin (mg)	Riboflavin (mg)	Niacin (mg)	Ascorbic acid (mg)
480	Waffles, made from mix, enriched, egg and milk added, 7-in. diam.	1 waffle	75	42	205	7	8	3	3	1	27	179	1.0	170	.11	.17	.7	Trace
481	Wheat, puffed, added nutrients	1 cup	15	3	55	2	Trace	—	—	—	12	4	.6	0	.08	.03	1.2	0
482	Wheat, shredded, plain	1 biscuit	25	7	90	2	1	—	—	—	20	11	.9	0	.06	.03	1.1	0
483	Wheat flakes, added nutrients	1 cup	30	4	105	3	Trace	—	—	—	24	12	1.3	0	.19	.04	1.5	0
	Wheat flours:																	
484	Whole-wheat, from hard wheats, stirred	1 cup	120	12	400	16	2	Trace	1	1	85	49	4.0	0	.66	.14	5.2	0
	All-purpose or family flour, enriched:																	
485	Sifted	1 cup	115	12	420	12	1	—	—	—	88	18	3.3[s]	0	.51[s]	.30[s]	4.0[s]	0
486	Unsifted	1 cup	125	12	455	13	1	—	—	—	95	20	3.6[s]	0	.55[s]	.33[s]	4.4[s]	0
487	Self-rising, enriched	1 cup	125	12	440	12	1	—	—	—	93	331	3.6[s]	0	.55[s]	.33[s]	4.4[s]	0
488	Cake or pastry flour, sifted	1 cup	96	12	350	7	1	—	—	—	76	16	.5	0	.03	.03	.7	0

FATS, OILS

No.	Food, approximate measure, and weight (in grams)	Measure	Grams	Water (%)	Food energy (cal)	Protein (g)	Fat (g)	Saturated (g)	Oleic (g)	Linoleic (g)	Carbohydrate (g)	Calcium (mg)	Iron (mg)	Vitamin A (I.U.)	Thiamin (mg)	Riboflavin (mg)	Niacin (mg)	Ascorbic acid (mg)
	Butter:																	
	Regular, 4 sticks per lb:																	
489	Stick	½ cup	113	16	810	1	92	51	30	3	1	23	0	3750[u]	—	—	—	0
490	Tablespoon (approx. 1/8 stick)	1 tbsp	14	16	100	Trace	12	6	4	Trace	Trace	3	0	470[u]	—	—	—	0
491	Pat (1-in. sq. 1/3-in. high; 90 per lb)	1 pat	5	16	35	Trace	4	2	1	Trace	Trace	1	0	170[u]	—	—	—	0
	Whipped, 6 sticks or 2, 8-oz containers per pound:																	
492	Stick	½ cup	76	16	540	1	61	34	20	2	Trace	15	0	2500[u]	—	—	—	0
493	Tablespoon (approx. 1/8 stick)	1 tbsp	9	16	65	Trace	8	4	3	Trace	Trace	2	0	310[u]	—	—	—	0
494	Pat (1¼-in. sq 1/3-in. high; 120 per lb)	1 pat	4	16	25	Trace	3	2	1	Trace	Trace	1	0	130[u]	—	—	—	0

[s] Iron, thiamin, riboflavin, and niacin are based on the minimum levels of enrichment specified in standards of identity promulgated under the Federal Food, Drug, and Cosmetic Act.

[t] Iron, thiamin, and niacin are based on the minimum levels of enrichment specified in standards of identity promulgated under the Federal Food, Drug, and Cosmetic Act. Riboflavin is based on unenriched rice. When the minimum level of enrichment for riboflavin specified in the standards of identity becomes effective the value will be 0.12 milligram per cup of parboiled rice and of white rice.

[u] Year-round average.

Table 1 (continued)

No.	Food, Approximate Measure, and Weight (in Grams)			Water (%)	Food Energy (kcal)	Protein (g)	Fat (g)	Fatty Acids			Carbohydrate (g)	Calcium (mg)	Iron (mg)	Vitamin A value (I.U.)	Thiamin (mg)	Riboflavin (mg)	Niacin (mg)	Ascorbic acid (mg)
								Saturated (total) (g)	Unsaturated Oleic (g)	Unsaturated Linoleic (g)								
	FATS, OILS—Continued																	
	Fats, cooking:																	
495	Lard	1 cup	205	0	1850	0	205	78	94	20	0	0	0	0	0	0	0	0
496		1 tbsp	13	0	115	0	13	5	6	1	0	0	0	0	0	0	0	0
497	Vegetable fats	1 cup	200	0	1770	0	200	50	100	44	0	0	0	—	0	0	0	0
498		1 tbsp	13	0	110	0	13	3	6	3	0	0	0	—	0	0	0	0
	Margarine:																	
	Regular, 4 sticks per pound:																	
499	Stick	½ cup	113	16	815	1	92	17	46	25	1	23	0	3750[v]	—	—	—	0
500	Tablespoon (approx. 1/8 stick)	1 tbsp	14	16	100	Trace	12	2	6	3	Trace	3	0	470[v]	—	—	—	0
501	Pat (1-in. sq 1/3-in. high; 1 pat 90 per lb)	1 pat	5	16	35	Trace	4	1	2	1	Trace	1	0	170[v]	—	—	—	0
	Whipped, 6 sticks per lb:																	
502	Stick	½ cup	76	16	545	1	61	11	31	17	Trace	15	0	2500[v]	—	—	—	0
	Soft, 2 8-oz tubs per lb:																	
503	Tub	1 tub	227	16	1635	1	184	34	68	68	1	45	0	7500[v]	—	—	—	0
504	Tablespoon	1 tbsp	14	16	100	Trace	11	2	4	4	Trace	3	0	470[v]	—	—	—	0
	Oils, salad or cooking:																	
505	Corn	1 cup	220	0	1945	0	220	22	62	117	0	0	0	—	0	0	0	0
506		1 tbsp	14	0	125	0	14	1	4	7	0	0	0	—	0	0	0	0
507	Cottonseed	1 cup	220	0	1945	0	220	55	46	110	0	0	0	—	0	0	0	0
508		1 tbsp	14	0	125	0	14	4	3	7	0	0	0	—	0	0	0	0
509	Olive	1 cup	220	0	1945	0	220	24	167	15	0	0	0	—	0	0	0	0
510		1 tbsp	14	0	125	0	14	2	11	1	0	0	0	—	0	0	0	0
511	Peanut	1 cup	220	0	1945	0	220	40	103	64	0	0	0	—	0	0	0	0
512		1 tbsp	14	0	125	0	14	3	7	4	0	0	0	—	0	0	0	0
513	Safflower	1 cup	220	0	1945	0	220	18	37	165	0	0	0	—	0	0	0	0
514		1 tbsp	14	0	125	0	14	1	2	10	0	0	0	—	0	0	0	0
515	Soybean	1 cup	220	0	1945	0	220	33	44	114	0	0	0	—	0	0	0	0
516		1 tbsp	14	0	125	0	14	2	3	7	0	0	0	—	0	0	0	0

No.	Food, approximate measure		Grams	Water (%)	Food energy (cal)	Protein (g)	Fat (g)	Saturated fatty acids (g)	Unsaturated Oleic (g)	Unsaturated Linoleic (g)	Carbohydrate (g)	Calcium (mg)	Iron (mg)	Vitamin A (I.U.)	Thiamin (mg)	Riboflavin (mg)	Niacin (mg)	Ascorbic acid (mg)
	Salad dressings:																	
517	Blue cheese	1 tbsp	15	32	75	1	8	2	2	4	1	12	Trace	30	Trace	.02	Trace	Trace
	Commercial, mayonnaise type:																	
518	Regular	1 tbsp	15	41	65	Trace	6	1	1	3	2	2	Trace	30	Trace	Trace	Trace	—
519	Special dietary, low-calorie	1 tbsp	16	81	20	Trace	2	Trace	Trace	1	1	3	Trace	40	Trace	Trace	Trace	—
	French:																	
520	Regular	1 tbsp	16	39	65	Trace	6	1	1	3	3	2	.1	—	—	—	—	—
521	Special dietary, lowfat with artificial sweeteners	1 tbsp	15	95	Trace	Trace	Trace	—	—	—	Trace	2	.1	—	—	—	—	—
522	Home cooked, boiled	1 tbsp	16	68	25	1	2	1	1	Trace	2	14	.1	80	.01	.03	Trace	Trace
523	Mayonnaise	1 tbsp	14	15	100	Trace	11	2	2	6	Trace	3	.1	40	Trace	.01	Trace	—
524	Thousand island	1 tbsp	16	32	80	Trace	8	1	2	4	3	2	.1	50	Trace	Trace	Trace	Trace
	SUGARS, SWEETS																	
	Cake icings:																	
525	Chocolate made with milk and table fat	1 cup	275	14	1035	9	38	21	14	1	185	165	3.3	580	.06	.28	.6	1
526	Coconut (with boiled icing)	1 cup	166	15	605	3	13	11	1	Trace	124	10	.8	0	.02	.07	.3	0
527	Creamy fudge from mix with water only	1 cup	245	15	830	7	16	5	8	3	183	96	2.7	Trace	.05	.20	.7	Trace
528	White, boiled	1 cup	94	18	300	1	0	—	—	—	76	2	Trace	0	Trace	.03	Trace	0
	Candy:																	
529	Caramels, plain or chocolate	1 oz	28	8	115	1	3	2	1	Trace	22	42	.4	Trace	.01	.05	.1	Trace
530	Chocolate, milk, plain	1 oz	28	1	145	2	9	5	3	Trace	16	65	.3	80	.02	.10	.1	Trace
531	Chocolate-coated peanuts	1 oz	28	1	160	5	12	3	6	2	11	33	.4	Trace	.10	.05	2.1	Trace
532	Fondant; mints, uncoated; candy corn	1 oz	28	8	105	Trace	1	—	—	—	25	4	.3	0	Trace	Trace	Trace	0
533	Fudge, plain	1 oz	28	8	115	1	4	2	1	Trace	21	22	.3	Trace	.01	.03	.1	Trace
534	Gum drops	1 oz	28	12	100	Trace	Trace	—	—	—	25	2	.1	0	0	Trace	Trace	0
535	Hard	1 oz	28	1	110	0	Trace	—	—	—	28	6	.5	0	0	0	0	0
536	Marshmallows	1 oz	28	17	90	1	Trace	—	—	—	23	5	.5	0	0	Trace	Trace	0
	Chocolate-flavored sirup or topping:																	
537	Thin type	1 fl oz	38	32	90	1	1	Trace	Trace	Trace	24	6	.6	Trace	.01	.03	.2	0
538	Fudge type	1 fl oz	38	25	125	2	5	3	2	Trace	20	48	.5	60	.02	.08	.2	Trace

v Based on the average vitamin A content of fortified margarine. Federal specifications for fortified margarine require a minimum of 15,000 I.U. of vitamin A per pound.

Table 1 (continued)

	Food, Approximate Measure, and Weight (in Grams)		Water (%)	Food Energy (kcal)	Protein (g)	Fat (g)	Fatty Acids			Carbohydrate (g)	Calcium (mg)	Iron (mg)	Vitamin A value (I.U.)	Thiamin (mg)	Riboflavin (mg)	Niacin (mg)	Ascorbic acid (mg)
							Saturated (total) (g)	Unsaturated Oleic (g)	Linoleic (g)								
	SUGARS, SWEETS–Continued																
	Chocolate-flavored beverage powder (approx. 4 heaping tsp per oz):																
539	With nonfat dry milk	1 oz	28	2	100	5	1	Trace	Trace	Trace	20	167	.5	10	.04	.21	.2	1
540	Without nonfat dry milk	1 oz	28	1	100	1	1	Trace	Trace	Trace	25	9	.6	—	.01	.03	.1	0
541	Honey, strained or extracted	1 tbsp	21	17	65	Trace	0	—	—	—	17	1	.1	Trace	Trace	.01	.1	Trace
542	Jams and preserves	1 tbsp	20	29	55	Trace	Trace	—	—	—	14	4	.2	Trace	Trace	.01	Trace	Trace
543	Jellies	1 tbsp	18	29	50	Trace	Trace	—	—	—	13	4	.3	Trace	Trace	.01	Trace	1
	Molasses, cane:																	
544	Light (first extraction)	1 tbsp	20	24	50	—	—	—	—	—	13	33	.9	—	.01	.01	Trace	—
545	Blackstrap (third extraction)	1 tbsp	20	24	45	—	—	—	—	—	11	137	3.2	—	.02	.04	.4	—
	Sirups:																	
546	Sorghum	1 tbsp	21	23	55	—	—	—	—	—	14	35	2.6	—	—	.02	Trace	—
547	Table blends, chiefly corn, light and dark	1 tbsp	21	24	60	0	0	—	—	—	15	9	.8	0	0	0	0	0
	Sugars:																	
548	Brown, firm packed	1 cup	220	2	820	0	0	—	—	—	212	187	7.5	0	.02	.07	.4	0
	White:																	
549	Granulated	1 cup	200	Trace	770	0	0	—	—	—	199	0	.2	0	0	0	0	0
550		1 tbsp	11	Trace	40	0	0	—	—	—	11	0	Trace	0	0	0	0	0
551	Powdered, stirred before measuring	1 cup	120	Trace	460	0	0	—	—	—	119	0	.1	0	0	0	0	0
	MISCELLANEOUS ITEMS																	
552	Barbecue sauce	1 cup	250	81	230	4	17	2	5	9	20	53	2.0	900	.03	.03	.8	13
	Beverages, alcoholic:																	
553	Beer	12 fl oz	360	92	150	1	0	—	—	—	14	18	Trace	—	.01	.11	2.2	—
	Gin, rum, vodka, whiskey:																	
554	80-proof	1½ fl oz jigger	42	67	100	—	—	—	—	—	Trace	—	—	—	—	—	—	—

No.	Food	Measure	Grams	Water (%)	Food energy (cal)	Protein (g)	Fat (g)	Saturated (g)	Oleic (g)	Linoleic (g)	Carbohydrate (g)	Calcium (mg)	Iron (mg)	Vitamin A (IU)	Thiamin (mg)	Riboflavin (mg)	Niacin (mg)	Ascorbic acid (mg)
555	86-proof	1½ fl oz jigger	42	64	105	—	—	—	—	—	Trace	—	—	—	—	—	—	—
556	90-proof	1½ fl oz jigger	42	62	110	—	—	—	—	—	Trace	—	—	—	—	—	—	—
557	94-proof	1½ fl oz jigger	42	60	115	—	—	—	—	—	Trace	—	—	—	—	—	—	—
558	100-proof	1½ fl oz jigger	42	58	125	—	—	—	—	—	Trace	—	—	—	—	—	—	—
	Wines:																	
559	Dessert	3½ fl oz glass	103	77	140	Trace	0	—	—	—	8	8	—	—	.01	.02	.2	—
560	Table	3½ fl oz glass	102	86	85	Trace	0	—	—	—	4	9	.4	—	Trace	.01	.1	—
	Beverages, carbonated, sweetened, nonalcoholic:																	
561	Carbonated water	12 fl oz	366	92	115	0	0	—	—	—	29	—	—	—	0	0	0	0
562	Cola type	12 fl oz	369	90	145	0	0	—	—	—	37	—	—	—	0	0	0	0
563	Fruit-flavored sodas and Tom Collins mixes	12 fl oz	372	88	170	0	0	—	—	—	45	—	—	—	0	0	0	0
564	Ginger ale	12 fl oz	366	92	115	0	0	—	—	—	29	—	—	—	0	0	0	0
565	Root beer	12 fl oz	370	90	150	0	0	—	—	—	39	—	—	—	0	0	0	0
566	Bouillon cubes, approx. ½ in.	1 cube	4	4	5	1	Trace	—	—	—	Trace	—	—	—	—	—	—	—
	Chocolate:																	
567	Bitter or baking	1 oz	28	2	145	3	15	8	6	Trace	8	22	1.9	20	.01	.07	.4	0
568	Semisweet, small pieces	1 cup	170	1	860	7	61	34	22	1	97	51	4.4	30	.02	.14	.9	0
	Gelatin:																	
569	Plain, dry powder in envelope	1 envelope	7	13	25	6	Trace	—	—	—	0	—	—	—	—	—	—	—
570	Dessert powder, 3-oz package	1 pkg	85	2	315	8	0	—	—	—	75	—	—	—	—	—	—	—
571	Gelatin dessert, prepared with water	1 cup	240	84	140	4	0	—	—	—	34	—	—	—	—	—	—	—
	Olives, pickled:																	
572	Green	4 medium or 3 extra large or 2 giant	16	78	15	Trace	2	Trace	2	Trace	Trace	8	.2	40	—	—	—	—
573	Ripe: Mission	3 small or 2 large	10	73	15	Trace	2	Trace	2	Trace	Trace	9	.1	10	Trace	Trace	—	—

Table 1 (continued)

	Food, Approximate Measure, and Weight (in Grams)		Water (%)	Food Energy (kcal)	Protein (g)	Fat (g)	Fatty Acids Saturated (total) (g)	Unsaturated Oleic (g)	Unsaturated Linoleic (g)	Carbohydrate (g)	Calcium (mg)	Iron (mg)	Vitamin A value (I.U.)	Thiamin (mg)	Riboflavin (mg)	Niacin (mg)	Ascorbic acid (mg)
	MISCELLANEOUS ITEMS—Continued																
	Pickles, cucumber:																
574	Dill, medium, whole, 3¾ in. long, 1¼ in. diam. 1 pickle	65	93	10	1	Trace	—	—	—	1	17	.7	70	Trace	.01	Trace	4
575	Fresh, sliced, 1½ in. diam., ¼ in. thick 2 slices	15	79	10	Trace	Trace	—	—	—	3	5	.3	20	Trace	Trace	Trace	1
576	Sweet, gherkin, small, whole, approx. 2½ in. long, ¾ in. diam. 1 pickle	15	61	20	Trace	Trace	—	—	—	6	2	.2	10	Trace	Trace	Trace	1
577	Relish, finely chopped, sweet 1 tbsp	15	63	20	Trace	Trace	—	—	—	5	3	.1	—	—	—	—	—
	Popcorn. See Grain Products.																
578	Popsicle, 3 fl oz size 1 popsicle	95	80	70	0	0	0	0	0	18	0	Trace	0	0	0	0	0
	Pudding, home recipe with starch base:																
579	Chocolate 1 cup	260	66	385	8	12	7	4	Trace	67	250	1.3	390	.05	.36	.3	1
580	Vanilla (blanc mange) 1 cup	255	76	285	9	10	5	3	Trace	41	298	Trace	410	.08	.41	.3	2
581	Pudding mix, dry form, 4 oz package 1 pkg	113	2	410	3	2	1	1	Trace	103	23	1.8	Trace	.02	.08	.5	0
582	Sherbet 1 cup	193	67	260	2	2	—	—	—	59	31	Trace	120	.02	.06	Trace	4
	Soups:																
	Canned, condensed, ready-to-serve:																
	Prepared with an equal volume of milk:																
583	Cream of chicken 1 cup	245	85	180	7	10	3	3	3	15	172	.5	610	.05	.27	.7	2
584	Cream of mushroom 1 cup	245	83	215	7	14	4	4	5	16	191	.5	250	.05	.34	.7	1
585	Tomato 1 cup	250	84	175	7	7	3	2	1	23	168	.8	1200	.10	.25	1.3	15
	Prepared with an equal volume of water:																
586	Bean with pork 1 cup	250	84	170	8	6	1	2	2	22	63	2.3	650	.13	.08	1.0	3
587	Beef broth, bouillon consomme 1 cup	240	96	30	5	0	—	—	—	3	Trace	.5	Trace	Trace	.02	1.2	—
588	Beef noodle 1 cup	240	93	70	4	3	1	1	1	7	7	1.0	50	.05	.07	1.0	Trace
589	Clam chowder, Manhattan type (with tomatoes, without milk) 1 cup	245	92	80	2	3	—	—	—	12	34	1.0	880	.02	.02	1.0	—

No.	Food	Measure	Grams	Water (%)	Food energy	Protein (g)	Fat (g)	Saturated	Oleic	Linoleic	Carbohydrate (g)	Calcium (mg)	Iron (mg)	Vitamin A (IU)	Thiamin (mg)	Riboflavin (mg)	Niacin (mg)	Vitamin C (mg)
590	Cream of chicken	1 cup	240	92	95	3	6	1	2	3	8	24	.5	410	.02	.05	.5	Trace
591	Cream of mushroom	1 cup	240	90	135	2	10	1	3	5	10	41	.5	70	.02	.12	.7	Trace
592	Minestrone	1 cup	245	90	105	5	3	—	—	—	14	37	1.0	2350	.07	.05	1.0	—
593	Split pea	1 cup	245	85	145	9	3	1	2	Trace	21	29	1.5	440	.25	.15	1.5	1
594	Tomato	1 cup	245	90	90	2	3	Trace	1	1	16	15	.7	1000	.05	.05	1.2	12
595	Vegetable beef	1 cup	245	92	80	5	2	—	—	—	10	12	.7	2700	.05	.05	1.0	—
596	Vegetarian	1 cup	245	92	80	2	2	—	—	—	13	20	1.0	2940	.05	.05	1.0	—
	Dehydrated, dry form:																	
597	Chicken noodle (2-oz package)	1 pkg	57	6	220	8	6	2	3	1	33	34	1.4	190	.30	.15	2.4	3
598	Onion mix (1½-oz package)	1 pkg	43	3	150	6	5	1	2	1	23	42	.6	30	.05	.03	.3	6
599	Tomato vegetable with noodles (2½-oz pkg)	1 pkg	71	4	245	6	6	2	3	1	45	33	1.4	1700	.21	.13	1.8	18
	Frozen, condensed:																	
	Clam chowder, New England type (with milk, without tomatoes):																	
600	Prepared with equal volume of milk	1 cup	245	83	210	9	12	—	—	—	16	240	1.0	250	.07	.29	.5	Trace
601	Prepared with equal volume of water	1 cup	240	89	130	4	8	—	—	—	11	91	1.0	50	.05	.10	.5	—
	Cream of potato:																	
602	Prepared with equal volume of milk	1 cup	245	83	185	8	10	5	3	Trace	18	208	1.0	590	.10	.27	.5	Trace
603	Prepared with equal volume of water	1 cup	240	90	105	3	5	3	2	Trace	12	58	1.0	410	.05	.05	.5	—
	Cream of shrimp:																	
604	Prepared with equal volume of milk	1 cup	245	32	245	9	16	—	—	—	15	189	.5	290	.07	.27	.5	Trace
605	Prepared with equal volume of water	1 cup	240	38	160	5	12	—	—	—	8	38	.5	120	.05	.05	.5	—
	Oyster stew:																	
606	Prepared with equal volume of milk	1 cup	240	83	200	10	12	—	—	—	14	305	1.4	410	.12	.41	.5	Trace
607	Prepared with equal volume of water	1 cup	240	90	120	6	8	—	—	—	8	158	1.4	240	.07	.19	.5	—
608	Tapioca, dry quick-cooking	1 cup	152	13	535	1	Trace	—	—	—	131	15	.6	0	0	0	0	0
	Tapioca desserts:																	
609	Apple	1 cup	250	70	295	1	Trace	—	—	—	74	8	.5	30	Trace	Trace	Trace	Trace
610	Cream pudding	1 cup	165	72	220	8	8	4	3	Trace	28	173	.7	480	.07	.30	.2	2

Table 1 (continued)

| | Food, Approximate Measure, and Weight (in Grams) | | Water (%) | Food Energy (kcal) | Protein (g) | Fat (g) | Fatty Acids | | | Carbohydrate (g) | Calcium (mg) | Iron (mg) | Vitamin A value (I.U.) | Thiamin (mg) | Riboflavin (mg) | Niacin (mg) | Ascorbic acid (mg) |
							Saturated (total) (g)	Unsaturated Oleic (g)	Linoleic (g)								
	MISCELLANEOUS ITEMS—Continued																
611	Tartar sauce	1 tbsp 14	34	75	Trace	8	1	1	4	1	3	.1	30	Trace	Trace	Trace	Trace
612	Vinegar	1 tbsp 15	94	Trace	Trace	0	—	—	—	1	1	.1	—	—	—	—	—
613	White sauce, medium	1 cup 250	73	405	10	31	16	10	1	22	288	.5	1150	.10	.43	.5	2
	Yeast:																
614	Baker's, dry, active	1 pkg 7	5	20	3	Trace	—	—	—	3	3	1.1	Trace	.16	.38	2.6	Trace
615	Brewer's, dry	1 tbsp 8	5	25	3	Trace	—	—	—	3	17	1.4	Trace	1.25	.34	3.0	Trace
	Yogurt. See Milk, Cheese, Cream, Imitation Cream.																

Appendix B
Zinc Content of Foods[a]

Appendix B Zinc Content of Foods[a]

(Data are given to two decimal places, if food contains less than 0.1 mg zinc)

Item No.	Food, approximate measure, and weight (in grams)		Zinc g	Zinc mg
1	Apples, raw	1 medium	180	0.08
2	Applesauce, unsweetened	1 cup	244	.3
3	Bananas, raw	1 medium	119	.3
	Beans, common, mature, dry:			
4	Raw	1 cup	190	5.3
5	Boiled, drained	1 cup	185	1.8
	Beans, lima, mature, dry:			
6	Raw	1 cup	180	5.0
7	Boiled, drained	1 cup	190	1.7
	Beans, snap, green:			
8	Raw, cut into 1–2 in. lengths	1 cup	110	.4
9	Boiled, drained, cut and French style	1 cup	125	.4
10	Canned, solids and liquid	1 cup	239	.6
11	Canned, drained solids	1 cup	135	.4
	Beef, separable lean:			
13	Cooked, dry heat	3 oz	85	4.9
14	Cooked, moist heat	3 oz	85	5.3
17	Beef, ground, cooked	3 oz	85	3.8
	Beverages, carbonated, nonalcoholic:			
18	12 fl oz	1 bottle	367	.01
19	12 fl oz	1 can	367	.3
	Breads:			
20	Rye	1 slice	25	.4
21	White	1 slice	28	.2
22	Whole wheat	1 slice	28	.5
	Butter, 4 sticks per lb:			

Item No.	Food, approximate measure, and weight (in grams)		Zinc g	Zinc mg
	Drumstick:			
35b	Meat only	1 drumstick	45	1.3
37	Meat and skin	1 drumstick	54	1.4
	Chickpeas, mature, dry:			
44	Raw	1 cup	200	5.4
45	Boiled, drained	1 cup	146	2.0
46	Chocolate sirup, 1 fl oz	2 tbsp.	38	.3
	Clams:			
48	Soft shell, cooked	3 oz	85	1.4
	Hard shell:			
49	Raw	4 cherry-stones or 5 little-necks	70	1.1
50	Cooked	4 or 5 clams	62	1.0
51	Surf, canned, solids and liquids, can size 211 × 300	1 can	220	2.7
	Cocoa, dry powder:			
52a	Approx. 5¼ tbsp	1 oz	28	1.6
52b		1 tbsp.	5	.3
	Coffee:			
53	Dry, instant	1 tbsp.	2.5	.02
54	Fluid beverage, 6 fl oz	1 cup	180	.05
55	Cookies (1⅞ × ¼ in.)	10 cookies	30	.08
	Corn, sweet, yellow:			
58	Boiled, drained	1 cup	165	.7

Item No.	Food, approximate measure, and weight (in grams)		Zinc g	Zinc mg
	Eggs, fresh (cont'd.)			
77	Yolk	1 large	17	0.5
78	Whole	1 large	50	.5
	Farina, regular:			
79	Dry form	1 cup	180	1.0
80	Cooked	1 cup	245	.2
	Fish, white varieties, flesh only:			
82	Fillet, cooked	3 oz	85	.9
83	Steak, cooked	3 oz	85	.7
	Gizzard, cooked, drained, diced:			
85	Chicken	1 cup	145	6.2
87	Turkey	1 cup	145	6.0
88	Granola	1 oz	28	.6
	Heart, cooked, drained, diced:			
90	Chicken	1 cup	145	6.9
92	Turkey	1 cup	145	7.0
93	Ice cream	1 cup	133	.6
	Lamb, separable lean:			
95	Cooked, dry heat	3 oz	85	3.7
96	Cooked, moist heat	3 oz	85	4.2
	Lard:			
98a		1 cup	205	.4
98b		1 tbsp	13	.03
	Lentils, mature, dry:			
99	Raw	1 cup	190	5.9
100	Boiled, drained	1 cup	200	2.0
	Lettuce, head or leaf:			
101a	Approx. ⅙ head	1 wedge	90	.4
101b	Loose leaf, chopped	1 cup	55	.2
	Liver, cooked:			

Appendix B Zinc Content of Foods[a] (Continued)
(Data are given to two decimal places, if food contains less than 0.1 mg zinc)

Item No.	Food, approximate measure, and weight (in grams)		g	mg
23a		1 cup	227	.2
23b		1 tbsp	14	.01
	Cabbage, common:			
24	Raw, shredded finely	1 cup	90	.3
25	Shredded, boiled, drained	1 cup	145	.6
	Cake, white, without icing, (3 × 3 × 2 in.):			
26		1 piece	86	.2
	Carrots:			
27	Raw	1 medium	72	.3
28	Cooked or canned, drained solids	1 cup	155	.5
29	Cheese, cheddar	1 slice	13	.5
	Chicken, broiler-fryer, cooked, dry heat:			
	Breast:			
31	Meat only	½ breast	85	.7
33	Meat and skin	½ breast	96	.9
	Drumstick, thigh,			
35a	back, meat only	3 oz	85	2.4
61	Canned, vacuum pack	1 cup	210	.8
62	Corn chips	1 oz	28	.4
63	Corn grits, dry form	1 cup	160	.7
64	Corn flakes	1 oz	28	.08
	Cornmeal, white or yellow:			
65	Bolted, dry form	1 cup	122	2.1
	Degermed:			
66	Dry form	1 cup	138	1.2
67	Cooked	1 cup	240	.3
	Cowpeas (blackeyes):			
69	Raw	1 cup	170	4.9
70	Boiled, drained	1 cup	250	3.0
72	Crabs, steamed, pieces	1 cup	155	6.7
	Crackers:			
73	Graham (2½ × 2½ in.)	2 squares	14	.2
74	Saltines	10 crackers	28	.1
75	Doughnuts (3¼ in. diam.)	1 doughnut	42	.2
	Eggs, fresh:			
76	White	1 large	33	<.01
103	Beef	2 oz	57	2.9
105	Calf	2 oz	57	3.5
107	Chicken, chopped	1 cup	140	4.7
109	Turkey, chopped	1 cup	140	4.7
111	Lobster, cooked cubed	1 cup	145	3.1
	Macaroni, cooked, tender:			
113a	Measured hot	1 cup	140	.7
113b	Measured cold	1 cup	105	.5
	Margarine:			
114a		1 cup	227	.5
114b		1 tbsp	14	.03
	Milk:			
115	Fluid	1 cup	244	.9
116	Canned, evaporated	1 cup	252	1.9
117	Dry, nonfat	1 cup	68	3.1
	Oatmeal or rolled oats:			
	Dry form:			
118a		1 oz	80	2.7
118b		1 oz	28	1.0
119	Cooked	1 cup	240	1.2

a Edible part of common household units. Measure and weight apply to edible part of food only.
Provisional table prepared by E. W. Murphy, B. W. Willis, and B. K. Watt CFEI, ARS, USDA. Hyattsville, Md. 20782. 1974.

Appendix B Zinc Content of Foods, Edible Part of Common Household Units[a]
(Data are given to two decimal places, if food contains less than 0.1 mg. zinc)

Item No.	Food, approximate measure, and weight (in grams)		g	mg
120	Oat cereal, puffed	1 oz	28	0.8
121	Oil, salad or cooking	1 cup	218	.4
	Onions:			
122a	Mature, chopped	1 cup	170	.6
122b	Young green, chopped	1 cup	100	.3
123	Oranges, raw, 2⅝ in. diam.	1 orange	131	.2
	Orange juice:			
124	Canned, unsweetened	1 cup	249	.2
125	Fresh or frozen	1 cup	248	.05
	Oysters:			
	Atlantic:			
	Pork, cooked, separable lean (cont'd.):			
146	Ham or picnic	3 oz	85	3.4
148	Loin	3 oz	85	2.6
	Potatoes:			
150	Raw, peeled, 2½ in. diam.	1 medium	112	.4
	Pared before cooking,			
151a	boiled, drained	1 medium	112	.3
151b	Boiled in skin, drained, pared	1 medium	136	.4
	Rice:			
	Brown:			
	Spinach:			
171	Raw, chopped	1 cup	55	0.5
172	Boiled, drained	1 cup	180	1.3
	Canned:			
173	Solids and liquid	1 cup	232	1.5
174	Drained solids	1 cup	205	1.6
175	Sugar, white, granulated	1 cup	200	.1
177	Tea, fluid beverage, 6 fl oz	1 cup	177	.04
	Tomatoes, ripe:			
178	Raw, 2⅗ in. diam.	1 medium	123	.2

Appendix B Zinc Content of Foods, Edible Part of Common Household Units[a] (Continued)

(Data are given to two decimal places, if food contains less than 0.1 mg zinc)

Item No.	Food, approximate measure, and weight (in grams)		Zinc g	mg
126a	Raw, drained, 12 fl oz can, 18-27 Select or 27-44 Standard oysters	1 can	340	254.3
126b	Frozen, solids and liquid, 12 fl oz can	1 can	360	268.9
	Pacific:			
127a	Raw, drained, 12 fl oz can, 6-9 medium or 9-13 small oysters	1 can	340	30.6
127b	Frozen, solids and liquid, 12 fl oz	1 can	360	32.4
	Peaches:			
128	Raw, peeled, 2½ in. diam.	1 medium	100	.2
129	Canned, drained, slices	1 cup	220	.3
131	Peanuts, roasted	1 tbsp	9	.3
132	Peanut butter	1 tbsp	16	.5
	Peas, green, immature:			
133	Raw or frozen	1 cup	145	1.2
134	Boiled, drained	1 cup	160	1.2
135	Canned, drained solids	1 cup	170	1.3
	Peas, green, mature seeds, dry:			
136	Raw	1 cup	200	6.4
137	Boiled, drained	1 cup	200	2.1
	Popcorn:			
138	Unpopped	1 cup	205	7.9
	Popped:			
139	Plain, large kernel	1 cup	6	.2
140	With oil and salt	1 cup	9	.3
	Pork, cooked, dry heat, separable lean:			
142	Trimmed lean cuts	3 oz	85	3.2
144	Boston butt	3 oz	85	3.8

Item No.	Food, approximate measure, and weight (in grams)		Zinc g	mg
152	Dry form	1 cup	185	3.4
153	Cooked, measured hot	1 cup	195	1.2
	White, regular, long-grain:			
154	Dry form	1 cup	185	2.5
	Cooked:			
155a	Measured hot	1 cup	205	.8
155b	Measured cold	1 cup	145	.6
	White, parboiled:			
156	Dry form	1 cup	185	2.1
	Cooked:			
157a	Measured hot	1 cup	175	.6
157b	Measured cold	1 cup	145	.5
	White, precooked, quick:			
158	Dry form	1 cup	95	.7
	Cooked:			
159a	Measured hot	1 cup	165	.4
159b	Measured cold	1 cup	130	.3
160	Cereal, ready-to-eat	1 oz	28	.4
161	Rolls, hamburger, 3½ in. diam.	1 roll	40	.2
162	Salad dressing	1 tbsp	15	.03
163	Salmon, canned, solids and liquid	1 cup	220	2.1
	Sausages and cold cuts:			
164	Bologna, beef, 4½ in. diam., 1 oz	1 slice	28	.5
165	Braunschweiger, 1 oz	1 slice	28	.8
	Frankfurters:			
166	Made with beef, 10 per lb	1 frank	45	.9
167	Made with beef and pork, 10 per lb	1 frank	45	.7
	Shrimp:			
169	Boiled, peeled, deveined, 33 per lb	6 shrimp	84	1.7
170	Canned, drained, solids	1 cup	128	2.7

Item No.	Food, approximate measure, and weight (in grams)		Zinc g	mg
179	Boiled	1 cup	241	.5
180	Canned, solids and liquid	1 cup	241	.5
	Tunafish, canned in oil:			
181	Chunk style, solids and liquid, can size 307 × 113, 6½ oz can	1 can	184	1.7
182a	Drained solids, can size 307 × 113, 6½ oz	1 can	157	1.8
182b	Drained solids	1 cup	160	1.8
184	Turkey, cooked, dry heat, meat only: Light meat	3 oz	85	1.8
186	Dark meat	3 oz	85	3.7
	Veal, separable lean:			
192	Cooked, dry heat	3 oz	85	3.5
193	Cooked, moist heat	3 oz	85	3.6
	Wheat flours:			
	Whole, stirred,			
199	spooned into cup	1 cup	120	2.9
	All-purpose, sifted,			
201	spooned into cup, standard granulation	1 cup	115	.8
	Bread flour, sifted,			
202	spooned into cup, standard granulation	1 cup	115	.9
	Cake flour, sifted,			
203	spooned into cup	1 cup	96	.3
	Wheat cereal, wholemeal:			
206a	Dry form	1 cup	125	4.5
206b	Dry form	1 oz	28	1.0
207a	Cooked	1 cup	245	1.2
207b	Cooked, from 1 oz dry	1 cup	216	1.0
	Wheat cereals, ready-to-eat:			
208	Bran flakes, 40%	1 oz	28	1.0
209	Flakes	1 oz	28	.6
210	Germ, toasted	1 tbsp	6	.9
211	Puffed	1 oz	28	.7
212	Shredded	1 oz	28	.8

[a] Measure and weight apply to edible part of food only.

Appendix C
Foods that are Important Sources of Nutrients

Foods are listed in descending order for each nutrient according to the percentage of the U.S. RDA they provide. Consider the amount of food specified. It may not be the same as the amount you usually eat.

Percentages have been rounded off to the nearest percentage that would be shown on labels.

Consider a food superior to another food as the source of a nutrient only if it provides a substantially higher percentage of the U.S. RDA. Labeling regulations allow a manufacturer to claim that his food is superior to another food only if it contains at least 10 percent more of the U.S. RDA per serving specified on the label.

VITAMIN A

Food	Percentage of U.S. RDA		Amount of food
MEAT AND MEAT ALTERNATES:			
Liver, beef	910	....	3 oz
Liver, calf	560	....	3 oz
Liver, hog	250	....	3 oz
Liver, chicken	60	....	1 oz
Chicken or turkey potpie, home recipe	60	....	⅓ of 9-in. pie
Beef and vegetable stew	50	....	1 cup
VEGETABLES AND FRUIT:			
Carrots, canned	470	....	1 cup
Sweetpotatoes, mashed	400	....	1 cup
Carrots, cooked	330	....	1 cup
Spinach, canned	330	....	1 cup
Pumpkin, canned	310	....	1 cup
Sweetpotatoes, pieces, canned	310	....	1 cup
Collards, cooked	300	....	1 cup
Peas and carrots, cooked	300	....	1 cup
Spinach, cooked	290	....	1 cup
Dandelion greens, cooked	250	....	1 cup
Carrots, raw, grated	240	....	1 cup
Sweetpotatoes, boiled in skin	240	....	Medium potato
Turnip greens, canned, solids and liquid	220	....	1 cup
Cress, garden, cooked	210	....	1 cup
Chard, Swiss, cooked	190	....	1 cup
Mango, raw	190	....	1 fruit (⅔ lb)
Cantaloupe, raw	180	....	½ of 5-in.-diam. melon
Kale, cooked	180	....	1 cup
Mustard greens, cooked from frozen	180	....	1 cup
Sweetpotatoes, baked in skin	180	....	Medium potato
Turnip greens, cooked	180	....	1 cup
Vegetables, mixed, cooked	180	....	1 cup
Squash, winter, baked	170	....	1 cup
Mustard greens, cooked	160	....	1 cup
Apricots, dried, cooked	150	....	1 cup
Beet greens, cooked	150	....	1 cup
Cabbage, spoon, cooked	110	....	1 cup
Sweetpotatoes, candied	110	....	3-oz piece
Broccoli, chopped, cooked from frozen	100	....	1 cup
Apricots, canned	90	....	1 cup
Broccoli, cooked	90	....	Medium stalk
Spinach, raw, chopped	90	....	1 cup
Apricots, dried, uncooked	80	....	10 medium halves
Broccoli, cut, cooked	80	....	1 cup
Melon balls, frozen, in sirup	70	....	1 cup
Pepper, red	70	....	1 pod
Apricots, raw	60	....	3 fruits
Peaches, dried, cooked	60	....	1 cup
Plums, canned	60	....	1 cup
Carrots, strips, raw	60	....	6–9 strips (2½–3 in. long)
Papaya, raw, cubed	50	....	1 cup
Tomatoes, cooked	50	....	1 cup
Watermelon, raw	50	....	4 x 8-in. wedge (2 lb)
CEREAL AND BAKERY PRODUCTS:			
Pie, pumpkin	80	....	4¾-in. sector
Pie, sweet potato	70	....	4¾-in. sector
MISCELLANEOUS:			
Soup:			
Vegetable, with beef broth	60	....	1 cup
Vegetable, vegetarian	60	....	1 cup
Vegetable beef	60	....	1 cup
Apricot nectar	50	....	1 cup

VITAMIN C

Food	Percentage of U.S. RDA		Amount of food
MEAT AND MEAT ALTERNATES:			
Peppers, stuffed	120	....	1 pepper (6.5 oz)
Lobster salad	80	....	A salad[a]
Chop suey, with beef and pork, home recipe	60	....	1 cup
Liver, calf	50	....	3 oz

[a] Prepared with lobster, onion, sweet pickle, celery, eggs, salad dressing (mayonnaise type), and tomatoes.

VEGETABLES AND FRUIT:

Broccoli, cooked	270	Medium stalk
Pepper, red, raw	250	1 pod
Collards, cooked	240	1 cup
Broccoli, cut, cooked	230	1 cup
Brussels sprouts, cooked	230	1 cup
Strawberries, frozen, sweetened	230	1 cup
Pepper, green, cooked	220	1 cup
Orange juice, fresh	210	1 cup
Orange juice, from frozen or canned concentrate	200	1 cup
Broccoli, chopped, cooked from frozen	180	1 cup
Kale, cooked	170	1 cup
Turnip greens, cooked	170	1 cup
Orange juice, canned	170	1 cup
Peaches, frozen	170	1 cup
Pepper, green, raw	160	1 pod
Grapefruit juice, fresh or from frozen unsweetened concentrate	160	1 cup
Canataloupe, raw	150	½ of 5-in. diam. melon
Orange sections, raw	150	1 cup
Strawberries, raw	150	1 cup
Grapefruit sections, raw, white or pink	140	1 cup
Grapefruit juice, canned, unsweetened	140	1 cup
Grapefruit juice, from frozen sweetened concentrate	140	1 cup
Grapefruit sections, canned, sirup pack	130	1 cup
Grapefruit juice, canned, sweetened	130	1 cup
Papaya, raw, cubed	130	1 cup
Grapefruit sections, canned, water pack	120	1 cup
Mango, raw	120	1 fruit (⅔ lb)
Cauliflower, cooked	120	1 cup
Cauliflower, raw	110	1 cup
Mustard greens, cooked	110	1 cup
Orange, raw	110	2⅝-in.-diam. orange
Tangerine juice, from frozen concentrate	110	1 cup
Tomatoes, cooked	100	1 cup
Raspberries, red, frozen	90	1 cup
Tangerine juice, canned	90	1 cup
Cabbage, cooked	80	1 cup
Cress, garden, cooked	80	1 cup
Spinach, cooked	80	1 cup
Strawberries, canned	80	1 cup
Cabbage, raw, finely shredded	70	1 cup
Cabbage, red, raw, shredded	70	1 cup
Rutabagas, cooked	70	1 cup
Tomatoes, raw	70	3-in.-diam. tomato
Turnip greens, canned, solids and liquid	70	1 cup
Tomato juice, canned or bottled	70	1 cup
Sauerkraut juice	70	1 cup
Grapefruit, white or pink, raw	70	½ medium fruit
Lemons, raw	70	1 lemon
Asparagus, pieces, cooked or canned	60	1 cup
Cabbage, common or savoy, raw, coarsely shredded	60	1 cup
Okra, sliced, cooked	60	1 cup
Peas, green, cooked	60	1 cup
Sauerkraut, canned	60	1 cup
Sweetpotatoes, canned, mashed	60	1 cup
Turnips, cooked	60	1 cup
Coleslaw	60	1 cup
Honeydew melon, raw	60	2 x 7-in. wedge (⅒ lb)
Loganberries, raw	60	1 cup
Melon balls, frozen, sirup pack	60	1 cup
Beans, lima, Fordhook, cooked from frozen	50	1 cup
Beans, lima, immature seeds, cooked	50	1 cup
Mustard greens, cooked from frozen	50	1 cup
Potato, baked in skin	50	Medium potato
Spinach, canned	50	1 cup
Blackberries, raw	50	1 cup
Raspberries, red, raw	50	1 cup
Watermelon, raw	50	4 x 8-in. wedge (2 lb)
Pineapple juice, from frozen concentrate	50	1 cup

CEREAL AND BAKERY PRODUCTS:

Spanish rice	60	1 cup
Pie, strawberry	50	4¾-in. sector

MISCELLANEOUS:

Orange juice, from dehydrated crystals	180	1 cup

461

Grapefruit juice, from dehydrated crystals	150	1 cup
Cranberry juice cocktail	70	1 cup
Grape juice drink, canned	70	1 cup
Orange-apricot juice drink	70	1 cup
Pineapple-orange juice drink	70	1 cup
Pineapple-grapefruit juice drink	70	1 cup

THIAMIN

Food	Percentage of U.S. RDA	Amount of food
MEAT AND MEAT ALTERNATES:		
Sunflower seeds	190	1 cup
Pork, loin, chopped, lean	100	1 cup
Brazilnuts, shelled	90	1 cup
Pork, fresh or cured, ham or shoulder, chopped, lean	60	1 cup
Pork loin, sliced, lean only	60	3 oz
Pecans, halves	60	1 cup
Pork, loin, sliced, lean and fat	50	3 oz
Pork, loin chop, lean and fat	50	2.7 oz
Pork, fresh or cured, ham or shoulder, ground, lean	45	1 cup
Pork, loin chop, lean	40	2 oz
Cashew nuts, whole kernels, roasted	40	1 cup
Filberts, whole kernels, shelled	40	1 cup
Pork, fresh or cured, ham or shoulder, sliced, lean	35	3 oz
Pork, cured, shoulder, sliced, lean and fat	30	3 oz
Pork, fresh, ham or shoulder, sliced, lean and fat	30	3 oz
Kidney, beef	30	3 oz
Peanuts	30	1 cup
Pork, cured, ham, sliced, lean and fat	25	3 oz
Spareribs	25	3 oz
Spaghetti (enriched) with cheese, canned	25	1 cup
Cowpeas, dry, cooked	25	1 cup
Soybeans, dry, cooked	25	1 cup
Almonds, whole, shelled	25	1 cup
Chestnuts, shelled	25	1 cup
Pumpkin kernels	25	1 cup
Walnuts, English, chopped	25	1 cup
Liver, hog	20	3 oz
Beef potpie, home-prepared from enriched flour	20	$\frac{1}{3}$ of 9-in. pie
Chicken or turkey potpie, home-prepared from enriched flour	20	$\frac{1}{3}$ of 9-in. pie
Chop suey, with beef and pork, home recipe	20	1 cup
Beans, navy (pea), dry, cooked	20	1 cup
Peas, split, dry, cooked	20	1 cup
Walnuts, black, chopped	20	1 cup
Bacon, Canadian	15	1 slice
Lamb, leg or shoulder, chopped, lean	15	1 cup
Heart, beef, sliced	15	3 oz
Liver, calf or beef	15	3 oz
Polish sausage	15	2.4-oz link
Pork sausage	15	1-oz patty or 2 links
Crab, deviled	15	1 cup
Lobster salad	15	A salad[b]
Macaroni (enriched) and cheese, home recipe	15	1 cup
Spaghetti (enriched) with cheese, home recipe	15	1 cup
Spaghetti (enriched) with meatballs, home recipe	15	1 cup
Beans, canned, with pork and tomato sauce	15	1 cup
Beans, lima, Great Northern, or kidney, dry, cooked	15	1 cup
VEGETABLES AND FRUIT:		
Cowpeas, cooked	35	1 cup
Peas, green, cooked	30	1 cup
Peas and carrots, cooked	20	1 cup
Beans, lima, fresh, cooked	20	1 cup
Asparagus, pieces, cooked	15	1 cup
Collards, cooked	15	1 cup
Cowpeas, canned, solids and liquid	15	1 cup
Okra, sliced, cooked	15	1 cup
Soybeans, sprouted seeds, raw or cooked	15	1 cup
Turnip greens, cooked	15	1 cup
Vegetables, mixed, cooked	15	1 cup
Potato salad, with cooked salad dressing	15	1 cup
Orange juice, fresh or from unsweetened frozen or canned concentrate	15	1 cup
Pineapple, canned, water or sirup pack	15	1 cup

[b] Prepared with lobster, onion, sweet pickle, celery, eggs, salad dressing (mayonnaise type), and tomatoes.

Food	Percentage of U.S. RDA		Amount of food
Pineapple, frozen, sweetened	15	....	1 cup

CEREAL AND BAKERY PRODUCTS:

Food			
Hoagie roll, enriched	35	....	11½-in.-long roll
Cereal, ready-to-eat (check label)	25	....	1 oz
Hard roll, enriched	15	....	1 roll (1.8 oz)
Spoonbread	15	....	1 cup
Oatmeal, cooked	15	....	1 cup
Oat and wheat cereal, cooked	15	....	1 cup
Macaroni, enriched, cooked	15	....	1 cup
Noodles, enriched, cooked	15	....	1 cup
Spaghetti, enriched, cooked	15	....	1 cup
Rice, white, enriched, cooked	15	....	1 cup
Gingerbread, with enriched flour	15	....	⅑ of 9-in.-square cake
Pie, pecan	15	....	4¾-in. sector

MISCELLANEOUS:

Food			
Orange juice, from dehydrated crystals	15	....	1 cup
Soup, split pea	15	....	1 cup
Bread pudding, with enriched bread	15	....	1 cup

RIBOFLAVIN

Food	Percentage of U.S. RDA		Amount of food

MILK AND MILK PRODUCTS:

Food			
Cheese, cottage	35	....	1 cup
Milk, partially skimmed	30	....	1 cup
Malted beverage	30	....	1 cup
Custard, baked	30	....	1 cup
Milk, whole or skim	25	....	1 cup
Milk, nonfat dry, reconstituted	25	....	1 cup
Buttermilk	25	....	1 cup
Chocolate drink	25	....	1 cup
Cocoa	25	....	1 cup
Ice milk, soft-serve	25	....	1 cup
Pudding, from mixes, with milk	25	....	1 cup
Pudding, vanilla, home recipe	25	....	1 cup
Rennin desserts	25	....	1 cup
Yogurt	25	....	1 cup
Ice cream, soft-serve	20	....	1 cup
Pudding, chocolate, home recipe	20	....	1 cup
Tapioca cream	20	....	1 cup

MEAT AND MEAT ALTERNATES:

Food			
Kidney, beef	240	....	3 oz
Liver, hog	220	....	3 oz
Liver, beef or calf	210	....	3 oz
Almonds, whole	80	....	1 cup
Fish loaf	60	....	4⅛ x 2½ x 1-in. slice
Heart, beef, sliced	60	....	3 oz
Almonds, sliced	50	....	1 cup
Liver, chicken	40	....	1 oz
Beef, dried, chipped, creamed	30	....	1 cup
Welsh rarebit	30	....	1 cup
Lamb, leg or shoulder, chopped, lean	25	....	1 cup
Pork, fresh, ham or loin, chopped, lean	25	....	1 cup
Veal, stewed or roasted, chopped	25	....	1 cup
Braunschweiger	25	....	1 oz
Chicken a la king, home recipe	25	....	1 cup
Macaroni (enriched) and cheese, home recipe	25	....	1 cup
Beef, chuck or rump, chopped, lean	20	....	1 cup
Lamb, leg or shoulder, chopped, lean and fat	20	....	1 cup
Pork, cured, ham or shoulder, chopped, lean	20	....	1 cup
Pork, fresh, shoulder, chopped	20	....	1 cup
Pork, fresh, ham or shoulder, ground, lean	20	....	1 cup
Veal, loin, chopped	20	....	1 cup
Veal, rib, ground	20	....	1 cup
Turkey, dark meat, chopped	20	....	1 cup
Chicken or turkey potpie, home-prepared from enriched flour	30	....	⅓ of 9-in. pie
Chop suey with beef and pork, home recipe	20	....	1 cup
Pepper, stuffed	20	....	1 pepper (6.5 oz)
Spaghetti (enriched) with meatballs, home recipe	20	....	1 cup

VEGETABLES AND FRUIT:

Food			
Broccoli, cooked	20	....	Medium stalk
Broccoli, cut, cooked	20	....	1 cup
Corn pudding	20	....	1 cup
Collards, cooked	20	....	1 cup
Turnip greens, cooked	20	....	1 cup
Avocado, Florida, raw	20	....	½ fruit

Avocado, Florida or California, raw, cubed	20	1 cup
CEREAL AND BAKERY PRODUCTS:		
Cereals, ready-to-eat (check label)	25	1 oz
Spoonbread	25	1 cup
Hoagie roll, enriched	20	11½-in.- long roll
MISCELLANEOUS:		
Bread pudding, with enriched bread	35	1 cup
Oyster stew, home recipe..	25	1 cup
Rice pudding	20	1 cup
Soup, cream of mushroom, with milk	20	1 cup

NIACIN

Food	Percentage of U.S. RDA	Amount of food
MEAT AND MEAT ALTERNATES:		
Peanuts	120	1 cup
Liver, hog	100	3 oz
Chicken, light meat, chopped	80	1 cup
Turkey, light meat, chopped	80	1 cup
Liver, calf or beef	70	3 oz
Chicken, breast	60	½ breast (3.3 oz)
Chicken, stewed, dark meat, chopped	60	1 cup
Veal rib, chopped	60	1 cup
Tuna, canned in water	60	3 oz
Chicken, roasted, light meat, sliced	50	3 oz
Turkey, canned	50	1 cup
Rabbit, domesticated	50	3 oz
Tuna, canned in oil, drained	50	3 oz
Tuna salad	50	1 cup
Lamb, leg, chopped, lean.	45	1 cup
Kidney, beef	45	3 oz
Pork, loin, chopped, lean..	45	1 cup
Veal, stewed, chopped	45	1 cup
Veal, rib, ground	45	1 cup
Chicken, canned	45	1 cup
Chicken, stewed, light meat, sliced	45	3 oz
Turkey, light meat, sliced..	45	3 oz
Swordfish, broiled	45	3 oz
Chicken, broiled	40	3 oz
Goose	40	3 oz
Lamb, shoulder, chopped, lean	40	1 cup
Pork, fresh, ham, chopped, lean	40	1 cup
Veal, loin, chopped	40	1 cup
Turkey potpie, home-prepared from enriched flour	40	⅓ of 9-in. pie
Salmon steak, broiled or baked	40	3 oz
Sunflower seeds	40	1 cup
Beef, rump, chopped, lean	35	1 cup
Pork, fresh or cured, shoulder, chopped, lean	35	1 cup
Veal, rib, sliced	35	3 oz
Heart, beef, sliced	35	3 oz
Chicken, stewed, dark meat, sliced	35	3 oz
Chicken, roasted, dark meat, chopped	35	1 cup
Halibut, broiled	35	3 oz
Mackerel, broiled	35	3 oz
Rockfish, oven-steamed....	35	3 oz
Shad, baked	35	3 oz
Beef, chuck, chopped	30	1 cup
Beef, rump, ground, lean..	30	1 cup
Pork, cured, ham, chopped, lean	30	1 cup
Pork, cured, shoulder, ground, lean	30	1 cup
Pork, loin, sliced, lean......	30	3 oz
Chicken fricassee, home recipe	30	1 cup
Turkey, dark meat, chopped	30	1 cup
Salmon, pink, canned	30	3 oz
Beef potpie, home-prepared from enriched flour	30	⅓ of 9-in. pie
Beef, chuck, ground, lean.	25	1 cup
Beef, steak (club, porterhouse, T-bone, or sirloin), lean	25	3 oz
Beef, steak (round)	25	3 oz
Ground beef	25	3 oz
Lamb, leg, sliced	25	3 oz
Lamb, loin chop, lean and fat	25	3.5 oz
Lamb, shoulder, sliced, lean	25	3 oz
Pork, cured, ham, ground, lean	25	3 oz
Pork, fresh, ham, sliced, lean	25	3 oz
Pork, loin chop, lean and fat	25	2.7 oz
Pork, loin, sliced, lean and fat	25	3 oz
Veal, stewed, sliced	25	3 oz
Veal, loin or cutlet	25	3 oz

Food	Percentage of U.S. RDA		Amount of food
Chicken, roasted, dark meat, sliced	25	....	3 oz
Chicken a la king, home recipe	25	....	1 cup
Chicken potpie, home-prepared from enriched flour	25	....	⅓ of 9-in. pie
Salmon, red, canned.........	25	....	3 oz
Salmon rice loaf...............	25	....	6-oz piece
Sardines, canned, drained.	25	....	3 oz
Beef and vegetable stew, home recipe	25	....	1 cup
Chop suey, with beef and pork, home recipe	25	....	1 cup
Corned beef hash, canned	25	....	1 cup
Peppers, stuffed...............	25	....	1 pepper (6.5 oz)
Spaghetti (enriched) with cheese, canned	25	....	1 cup
Beef, chuck, sliced............	20	....	3 oz
Beef, rump, sliced............	20	....	3 oz
Beef, rib, sliced, lean and fat	20	....	3 oz
Beef, flank steak	20	....	3 oz
Beef, plate, lean..............	20	....	3 oz
Beef, steak (club, porter-house, T-bone, or sirloin), lean and fat	20	....	3 oz
Lamb, rib chop, lean and fat	20	....	3.2 oz
Lamb, loin chop, lean.......	20	....	2.3 oz
Lamb, shoulder, sliced, lean and fat	20	....	3 oz
Pork, cured, ham, sliced, lean	20	....	3 oz
Pork, fresh, ham, sliced, lean and fat	20	....	3 oz
Pork, fresh or cured, shoulder sliced	20	....	3 oz
Pork, loin chop, lean.........	20	....	2 oz
Chicken, thigh..................	20	....	2.3-oz piece
Turkey, dark meat, sliced..	20	....	3 oz
Chicken and noodles, home recipe	20	....	1 cup
Chow mein, home recipe..	20	....	1 cup
Spaghetti (enriched) with meatballs, home recipe	20	....	1 cup
Lobster salad	20	....	A salad[c]
Lobster Newburg..............	20	....	1 cup
Crab, deviled...................	20	....	1 cup
VEGETABLES AND FRUITS:			
Dates, pitted, chopped......	20	....	1 cup

[c] Prepared with lobster, onion, sweet pickle, celery, eggs, salad dressing (mayonnaise type), and tomatoes.

Food	Percentage of U.S. RDA		Amount of food
Peaches, dried, cooked, unsweetened	20	....	1 cup
Peas, green, cooked..........	20	....	1 cup
CEREAL AND BAKERY PRODUCTS:			
Hoagie roll, enriched........	25	....	11½-in.-long roll
Cereals, ready-to-eat (check label)	20	....	1 oz

CALCIUM

Food	Percentage of U.S. RDA		Amount of food
MILK AND MILK PRODUCTS:			
Cheese, Parmesan, grated	40	....	1 oz
Milk, partially skimmed	35	....	1 cup
Pudding, uncooked, from mix	35	....	1 cup
Milk, whole or skim..........	30	....	1 cup
Milk, nonfat dry, reconstituted	30	....	1 cup
Buttermilk.......................	30	....	1 cup
Chocolate drink, made from whole milk	30	....	1 cup
Cocoa.............................	30	....	1 cup
Malted beverage	30	....	1 cup
Custard, baked	30	....	1 cup
Pudding, vanilla, home recipe	30	....	1 cup
Rennin desserts................	30	....	1 cup
Yogurt, made from partially skimmed milk	30	....	1 cup
Chocolate drink, made from skim milk	25	....	1 cup
Cheese, cottage, creamed.	25	....	1 cup
Cheese, Swiss..................	25	....	1 oz
Yogurt, made from whole milk	25	....	1 cup
Ice cream or ice milk, soft-serve	25	....	1 cup
Pudding, cooked, from mix, with milk	25	....	1 cup
Pudding, chocolate, home recipe	25	....	1 cup
Cheese, American, process	20	....	1 oz
Cheese, Cheddar, natural.	20	....	1 oz
Cheese, cottage, uncreamed	20	....	1 cup
Ice cream or ice milk, hardened	20	....	1 cup
MEAT AND MEAT ALTERNATES:			
Welsh rarebit...................	60	....	1 cup
Sardines, canned, drained.	35	....	3 oz
Macaroni (enriched) and cheese, home recipe	35	....	1 cup
Potatoes au gratin............	30	....	1 cup

465

Food	%	Amount
Beef, dried, chipped, creamed	25	1 cup
Cheese souffle	20	1 cup
Lobster Newburg	20	1 cup
Macaroni (enriched) and cheese, canned	20	1 cup

VEGETABLES AND FRUIT:

Collards, cooked	35	1 cup
Cabbage, spoon, cooked	25	1 cup
Spinach, canned	25	1 cup
Turnip greens	25	1 cup
Kale, cooked	20	1 cup
Mustard greens, cooked	20	1 cup
Rhubarb, cooked	20	1 cup

CEREAL AND BAKERY PRODUCTS:

Spoonbread	25	1 cup
Farina, enriched, instant	20	1 cup

MISCELLANEOUS:

Bread pudding	30	1 cup
Oyster stew, home recipe	30	1 cup
Rice pudding	25	1 cup
Soup, with milk:		
Green pea	20	1 cup
Cream of celery	20	1 cup
Cream of mushroom	20	1 cup
Cream of asparagus	20	1 cup

IRON

Food	Percentage of U.S. RDA	Amount of food
MEAT AND MEAT ALTERNATES:		
Liver, hog	140	3 oz
Pumpkin kernels	90	1 cup
Liver, calf	70	3 oz
Kidney, beef	60	3 oz
Sunflower seeds	60	1 cup
Liver, beef	40	3 oz
Walnuts, black, chopped	40	1 cup
Clams, canned, drained, chopped	35	1 cup
Beans, lima, dry, cooked	35	1 cup
Beans, with pork and sweet sauce, canned	35	1 cup
Almonds, whole, shelled	35	1 cup
Beef, chuck or rump, chopped, lean	30	1 cup
Pork, cured, shoulder, chopped, lean	30	1 cup
Pork, fresh, ham or loin, chopped, lean	30	1 cup
Heart, beef, sliced	30	3 oz
Clams, raw	30	4 or 5 clams
Beef potpie, home-prepared from enriched flour	30	$\frac{1}{3}$ of 9-in. pie
Beans, navy (pea), dry, cooked	30	1 cup
Beans, white, dry, canned, solids and liquid	30	1 cup
Cashew nuts, whole kernels, roasted	30	1 cup
Beef, chuck or rump, ground, lean	25	1 cup
Pork, cured, ham, chopped, lean	25	1 cup
Pork, fresh, shoulder, chopped	25	1 cup
Pork, fresh, ham, ground, lean	25	1 cup
Veal, chopped	25	1 cup
Chicken or turkey potpie, home-prepared from enriched flour	25	$\frac{1}{3}$ of 9-in. pie
Chile con carne with beans, canned	25	1 cup
Chop suey, with beef and pork, home recipe	25	1 cup
Corned beef hash, canned	25	1 cup
Beans, Great Northern or red kidney, dry, cooked	25	1 cup
Beans, red kidney, dry, canned, solids and liquid	25	1 cup
Lentils, dry, cooked	25	1 cup
Soybeans, dry, cooked	25	1 cup
Beans, with frankfurters, canned	25	1 cup
Beans, with pork and tomato sauce, canned	25	1 cup
Beef, chuck, sliced, lean	20	3 oz
Beef, flank steak	20	3 oz
Beef, plate, lean	20	3 oz
Beef, steak, sirloin, lean	20	3 oz
Pork, cured, ham or shoulder, ground, lean	20	1 cup
Pork, fresh, shoulder, ground, lean	20	1 cup
Pork, fresh, ham, sliced, lean	20	3 oz
Pork, loin, sliced, lean	20	3 oz
Turkey, dark meat, chopped	20	1 cup
Veal, rib, ground	20	1 cup
Peppers, stuffed	20	1 pepper (6.5 oz)
Spaghetti (enriched) in tomato sauce, with meatballs; canned or home-prepared	20	1 cup
Cowpeas, dry, cooked	20	1 cup
Peas, split, dry, cooked	20	1 cup
Beef, chuck, lean and fat, sliced	15	3 oz

Beef, corned	15	3 oz
Beef, plate, lean and fat	15	3 oz
Beef, rump, sliced	15	3 oz
Beef, rib, sliced, lean	15	3 oz
Beef, steak (round)	15	3 oz
Beef, steak (club, porterhouse, or T-bone), lean	15	3 oz
Beef, steak (sirloin), lean and fat	15	3 oz
Ground beef	15	3 oz
Lamb, shoulder, chopped, lean	15	1 cup
Lamb, leg, chopped	15	1 cup
Pork, cured, shoulder, sliced	15	3 oz
Pork, cured, ham, sliced, lean	15	3 oz
Pork, fresh, loin or ham, sliced, lean and fat	15	3 oz
Pork, loin chop, lean and fat	15	2.7 oz
Pork, fresh, shoulder, sliced	15	3 oz
Veal, sliced	15	3 oz
Veal, cutlet or loin	15	3 oz
Beef and vegetable stew, home recipe	15	1 cup
Chicken, dark meat, chopped	15	1 cup
Chicken, canned	15	1 cup
Spaghetti (enriched) with tomato sauce and cheese, canned	15	1 cup
Turkey, canned	15	1 cup
Chow mein, chicken, home recipe	15	1 cup
Chicken a la king, home recipe	15	1 cup
Crab, deviled	15	1 cup
Sardines, canned	15	3 oz
Shrimp, canned	15	3 oz
Lobster salad	15	A salad[d]
Tuna salad	15	1 cup

VEGETABLES AND FRUIT:

Peaches, dried, uncooked	60	1 cup
Prune juice, canned	60	1 cup
Dates, pitted, chopped	30	1 cup
Raisins, seedless	30	1 cup
Spinach, canned	30	1 cup
Asparagus, pieces, canned	25	1 cup
Beans, lima, canned	25	1 cup
Beans, lima, fresh or frozen, baby, cooked	25	1 cup
Apricots, dried, cooked	25	1 cup

[d] Prepared with lobster, onion, sweet pickle, celery, eggs, salad dressing (mayonnaise type), and tomatoes.

Peaches, dried, cooked	25	1 cup
Cowpeas, cooked	20	1 cup
Cowpeas, canned, solids and liquid	20	1 cup
Peas, green, canned	20	1 cup
Spinach, cooked	20	1 cup
Turnip greens, canned, solids and liquid	20	1 cup
Prunes, dried, cooked	20	1 cup
Beans, lima, Fordhook, cooked	15	1 cup
Beet greens, cooked	15	1 cup
Chard, Swiss, cooked	15	1 cup
Mustard greens, fresh or frozen, cooked	15	1 cup
Peas, green, cooked	15	1 cup
Sauerkraut juice	15	1 cup
Vegetables, mixed, cooked	15	1 cup
Boysenberries, canned	15	1 cup
Plums, canned, water or syrup pack	15	1 cup
Prunes, dried, uncooked	15	10 prunes

CEREAL AND BAKERY PRODUCTS:

Farina, instant, enriched, cooked	90	1 cup
Farina, regular and quick-cooking, enriched, cooked	70	1 cup
Hoagie roll, enriched	40	$11\frac{1}{2}$-in.-long roll
Cereals, ready-to-eat (check label)	20	1 oz
Cottage pudding with enriched flour and chocolate sauce	20	$\frac{1}{6}$ of 8-in.-square cake
Gingerbread, with enriched flour	20	$\frac{1}{9}$ of 9-in.-square cake
Pie, pecan	20	$4\frac{3}{4}$-in. sector
Coffeecake, with enriched flour	15	2.5 oz piece
Cottage pudding, with enriched flour and strawberry sauce	15	$\frac{1}{6}$ of 8-in. square cake
Hard roll, enriched	15	1 roll (1.8 oz)
Spoonbread	15	1 cup

MISCELLANEOUS:

Bread pudding, with raisins and enriched bread	20	1 cup
Oyster stew, home recipe	20	1 cup
Molasses, blackstrap	20	1 tbsp
Apple brown betty, with enriched bread	15	1 cup
Sirup, sorghum	15	1 tbsp

Appendix D
Vitamin Structures

Vitamin A (Retinol)

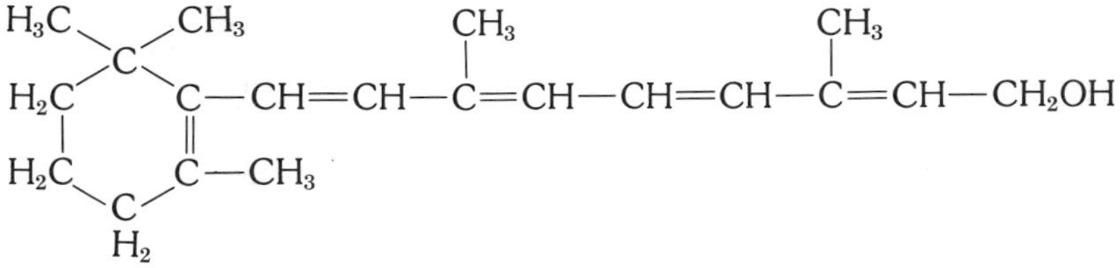

$$H_3C-C-CH=CH-C=CH-CH=CH-C=CH-CH_2OH$$

Vitamin D (Calciferol)

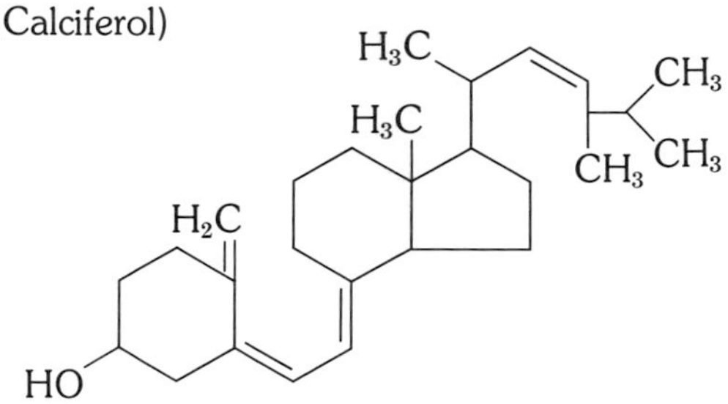

Vitamin E (α-Tocopherol)

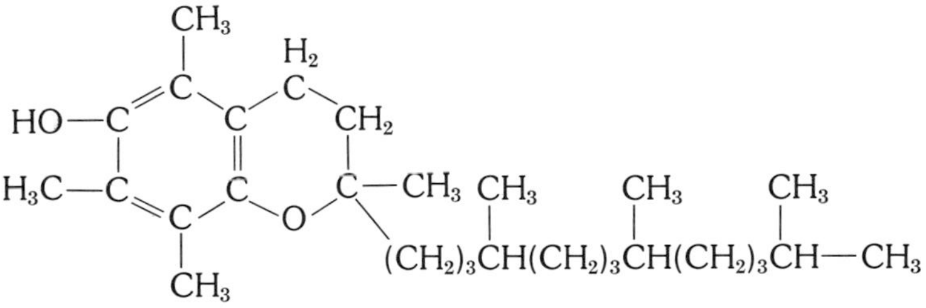

$$HO-C \quad C \quad CH_2$$
$$H_3C-C \quad C \quad C-CH_3 \quad CH_3 \quad CH_3 \quad CH_3$$
$$(CH_2)_3CH(CH_2)_3CH(CH_2)_3CH-CH_3$$

Vitamin K (Phylloquinone)

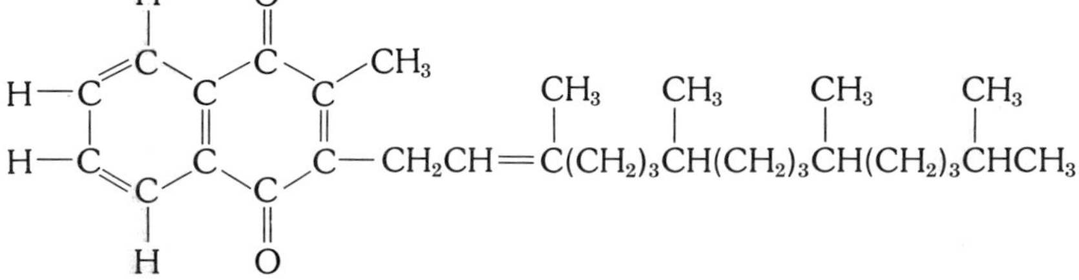

$$-CH_2CH=C(CH_2)_3CH(CH_2)_3CH(CH_2)_3CHCH_3$$

Thiamin (Thiamin hydrochloride)

$$H_3C-C \underset{\underset{H}{\overset{\displaystyle \|}{\text{N}}}{\overset{N=}{}}}{} C-NH_3^+ Cl^- \quad \underset{}{\overset{S}{}} CH \quad C-CH_2CH_2OH$$

$$\text{H}_3\text{C}-\text{C} \quad \text{C}-\text{NH}_3^+ \text{ Cl}^- \qquad \text{CH} \quad \text{C}-\text{CH}_2\text{CH}_2\text{OH}$$

$$\text{N} \quad \text{C}-\text{CH}_2-\text{N}_+-\text{C}-\text{CH}_3$$

$$\text{Cl}^-$$

Riboflavin

$$\text{CH}_2-\text{CHOH}-\text{CHOH}-\text{CHOH}-\text{CH}_2\text{OH}$$

$$\text{H}_3\text{C}-\text{C} \quad \text{C} \quad \text{N} \quad \text{N} \quad \text{C}=\text{O}$$

$$\text{H}_3\text{C}-\text{C} \quad \text{C} \quad \text{C} \quad \text{NH}$$

$$\text{H} \qquad \text{O}$$

Niacin

$$\underset{}{\overset{O}{\overset{\|}{\text{C}}}}-\text{OH}$$

Vitamin B$_6$ (Pyridoxine)

$$\text{CH}_2\text{OH}$$

$$\text{HO}-\text{C} \quad \text{C} \quad \text{C}-\text{CH}_2\text{OH}$$

$$\text{CH}_3-\text{C} \quad \text{N} \quad \text{C}-\text{H}$$

Pantothenic Acid

$$\text{HO}-\underset{\underset{H}{|}}{\overset{\overset{H}{|}}{\text{C}}}-\underset{\underset{CH_3}{|}}{\overset{\overset{CH_3}{|}}{\text{C}}}-\underset{}{\overset{\overset{OH}{|}}{\text{C}}}-\underset{}{\overset{\overset{O}{\|}}{\text{C}}}-\underset{}{\overset{\overset{H}{|}}{\text{N}}}-\underset{\underset{H}{|}}{\overset{\overset{H}{|}}{\text{C}}}-\underset{\underset{H}{|}}{\overset{\overset{H}{|}}{\text{C}}}-\underset{}{\overset{\overset{O}{\|}}{\text{C}}}-\text{OH}$$

Biotin

$$\underset{}{\overset{O}{\overset{\|}{\text{C}}}}$$

$$\text{H}-\text{N} \qquad \text{N}-\text{H}$$

$$\text{H}-\text{C} \qquad \text{C}-\text{H}$$

$$\text{H}_2\text{C} \qquad \text{C} \qquad \text{CH}_2-\text{CH}_2-\text{CH}_2-\text{COOH}$$

$$\text{S} \qquad \text{H}$$

Folacin

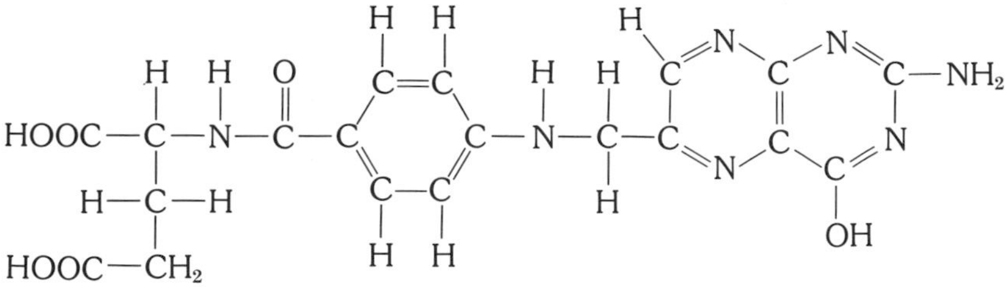

Vitamin B$_{12}$ (Cobalamin)

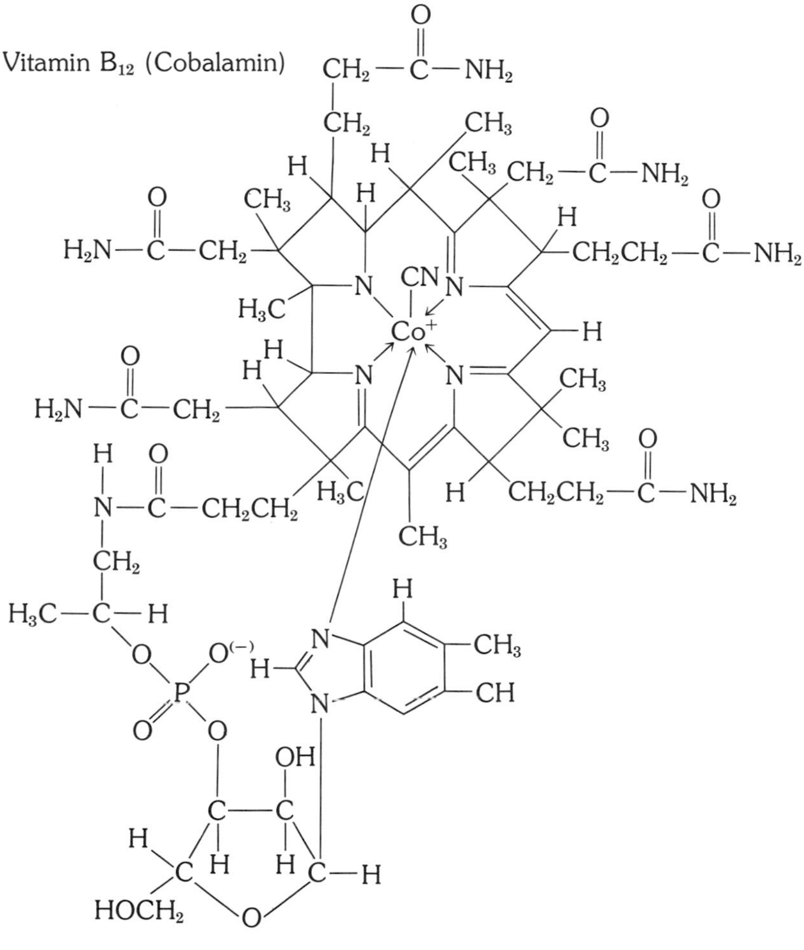

Ascorbic Acid (Vitamin C)

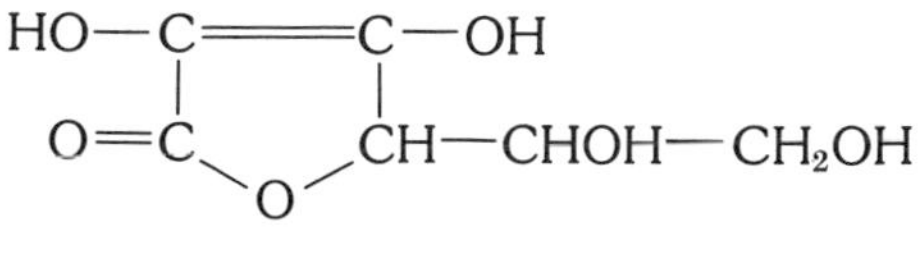

Appendix E
Amino Acid Structures

Methionine

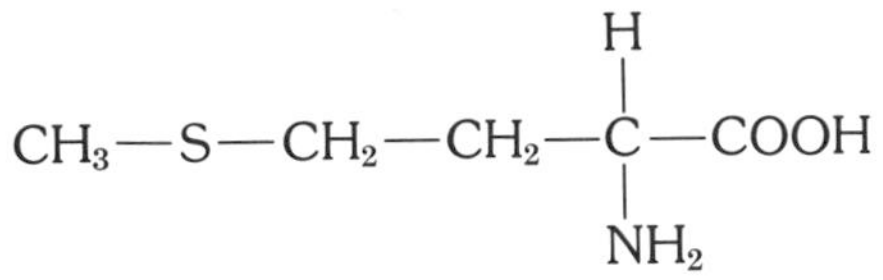

$$CH_3-S-CH_2-CH_2-\underset{\underset{NH_2}{|}}{\overset{\overset{H}{|}}{C}}-COOH$$

Threonine

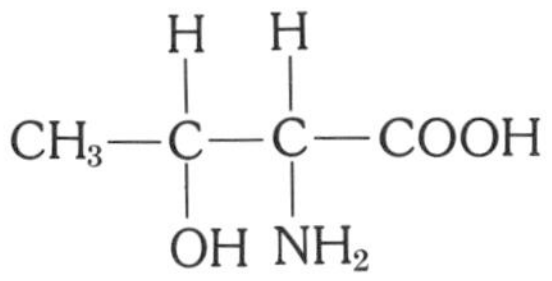

$$CH_3-\underset{\underset{OH}{|}}{\overset{\overset{H}{|}}{C}}-\underset{\underset{NH_2}{|}}{\overset{\overset{H}{|}}{C}}-COOH$$

Tryptophan

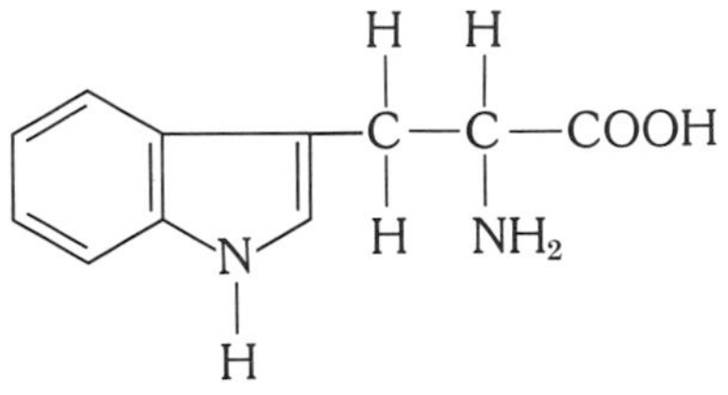

$$\underset{\underset{H}{|}}{N}\diagup\diagdown\quad\underset{\underset{H}{|}}{\overset{\overset{H}{|}}{C}}-\underset{\underset{NH_2}{|}}{\overset{\overset{H}{|}}{C}}-COOH$$

Isoleucine

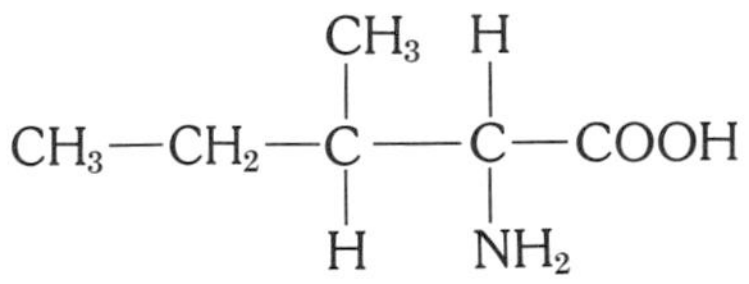

$$CH_3-CH_2-\underset{\underset{H}{|}}{\overset{\overset{CH_3}{|}}{C}}-\underset{\underset{NH_2}{|}}{\overset{\overset{H}{|}}{C}}-COOH$$

Leucine

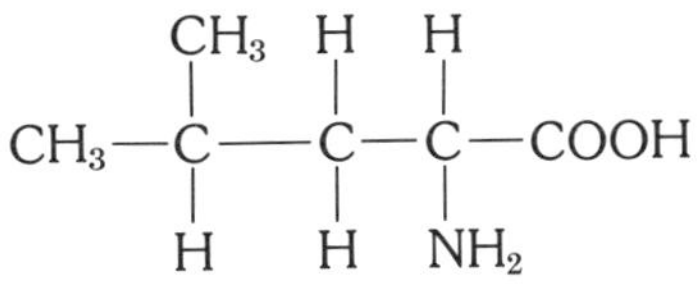

$$CH_3-\underset{\underset{H}{|}}{\overset{\overset{CH_3}{|}}{C}}-\underset{\underset{H}{|}}{\overset{\overset{H}{|}}{C}}-\underset{\underset{NH_2}{|}}{\overset{\overset{H}{|}}{C}}-COOH$$

Lysine

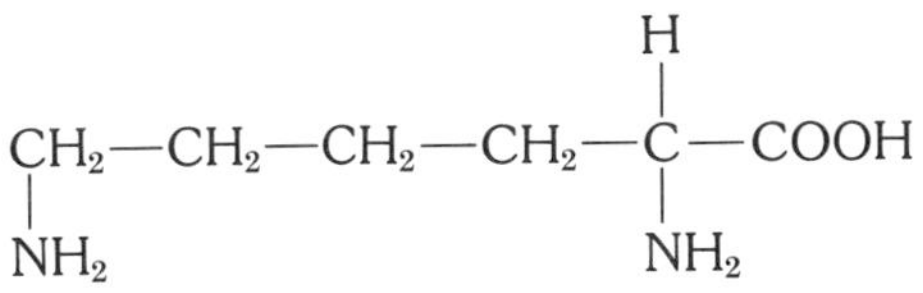

$$\underset{\underset{NH_2}{|}}{CH_2}-CH_2-CH_2-CH_2-\underset{\underset{NH_2}{|}}{\overset{\overset{H}{|}}{C}}-COOH$$

Valine

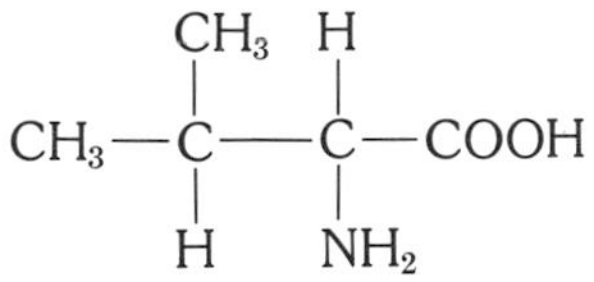

$$CH_3-\underset{\underset{H}{|}}{\overset{\overset{CH_3}{|}}{C}}-\underset{\underset{NH_2}{|}}{\overset{\overset{H}{|}}{C}}-COOH$$

Phenylalanine

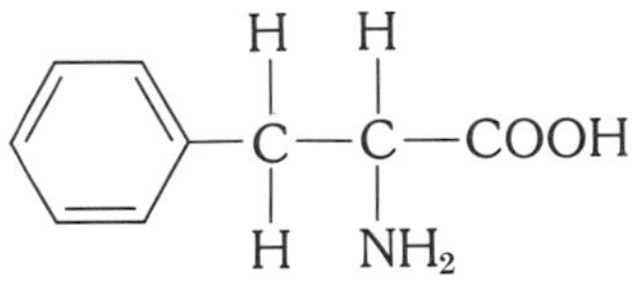

$$\diagup\diagdown\diagdown-\underset{\underset{H}{|}}{\overset{\overset{H}{|}}{C}}-\underset{\underset{NH_2}{|}}{\overset{\overset{H}{|}}{C}}-COOH$$

Histidine

$$\overset{\overset{H}{|}}{C}\diagup\diagdown\\ N\quad NH\\ H-C=\underset{}{C}-CH_2-\underset{\underset{NH_2}{|}}{\overset{\overset{H}{|}}{C}}-COOH$$

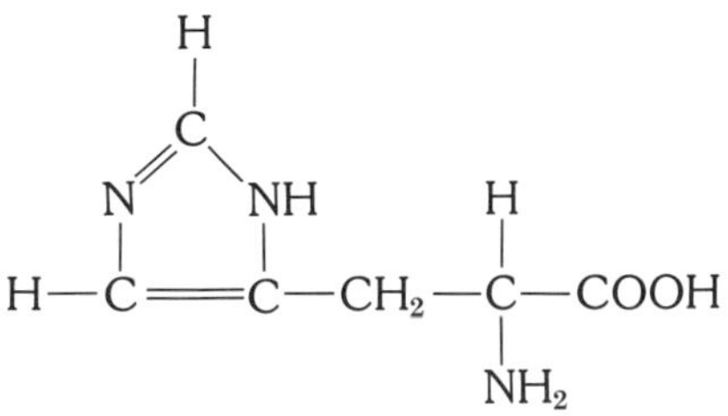

Glycine

$$H-\underset{\underset{NH_2}{|}}{\overset{\overset{H}{|}}{C}}-COOH$$

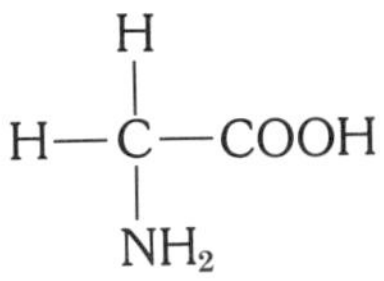

Alanine

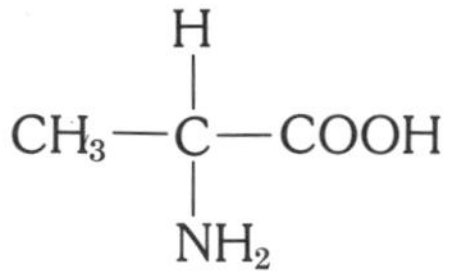

$$CH_3 - \underset{\underset{NH_2}{|}}{\overset{\overset{H}{|}}{C}} - COOH$$

Serine

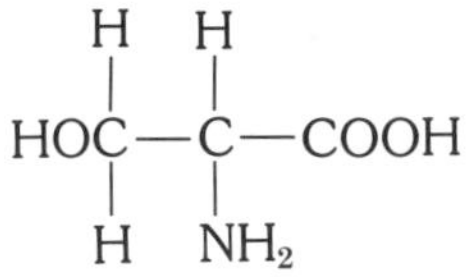

$$HO\overset{\overset{H}{|}}{\underset{\underset{H}{|}}{C}} - \underset{\underset{NH_2}{|}}{\overset{\overset{H}{|}}{C}} - COOH$$

Tyrosine

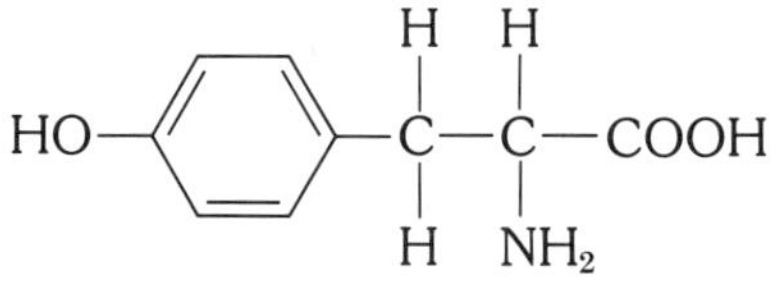

$$HO - \bigcirc - \underset{\underset{H}{|}}{\overset{\overset{H}{|}}{C}} - \underset{\underset{NH_2}{|}}{\overset{\overset{H}{|}}{C}} - COOH$$

Proline

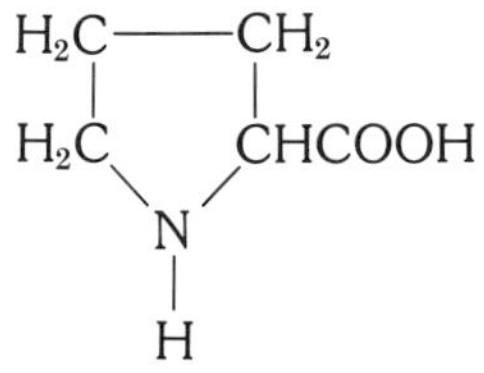

$$\begin{array}{c} H_2C - CH_2 \\ H_2C \quad\; CHCOOH \\ \diagdown \;N\; \diagup \\ | \\ H \end{array}$$

Hydroxyproline

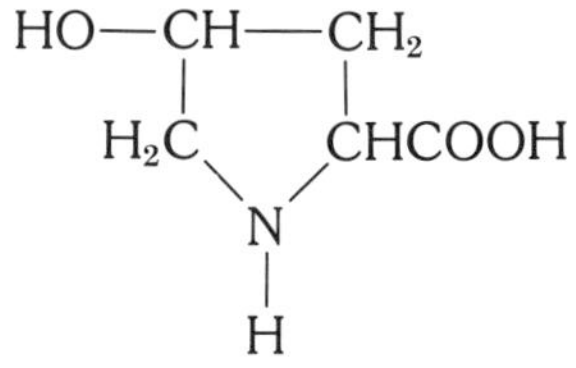

$$\begin{array}{c} HO - CH - CH_2 \\ H_2C \quad\; CHCOOH \\ \diagdown \;N\; \diagup \\ | \\ H \end{array}$$

Arginine

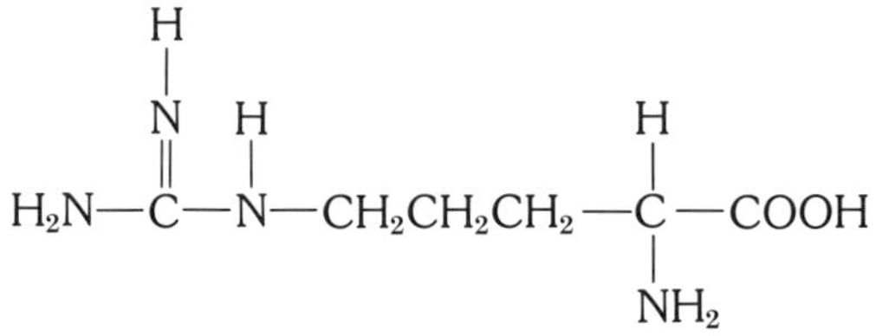

$$\underset{\underset{}{}}{H_2N} - \overset{\overset{N}{\|}}{\underset{}{C}} - \underset{\underset{}{}}{N} - CH_2CH_2CH_2 - \underset{\underset{NH_2}{|}}{\overset{\overset{H}{|}}{C}} - COOH$$

(with $\overset{H}{|}$ on the first N and $\overset{}{H}$ on the second N)

Aspartic acid

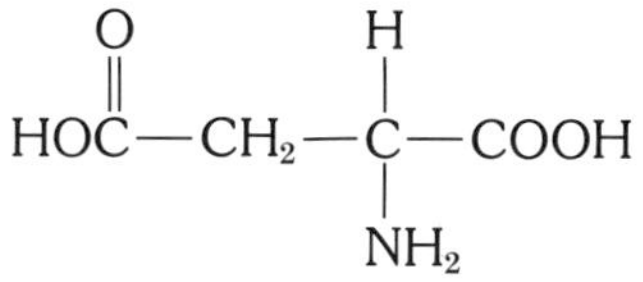

$$\overset{\overset{O}{\|}}{HOC} - CH_2 - \underset{\underset{NH_2}{|}}{\overset{\overset{H}{|}}{C}} - COOH$$

Glutamic acid

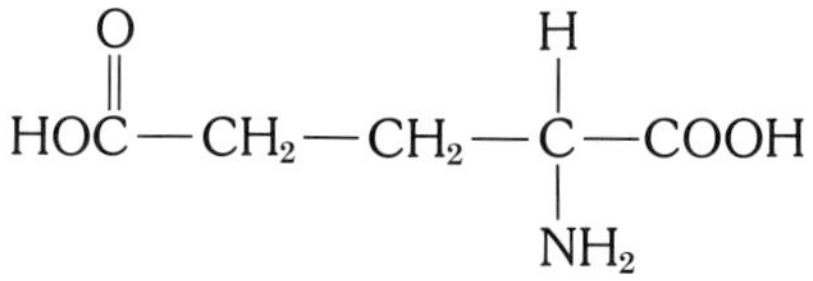

$$\overset{\overset{O}{\|}}{HOC} - CH_2 - CH_2 - \underset{\underset{NH_2}{|}}{\overset{\overset{H}{|}}{C}} - COOH$$

Cysteine

$$HS - CH_2 - \underset{\underset{NH_2}{|}}{\overset{\overset{H}{|}}{C}} - COOH$$

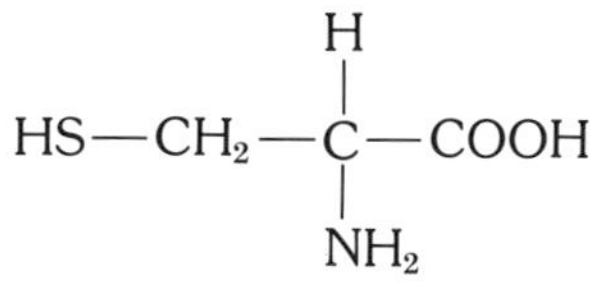

Cystine

$$S - CH_2 - \underset{\underset{NH_2}{|}}{\overset{\overset{H}{|}}{C}} - COOH$$

$$S - CH_2 - \underset{\underset{NH_2}{|}}{\overset{\overset{H}{|}}{C}} - COOH$$

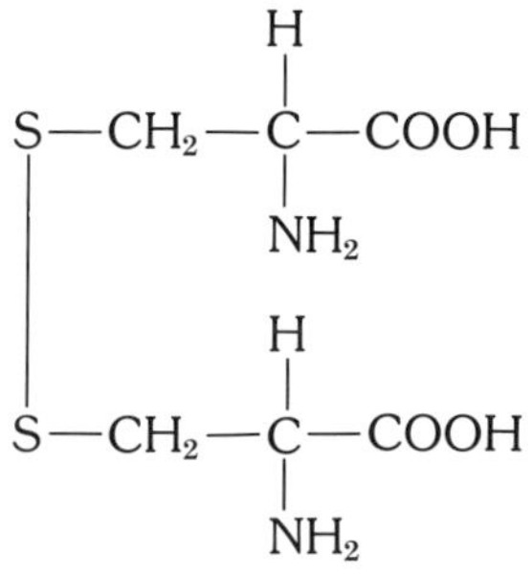

Appendix F
Selected Dietary Standards

Nation	Sex	kcal	Protein (g)	Calcium (g)	Iron (mg)	A (I.U.)	Vitamins[a] Thiamin (mg)	Riboflavin (mg)	Niacin (mg)	C (mg)
FAO[b,c]	M	3200	46[d]	0.4 to 0.5	10	750[e]	1.3[f]	1.8[g]	21.1[h]	
	F	2300	39	0.4 to 0.5	18	750	0.9	1.3	15.2	
Canada[i,j]	M	2850	50[k]	0.5	6	3700[l]	0.9	1.4	9	30
	F	2400	39	0.5	10	3700	0.7	1.2	7	30
United Kingdom[m,n]	M	2750	75[o]	0.8	12	750[e]	1.0	1.7	12[p]	30
	F	2200	55	0.5	12	750[e]	1.0	1.3	10	30
Austra-lia[q,r]	M	2900	70[s]	0.4 to 0.8	10	2500[t]	1.2	1.5	18[u]	30
	F	2100	58	0.4 to 0.8	10	2500	0.8	1.1	14	30
United States[v,w]	M	2700	56	0.8	10	5000	1.4	1.6	18[x]	45
	F	2000	46	0.8	18	5000	1.0	1.2	13	45

[a] Vitamin A figures are those for vitamin A activity; niacin figures are niacin equivalents.

[b] FAO figures are from: FAO Nutr. Stud. No. 15. *Calorie Requirements.* Rome. 1957; FAO/WHO FAO Nutr. Meet. Rep. Ser. No. 37. *Protein Requirements.* 1965; FAO/Nutr. Meet. Rep. Ser. No. 30. *Calcium Requirements.* 1962; FAO Nutr. Rep. No. 41. *Requirements of Vitamin A, Thiamine, Riboflavin, and Niacin.* 1967.

[c] Values are for persons aged 25 and weighing 65 kg, leading moderately active ("employed 8 hours in an occupation which is not sedentary, but does not involve more than occasional periods of hard physical labor . . . engaged either in general household duties or in light industry . . . Her daily activities include walking for about 1 hour and 1 hour of active recreation").

[d] Practical value to cover the needs of all but a small fraction of population. Value is 0.71 g/kg: body weight.

[e] 750 μg retinol (1 μg beta carotene = 0.167 μg retinol).

[f] 0.4 mg/1000 kcal.

[g] 0.55 mg/1000 kcal.

[h] 6.6 niacin equivalents/1000 kcal.

[i] Recommended Daily Intakes of Nutrients Adequate for the Maintenance of Health among the Majority of Canadians. *Can. Bull. Nutr. 6:* 1. 1964.

[j] Values are for persons aged 25; males weighing 72 kg and females weighing 57 kg. Activity level for these figures is moderate.

[k] Normal mixed Canadian diets.

[l] Mixed Canadian diet supplying both vitamin A and provitamin A (carotene).

[m] Dept. of Health and Social Security: Report on Public Health and Medical Subjects, No. 120. London. 1969.

[n] Values are for persons over age 20; males weighing 65 kg, females weighing 56 kg. Activity level is medium.

[o] Protein recommendation is in relation to caloric intake; calculated on basis that not less than 11 percent of the calories for moderately active people should come from protein.

[p] Value is for preformed vitamin only.

[q] Dietary Allowances for Australians. 1965 revision. *Med. J. Australia. 1:* 1041. 1965.

[r] Values are for persons aged 25; male weighing 70 kg, female weighing 58 kg. Activity level is comparable to that of FAO, with the temperature being 18°C annually compared with 10°C for FAO calculations.

(continued)

ˢ Calculated on the basis of protein contributing between 10 and 12 percent of the total calories.

ᵗ Calculated with the value of 3 I.U. carotene = 1 I.U. vitamin A activity.

ᵘ Preformed niacin + (protein in grams times 0.16).

ᵛ National Academy of Sciences. ***Recommended Dietary Allowances.*** Washington, D.C. 1974.

ʷ Values are for persons aged 22; male weighing 70 kg, female weighing 58 kg. Activity level is normal.

ˣ Dietary sources of niacin and tryptophan (60 mg tryptophan + 1mg niacin) are included.

Absorption—The passage of digestive products from the gastrointestinal tract into the blood or lymphatic systems.

Acid—A sour compound capable of reacting with an alkali. On the pH scale, a substance with a pH between 1 and 7.

Acid-base balance—The equilibrium or relationship between acidic and alkaline compounds in the body.

Additives—Accidental or intentional substances incorporated in processed foods.

Alkaline—Basic in reaction. pH ranging between 7 and 14.

Amino acid—Organic molecules containing carbon, hydrogen, oxygen, and nitrogen. The structural unit of protein. Contains an amino group (—NH$_2$) and a carboxyl or acidic group (—COOH).

Amylase—Enzyme that breaks down starch.

Amylopectin—The branched chain component of starch.

Amylose—The straight chain component of starch.

Anabolism—The synthesis of new compounds in the body.

Antibody—A substance that combats specific disease-producing organisms and foreign matter to give immunity to the disease for a period of time.

Anorexia—Loss of appetite.

Antihemorrhagic—Protecting against hemorrhage. A function of vitamin K.

Antioxidant—A substance that is easily oxidized itself so that it protects other substances against oxidation.

Antirachitic—Protecting against rickets. Describes a role of vitamin D.

Antiscorbutic—Protecting against scurvy. Describes a role of ascorbic acid.

Antivitamin—A substance that has such a similar structure to a vitamin that it substitutes for the vitamin, but in so doing, prevents the vitamin from performing its essential function.

Apatite—The crystalline structural matrix in bones and teeth. Contains calcium, phosphate, and other ions such as hydroxyl or fluoride.

Apoenzyme—The protein component of an enzyme.

Arteriosclerosis—Disease characterized by hardening and thickening of the walls of the arteries.

Ascorbic acid—Vitamin C.

Atherosclerosis—A type of arteriosclerosis in which mushy deposits of fatty substances (cholesterol) partially obstruct blood flow.

Avidin—A substance in raw egg white that acts as an antagonist of the B vitamin, biotin.

Basal metabolic rate—The rate at which the body uses energy for maintaining minimal bodily functions, such as body temperature, respiration, and heart beat when at rest.

Basal metabolism—The energy required to maintain cellular activity, respiration, and circulation in the resting, fasting body.

Base—An alkaline substance that can react with acids to neutralize the acid.

Basic Four—The food plan outlining the milk, meat, fruits and vegetables, and breads and cereals that need to be included in the diet on a daily basis to give variety to the diet and thus provide a healthful balance of nutrients.

Beriberi—A disease that develops when thiamin is inadequate in the diet.

Biotin—One of the B vitamins.

Blood serum—The fluid, colorless plasma of blood from which the blood cells, clotting factor, and fibrin have been removed.

Buffer—A substance that can neutralize acids or bases to minimize any change in the pH of a solution.

Calciferol—Vitamin D.

calorie—The heat required to raise the temperature of 1 gram of water (at 1 atmosphere of pressure) 1 centigrade degree.

Calorie—The heat required to raise the temperature of 1 kilogram of water (at 1 atmosphere of pressure) 1 centigrade degree; also called a kilocalorie.

Carbohydrates—Organic compounds composed of carbon, hydrogen, and oxygen, the hydrogen/oxygen ratio being that of water.

Carotene—Yellow pigments that act as provitamin A; that is, they are converted into vitamin A in the body.

Catabolism—The breakdown of complex compounds to simpler compounds in the body.

Catalyst—A compound that alters (usually speeds up) the speed of a chemical reaction without being changed by the reaction.

Cellulose—A polysaccharide that provides roughage, but is not digested by man.

Cheilosis—Condition of lesions on the lips and cracks at the corners of the mouth, due primarily to a lack of riboflavin in the diet.

Cholesterol—A steroid alcohol.

Choline—A compound required for fat transport to prevent fatty liver and frequently considered as one of the B-complex vitamins.

Chylomicron—Very small emulsified lipoproteins that transport fat in the blood.

Cobalamin—Vitamin B_{12}.

Coenzyme—A component of an enzyme system. (usually containing a vitamin) that is required for the activity of the enzyme.

Collagen—Principal protein of connective tissue, including matrix of bone and dentin.

Colostrum—The first thin, rather yellow fluid that is produced by the mammary glands during the first few days of lactation.

Deamination—The removal of the amino group from an amino acid.

Decalcification—The removal of calcium from bones or teeth.

Dentin—Calcareores material, principal mass of tooth.

Dermatitis—Inflammation of the skin.

Disaccharide—Carbohydrates that break down to two monosaccharide molecules during digestion. Examples are sucrose, maltose, and lactose.

DNA—Desoxyribonucleic acid. The material in the cell that contains genetic codes.

Eclampsia—Severe indication of toxemia in pregnancy; symptoms include convulsions.

Edema—Accumulation of fluid in the tissues.

Embryo—The developing being, from implantation of the sperm in the ova through the second month of pregnancy (in the human).

Emulsify—To disperse small droplets of one liquid in a liquid with which it is immiscible. An example is a dispersion of small fat droplets in an aqueous medium.

Endemic—Occurring with some constancy in a region.

Endocrine gland—Gland in the body that secretes hormones in the body.

Endosperm—The portion of a grain in which the food for the seed to grow is stored. Contains mostly starch and some protein.

Enzyme—Proteins that catalyze reactions in the body. The names of enzymes frequently end with the suffix -ase, such as sucrase, the enzyme effecting the breakdown of sucrose.

Epithelium—The outer layer of skin and mucous membranes.

Erythrocyte—Red blood cell. Formation of erythrocytes is called erythropoiesis.

Essential amino acid—An amino acid needed for growth and maintenance of the body and which must be supplied in the diet.

Etiology—Study of the cause of disease or disorder.

Fatty acid—An organic acid that can combine with glycerol.

Ferritin—Storage form of iron in combination with protein.

Fetus—The developing, unborn animal. With humans this usually designates the period from the third month of pregnancy to birth.

Fiber (crude)—Insoluble organic material remaining from plants after prolonged acid and base hydrolysis.

Fiber (dietary)—Generic term that includes those plant constituents, mostly carbohydrates, which are not digestible by humans.

Flavin-adenine dinucleotide (Fad)—Coenzyme required for normal cellular respiration. Contains riboflavin.

Flavoprotein—Protein containing riboflavin. Functions in the Krebs cycle.

Fluoridation (and defluoridation)—Adjustment of fluoride to the level of one part fluoride per million parts of water, a measure that increases resistance to dental caries among children and may strengthen the bones of adults.

Folacin—One of the B vitamins.

Fructose—A monosaccharide.

Galactose—A monosaccharide.

Gestation—Pregnancy.

Glucagon—Pancreatic hormone that releases glucose stores from the liver.

Gluconeogenesis—Formation of glucose from a substance such as an amino acid or other noncarbohydrate material.

Glucose—A monosaccharide; the sugar of the blood.

Glyceride—Fatty compound formed when glycerol and fatty acids are combined.

Glycogen—The storage form of carbohydrate in animals and man. Comparable to starch in plants.

Goiter—Enlargement of the thyroid gland. Visible as a swelling in the throat.

Gossypol—Toxic phenolic pigment in cottonseed.

Heme—The iron-containing, colored component of hemoglobin. Porphyrin (ring) structure combined with iron.

Hormone—A compound secreted by an endocrine gland that influences the functioning of an organ in another part of the body.

Hydrogenation—The controlled addition of hydrogen to an unsaturated fatty acid. This process changes the melting point, thus producing solid fats from oils, depending on the extent of hydrogenation.

Hydrolysis—The chemical splitting of a compound into smaller molecules by the addition of water (as H^+ and OH^-).

Hydroxyapatite—Complex crystal lattice of variable composition which makes up mineral component of enamel, dentin, and bone.

Hypercalcemia—Too much calcium in the blood.

Hypervitaminosis—A condition caused by excessively high intake of a vitamin, particularly an excess of vitamin A or vitamin D.

Hypothalamus—A part of the mid-brain.

Joule—Unit of energy; 1 kcal = 4.18 kilojoules.

Keratin—An insoluble protein in the epidermis, hair, and nails.

Ketogenic—Substances that can be converted to ketone bodies (acetone, acetoacetic acid, and β-hydroxybutyric acid) during metabolism. Fatty acids and some amino acids are ketogenic compounds.

Kilocalorie—The amount of heat required to raise 1 kilogram of water (at 1 atmosphere of pressure) 1 centigrade degree, same as a Calorie (spelled with a capital C).

Kwashiorkor—Severe protein deficiency condition in children.

Lactation—Production of milk.

Linoleic acid—An essential fatty acid.

Lipase—Enzyme that digests fats.

Lipids—Organic compounds composed of carbon, hydrogen, and oxygen and generally immiscible with water. Fat or fatlike substances.

Lipoprotein—Compound composed of a lipid and a protein.

Macrocytic anemia—Abnormally large blood cells.

Marasmus—Condition of wasting due to very restricted caloric intake.

Matrix—Framework.

Megaloblastic anemia—Anemia in which red blood cells are enlarged and fail to mature.

Melanin—Dark pigments in the skin and hair.

Metabolism—Chemical changes involved in the utilization of nutrients and the functioning of the body. General term for both anabolism and catabolism.

Mitochondria—Rod-shaped organelles in cells in which energy-releasing reactions take place.

Monoglyceride—Compound consisting of one fatty acid attached to glycerol.

Monosaccharide—Carbohydrate in its simplest form. Examples are fructose, glucose, and galactose.

Monounsaturated—Fatty acid containing one double bond.

Niacin—One of the B vitamins.

Nicotinamide adenine dinucleotide (NAD)—Coenzyme containing niacin and functioning in energy release from food.

Night blindness—Limited ability to adapt to changes in light intensity.

Nucleotide—Organic compound composed of a phosphorylated sugar and a pyrimidine or purine base.

Obesity—Condition of being 20 percent or more above desirable weight.

Opsin—The protein that combines with retinal to form rhodopsin.

Organelle—A specialized structure in a cell.

Osmotic pressure—The force on a semipermeable membrane that enables a solvent to pass through the membrane when the concentration of solutes on both sides of the membrane is different.

Ossification—The formation of bone.

Osteomalacia—Adult counterpart of rickets, in which inadequate calcium and phosphorus are absorbed from the intestine to maintain normal bone structure.

Osteoporosis—Prolonged chronic reduction in bone mass in which either or both reduced bone formation or accelerated resorption may occur. Cause is unknown.

Oxidation—The loss of electrons. Combining with oxygen or removing hydrogen.

Pantothenic acid—One of the B vitamins.

Pellagra—A disease due to a deficiency of niacin.

Peptide—A molecule composed of amino acids, smaller than protein.

Peristalsis—Motions of the alimentary tract to move the food through the tract.

pH—Negative logarithm of the effective hydrogen ion concentration. A means of expressing relative acidity or alkalinity, with pH 7 representing neutrality, numbers less than 7 are acidic, greater than 7 are alkaline.

Phenylketonuria (PKU)—Condition in which phenylalanine (an amino acid) is not metabolized properly because of an inborn error, and thus accumulates in the blood, causing brain damage early in life.

Phospholipid—A fat containing phosphate and a nitrogenous substance in place of one of the fatty acids.

Protease—Enzyme that digests protein.

Protein—Organic compound composed of amino acids, contains carbon, hydrogen, oxygen, nitrogen, and sometimes other elements, too.

Protein-calorie malnutrition (PCM)—Condition caused by inadequate intake of both protein and calories.

Pyridoxine—Vitamin B_6.

Retinal—Aldehyde form of vitamin A.

Retinol equivalent—Unit of vitamin A activity = 3.33 I. U. retinol.

Riboflavin—One of the B vitamins.

Ribosome—Organelle in which protein synthesis takes place in the cell.

Rickets—Deficiency condition caused by lack of vitamin D which is needed for absorption of calcium.

Scurvy—A disease caused by a lack of ascorbic acid (vitamin C).

Syndrome—Group of symptoms occurring together.

Synthesis—Formation of organic compounds.

Thiamin—One of the B vitamins.

Thyroxine—Hormone containing iodine that is secreted by the thyroid gland.

Tocopherol—A substance that has vitamin E activity.

Transamination—Transfer of the amino group from an amino acid to another compound to make a new amino acid. Only nonessential amino acids can be formed by transamination.

Transferrin—Protein compound, the form in which iron is transported.

Transketolase—Enzyme containing TPP (thiamin pyrophosphate) that is needed for formation of five-carbon sugar (ribose) in DNA and RNA.

Vitamin A—Fat-soluble vitamin.

Vitamin B_6—Water-soluble B vitamin.

Vitamin B$_{12}$—Water-soluble B vitamin.

Vitamin C—Water-soluble vitamin, commonly called ascorbic acid.

Vitamin D—Fat-soluble vitamin.

Vitamin E—Fat-soluble vitamin.

Vitamin K—Fat-soluble vitamin.

Xerophthalmia—A disease of the eye caused by a lack of vitamin A and frequently resulting in blindness.

Photography Credits

Frontispiece Carl Frank/Photo Researchers

Chapter One Opener, Mimi Forsyth/Monkmeyer. 5, 8 & 9, National Dairy Council. 17, Wheat Flour Institute.

Chapter Two Opener, WHO. 31, FAO. 32, National Marine Fisheries Service. 36, Hiroji Kubota/Magnum. 38, William Mares/Monkmeyer. 44, UN. 45 & 47, USDA. 48, FAO. 49 (top), USDA. 49 (bottom), Ben Rose. 50 (a) Courtesy of the Controller of H. M. Stationery Office (U.K.) Crown Copyright. From the Department of Agriculture & Fisheries for Scotland Marine Laboratory. 51 (b) Courtesy Blount Marine Corporation, Rhode Island. 51 (c) Courtesy Australian Information Service. 52, Sovfoto/Eastfoto.

Chapter Three Opener, Ken Heyman. 62, Courtesy Dr. Donald McLarren, American University of Beirut, Lebanon. 66, Burk Uzzle/Magnum. 68 & 72, Ken Heyman. 73 & 75, USDA. 77, Michal Heron/Monkmeyer.

Chapter Four Opener, Mimi Forsyth/Monkmeyer. 83 (a), (b), & (c), Courtesy William Sheldon, M.D. From *Atlas of Men: A Guide for Somatotyping the Adult Male At All Ages,* Hafner, 1970. 85, National Institute of Health. 86, Courtesy Professor P. Teitelbaum, University of Pennsylvania. 92, Courtesy Cambridge Scientific Industries, Cambridge, Maryland. 106, Mitchell Payne/Jeroboam. 109, Mimi Forsyth/Monkmeyer.

Chapter Five Opener, Hugh Rogers/Monkmeyer. 118, Hugh Rogers/Monkmeyer. 119, Dennis Stock/Magnum. 123, Crista Armstrong/Rapho-Photo Researchers. 124, Grant Hailman. 126, *Journal of Nutrition.* Reprinted by permission from S. M. Picardi and E. R. Pariser, "Food and Nutrition Minicourses for 11th and 12th Grades," *Journal of Nutrition Education,* 7 (No. 1): 25–29, January/March 1975; © Society for Nutrition Education, 1975. 129, Bruce Roberts/Rapho-Photo Researchers.

Chapter Six Opener, Salvatore Guida and Nickola Sargent, New York. 144, Courtesy Jeanne M. Riddle, Ph.D., Wayne State University School of Medicine. 145, (a), Luis Biempica, M.D., Albert Einstein College of Medicine. 145 (b), Jeanne M. Riddle, Ph.D., Wayne State University School of Medicine.

Chapter Seven Opener, Salvatore Guida and Nickola Sargent, New York.

Chapter Eight Opener, Thomas Hopker/Woodfin Camp. 170, Ken Kay/DPI. 172, John Oldencamp/*Psychology Today.* 181, WHO. 182, UNICEF, photo by Jack Lind.

Chapter Nine Opener, Mimi Forsyth/Monkmeyer.

Chapter Ten Opener, Eric V. Gravé (Sodium chloride crystals from a human tear.) 208 & 210, Courtesy The Upjohn Company, Kalamazoo, Michigan. 213, Courtesy The Center for Disease Control, Atlanta, Georgia.

Chapter Eleven Opener, Manfred Kage/Peter Arnold (Crystals of vitamin

B$_6$.) 240, Courtesy Hoffman-LaRoche. 242, Bruce Roberts/Rapho-Photo Researchers. 243, Courtesy *Nutrition Today,* from Teaching Aid on Nutritional Diagnosis. 244, Courtesy The Upjohn Company, Kalamazoo, Michigan. 251, Courtesy The Children's Hospital Medical Center, Boston, Massachusetts. From Wolback, Jollife, Tisdale & Cannon, "Clinical Nutrition," Paul B. Hoeber, Inc., New York, 1950. 252, Courtesy Armed Forces Institute of Pathology. 256, Courtesy The Center for Disease Control, Atlanta, Georgia. 260 & 264, Courtesy Dr. R. H. Kampmeier, Vanderbilt University. 275, Courtesy The Center for Disease Control, Atlanta, Georgia.

Chapter Twelve Opener, Courtesy Carnegie Institution of Washington. 287, 288 & 289, Courtesy Lucille S. Hurley, Department of Nutrition, University of California, Davis. 297, Hanna Schreiber/Rapho-Photo Researchers. 305, Leonard Freed/Magnum.

Chapter Thirteen Opener, Suzanne Szasz. 315, Jan Lukas/Rapho-Photo Researchers. 320, Lew Merrim/Monkmeyer. 323, Marvin E. Newman/ Woodfin Camp.

Chapter Fourteen Opener, Charles Gatewood/Magnum. 331, Hays/ Monkmeyer. 333, David Powers/Jeroboam. 335, AID. 336, Hanna Schreiber/Rapho-Photo Researchers. 337, Suzanne Szasz. 339, Hella Hammid/Rapho-Photo Researchers. 340, Peeter Vilms/Jeroboam.

Chapter Fifteen Opener, Christa Armstrong/Rapho-Photo Researchers. 346, USDA. 347, Courtesy Campbell Soup Company. 348, USDA. 349, Van Bucher/Photo Researchers. 351, Hugh Rogers/Monkmeyer. 353, Bob Combs/Rapho-Photo Researchers. 357, George Whiteley/Photo Researchers.

Chapter Sixteen Opener, Myron Wood/Photo Researchers. 364, Kenneth Murray/Nancy Palmer. 369, Rollie McKenna. 372, G. Gillette/Photo Researchers. 374, Ken Heyman. 375 (left), James Motlow/Jeroboam. 375 (right), Winston Vargas/Photo Researchers. 376, Sybil Shelton/Monkmeyer. 379, Courtesy Campbell Soup Company. 381, Ken Heyman.

Chapter Seventeen Opener, Gerry Cranham/Photo Researchers. 392, Courtesy Campbell Soup Company. 401, David Kramer/Photo Researchers. 404, Salvatore Guida and Nickola Sargent, New York.

Chapter Eighteen Opener, Susan S. Perry/Woodfin Camp. 409 & 410, Salvatore Guida and Nickola Sargent, New York. 411, Ellis Herwig/Stock, Boston. 413 (top), Hank Lebo/Jeroboam. 413 (bottom), Jack & Betty Cheetham/Magnum. 414, Salvatore Guida and Nickola Sargent, New York. 415, George W. Gardner.

Index